Eighth Edition

Advanced Fitness Assessment
and
Exercise Prescription

Ann L. Gibson, PhD

University of New Mexico

Dale R. Wagner, PhD

Utah State University

Vivian H. Heyward, PhD

University of New Mexico, Professor Emerita

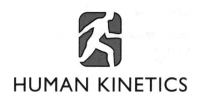

HUMAN KINETICS

Library of Congress Cataloging-in-Publication Data

Names: Gibson, Ann L., [date]- author. | Wagner, Dale R., 1966- author. |
Heyward, Vivian H., author.
Title: Advanced fitness assessment and exercise prescription / Ann L. Gibson,
PhD, University of New Mexico, Dale R. Wagner, PhD, Utah State University,
Vivian H. Heyward, PhD, University of New Mexico.
Description: Eighth Edition. | Champaign, Illinois : Human Kinetics, [2019] |
Previous edition: 2014. | Includes bibliographical references and index. |
Identifiers: LCCN 2018008261 (print) | LCCN 2018009017 (ebook) | ISBN
9781492563549 (enhanced ebook) | ISBN 9781492561347 (print)
Subjects: LCSH: Physical fitness--Testing. | Exercise tests. | Health.
Classification: LCC GV436 (ebook) | LCC GV436 .H48 2019 (print) | DDC
613.7--dc23
LC record available at https://lccn.loc.gov/2018008261

ISBN: 978-1-4925-6134-7 (print)

The web addresses cited in this text were current as of July 2018, unless otherwise noted.

Senior Acquisitions Editor: Michelle Maloney; **Senior Developmental Editor:** Cynthia McEntire; **Senior Managing Editor:**
Amy Stahl; **Copyeditor:** Patricia L. MacDonald; **Indexer:** Rebecca McCorkle; **Permissions Manager:** Martha Gullo; **Graphic
Designers:** Sean Roosevelt and Whitney Milburn; **Cover Designer:** Keri Evans; **Cover Design Associate:** Susan Rothermel
Allen; **Photographs (interior):** © Human Kinetics, unless otherwise noted; **Photo Asset Manager:** Laura Fitch; **Photo Pro-
duction Manager:** Jason Allen; **Senior Art Manager:** Kelly Hendren; **Illustrations:** © Human Kinetics; **Printer:** Walsworth

We thank the Exercise Physiology Laboratory at the University of New Mexico, Albuquerque, New Mexico, for assistance in
providing the location for the photo shoot for this book.

Human Kinetics books are available at special discounts for bulk purchase. Special editions or book excerpts can also be created
to specification. For details, contact the Special Sales Manager at Human Kinetics.

The video contents of this product are licensed for educational public performance for viewing by a traditional (live) audience,
via closed circuit television, or via computerized local area networks within a single building or geographically unified campus.
To request a license to broadcast these contents to a wider audience—for example, throughout a school district or state, or on a
television station—please contact your sales representative (**www.HumanKinetics.com/SalesRepresentatives**).

Printed in the United States of America   10   9   8   7   6   5

The paper in this book is certified under a sustainable forestry program.

Human Kinetics
1607 N. Market St.
Champaign, IL 61820
Website: www.HumanKinetics.com

In the United States, email info@hkusa.com or call 800-747-4457.
In Canada, email info@hkcanada.com.
In the United Kingdom/Europe, email hk@hkeurope.com.

For information about Human Kinetics' coverage in other areas of the world,
please visit our website: **www.HumanKinetics.com**

E7227

Eighth Edition

Advanced Fitness Assessment
and
Exercise Prescription

Contents

Video Contents

We continue to offer online streaming video in this eighth edition, including over 70 videos of content demonstrating key concepts from the book, such as assessments, procedures, tips, stretches, and exercises. You can access the online video by visiting www.HumanKinetics.com/AdvancedFitnessAssessment AndExercisePrescription. If you purchased a new print book, follow the instructions on the orange-framed page at the front of your book. That page includes access steps and the unique key code that you'll need the first time you visit the *Advanced Fitness Assessment and Exercise Prescription* website. If you purchased an e-book from HumanKinetics.com, follow the access instructions that were emailed to you after your purchase. If you have purchased a used book, you can purchase access to the online video separately by following the links at www.HumanKinetics.com/AdvancedFitnessAssessmentAndExercisePrescription.

Once at the *Advanced Fitness Assessment and Exercise Prescription* website, select Online Video in the ancillary items box in the upper-left corner of the screen. You'll then see an Online Video page with information about the video. Select the link to open the online video web page. From the online video page, you can select the chapter and then the desired video, numbered as they are in the text.

Following is a list of the clips in the online video.

Preface

Exercise professionals need to have extensive knowledge and technical skills in order to work safely and effectively. Historically, individuals working in exercise settings, such as health and fitness clubs, were not necessarily required to have specialized education and training in exercise science. However, survey research indicates that a bachelor's degree in exercise science and certification from the American College of Sports Medicine (ACSM) or National Strength and Conditioning Association (NSCA) are strong predictors of a personal trainer's knowledge (Malek et al. 2002). To carry the U.S. Bureau of Labor and Statistics' job title of "exercise physiologist," one must have earned the minimum of a bachelor's degree (Simpson 2015). There is also a growing trend within health care facilities to require their exercise physiologists to hold a master's degree (Collora 2017); this corroborates Wagner's (2014) finding that a master's degree is commonly held by exercise physiologists working in clinical settings (69% of 140 survey respondents).

A global survey of fitness trends for 2018 revealed that "educated, certified, and experienced fitness professionals" is ranked number 6 in importance, and this has been a top 10 concern since the annual survey began more than a decade ago (Thompson 2017). These findings suggest that formal education and certification by professional organizations should be required for personal fitness trainers and exercise science professionals. Their knowledge and skills are instrumental in preparticipation screening, cardiorespiratory fitness testing, muscular fitness testing, flexibility assessment, results interpretation, and scientifically sound exercise prescription design. To promote exercise science as a profession, issues surrounding accreditation, certification, national boards, and licensure need to be understood and addressed.

ACCREDITATION

Organizations and programs are awarded accreditation by meeting or exceeding standards established by an independent third-party accrediting agency. Although no single accrediting agency exists for health and fitness and clinical exercise science programs, exercise science professionals seem to agree that some form of regulation is needed.

Independent third-party accrediting agencies such as the Commission on Accreditation of Allied Health Education Programs (CAAHEP) and the National Commission for Certifying Agencies (NCCA) may serve this purpose. The CAAHEP accredits academic programs—graduate programs in exercise physiology, baccalaureate programs in exercise science, and certificate and associate degree programs for personal fitness trainers. Also, the American Society of Exercise Physiologists (ASEP) has developed standards for the profession of exercise physiology as well as accreditation standards for universities and colleges offering academic degrees in exercise science (ASEP 2018). The NCCA accredits certification programs; many organizations that provide professional credentialing or licensing exams in the allied health professions are accredited through the NCCA (ACSM 2004).

CERTIFICATION

Fitness and exercise science professionals obtain certification by passing examinations developed by professional organizations. These organizations typically offer education and training programs, administer their own examinations (written and practical), and issue certifications to individuals passing the examinations. These certifications are generally issued for a 2 to 3 yr period; certification is maintained by taking continuing education courses and earning continuing education credits. Some certification programs are accredited by third-party agencies like the NCCA.

More than 75 organizations offer over 250 certifications for exercise science and fitness professionals (Cohen 2004; Pierce and Herman 2004). Given that there is no governing entity to oversee the development of certification examinations and eligibility requirements, inequalities exist among the certifications available to exercise science professionals. Some certification programs are more rigorous than others, having stringent eligibility requirements; others may or may not be accredited by a third-party accrediting agency like the NCCA. To address the inequality among certification programs, the NCCA formally reviews applications for the accreditation of certification programs. In 2004, the International Health, Racquet, and Sportsclub Association (IHRSA) recommended that all health clubs belonging to their organization hire only personal fitness trainers certified by an NCCA-accredited organization or agency. Wagner (2014) reported results from a survey of 589 exercise physiologists and indicated that 69% of the respondents held one certification while 28% held two or more. Nevertheless, not all exercise science and fitness certifications are equal. This leads to confusion for the consumer in terms of knowing who is and who is not highly trained and qualified as an exercise professional. It also complicates selecting the most appropriate certification for yourself. Some agencies sponsor certification programs primarily for financial gain, while others certify professionals in order to promote exercise science as a profession.

Table 1 lists some of the organizations that offer certifications accredited by the NCCA. Additionally, the Coalition for the Registration of Exercise Professionals (CREP), a not-for-profit corporation composed of organizations that offer NCCA-accred- ited exercise certifications, established a registry of professionals in the United States certified by any of six organizations (www.usreps.org). This website is a convenient means for locating professionals by location, certification, or name. Registries are also available for the United Kingdom (www.exerciseregister.org), Europe (www.europeactive.eu/why-ereps), and New Zealand (www.reps.org.nz).

NATIONAL BOARDS

Some professional organizations in the fitness industry believe there should be alternatives to accreditation of certification programs by the NCCA or other third-party agencies. In the United States, one such alternative was the establishment of National Board examinations for fitness professionals. Unlike the multitude of certification examinations developed by individual organizations and agencies, National Boards are standardized tests to assess the knowledge, skill, and competence of professionals. Most medical and allied health professions utilize National Boards.

In 2003, the National Board of Fitness Examiners (NBFE) was founded as a nonprofit organization with the twin purposes of defining scopes of practice for all fitness professionals and determining standards of practice for various fitness professionals, including floor instructors, group exercise instructors, personal fitness trainers, specialists in youth and senior fitness, and medical exercise specialists.

Table 1 Selected Organizations Associated With National Commission for Certifying Agencies (NCCA) and National Board of Fitness Examiners (NBFE)

NCCA affiliates	NBFE affiliates
American Council on Exercise (ACE)	Aerobics and Fitness Association of America (AFAA)
American College of Sports Medicine (ACSM)	American Aerobic Association International/International Sports Medicine Association (AAAI/ISMA)
Cooper Institute for Aerobics Research	International Sports Sciences Association (ISSA)
National Exercise and Sports Trainers Association (NESTA)	National Association for Fitness Certification (NAFC)
National Exercise Trainers Association (NETA)	National Council for Certified Personal Trainers (NCCPT)
National Federation of Professional Trainers (NFPT)	National Exercise and Sports Trainers Association (NESTA)
National Strength and Conditioning Association (NSCA)	National Gym Association (NGA)
International Fitness Professionals Association (IFPA)	National Personal Training Institute (NPTI)
National Council on Strength and Fitness (NCSF)	National Strength Professionals Association (NSPA)
National Academy of Sports Medicine (NASM)	

The NBFE established national standards of excellence that certifying organizations and colleges or universities may adopt. The written portion of the National Boards for personal fitness trainers is now offered through the NBFE (for additional information, visit www.NBFE.org). The practical portion of this exam is still being developed and validated under the supervision of the National Board of Medical Examiners (NBME). The NBME and the NBFE are engaged in preliminary discussions and planning that will allow certification organizations to assist in the delivery of practical exams for personal trainers.

To be eligible to sit for the National Boards, personal fitness trainers must successfully complete a personal training certification program from an approved NBFE affiliate. Affiliate status is available to qualified groups from the areas of medicine, certification organizations, fitness professionals, health clubs, and higher education. In the future, the NBFE's National Boards may be used by certifying organizations, colleges and universities, and U.S. state licensing programs to test the knowledge, skill, and competence of fitness professionals (American Fitness Professionals and Associates 2004). Table 1 lists some of the organizations offering personal training certifications affiliated with the NBFE.

LICENSURE

Although many practitioners in the fitness and exercise science fields agree that certification ensures professional competency, other professionals believe that licensure is better suited for protecting consumers and for enhancing the credibility and professionalism of exercise science and fitness professionals (Eickhoff-Shemek and Herbert 2007). For the first time in the 12 yr history of the worldwide survey of fitness trends, licensure for fitness professionals broke into the top 20 trends (number 16 for 2018) (Thompson 2017). In the United States, licensure is decided at the state level; therefore, requirements may vary from state to state. Louisiana was the first state to pass a law requiring licensure of all clinical exercise physiologists (Herbert 1995). Licensure of clinical exercise physiologists has also been considered in Maryland, Massachusetts, Michigan, North Carolina, Texas, and Utah (Clinical Exercise Physiology Association, 2013). Several states including Georgia, Maryland, Massachusetts, New Jersey, Nevada, Oregon, and the District of Columbia have considered licensure for personal trainers (Eickhoff-Shemek and Herbert 2008b; Herbert 2004; Thompson 2017).

To promote exercise science and exercise physiology as a profession, the ASEP is working with exercise professionals throughout the United States to develop uniform state licensure requirements for exercise physiologists. Licensure would place exercise physiologists and personal trainers on a par with other allied health professionals (e.g., nurses, nutritionists, physical therapists, and occupational therapists) who are required to have licenses to practice. Licensed fitness professionals may be more likely to obtain referrals from health care professionals and to receive reimbursement for services from third parties (e.g., insurance companies).

Along with advantages, added responsibilities and disadvantages are associated with state licensure. Licensure may limit the scope of practice and services that exercise professionals are currently able to provide to the public. For example, Louisiana licensure law requires clinical exercise physiologists to work under the direction of a licensed physician. Also, the costs of licensure, continuing education for licensure, and professional liability insurance may be more expensive compared with the cost of certifications. Professionals moving from state to state may be required to obtain another license because each state could require different credentials for licensure (Eickhoff-Shemek and Herbert 2008a, 2008b).

STATUTORY CERTIFICATION

Instead of licensure, some American states use statutory certification for allied health professionals. Statutory certification regulates what titles professionals can use and the qualifications needed to obtain these titles. Only certified professionals with the required credentials are allowed to use the specific title (e.g., certified nutritionist). Other professionals without the necessary credentials can still practice in the state but must use a different title. This approach could be promoted by the fitness and exercise professions to prevent the use of titles, such as personal trainer or exercise physiologist, by individuals having no formal education or professional certifications.

All these approaches demonstrate the pressing need to get a handle on certifications for exercise professionals so we can gain control of who is practicing in our field. This will ensure the safety of exercise program participants and enable individuals working in the fitness field to be recognized as exercise science professionals. Until these issues are resolved and a list of accredited certification agencies and organizations is finalized, you should select a professional certification that matches your level of education and career goals. For more information about certification programs, visit the websites of those professional certifying organizations.

Many advantages are associated with obtaining either state licensure or certification with professional organizations. You will have a better chance of finding a job in the health and fitness field because many employers are now hiring only professionally certified health and fitness instructors. Certification by reputable professional organizations upgrades the quality of the typical person working in the field and assures employers and their clientele that employees have mastered the knowledge and skills needed to be competent exercise science professionals. Hence, the likelihood of lawsuits resulting from negligence or incompetence may be lessened. Also, certification and licensure help validate exercise specialists as health professionals who are equally deserving of the respect afforded to professionals in other allied health professions. Individuals holding a Registered Clinical Exercise Physiologist (RCEP) or Certified Clinical Exercise Physiologist (CEP) certification now have a National Provider Identifier code that may be used for service reimbursement from insurance companies. For more information on this development, visit the website of the Clinical Exercise Physiology Association (www.acsm-cepa.org).

Acknowledgments

The first edition of this textbook was titled *Designs for Fitness* and was published by Burgess Publishing in 1984. It was a softcover book of about 200 pages. Dr. Swede Schoeller took the photos for that edition. Eileen Fletcher, our department secretary, typed the manuscript on her Smith-Corona.

The second edition was published by Human Kinetics in 1991. This edition was a hardcover book consisting of 350 pages. For this edition, Linda K. Gilkey took the photos. For the first time, the manuscript was typed using a DOS word processing system, by department secretary Sandi Travis.

In 1998, the third edition was published by Human Kinetics. The book grew in size from a 7" × 9" format to an 8.5" × 11" format. Once again, Linda K. Gilkey took the photos, and the computer graphics were done by Dr. Robert Robergs, Dr. Brent Ruby, and Dr. Peter Egan.

The fourth edition, published by Human Kinetics in 2002, was 370 pages. Our colleagues Dr. Christine Mermier, Dr. Virginia Wilmerding, Dr. Len Kravitz, and Dr. Donna Lockner shared their excellent ideas and expertise. The developmental editors, Elaine Mustain and Maggie Schwarzentraub, meticulously edited this edition.

In 2006, the fifth edition was released. For this edition, the total number of pages increased to 425, and Human Kinetics updated all the photos. Sarah Ritz did an excellent job organizing and taking these photos. Dr. Dale Wagner contributed the test question bank that accompanied this edition.

The sixth edition was released in May 2010. For the first time, this book was also published as an ebook. The book expanded to 465 pages. Dr. Dale Wagner updated the test question bank, and Dr. Ann Gibson prepared the slides for the presentation package.

The seventh edition, published in 2014 by Human Kinetics, was coauthored with Dr. Ann Gibson. In addition to being published as an ebook, the 537-page seventh edition was supplemented with instructional videos.

The eighth edition is coauthored with Dr. Ann Gibson and Dr. Dale Wagner. Dr. Wagner's extensive background as a researcher and professor of exercise science has been invaluable in updating and revising this edition. We also acknowledge Cynthia McEntire, our Human Kinetics developmental editor, Martha Gullo, who obtained the publication permissions for this edition, and Amy Stahl, the senior managing editor assigned to this edition.

Many individuals have contributed to the continued success of *Advanced Fitness Assessment and Exercise Prescription*. We are indebted to each person who played a role in the metamorphosis of this book.

CHAPTER 1

Physical Activity, Health, and Chronic Disease

KEY QUESTIONS

▶ Are adults in the United States and other countries getting enough physical activity?

▶ How does physical inactivity differ from sedentarism?

▶ What diseases are associated with a sedentary lifestyle, and what are the major risk factors for these diseases?

▶ What are the benefits of regular physical activity in terms of disease prevention and healthy aging?

▶ How does physical activity improve health?

▶ How much physical activity is needed for improved health benefits?

▶ What kinds of physical activities are suitable for typical people, and how often should they exercise?

Although physical activity plays an important role in preventing chronic diseases and reducing the hazardous effects of extended periods of sitting time, an alarming percentage of adults in the United States report no physical activity during leisure time. One of the national health objectives for the year 2020 is to increase to 47.9% the proportion of people aged 18 yr and older who regularly (preferably daily) engage in moderate physical activity at least 30 min per day (U.S. Department of Health and Human Services 2010). According to a U.S. national survey, in 2014 only a small percentage (21.5%) of adults over the age of 18 met the 2008 federal physical activity guidelines for adults in terms of both aerobic and muscle strengthening activities. Slightly more than half (53.2%) met either the aerobic activity or the muscle-strengthening guidelines, but not both (Centers for Disease Control and Prevention 2015a). Generally, women (50%) are less likely to meet the full aerobic and muscle-strengthening recommendations than men (43.4%), and older (≥65 yr) adults are less likely (58.7%) to meet them than younger (18-24 yr) adults (40.8%) (Centers for Disease Control and Prevention 2015a).

Physical inactivity, the failure to meet the recommended physical activity guidelines, is not just a problem in the United States; it is a global issue and the fourth leading cause of global mortality (World Health Organization 2010). Cardiovascular diseases, diabetes, obesity, chronic respiratory disorders, and cancers as a group of **noncommunicable diseases (NCDs)** are the leading causes of death worldwide. These chronic conditions are heavily influenced by poor lifestyle factors including physical inactivity and unhealthy diet (World Medical Association 2017). NCDs accounted for approximately 52% of worldwide deaths occurring before age 70 in 2012 (World Health Organization 2016d). Physical inactivity became a targeted priority of the World Health Organization's Global Action Plan for 2013-2020 (World Health Organization 2013); a global goal was set to reduce physical inactivity levels by 10% by the year 2025 (Sallis et al. 2016).

Results from survey data collected from 146 countries representing all income levels estimated that 23% of the global adult (≥15 yr) population was physically inactive in 2016. However, an 8% decrease in physical inactivity between 2012 and

USING TECHNOLOGY TO INCREASE PHYSICAL ACTIVITY AT WORK

Active workstations (e.g., treadmill desks or pedal desks) and adjustable-height work surfaces that allow employees to stand (sit-stand desks) are becoming more commonplace. They provide a means to reduce prolonged periods of sitting. Some employees have their own active workstations, while others have access to one located in a common area. A recent review of studies about active workstations (Cao et al. 2016) indicates that the calories burned may increase two- to fourfold for employees who change from sitting in a chair (~70-90 kcal·h^{-1}) to active workstations. Additionally, daily step counts and physical activity (min/day) increase dramatically for those using active workstations during the workday. Crandall and colleagues (2016) found that using sit-stand workstations reduces sitting time by approximately 85 min/day. They also reported that employees using a shared treadmill desk accumulate slightly fewer than 9,000 steps·day^{-1} while at work. Ongoing longitudinal research in this area may identify long-term effects of using active workstations on employee health. Currently, these effects are not well documented.

2016 may be less reflective of changes in activity levels than in updated physical activity recommendations (150 min of moderate-intensity activity or 75 min of vigorous-intensity activity per week, or combination thereof). The current recommendations changed the frequency of exercise bouts from 5 days per week (moderate-intensity) or 3 days per week (vigorous-intensity) to weekly totals of minutes. The prevalence of physical inactivity ranges from approximately 38% in the eastern Mediterranean countries to a low of 14.8% in southeast Asia; by World Bank income classification, the low- and lower-middle-income countries were more physically active than their upper-middle- and high-income counterparts (Sallis et al. 2016). In England and Scotland, more than 65% of men and at least 50% of women met the government's physical activity guidelines in 2012 (British Heart Foundation 2015a). However, only 18% of Canadian adults responding to the 2014-2015 Canadian Health Measures Survey met the recommendation of 150 minutes of moderate-to-vigorous intensity activity in bouts lasting at least 10 minutes (Statistics Canada 2017). Thus, as an exercise specialist, you face the challenge of educating and motivating your clients to incorporate physical activity as a regular part of their lifestyles and to reduce the amount of time spent being seated (Benatti and Ried-Larsen 2015; Bergouignan et al. 2016; Levine 2015; Same et al. 2016).

This chapter deals with the physical activity trends, risk factors associated with chronic noncommunicable diseases, the role of regular exercise and physical activity in disease prevention and health, physical activity guidelines and recommendations for improved health, and the importance of including exercise and physical activity as one of the vital signs (i.e. heart rate, blood pressure, etc.) monitored during annual visits to the doctor. For definitions of terminology used in this chapter, see the glossary.

PHYSICAL ACTIVITY, HEALTH, AND DISEASE: AN OVERVIEW

Technological advances affecting nearly every facet of life have substantially lessened work-related physical activity as well as the energy expenditure required for performing activities of daily living like cleaning the house, washing clothes and dishes, mowing the lawn, and traveling to work. What would have once required an hour of physical work now can be accomplished in just a few seconds by pushing a button or setting a dial. Survey results from 23 low-income and 25 upper-middle-income countries suggest that access to modern technological conveniences underlies an inverse relationship between both education level and financial assets with the prevalence of physical inactivity (Allen et al. 2017). The unfortunate fact is, however, that many individuals do not engage in physical activity during their leisure time and sit too much at work and after hours.

Although the human body is designed for movement and strenuous physical activity, exercise is not part of the average person's lifestyle. Industrialization and urbanization have led to increased

sedentarism and sedentary behaviors (performing activities of ≤1.5 METs while in a sitting or reclining posture) (Benatti and Ried-Larsen 2015; Sedentary Behaviour Research Network 2012). One cannot expect the human body to function optimally and to remain healthy for extended periods if it is abused or is not used as intended.

Physical inactivity is recognized as a major contributor to the physical and economic burden of disease nationally and globally. The identification of physical inactivity as the fourth leading risk factor for mortality supports what experts noted nearly a decade ago—physical inactivity may well be the most important public health problem in the 21st century (Blair 2009). To highlight this, a global action plan was developed to increase the number of people meeting the recommended weekly amount of physical activity by 10% (World Health Organization 2013). The World Health Organization (2014) reported that physical inactivity causes an estimated 3.2 million deaths annually. Data from large cohort studies conducted around the world were pooled and analyzed; resulting estimations revealed that between 6% and 10% of coronary heart disease, type

2 diabetes, and breast and colon cancers are due to physical inactivity (Lee et al. 2012). As a risk factor, physical inactivity is basically equivalent to the combined risk of smoking and obesity. Sedentarism has repeatedly been identified as an independent risk factor associated with an increased risk for all-cause mortality and metabolic and heart disorders (Benatti and Ried-Larsen 2015). Individuals who do not exercise regularly and sit too much are at greater risk for developing chronic noncommunicable diseases such as those in figure 1.1.

For years, exercise scientists as well as health and fitness professionals have maintained that regular physical activity is the best defense against the development of many diseases, disorders, and illnesses. The importance of regular physical activity in maintaining a high quality of life and in preventing disease and premature death received recognition as a national health objective in the first U.S. surgeon general's report on physical activity and health (U.S. Department of Health and Human Services 1996). This report identified physical inactivity as a serious nationwide health problem, provided clear-cut scientific evidence linking physical activity to

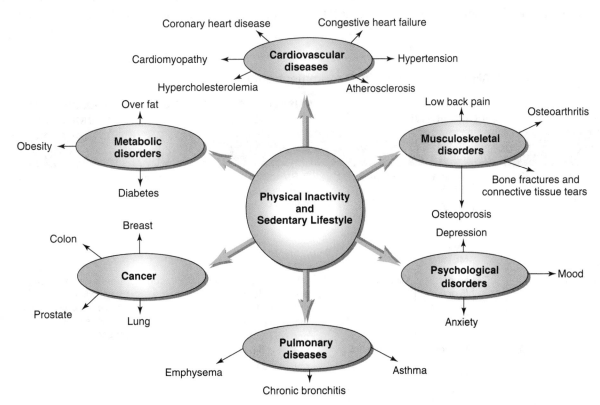

FIGURE 1.1   Role of physical activity and exercise in disease prevention and rehabilitation.

numerous health benefits, presented demographic data describing physical activity patterns and trends in the U.S. population, and made physical activity recommendations for improved health. In 1995, the CDC and the American College of Sports Medicine (ACSM) recommended that every U.S. adult should accumulate 30 min or more of moderate-intensity physical activity on most, preferably all, days of the week (Pate et al. 1995). This recommendation has since been adopted by many international organizations.

Since 1995, new scientific evidence increased our understanding of the benefits of physical activity for improved health and quality of life. In light of these findings, the American Heart Association (AHA) and the ACSM updated physical activity recommendations for healthy adults and older adults (Haskell et al. 2007; Nelson et al. 2007). These recommendations address how much and what type of physical activity are needed to promote health and reduce the risk of chronic disease in adults. Table 1.1 summarizes the ACSM and AHA physical activity recommendations for adults.

The recommended amounts of physical activity are in addition to routine activities of daily living (ADLs) such as housework, cooking, shopping, and walking around the home or from the parking lot.

The intensity of exercise is expressed as a metabolic equivalent of task (MET). An MET is the ratio of the person's working (exercising) metabolic rate to the resting metabolic rate, with 1 MET defined as the energy cost of sitting quietly. Moderate-intensity aerobic activity (3.0-6.0 METs or 5 or 6 on a 10-point perceived exertion scale) is operationally defined as activity that noticeably increases heart rate and lasts more than 10 min (e.g., brisk walking at 3.0-4.0 mph [4.8-6.4 km·hr^{-1}]). Vigorous-intensity activity (>6.0 METs or 7 or 8 on a 10-point perceived exertion scale) causes rapid breathing and increases heart rate substantially (e.g., jogging or running at 4.5 mph [7.2 km·hr^{-1}] or higher). For adults (18-65 yr) and older adults (>65 yr), the ACSM recommends a minimum of 150 min of moderate-intensity aerobic activity per week or 75 min of vigorous-intensity aerobic exercise per week. It is also recommended that these totals be spread over the course of a week to avoid injury). They also recommend moderate- to high-intensity (8- to 12-repetition maximum [RM] for adults and 10-RM to 15-RM for older adults) resistance training for a minimum of 2 nonconsecutive days per week. Balance and flexibility exercises are also suggested for older adults.

Table 1.2 summarizes the physical activity guidelines (U.S. Department of Health and Human

Table 1.1 ACSM/AHA Physical Activity Recommendations

	AEROBIC ACTIVITIES[a]				MUSCLE-STRENGTHENING ACTIVITIES		FLEXIBILITY AND BALANCE ACTIVITIES
Population group	Duration[b] (min/day)	Intensity	Frequency (days/wk)	Sets	Intensity or # of exercises	Frequency (days/wk)	
Healthy adults 18-65 yr	30	Moderate (3.0-6.0 METS)	Minimum 5	1	8-RM to 12-RM; 8-10 exercises for major muscle groups	≥2 nonconsecutive days	No specific recommendation
	20	Vigorous (>6.0 METS)	Minimum 3				
Older adults >65 yr	30	Moderate (5 or 6 on 10 pt. scale)	Minimum 5	1	10-RM to 15-RM; 8-10 exercises for major muscle groups; Moderate intensity (5 or 6 on 10 pt. scale) Vigorous intensity (7 or 8 on 10 pt. scale)	2 nonconsecutive days	For flexibility at least 2 days/wk for at least 10 min each day; include balance exercises for those at risk for falls
	20	Vigorous (7 or 8 on 10 pt. scale)	Minimum 3				

[a]Combinations of moderate and vigorous intensity may be performed to meet recommendation (e.g., jogging 20 min on 2 days and brisk walking on 2 other days).

[b]Multiple bouts of moderate-intensity activity, each lasting at least 10 min, can be accumulated to meet the minimum duration of 30 min.

Table 1.2 2008 Physical Activity Guidelines for Americans

Population group	AEROBIC ACTIVITIES			MUSCLE-STRENGTHENING ACTIVITIES			BONE-STRENGTHENING ACTIVITIES	FLEXIBILITY AND BALANCE ACTIVITIES
	Duration	Intensity*	Frequency	Sets	Intensity*	Frequency		
Children and adolescents 6-17 yr	≥60 min	Moderate Vigorous	Daily 3 days/wk		Moderate to high	3 days/wk	3 days/wk	
Adults 18-64 yr								
Inactive	60-150 min/wk	Light (1.1-2.9 METs) to moderate (3.0-5.9 METs)		1	Light to moderate	1 day/wk		All adults should stretch to maintain flexibility for regular physical activity (PA) and activities of daily living (ADLs).
Active	150-300 min/wk or 75-150 min/wk	Moderate (3.0-5.9 METs) Vigorous (≥6.0 METs)		≥1	Moderate to high 8-RM to 12-RM	≥2 days/wk		
Highly active	>300 min/wk >150 min/wk	Moderate (3.0-5.9 METs) Vigorous (≥6.0 METs)		2 or 3	Moderate to high	≥2 days/wk		
Older adults ≥65 yr								
Inactive	150 min/wk	Light (RPE = 3 or 4) to moderate (RPE = 5 or 6)	5 days/wk	1	Light (RPE = 3 or 4) to moderate (RPE = 5 or 6)	2 or 3 days/wk		Older adults should stretch to maintain flexibility for regular PA and ADLs. ≥3 days/wk balance
Active	150-300 min/wk or 75-150 min/wk	Moderate (RPE = 5 or 6) Vigorous (RPE = 7 or 8)	≥3 days/wk	≥1	Moderate (RPE = 5 or 6) to high (RPE = 7 or 8) 8-RM to 12-RM	≥2 days/wk, nonconsecutive days		

*Intensity is expressed in METs and repetition maximums (RM) for adults; for older adults, intensity is expressed as a rating of perceived exertion (RPE; 0-10 scale) and RM.

HEALTH BENEFITS OF PHYSICAL ACTIVITY

Lower risk of

- dying prematurely;
- coronary artery disease;
- stroke;
- type 2 diabetes and metabolic syndrome;
- high blood pressure;
- adverse blood lipid profile;
- colon, breast, lung, and endometrial cancers; and
- hip fractures.

Reduction of

- abdominal obesity and
- feelings of depression and anxiety.

Helps in

- weight loss, weight maintenance, and prevention of weight gain;
- prevention of falls and improved functional health for older adults;
- improved cognitive function;
- increased bone density; and
- improved quality of sleep.

Data from U.S. Department of Health and Human Services 2008.

Services 2008) for children and adolescents (6-17 yr), adults (18-64 yr), and older adults (≥65 yr). The key message in these guidelines is that for substantial health benefits, adults should engage in aerobic exercise at least 150 min/wk at a moderate intensity or 75 min/wk at a vigorous intensity or an equivalent combination thereof. In addition, adults of all ages should do muscle-strengthening activities at least 2 days/wk. In addition to stretching to support physical activity and activities of daily living, those who are at risk for falling should also perform balance exercises. Children should do at least 60 min of physical activity every day. Most of the 60 min per day should be either moderate or vigorous aerobic activity and should include vigorous aerobic activities at least 3 days/wk. Part of the 60 min or more of daily physical activity should be muscle-strengthening activities (at least 3 days/wk) and bone-strengthening activities (at least 3 days/wk).

The term **exercise deficit disorder (EDD)** has been used to identify children who do not attain at least 60 min of moderate- to vigorous-intensity physical activity (MVPA) on a daily basis (Faigenbaum and Myer 2011). Children with EDD are at an increased risk for developing harmful health effects in their adolescent and adult years due to a physically inactive lifestyle (Stracciolini, Myer, and Faigenbaum 2013). For example, results from a study that monitored children for 14 yr revealed that those who maintained their active childhood MVPA levels through adolescence were less likely to become obese as young adults (Kwon et al. 2015).

Exercising 150 min/wk equates to expending approximately 1,000 kcal·wk^{-1}. Results from a meta-analysis (Sattelmair et al. 2011) indicated that individuals meeting the 2008 physical activity guidelines decrease their risk for coronary heart disease by 14% compared with those reporting no leisure-time physical activity (LTPA). Participating in regular physical activity and exercise on a daily basis provides numerous preventative benefits for no fewer than 25 chronic medical conditions (Warburton and Breden 2016) such as cardiovascular disease, hypertension, diabetes, stroke, dementia, and several types of cancer. Disease risk is further reduced when moderate-intensity physical activity (150-180 min/wk) is performed throughout the week (i.e., 30 min/day on 5 days/wk) and in bouts lasting at least 10 min as opposed to in one single session (Kesäniemi et al. 2010).

Sattelmair and colleagues (2011) reported that 300 min/wk of moderate-intensity physical activity results in a 20% reduction in the risk for coronary heart disease (CHD). Furthermore, a review of studies on asymptomatic adults (19-65 yr) revealed that 90 min of vigorous-intensity physical activity accumulated throughout the week (90 min/wk) in increments of no fewer than 10 min reduces the risk of all-cause mortality by 30%, as well as the risk for cardiovascular disease (CVD), hypertension, stroke, type 2 diabetes, and breast and colon cancer (Kesäniemi et al. 2010).

In 2009, an international consensus conference was convened to review Canada's *Physical Activity Guide to Healthy Active Living* (Health Canada 2003). The consensus panel recommended that asymptomatic Canadian adults (19-65 yr) accumulate 150 min/wk of moderate-intensity physical activity or 90 min/wk of vigorous-intensity activity as a primary prevention against cardiovascular disease, stroke, hypertension, colon cancer, breast cancer, type 2 diabetes, and osteoporosis. They also recommended multiple exercise sessions in a week, with each session lasting a minimum of 10 min (Kesäniemi et al. 2010). In addition to the aerobic exercise, they recommended strength activities (2-4 days/wk) and flexibility activities (4-7 days/wk). The duration of the activity depends on the intensity or effort: Perform light activities (e.g., walking, video gaming that promotes light effort, gardening, carrying small children, or hairstyling) for 60 min, moderate activities (e.g., brisk walking, swimming, vacuuming, moving furniture, or chopping wood) for 30 to 60 min, and vigorous activities (e.g., jogging, hockey, wheelchair basketball, felling large trees, or rollerblading) for 20 to 30 min.

Improvements in health benefits depend on the volume (i.e., combination of frequency, intensity, and duration) of physical activity. This is known as the **dose-response relationship** (Loprinzi 2015). Because of the dose-response relationship between physical activity and health, even a low level of MVPA each week is better than none; doses less than one-half of the recommended guidelines may lead to notable health benefits for those with elevated risks for chronic conditions and premature mortality (Warburton and Breden 2016). Exceeding the minimum recommended MVPA dose by a factor of 5 (i.e., 750 min/wk or ≥10,000 MVPA MET-min/mo) may confer the greatest reduction in all-cause mortality risk; no additional mortality-related benefit is associated with a dose 10 times higher than recommended (Arem et al. 2015; Loprinzi 2015). MVPA MET-min/mo is easily computed by multiplying the respective MET level for the specific activities (see appendix E.3) by the number of minutes one engages in those MVPA activities within a month.

Figure 1.2 illustrates the general dose-response relationship between the volume of physical activity participation and selected health benefits (e.g., muscular strength and aerobic fitness) that do not require a minimal threshold intensity for improvement. The volume of physical activity participation needed for the same degree of relative improvement (%) varies among health benefit indicators. For example, to improve triglycerides from 0% to 40% requires 250 kcal·wk[-1] of physical activity compared with 1,800 kcal·wk[-1] for the same relative improvement (0%-40%) in high-density lipoprotein (HDL; see figure 1.2). It appears that aerobic-style activities that can be maintained for longer periods (e.g., bicycling, dancing, jogging) are positively related to beneficial

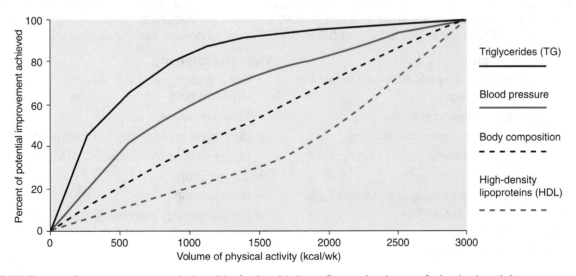

FIGURE 1.2 Dose-response relationship for health benefits and volume of physical activity.

Courtesy of N. Gledhill and V. Jamnik of York University School of Kinesiology and Health Science.

changes in HDL (Loprinzi 2015). Jogging at a slow or average pace ≤3 days/wk for a total of 60 to 150 min/wk confers a favorable increase in heart function and a similar decrease in mortality, whereas decades-long strenuous endurance training routines (≥12 METs) in preparation for extreme endurance competitions may actually damage the cardiovascular system (Schnohr et al. 2015). Therefore, too much physical activity, defined as engaging in 5 hr of structured high-intensity activity per week, may be associated with negative health consequences or overuse injuries.

Although no specific dose of sedentary behavior has been found, a direct linear relationship between total daily time in sedentary behavior and negative health indicators associated with metabolic syndrome (high triglycerides, high fasting blood glucose, and low HDL-C) has been reported (Gennuso et al. 2015). Each 60 min increase in daily time spent being sedentary is associated with a 9% increase in the odds of satisfying the criteria for metabolic syndrome (Gennuso et al. 2015).

Although the physical activity guideline—a minimum of 150 min of moderate- to vigorous-intensity aerobic activity weekly, preferably performed on a daily basis—reduces disease risk, additional physical activity is needed to mitigate weight gain over time (Moholdt et al. 2014). Levine (2015) describes how standing and walking double the energy expended as compared with sitting; he also illustrates how office workers can expend approximately 1,000 kcal·day^{-1} and increase time spent being active by incorporating walking meetings and short activity breaks in the typical business day. In 2002, the Institute of Medicine (IOM) recommended 60 min of daily moderate-intensity physical activity. In the IOM report, the expert panel stated that 30 min of daily physical activity is insufficient to maintain a healthy body weight and to fully reap its associated health benefits. The IOM recommendation addresses the amount of physical activity necessary to maintain a healthy body weight and to prevent unhealthful weight gain (Brooks et al. 2004). The IOM recommendation of 60 min of daily physical activity is consistent with recommendations for preventing weight gain made by other organizations (i.e., Health Canada, International Association for the Study of Obesity, and World Health Organization) (Brooks et al. 2004).

EXAMPLES OF MODERATE-INTENSITY AND VIGOROUS-INTENSITY AEROBIC ACTIVITIES

This list provides several examples of moderate- and vigorous-intensity aerobic activities. Some activities can be performed at varied intensities. This list is not all-inclusive; examples are provided to help people make choices. For a detailed list of energy expenditures (METs) for conditioning exercises, sports, and recreational activities, see appendix E.3 and http://links.lww.com/MSS/A82. Generally, light activity is defined as <3.0 METs, moderate activity as 3.0 to 6.0 METs, and vigorous activity as >6.0 METs.

Moderate Intensity

- Walking briskly (3.0 mph [4.8 km·hr^{-1}] or faster, but not race walking)
- Skateboarding (noncompetitive)
- Water aerobics and water calisthenics
- Bicycling slower than 10 mph (16 km·hr^{-1})
- Tennis (doubles)
- Ethnic and cultural dancing (e.g., Middle Eastern, salsa, merengue, swing)
- General gardening
- Yoga (e.g., hatha, power)

Vigorous Intensity

- Race walking, jogging, running, or vigorous lap swimming
- Tennis (singles)
- Dancing (e.g., folk, line, competitive ballroom)
- Bicycling 10 mph (16 km·hr^{-1}) or faster
- Jumping rope
- Backpacking
- Circuit training (resistance based with some aerobics and minimal rest intervals)

Data from http://links.lww.com/MSS/A82 (accessed June 28, 2018).

The bottom line is that 150 min/wk of moderate-intensity physical activity provides substantial health benefits but may be insufficient to prevent weight gain for many individuals. It is a good initial goal and a sufficient amount of activity to move individuals from a sedentary to low physical activity level (Brooks et al. 2004). As individuals adopt regular physical activity and improve their lifestyle and fitness, they should increase the duration of daily physical activity to a level (60 min) that prevents short-term weight gain and provides additional health benefits. Progression to daily engagement in physical activity, inclusive of resistance training, for 60 to 90 min is important for long-term weight maintenance after weight loss (Bray et al. 2016; Ryan and Heaner 2014). Although there appears to be little overall effect on long-term weight loss based on exercise type (aerobic vs. resistance) or intensity (lower vs. higher), the reduced time requirement for equivalent energy expenditure of high-intensity exercise as compared with low-intensity exercise may increase exercise adherence and, hence, weight maintenance (Bray et al. 2016).

The Exercise and Physical Activity Pyramid illustrates a balanced plan of physical activity and exercise to promote health and to improve physical fitness (see figure 1.3). Encourage your clients to engage in physical activities around the home and workplace on a daily basis to establish a foundation (base of pyramid) for an active lifestyle. Strategies for increasing energy expenditure in the workplace are built on encouraging active breaks from sitting in order to move around (e.g., step in place, walk laps around the office, perform light calisthenics,

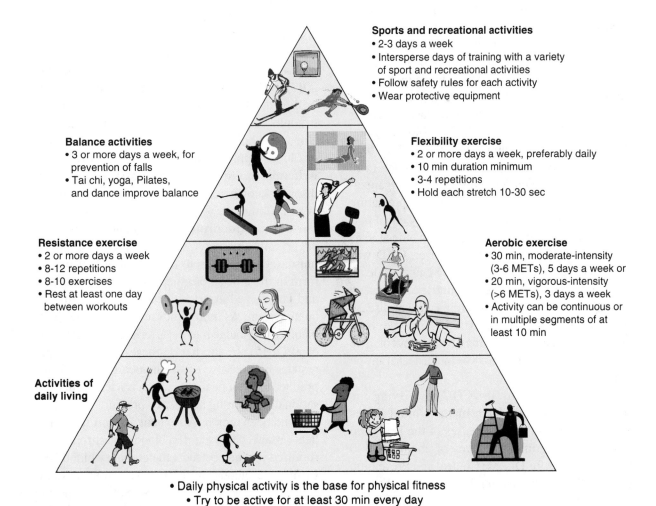

Sports and recreational activities
- 2-3 days a week
- Intersperse days of training with a variety of sport and recreational activities
- Follow safety rules for each activity
- Wear protective equipment

Balance activities
- 3 or more days a week, for prevention of falls
- Tai chi, yoga, Pilates, and dance improve balance

Flexibility exercise
- 2 or more days a week, preferably daily
- 10 min duration minimum
- 3-4 repetitions
- Hold each stretch 10-30 sec

Resistance exercise
- 2 or more days a week
- 8-12 repetitions
- 8-10 exercises
- Rest at least one day between workouts

Aerobic exercise
- 30 min, moderate-intensity (3-6 METs), 5 days a week or
- 20 min, vigorous-intensity (>6 METs), 3 days a week
- Activity can be continuous or in multiple segments of at least 10 min

Activities of daily living

- Daily physical activity is the base for physical fitness
- Try to be active for at least 30 min every day

FIGURE 1.3 The Exercise and Physical Activity Pyramid.

Adapted by permission from "Exercise and Activity Pyramid," Metropolitan Life Insurance Company, 1995.

walk down the hall to a colleague's office instead of calling or e-mailing to deliver a message, climb a flight of stairs to get a drink of water or use the restroom). Your clients should perform aerobic activities a minimum of 3 days/wk; they should do weight-resistance exercises and flexibility or balance exercises at least 2 days/wk. Recreational sport activities (middle levels of pyramid) are recommended to add variety to the exercise plan. High-intensity training and competitive sport (top of pyramid) require a solid fitness base and proper preparation to prevent injury; most adults should engage in these activities sparingly.

CARDIOVASCULAR DISEASE

Cardiovascular disease (CVD) is projected to cause more than 26 million deaths by 2030 (World Health Organization 2011b). CVD caused 17.9 million deaths (46% of the deaths attributed to all noncommunicable diseases) worldwide in 2015. Of the deaths due to CVD in 2015, the combination of stroke and ischemic heart disease accounted for the great majority (85%) (GBD 2015 Mortality and Causes of Death Collaborators 2016). More than 75% of cardiovascular deaths occurred in low- and middle-income countries (World Health Organization 2016a). CVD is the principal cause of premature death in Europe, accounting for a nearly equal percentage of all deaths before age 75 in women (36%) and men (35%). Interestingly, however, CVD was surpassed by cancer as the leading cause of death in several Western European countries (Townsend et al. 2016). CVD is also a leading cause of disease burden in developing low- and middle-income countries; deaths due to CVD range from a low of 10% in sub-Saharan Africa to 58% in Eastern Europe (Wagner and Brath 2012).

In a 2015 report by the CDC identifying the underlying causes of death in the United States between 1999 and 2003, diseases of the heart and blood vessels claimed the lives of about 610,000 people (Centers for Disease Control and Prevention 2015a). CVD accounted for 25% of all deaths (one out of every four) in the United States. Extrapolating to 2014 levels, the CDC estimated that more than 92 million Americans have some form of CVD such as hypertension (~86 million), CHD (27.6 million), or stroke (7.2 million) (American Heart Association 2017). Among American adults 20 yr of age or older, the estimated age-adjusted prevalence of coronary heart disease is higher for black men and women compared with Hispanic and white men and women (American Heart Association 2017).

One myth about CVD is that it is much more prevalent in men than in women. Between 2011 and 2014, the prevalence of CVD in adult women (35.9%) and men (37.7%) in the United States was similar (American Heart Association 2017). Nearly 399,000 females died from CVD in 2014 in the United States. Another misconception about CVD is that it afflicts only the older population. Although it is true that older people are at greater risk, more than 50% of the people in the United States with CVD are younger than 60 yr (American Heart Association 2017), and CVD ranks as the second-leading cause of death for children under age 15 (American Heart Association 2012).

The prevalence of American adults with CHD was 45.1% in 2014 (American Heart Association 2017). In Europe, CHD accounts for more than 1.7 million deaths, with nearly 19% of those occurring in adults below the age of 65 (Townsend et al. 2016). **Coronary heart disease (CHD)** is caused by a lack of blood supply to the heart muscle (**myocardial ischemia**) resulting from a progressive degenerative disorder known as **atherosclerosis**. Atherosclerosis is an inflammatory process involving a buildup of **low-density lipoprotein (LDL)** cholesterol, scavenger cells (monocytes), necrotic debris, smooth muscle cells, and fibrous tissue. This is how plaques form in the intima, or inner lining, of the medium- and large-sized arteries throughout the cardiovascular system. As more lipids and cells gather in the plaques, they bulge into the arterial lumen (Barquera et al. 2015). In the heart, these bulging plaques restrict blood flow to the myocardium and may produce **angina pectoris**, which is a temporary sensation of tightening and heavy pressure in the chest and shoulder region. A **myocardial infarction**, or heart attack, can occur if a blood clot (thrombus) or ruptured plaque obstructs the coronary blood flow. In this case, blood flow through the coronary arteries is usually reduced by more than 80%. The portion of the myocardium supplied by the obstructed artery may die and eventually be replaced with scar tissue.

CARDIOVASCULAR DISEASE RISK FACTORS

Epidemiological research indicates that many factors are associated with the risk of CVD. The greater the number and severity of risk factors, the greater the probability of CVD. The positive risk factors for CVD are

- age,
- family history,
- hypercholesterolemia,
- hypertension,
- tobacco use,
- diabetes mellitus or prediabetes,
- overweight and obesity, and
- physical inactivity.

An increased level ($\geq$60 mg·dl^{-1}) of high-density lipoprotein cholesterol, or **HDL-cholesterol (HDL-C)**, in the blood decreases CVD risk. If the HDL-C is high, you should subtract one risk factor from the sum of the positive factors when assessing your client's CVD risk.

PHYSICAL ACTIVITY AND CORONARY HEART DISEASE

Approximately 12% of CHD deaths in the United States can be attributed to a lack of physical activity (American Heart Association 2017). As cited in American Heart Association (2017), the percentage of physically inactive people worldwide in 2012 (35%) surpassed the percentage of those who smoked (26%); however, Sallis and colleagues (2016), reported the global percentage of physically inactive adults to be closer to 23%. As an exercise scientist, you must educate your clients about the benefits of physical activity and regular exercise for preventing CHD. Physically active people have lower incidences of myocardial infarction and mortality from CHD and tend to develop CHD at a later age compared with their sedentary or less active counterparts (American Heart Association 2017). Leading a physically active lifestyle and sitting less than 4 hr a day may reduce cardiovascular disease mortality rates by 23% to 74% (Ekelund et al. 2016). Alternatively, in their analysis of multiple studies investigating

sedentary behavior and incidence of CVD, Biswas and associates (2015) reported an increase in odds ranging from 6% to more than doubled.

Physical activity, just like sedentary behavior and cardiorespiratory fitness levels, exerts its effect independently of other risk factors related to premature death from CHD and all causes (Bouchard, Blair, and Katzmarzyk 2015). Another conclusion about the independent effect of sedentary behavior (Carter et al. 2017) is that evidence increasingly points to the likely link between sedentarism and its ability to further exacerbate the traditional, modifiable CV risk factors (Benatti and Ried-Larsen 2015; Bergouignan et al. 2016; Same et al. 2016). Also, in a meta-analysis of studies dealing with the dose-response effects of physical activity and cardiorespiratory fitness on CVD and CHD risk, Williams (2001) reported that cardiorespiratory fitness and physical activity have significantly different relationships to CVD and CHD risk. Although physical fitness and physical activity each lower the risk of developing CVD and CHD, the reduction in relative risk was almost twice as great for cardiorespiratory fitness as for physical activity. These findings suggest that in addition to physical activity level, low cardiorespiratory fitness level should be considered a potential risk factor for CHD (U.S. Department of Health and Human Services 2008).

HYPERTENSION

Hypertension, or high blood pressure, is a chronic, persistent elevation of blood pressure. Individuals with this diagnosis are often prescribed antihypertensive medicine. **Elevated blood pressure** is the term used to identify systolic blood pressure (SBP) values between 120 and 129 mmHg, even if diastolic blood pressure (DBP) is lower than 80 mmHg. **Stage 1 hypertension** describes a value of 130 to 139 mmHg for SBP or a DBP value of 80 to 89 mmHg; **stage 2 hypertension** denotes SBP values $\geq$140 mmHg or DBP values $\geq$ 90 mmHg (Whelton et al. 2017). An expanded link exists between hypertension and several forms of CVD (Rapsomaniki et al. 2014). The World Health Organization (2011b) identified hypertension as the leading cardiovascular risk factor, attributing 13% of deaths worldwide to high blood pressure. If not kept in check, hypertension becomes a primary risk factor for stroke, heart attacks, heart and kidney failure, dementia, and blindness (World Health Organization 2014). In the United States, hypertension attributes to about 40% of all adult deaths from CVD (Yang et al. 2012).

In 2014, about 22% of the global adult population (≥18 yr of age) had hypertension (World Health Organization 2014). As of 2015, hypertension is more prevalent in low-income countries in sub-Saharan Africa and south Asia than in high-income countries; however, elevated blood pressure continues to be problematic in Eastern and Central Europe (NCD Risk Factor Collaboration 2017). With an estimated 1.4 billion adult diagnoses worldwide, hypertension is touted as being the leading preventable cause of death before age 70. Its prevalence is lower in high-income countries (28.5%) as compared with low- and middle-income countries (31.5%), which reflects differences in awareness levels as well as treatment and control of the condition (Mills et al. 2016). Nearly one out of every three adults has blood pressure values in the elevated rage (Centers for Disease Control and Prevention 2016). In the United Kingdom, approximately 14% of adults are hypertensive, with Northern Ireland having a lower prevalence compared with England and Scotland (British Heart Foundation 2015b). In comparison, the prevalence of hypertension is estimated to be higher for adults in Latin America and the Caribbean (~39%) than for the Pacific and East Asian region (~36%), Europe and Central Asia (~32%), South Asia (~29%), and Africa (~27%) (Sarki et al. 2015).

In the United States, more men than women are hypertensive prior to age 65; after that the percentage of hypertensive women surpasses that of their male counterparts (American Heart Association 2017). Up to age 45 yr, the percentage of American men with hypertension (11%-23%) is slightly higher than that of women (8%-23%). Between ages 45 and 54 yr, the prevalence of hypertension is similar for men (36.1%) and women (33.2%). Likewise, for those between 55 and 64 yr, men have a slightly higher (57.6%) prevalence of hypertension than do women (~55.5%). After age 65, the percentage of women (65.8%) with high blood pressure is somewhat higher than that of men (63.6%). Women with hypertension have a 3.5 times greater risk of developing CHD than do women who have normal blood pressure (**normotensive**). Also, the prevalence of high blood pressure for blacks in the United States (45.5%) is among the highest in the world and is substantially greater than that of American Indians or Alaskan Natives, Asians or Pacific Islanders, Hispanics, and whites in the United States (American Heart Association 2017). Table 1.3 summarizes the risk factors associated with developing hypertension.

For individuals with elevated blood pressure values, healthy lifestyle changes and periodic BP reassessments are recommended as part of the treatment plan. For people whose blood pressure is in the stage 1 range, their risk for stroke and CVD within the next 10 yr should be assessed using the atherosclerotic cardiovascular disease risk calculator (http://static.heart.org/riskcalc/app/index.html#!/baseline-risk) (Whelton et al. 2017). Sharman, La Gerche, and Coombes (2015) combined data from studies investigating the effect of exercise on blood pressure values in people diagnosed with hypertension. They indicate that while both aerobic and resistance training can reduce blood pressure, aerobic training is the preferred method. Their study also reports on the combination of exercise and antihypertensive medications, with a cautionary note about monitoring postexercise blood pressure responses. Regular physical activity prevents hypertension and lowers blood pressure in younger and older adults who have normal, elevated, stage 1, or stage 2 values. Compared with normotensive individuals, training-induced changes in resting systolic and diastolic blood pressures (5-7 mmHg) are greater for hypertensive individuals who participate in endurance exercise. However, even modest reductions in blood pressure (2-3 mmHg) by endurance or resistance exercise training decrease CHD risk by 5% to 9%, stroke risk by 8% to 14%, and all-cause mortality by 4% in the general population (Pescatello et al. 2004). See Exercise Prescription for Individuals with Hypertension for an exercise prescription that the ACSM endorses to lower blood pressure in adults with hypertension.

Table 1.3 Summary of Factors Associated With Disease Risk

Factor	CHD	Type 2 diabetes	Hypertension	Hypercholesterolemia	Low back pain	Obesity	Osteoporosis	Cancer
Age	↑	↑	↑	↑	↑	↑	↑	↑
Gender	M > F[a]	F > M	F > M[b]	F > M[b]	F = M	F > M	F > M[b]	
Race	B > W > AA, AN > H	AI, AN, B, H > A, W	B > A, AI, H, W	B, H, W > A, AI		AI, B, H, W > A	A, W > AI, B, H	
Family history	↑	↑	↑	↑		↑	↑	↑
SES	→	→	→	→	→	→		↑
Alcohol use			↑	↑			↑	↑
Smoking	↑	↑	↑	↑			↑	↑
Nutrition								
Na+ intake			↑					
Ca++ intake/vitamin D							→	
Fat/cholesterol intake	↑		↑	↑		↑		↑
CHO intake		↑						
Intake > expenditure						↑		
Physical activity	→	→	→	→	→	→	→	→
Exercise amenorrhea							→	
Flexibility					→			
Muscular strength					→		→	
Skeletal frame size							→	
Other diseases								
Anorexia nervosa							↑	
Diabetes	↑							
Hypertension	↑							
Hypercholesterolemia	↑							
Obesity and overweight	↑	↑	↑	↑	↑			↑

↑ = Direct relationship; as factor increases, risk increases.

↓ = Indirect relationship; as factor increases, risk decreases.

CHD = coronary heart disease; CHO = carbohydrate; A = Asian; AI = American Indian; AN = Alaska Native; B = Black; H = Hispanic; W = White; Na = sodium; Ca = calcium; SES = socioeconomic status (reflects income and education levels).

[a]Males (M) at higher risk than females (F) up to age 55 yr.

[b]Menopausal females at higher risk than males.

EXERCISE PRESCRIPTION FOR INDIVIDUALS WITH HYPERTENSION

Mode: Primarily endurance activities supplemented by resistance exercises

Intensity: Moderate-intensity endurance (40%-60% $\dot{V}O_2R$),* rate of perceived exertion of 12-13, and resistance training (60%-80% 1-RM)

Duration: 30 min or more of continuous or accumulated aerobic physical activity per day, and a minimum of two sets (8-12 reps) of resistance training exercises for each major muscle group

Frequency: Most, preferably all, days of the week for aerobic exercise; 2 or 3 days/wk for resistance training

*$\dot{V}O_2R$ is the difference between the maximum and the resting rate of oxygen consumption. See the $\dot{V}O_2$ Reserve (MET) Method section in chapter 5 for more information.

Based on American College of Sports Medicine 2018.

HYPERCHOLESTEROL-EMIA AND DYSLIPIDEMIA

Hypercholesterolemia, an elevation of **total cholesterol (TC)** in the blood, is associated with increased risk for CVD. Hypercholesterolemia is also referred to as **hyperlipidemia**, which is an increase in blood lipid levels; **dyslipidemia** refers to an abnormal blood lipid profile. Approximately 18% of strokes and 56% of heart attacks are caused by high blood **cholesterol** (World Health Organization 2002a). Between 2011 and 2014, the number of adults (≥20 yr of age) having a TC value ≥240 mg·dl⁻¹ fell for all racial and ethnic subgroups; however, this decrease may be due to an increase in medication prescriptions instead of exercise or diet (American Heart Association 2017). Results from the longitudinal, biracial CARDIA study (Schneider et al. 2016) indicate that although TC dropped initially, values stabilized and appear to be reversing toward the end of the 25 yr observation period.

More than 94.6 million Americans age 20 yr and older have total blood cholesterol levels of 200 mg·dl⁻¹ or higher. According to data gathered between 2011 and 2014, 28.5 million American adults (≥20 yr) have TC levels classified as high risk (>240 mg·dl⁻¹); more women (16.4 million) than men (10.6 million) have TC levels equaling or exceeding 240 mg·dl⁻¹ (American Heart Association 2017). Of note, the prevalence of TC, when adjusted for age, decreased in the 2013-2014 period as compared with the 2011-2012 period for both men and women across the four major racial and ethnic groups; the one exception is a 2.6% increased prevalence for non-Hispanic Asian males. Compared with Western countries, the average TC levels for adults in China, Japan, and Indonesia are uniformly lower (190-207 mg·dl⁻¹) (American Heart Association 2001). Risk factors for hypercholesterolemia are identified in table 1.3.

LDLS, HDLS, AND TC

Cholesterol is a waxy, fatlike substance found in all animal products (meats, dairy products, and eggs). The body can make cholesterol in the liver and absorb it from the diet. Cholesterol is essential to the body, and it is used to build cell membranes, produce sex hormones, and form bile acids necessary for fat digestion. **Lipoproteins** are an essential part of the complex transport system that exchanges lipids among the liver, intestine, and peripheral tissues. Lipoproteins are classified by the thickness of the protein shell that surrounds the cholesterol. The four main classes of lipoproteins are **chylomicron**, derived from the intestinal absorption of triglycerides (TG); **very low-density lipoprotein (VLDL)**, made in the liver for the transport of triglycerides; low-density lipoprotein (LDL), a product of VLDL metabolism that serves as the primary transporter of cholesterol; and **high-density lipoprotein (HDL)**, involved in the reverse transport of cholesterol to the liver. The molecules of LDL are larger than those of HDL and therefore precipitate in the plasma and are actively transported into the vascular walls. Excess **LDL-cholesterol (LDL-C)** stimulates the formation of plaque in the intima of the coronary arteries. Plaque formation reduces the cross-sectional area and obstructs blood flow in these arteries, eventually producing a myocardial infarction. Therefore, LDL-C values less than 100 mg·dl⁻¹ are considered optimal for reducing CVD and CHD risk (National Cholesterol Education Program 2001). The prevalence of borderline high levels ($\geq$130 mg·dl^{-1} to <160 mg·dl^{-1}) of LDL-C is nearly identical for adult women (31%) and adult men (32.5%) in the United States (Roger et al. 2012).

The smaller HDL molecules are suspended in the plasma and protect the body by picking up excess cholesterol from the arterial walls and delivering it to the liver, where it is metabolized. HDL-cholesterol (HDL-C) values less than 40 mg·dl^{-1} are associated with a higher risk of CHD. Based on data collected between 2011 and 2014, 19% of men and women in the United States who are older than 20 yr have low (<40 mg·dl^{-1}) HDL-C levels (Zwald et al. 2017).

Individuals with low HDL-C or high TC levels (dyslipidemia) have a greater risk of heart attack. Those with lower HDL-C (<37 mg·dl^{-1}) are at higher risk regardless of their TC level. This emphasizes the importance of screening for both TC and HDL-C in adults.

PHYSICAL ACTIVITY AND LIPID PROFILES

Regular physical activity, especially habitual MVPA aerobic exercise, positively affects lipid metabolism and lipid profiles (Lin, Zhang, et al. 2015). Cross-sectional comparisons of lipid profiles in physically active and sedentary women and men suggest that physical fitness is inversely related to TC and the TC/HDL-C ratio (Despres and Lamarche 1994; Shoenhair and Wells 1995).

Data from 160 randomized controlled trials were pooled to examine the effects of aerobic exercise on cardiometabolic biomarkers such as lipids and lipoproteins in a large number of adults. Results show that compared with control groups, adults in moderate-intensity and vigorous-intensity aerobic exercise interventions, respectively, reduce TC (4.3 and 3.87 mg·dl^{-1}), LDL-C (3.09 and 4.64 mg·dl^{-1}), VLDL-C (1.93 and 7.35 mg·dl^{-1}), and TG (5.31 and 5.31 mg·dl^{-1}) and increase HDL-C (1.16 and 2.71 mg·dl^{-1}) (Lin, Zhang, et al. 2015). However, Lin and colleagues found no differences across exercise-intensity subgroups, which lends support to the premise that moderate- and vigorous-intensity exercise training confer similar favorable results for cardiometabolic health. A 1% reduction in TC has been shown to reduce the risk for CHD by 2%;

likewise, a 1% reduction in HDL-C increases CHD risk by 2% to 3% (Gordon et al. 1989). However, for individuals with hyperlipidemia, lifestyle changes (e.g., healthy diet) or pharmacologic interventions (e.g., statins), in addition to aerobic exercise, may be necessary for optimizing lipid and lipoprotein profiles (Kelley and Kelley 2006).

Increases in HDL-C in response to aerobic exercise appear to be related to the training dose (interaction of the intensity, frequency, and duration of each exercise session and the length of the training period), and they are less dramatic in women than in men. Across adult age ranges, those who met (17.7%) the physical activity guidelines ($\geq$150 min of MVPA per week) had higher HDL-C levels than did those American adults (21.0%) who did not meet the meet the guidelines. Interestingly, the prevalence of low HDL-C values decreased with increasing age for adults meeting the physical activity guidelines; for those $\geq$60 yr old, only 12.6% of the active seniors had low HDL-C values compared with approximately 19% for the younger age groups (Zwald et al. 2017). Based on results from a longitudinal study of biracial adults, a high level of aerobic fitness as a young adult in combination with a continued physically active lifestyle confers favorable results for blood lipid levels in the middle-age adult years (Sarzynski et al. 2015).

The research on the effect of resistance training on cholesterol levels continues to remain inconclusive. Ribeiro and associates (2016) reported improvements in HDL-C for the older, physically independent women (67.6 ± 5.1 yr) randomly assigned to 8 wk of traditional (three sets of 8-RM to 12-RM) or 8 wk of pyramid (12-RM/10-RM/8-RM) styles of resistance training. After a 12 wk washout period, the women switched training styles. There were numerous favorable responses, including increases in HDL-C, by the end of each 8 wk period; however, there were no differences between training styles. Similarly, 12 wk of a nonlinear resistance training program designed to increase strength significantly improved HDL-C and other variables compared with the normally active controls in a sample of adults (18-60 yr) living with HIV and taking prescribed highly active antiretroviral medications (Zanetti et al. 2016). Conversely, 16 wk of combined aerobic (30 min) and resistance (27 min) training produced no significant improvements in HDL-C in postmenopausal women as compared with those in the aerobic training (52 min) group (Rossi et al. 2016). It is possible that the resistance training portion of their combined group (three or four sets of 12-RM to 15-RM) may not have provided the exercise intensity needed to invoke significant changes in HDL-C in their postmenopausal sample.

TOBACCO

Although tobacco usage (e.g., cigarettes and cigars) is declining in the United States and other countries, there continues to be a steep increase worldwide (American Heart Association 2017). Ng and colleagues (2014) attribute the increase in the number of smokers to the world's population growth. The World Health Organization (2011) estimates there are approximately 1 billion smokers in the global population. According to age-standardized results for smoking prevalence (Ng et al. 2014), between 16.5% and 19.7% of men in the United States, Canada, Brazil, and Australia smoke, while 34.7% to 61.1% of men in Russia, China, Eastern Europe, Egypt, and Turkey smoke. The lowest prevalence (0.5%-2.6%) of female smokers is found in Africa, China, and the Persian Gulf, whereas the prevalence exceeds 25% in Austria, Chile, France, and Hungary. Of the 187 countries included in the study, the age-adjusted prevalence of men who smoke daily exceeds that of their female counterparts in all but one country: Sweden. Although the prevalence of tobacco usage is lower for women than men across the majority of the predominant race and ethnic groups in the United States, the prevalence is slightly higher for Native American and Alaskan Indian women and nearly equal for non-Hispanic white women compared with their respective male counterparts (American Heart Association 2017).

Approximately 13.7% of American women and 16.7% of American men currently smoke (American Heart Association 2017). Smoking cessation strategies in Canada, Iceland, Mexico, and Norway have cut smoking rates in half since 1980 (Ng et al. 2014) and may provide invaluable assistance for curbing tobacco use in other countries. In a study of school-aged adolescents (average age 15 yr) representing 50 schools in six European cities (Lorant et al. 2015), 17.4% of the 11,000 participants self-reported being a smoker. Even if people abstain from smoking tobacco, the risk of death from CHD increases by 30% in those exposed to environmental tobacco smoke at home or at work (American Heart Association 2004).

Smoking is one of the largest preventable causes of disease and premature death. Nearly 33% of CHD deaths are due to first- and secondhand exposure to smoke (American Heart Association 2017). Cigarette smoking is linked to CHD, stroke, and chronic obstructive pulmonary disease. It causes cancer of the lungs, larynx, esophagus, mouth, and bladder and is also associated with no fewer than eleven cancers (Carter et al. 2015). Compared with nonsmokers, smokers have more than twice the risk of heart attack and die, on average, at least 10 yr earlier (American Heart Association 2017). As mentioned previously, cigarette smoking is a major cause of stroke. It also multiplies the effect of CHD risk factors such as elevated blood lipid levels, diabetes mellitus, and untreated hypertension. Some researchers who study adults ≥55 yr of age are encouraging further investigations of the possible associations between smoking and deaths resulting from infections, respiratory diseases, prostate and breast cancer, intestinal ischemia, kidney failure, and hypertensive heart disease. The relative risk of dying from these conditions drops with each year subsequent to quitting (Carter et al. 2015). Additionally, although not well studied at this time, the inhaled vapors from electronic cigarettes deliver nicotine and other substances for which the health risks are not yet known.

When individuals stop smoking, their risk of CHD declines rapidly, regardless of how long or how much they have smoked. Although health benefits associated with smoking cessation happen within weeks or months, the relative risk of a former smoker dying from CHD approximates that of a nonsmoker within 10 yr of quitting (American Heart Association 2017).

DIABETES MELLITUS

Diabetes is a global epidemic with rising prevalence rates, especially in the low- and middle-income countries. Consequently, there is a commitment by world leaders to reduce, by one-third, the rates of premature mortality from diabetes and the other priority NCDs by 2030 (World Health Organization 2016b). As of 2014, an estimated 422 million adults (8.5%) worldwide have the disease (World Health Organization 2016b). Factors linked to this epidemic include urbanization, aging, physical inactivity, unhealthy diet, and obesity (Wagner and Brath 2012). At least 43% of the deaths attributable to elevated blood glucose levels occur in people younger than 70 yr of age (World Health Organization 2016b). **Diabetes** is a major contributor toward the development of CHD, stroke, specific cancers, kidney failure, and cognitive disability (World Health Organization 2016b). This increased risk of CHD and stroke is higher for women than men with diabetes for a variety of reasons: higher-level CVD risk factors and obesity at time of diagnosis, longer exposure to an elevated risk profile when in the prediabetic stage, and relative undertreatment following diagnosis (Peters, Huxley, and Woodward 2014). In the United States, diabetes was the seventh leading cause of death in 2010 (American Diabetes Association 2017).

In 2012, 29 million adults in the United States had type 2 diabetes, while 86 million ≥20 yr of age were identified as having prediabetes (American Diabetes Association 2017). In China and India, there are 138 million people with diabetes (Danaei et al. 2011). Danaei and colleagues (2011) also estimated that approximately 42 million people with diabetes are from Brazil, Indonesia, Japan, Mexico, and Pakistan. Furthermore, in 2008, they reported the highest prevalence of diabetes was found in countries located in Oceania, northern Africa, the Middle East, and the Caribbean. Conversely, the lowest prevalence of diabetes was in southeast Asia, east Africa, and Andean Latin America (Danaei et al. 2011).

The prevalence of diabetes for adults (≥20 yr) in the United States was 12.3%; 1.7 million people in this age group were diagnosed with diabetes for the first time in 2012 (Centers for Disease Control and Prevention 2014). Compared with white adults in the United States, the prevalence of diabetes and impaired blood glucose levels for blacks (13.2%), Hispanics (12.8%), and American Indians/Alaska Natives (15.9%) is higher (Centers for Disease Control and Prevention 2014). The age-adjusted prevalence of diabetes for American Indians and Alaska Native adults is region dependent; American Indians in southern Arizona have a prevalence of diabetes (24.1%) that is four times that of Alaska Natives (Centers for Disease Control and Prevention 2014).

Prediabetes, in addition to being a positive risk factor for CVD, is a medical condition identified by fasting blood glucose or glycated hemoglobin (**HbA1c**) levels that are above normal values but lower than the threshold for a diagnosis of diabetes. HbA1c is an indicator of the average blood glucose over the past 2 to 3 mo (Centers for Disease Control and Prevention 2014). Fortunately for the 86 million American adults (Centers for Disease Control and Prevention 2014) and others worldwide, prediabetes appears to respond favorably to weight loss, dietary changes, and increases in physical activity. The age-adjusted percentage of prediabetes in U.S. adults during the period 2009 to 2012 was nearly identical for non-Hispanic whites, non-Hispanic blacks, and Hispanics (35%, 39%, and 38%, respectively) (Centers for Disease Control and Prevention 2014).

Type 1 diabetes, formerly referred to as insulin-dependent diabetes mellitus (IDDM), usually occurs in children and adolescents but can develop at any age. **Type 2 diabetes**, previously known as non-insulin-dependent diabetes mellitus (NIDDM), is more common and no longer occurs primarily in middle-aged and elderly adults; 90% to 95% of individuals diagnosed with diabetes mellitus have type 2 diabetes (Centers for Disease Control and Prevention 2014). Risk factors for developing diabetes are presented in table 1.3. Type 1 diabetes may be caused by autoimmune, genetic, or environmental factors, but the specific cause is unknown. Unfortunately, although clinical trials are under way, there is currently no known way to prevent type 1 diabetes (World Health Organization 2016b). Healthy nutrition and increased physical activity, however, can reduce the risk of type 2 diabetes by as much as 67% in high-risk individuals (Sanz, Gautier, and Hanaire 2010). Regular physical activity, as part of a modest weight loss intervention, has reduced the risk of developing type 2 diabetes by a maximum of 58% for those in the high-risk category (Colberg et al. 2010). Too much body fat is recognized as the dominant risk factor for type 2 diabetes. Elevated waist circumferences and BMI values also increase the risk, but the associated risk varies by geographic region (World Health Organization 2016b).

The effect of exercise alone as an intervention for people with type 2 diabetes is not well known beyond its ability to improve glucose control (Handelsman et al. 2015). However, a minimum of 150 min/wk of MVPA is recommended and should include flexibility and strength training (Handelsman et al. 2015). Of note, though, for continued benefits, the exercise program needs to be performed regularly and include both strength and aerobic training to help those with type 2 diabetes achieve optimal health. Decreasing the time spent being sedentary, in addition to increasing daily physical activity, is a viable means of decreasing the risk for developing type 2 diabetes. As reported in a review of five studies, the pooled hazard of developing type 2 diabetes is nearly double for those reporting high amounts of sedentary time (Biswas et al. 2015). Although few adverse effects or diabetic complications resulting from exercise have been reported, being watchful for acute postexercise hypoglycemia and transient hyperglycemia is prudent (Colberg et al. 2010).

Research that associates physical activity with weight loss, fat loss, and glycemic control suggests that regular physical activity in accordance with the recommended guidelines reduces one's risk of developing type 2 diabetes (Colberg et al. 2010). In a small sample of overweight and obese participants, an intensive 6 mo nonrandomized lifestyle intervention consisting of exercise and behavioral weight loss counseling reduced baseline HbA1C values ($6.8 \pm 0.2\%$ to $6.2 \pm 0.3\%$), consequently precluding the need for medications to reduce blood glucose levels. Numerous other aspects (e.g., insulin levels, insulin resistance, blood pressure, body mass, body composition) were also favorably affected (Ades et al. 2015). The frequency of exercise is crucial for those with diabetes. If daily exercise is not possible, it should not be skipped 2 days in a row. Specific guidelines for prescribing exercise programs for people who have type 1 and type 2 diabetes are available elsewhere (American College of Sports Medicine 2018).

OBESITY AND OVERWEIGHT

Adult **overweight** and **obesity** are classified using the **body mass index (BMI)** (BMI = weight [kg] / height squared [m²]). According to traditional BMI values, individuals ≥20 yr of age with a BMI between 25 and 29.9 kg/m² are classified as overweight; those with a BMI of 30 kg/m² or more are classified as obese (Smith and Smith 2016). As the result of research on people from various population subgroups, more conservative BMI cut-points for identifying overweight (23-24.9 kg/m²) and obesity (≥25 kg/m²) have been identified for Asians and South Asians (Seidell and Halberstadt 2015). Consequently, as noted by Seidell and Halberstadt (2015), the prevalence of obesity in the world may be understated because many Asians would be erroneously classified based on BMI. Although BMI has utility as a simple index of obesity, it cannot account for relative fatness, and including some additional determination or estimation of abdominal fat distribution is recommended for understanding actual health risk (Seidell and Halberstadt 2015). The World Health Organization (2012b) defines overweight and obesity as having *abnormal or excessive fat accumulation that may impair health*. Regardless, overweight and obesity ranks as the fifth leading risk factor for death worldwide.

More than 2.1 billion people worldwide are classified as being overweight or obese (Smith and Smith 2016). Globally, more than 1 in 3 adults (≥18 yr) is overweight, and more than 1 in every 10 adults is obese (World Health Organization 2016b). The countries in the World Health Organization's Region of the Americas have the highest prevalence of obesity, while those countries categorized into the South-East Asian Region have the lowest (World Health Organization 2016b). In England, fairly equal percentages of men (24%) and women (27%) were categorized as obese based on BMI in 2014 (NHS Digital 2014). Self-reported heights and weights for the 48,000 Canadian adults responding to the Canadian Community Health Survey in 2012 were used to calculate BMI for the younger (age 30-59 yr) and older (age 60-80+ yr) age groups. Nearly 55% of the younger and 60% of the older group were overweight or obese (Cohen, Baker, and Ardern 2016). In 2014, China surpassed all other countries for adult obesity, with their obese men and women representing 16.3% and 12.4% of the world's sex-specific obesity prevalence; the United States ranked second for both sexes (men: 15.7%; women: 12.3%) (NCD Risk Factor Collaboration 2017). For a detailed report of changes in global BMI levels between 1975 and 2014 based on data from about 99% of the world's population, see the work of the NCD Risk Factor Collaboration group (2017).

In the United States, approximately 35% of adults are classified as obese, and one of every three children and adolescents falls into the overweight or obese categories (Smith and Smith 2016). The age-adjusted prevalence of obesity for American men is approximately 35% for whites and 12.6% for Asians, respectively; the obesity prevalence is approximately 38% for non-Hispanic black and Hispanic men. For American women, the age-adjusted prevalence of obesity based on BMI is 40.4%, 46.9%, 57.2%, and 12.4%, respectively, for white, Hispanic, black, and Asian women. For those having a BMI in the class 3 obesity range ($\geq$40 kg/m^2), the prevalence for both men and women across the four racial and ethnic groups ranged between 5.5% and 9.9%, with the exception being 16.8% for black women (Flegal et al. 2016). Asian adults in the United States continue to have a much lower prevalence of obesity compared with whites, blacks, and Hispanics (Flegal et al. 2016).

Childhood obesity ($\geq$95th percentile for sex and age) is also a global problem (see chapter 9). Overweight adolescents have a 70% chance of becoming overweight adults; this increases to 80% if one or both parents are overweight or obese (American Heart Association 2012). In England, 33% of boys and 35% of girls, ages 2 to 15 yr, were either overweight or obese (British Heart Foundation 2006). Similarly, in the United States, the prevalence of overweight and obesity in children and adolescents, ages 2 to 19 yr, was approximately 33% in 2014, with 17.2% being classified as obese (American Heart Association 2017). That year's prevalence of obesity in children increased with each age group and ranged from 9.4% (preschool children 2-5 yr) to 20.6% for adolescents (12-19 yr); the prevalence was 17.4% for grade school–aged children (American Heart Association 2017). The World Health Organization (2018b) reported that approximately 41 million children (0 to 5 yr) globally are either overweight or obese, and nearly 340 million children (5 – 19 yr) are overweight or obese). Table 1.3 summarizes factors associated with increased risk of obesity.

Excess body weight and fatness pose a threat to both the quality and duration of one's life. A rare longitudinal study spanning 40 yr tracked over 900

men to document changes in BMI and cardiometabolic outcomes (Xian et al. 2017). BMI trajectories were modeled based on assessments at ages 20, 40, 56, and 62 yr. Compared with the men who were normal weight in their 20s but attained an overweight BMI at age 62, those having normal-weight BMIs at baseline and ending with BMIs in the obese range (normal-obese) had significantly greater risks of hypertension, diabetes, dyslipidemia, and inflammation; the same is true for the men having baseline BMI values in the overweight range and entering the obesity level by age 40 and attaining the highest level of obesity ($\geq$40 kg/m^2) at age 62 (overweight-obese level 3). However, the overweight-obese level 3 group had more than three times the risk of hypertension, double the risk of inflammation, and a 60% higher risk of diabetes compared with the normal-obese group. Interestingly, there were no differences in the three groups for ischemic heart disease.

Although obesity is strongly associated with CHD risk factors such as hypertension, glucose intolerance, and hyperlipidemia, the contribution of obesity to CHD appears to be independent of the influence of obesity on these risk factors. Interestingly, an **obesity paradox** has been identified; paradoxically and counterintuitively, when investigating the short- and long-term prognosis for cardiovascular diseases, such as hypertension, atrial fibrillation, and heart failure, prognosis is improved for those who are overweight or mildly obese as compared with leaner clients (Lavie et al. 2014). For a comprehensive review of the effects of obesity on cardiac performance, cardiac remodeling, aerobic fitness level, and the obesity paradox, see the work of Lavie and colleagues (2014).

Obesity, the fifth leading cause of death, may be caused by genetic and environmental factors as well as gut biome. Although studies suggest that genetic factors contribute to some of the variation in body fatness, there has been no substantial change in the genotype of the American population since the 1960s (Hill and Melanson 1999). Nevertheless, in terms of prevalence, obesity varies across ethnic groups. Obesity clusters within families have been reported, as have heritability estimates. **Genome-wide association studies (GWASs)** are now under way, and upwards of 90 possible areas of genetic variation associated with obesity and BMI have been identified (Chen et al. 2017). Without any doubt, our environment and culture are additional key contributors to the increases being seen in the rates of obesity. In addition to the countless calorically dense food options we have and technological advancements that reduce energy expenditure through physical activity and manual labor, we are exposed daily to innumerable chemical compounds (e.g., pesticides, personal and home care products, food additives, industrial waste) that promote obesity through their interference with the endocrine system and metabolic pathway functions (Regnier and Sargis 2014).

As an exercise specialist, you play an important role in combating the obesity-related health epidemic by encouraging a physically active lifestyle, planning scientifically sound exercise programs, and consulting with your clients and trained nutrition professionals to formulate appropriate diets. Restricting caloric intake and increasing caloric expenditure through physical activity and exercise are effective ways of reducing body weight and fatness while normalizing blood pressure and blood lipid profiles.

METABOLIC SYNDROME

Metabolic syndrome (MetS) refers to a combination of CVD risk factors associated with hypertension, dyslipidemia, insulin resistance, and abdominal obesity. According to clinical criteria adopted by the National Cholesterol Education Program (2001), individuals with three or more CVD risk factors are classified as having metabolic syndrome (see table 1.4). Although there is some overlap, these criteria vary among different organizations such as the International Diabetes Federation (IDF), World Health Organization (WHO), European Group for the Study of Insulin Resistance (EGIR), American Association of Clinical Endocrinology (AACE), and American Heart Association/National Heart, Lung, and Blood Institute (AHA/NHLBI). A side-by-side comparison of similarities and differences in criteria is available in the article by O'Neill and O'Driscoll (2015). Body mass index is an acceptable criterion according to the World Health Organization; however, all of the other organizations use waist circumference as the reference for abdominal obesity. Sex- and ethnic-specific references for the waist circumference criteria are also now defined (O'Neill and O'Driscoll 2015). Alberti and colleagues (2009) present extensive information regarding the history of metabolic syndrome and the ongoing efforts of major organizations to reach a consensus on a single set of criteria. Likewise, Steinberger and associates (2009) highlight similar issues for determining metabolic syndrome in children and adolescents.

Data reviewed by O'Neill and O'Driscoll (2015) indicate that approximately 34% of the men and 35% of the women (≥20 yr) in the United States met the National Cholesterol Education Program's Adult Treatment Panel III (NCEP-ATPIII) criteria for metabolic syndrome, as did 17% of the men and 19% of the women of similar age living in India. O'Neill and O'Driscoll also present results from numerous studies of adults from Australia, China, Denmark, Ireland, and South Korea. By far, the prevalence of metabolic syndrome in adults is higher in adults from the United States, but disparate age ranges

Table 1.4 Risk Factors for Metabolic Syndrome

Risk factor	Risk criteria
Waist circumference	>102 cm (>40 in.) for men >88 cm (>35 in.) for women
Blood pressure (BP)	≥130 mmHg (systolic BP) or ≥85 mmHg (diastolic BP) or both
Fasting blood glucose	≥110 mg·dl⁻¹ or ≥6.1 mmol·L⁻¹
Triglycerides	≥150 mg·dl⁻¹ or ≥1.6 mmol·L⁻¹
HDL-C	<40 mg·dl⁻¹ or <1.04 mmol·L⁻¹ for men <50 mg·dl⁻¹ or <1.29 mmol·L⁻¹ for women

Note: Metabolic syndrome is defined as three or more risk factors.

Data from National Cholesterol Education Program 2001.

and sample sizes across the groups may interfere with further comparisons. Of interest, for the listed countries having prevalences identified by both NCEP-ATPIII and IDF criteria, the latter's prevalence is consistently higher for both sexes. Therefore, until a uniform definition of metabolic syndrome is agreed upon, it is possible that its global prevalence may be misestimated.

Other common study findings include that the prevalence of MetS increases with age and that physical inactivity plus unhealthy diet are key underlying factors. Metabolic syndrome increases the risk of stroke (by two- to fourfold), CVD (by threefold), myocardial infarction (by three- to fourfold), and type 2 diabetes (by fivefold) (Kaur 2014). Older adults ($\geq$60 yr) with MetS spend a larger percentage of time being sedentary and have longer bouts of being sedentary compared with those without a MetS diagnosis (Bankoski et al. 2011). Publications from genome-wide association studies focusing on MetS are growing in number and indicate that a combination of genes may underlie the linkages of independent factors (e.g., visceral adipose tissue, insulin resistance, hypertension) and the MetS condition (O'Neill and O'Driscoll 2015).

Age and BMI directly relate to metabolic syndrome (National Cholesterol Education Program 2001). The prevalence of MetS is higher (>40%) for older (>60 yr) adults than for younger (20-29 yr) adults (7%). Also, the prevalence of MetS is much higher for obese (BMI >30 kg/m^2) individuals (~50%) than for normal weight (BMI $\leq$25 kg/m^2) individuals (6.2%). Lifestyle must be modified in order to manage metabolic syndrome. The combination of healthy nutrition and increased physical activity is an effective way to increase HDL-C and to reduce blood pressure, body weight, waist circumference, triglycerides, and blood glucose levels.

CANCER

Cancer is a leading cause of death worldwide; it is also the second leading cause of death in the United States behind heart disease for adults and accidents for children in the age range of 1 to 14 yr (Siegel, Miller, and Jemal 2016). A systematic analysis of global cancer incidence indicates that cancer accounted for 8.7 million deaths in 2015 (Fitzmaurice et al. 2017). There is a sex-specific difference in the odds of developing cancer in a lifetime: one in three for men and one in four for women (Fitzmaurice et al. 2017). Siegel and colleagues (2016) estimated the number of cancer deaths in the United States; three of their top four estimates—for lung and bronchus, colorectal, and pancreatic cancer—are identical for men and women. The type of cancer second on the list is prostate for men and breast for women. Fortunately, the death rates for lung, breast, prostate, and colorectal cancers have decreased over the past 20 yr, with the decreases related to early detection and treatment as well as public awareness campaigns (Siegel, Miller, and Jemal 2016). The most common types of cancer vary by geographical region (Fitzmaurice et al. 2017; Siegel, Miller, and Jemal 2016) and for developing as opposed to developed countries (Fitzmaurice et al. 2017). The main risk factors for cancer are tobacco and alcohol use, unhealthy diet, physical inactivity, and infection-related risk factors, such as hepatitis and human papilloma virus (World Health Organization 2018a).

Globally, physical inactivity is one of the primary prevention targets for many chronic conditions; physical inactivity is a modifiable risk factor associated with increased risk of breast, colon, and endometrial cancers (Leitzmann et al. 2015). Specifically, physical inactivity is believed to cause 10% of colon and 9% of breast cancer cases in Europe; on the other hand, the risk of colon cancer decreases with increasing levels of physical activity (Leitzmann et al. 2015). Moore and colleagues (2016) investigated the association of leisure-time physical activity (LTPA) and multiple types of cancer in over 1.4 million people. They found that the highest levels of LTPA (90th percentile) were associated with a lower risk for 13 of the 26 cancers of interest. For 7 of those cancers, LTPA reduced the risk by at least 20% (Moore et al. 2016). Strong evidence also shows that physically active people with a cancer diagnosis may have higher survival rates than do inactive cancer patients.

Although the mechanisms through which physical activity reduces the risk of several cancers are not fully elucidated at this time, attention is being focused on steroid hormones, insulin resistance, growth factors, immune system function, and adipokines as well as body composition (Leitzmann et al. 2015). The American Cancer Society's 2017 guidelines for reducing the risk of cancer through diet and physically active lifestyles recommend that adults engage in 150 min/wk of moderate-intensity physical activity, 75 min/wk of vigorous-intensity physical activity, or an equivalent combination thereof beyond the normal activities of daily living. Children and adolescents are encouraged to engage in moderate or vigorous physical activity at least 60 min each day (American Cancer Society 2017). Additionally, maintaining a healthy body weight may be important for reducing cancer risk; 4.5 million cancer deaths worldwide in 2013 were attributed to being overweight or obese (Lauby-Secretan et al. 2016). Lauby-Secretan and associates (2016) concluded that lower body fat levels reduce the risk for the majority of cancers, although research on intentional weight loss to reduce cancer risk is lacking in humans. Studying associations between physical activity levels and 26 types of cancer, Moore and colleagues (2016) reported that the associations for most of the cancers they studied are independent of BMI.

MUSCULOSKELETAL DISEASES AND DISORDERS

Diseases and disorders of the musculoskeletal system, such as osteoporosis, osteoarthritis, bone fractures, connective tissue tears, and low back syndrome, are also related to physical inactivity and a sedentary lifestyle. Osteoporosis is a disease characterized by the loss of bone mineral content and bone mineral density due to factors such as aging, amenorrhea, malnutrition, menopause, and physical inactivity (see table 1.3 for osteoporosis risk factors). It is reported to affect approximately 200 million people worldwide (Pisani et al. 2016), 54 million of whom live in the United States (National Osteoporosis Foundation 2017). Osteoporosis usually remains silent until a fracture is sustained; consequently, it is becoming a major health issue for both men and women over the age of 50 (Willson et al. 2015)—with an osteoporotic fracture occurring every 3 sec worldwide—and has an associated high socioeconomic impact.

Although osteoporotic fractures may occur in any bone, a hip fracture is recognized as a surrogate measure of the health care burden and expense due to osteoporosis, especially for men and women ≥50 yr. Wrist fractures precede the most common osteoporotic fracture, vertebral fractures. For women, the risk of subsequent fractures in the hips and the extremities is also associated with a prior wrist fracture; however, this has been studied more internationally than in the United States (Crandall et al. 2015). Nevertheless, hip fractures are the most devastating (International Osteoporosis Foundation 2015). In a study of hip fractures in 63 countries around the world, Kanis and colleagues (2012) noted the highest incidence rates per 100,000 women in Denmark, Norway, and Sweden. The lowest are in Nigeria and South Africa. Age-standardized incidence rates of hip fractures in the men are highest in Denmark but lowest in Ecuador (Kanis et al. 2012).

Osteoporosis affects an estimated 75 million people in Europe, the United States, and Japan. Close to 12 million U.S. adults over the age of 50 have osteoporosis (Pisani et al. 2016). An estimated 1.5 million osteoporotic fractures occur each year in the United States, with the majority being sustained by postmenopausal women (Black and Rosen 2016). Nine percent of American men and women over the age of 50 have osteoporosis at either the hip (femur) or spine, but the prevalence of osteoporosis varies with age, sex, and ethnicity. Women continue to have a higher prevalence compared with men, as do older adults compared with younger adults. Compared with non-Hispanic whites, Mexican-Americans have a higher risk of osteoporosis or low bone mass, and non-Hispanic blacks have a lower risk (Looker et al. 2012).

Individuals with osteoporosis have values for bone mineral density (BMD) that are more than 2.5 standard deviations below the mean value for young adults. Osteopenia, or low bone mineral mass, is a precursor to osteoporosis. More than one of every two adults aged 50 or older has either osteoporosis or osteopenia (National Osteoporosis Foundation 2004). A racial difference in the prevalence of osteoporosis is evident, with African-Americans having the lowest and Asian-Americans the highest. Regardless, women have a higher prevalence of osteoporosis than do men, and this difference is especially evident with increasing age (Wright et al. 2017).

Kanis and colleagues (2005) developed a free online tool, called FRAX, to identify an individual's

10 yr risk of developing osteoporosis and experiencing a hip fracture. FRAX can be accessed at www.shef.ac.uk/FRAX. To use this tool, the client answers 12 questions about age, height, weight, prior fracture history, parental history of hip fracture, smoking, rheumatoid arthritis, alcohol consumption, and long-term use of glucocorticoids. If available, the bone mineral density of the femoral neck may be included to better refine the accuracy of these estimations, especially for women. However, the World Health Organization based its BMD T-score criterion at the femoral neck on a reference group of young women so that criterion is not directly applicable for men. The combination of FRAX score and qualifying fracture history is better at identifying osteoporosis in men over the age of 50 (Wright et al. 2017). The FRAX methodology is widely used around the world and has become integral to the formation of intervention guidelines. The United States created new thresholds for the purpose of guiding treatment plans for adults ≥40 yr with low bone mass.

A public-private partnership (National Bone Health Alliance, or NBHA) in the United States spawned a working group tasked with expanding the clinical criteria for diagnosing osteoporosis. Data from the 2005-2008 NHANES project formed the basis of the working group's efforts. Information from the predominantly Caucasian subjects in the 50+ yr age group resulted in a prevalence of osteoporosis that was lower than for those in the 80+ yr group (respectively, men: 16% and 46.3%; women: 29.9% and 88.1%) (Wright et al. 2017). The more conservative NBHA definition is based on a man ≥50 yr or a postmenopausal woman satisfying one of three criteria: traditional definition of low BMD at the hip or lumbar spine, a past site-specific low trauma fracture, or a FRAX score ≥ cut-point values for traditional intervention for low BMD. Compared with the corresponding prevalence of osteoporosis diagnoses based solely on low BMD or FRAX scores in the study by Wright and colleagues (2017), the prevalence of osteoporosis by NBHA criteria was higher.

Adequate calcium intake, vitamin D intake, and regular physical activity (especially of the weight-bearing modalities) help counteract age-related bone loss; however, there may be sex-specific dose-response differences, especially in terms of dietary supplementation (Willson et al. 2015).

Epidemiological studies show that the incidence of bone fracture is lower in those with higher levels of physical activity. According to a recent update (Daly 2017), walking, by itself, confers little if any effect on preventing muscle or bone loss. Likewise, Watson and colleagues (2015) comment on the continued paucity of evidence that moderate-intensity exercise is beneficial as an osteoporosis treatment targeting the hip and low spine. For example, in a group of middle-aged Chinese adults, 12 wk of moderate-intensity exercise (tai chi or self-paced walking) produced no significant change in BMD as compared to the control group (Hui et al. 2015).

Vigorous-intensity activity, on the other hand, is associated with changes at the femoral neck of 70 yr olds, whereas light- to moderate-intensity activity strengthens the tibia (Johansson, Nordström, and Nordström 2015). According to preliminary results from a sample of postmenopausal women with low to very low bone mass, a supervised 8 mo (30 min/day, 2 days/wk) high-intensity progressive resistance training program targeting the skeletal system results in statistically significant and injury-free improvements in posture, BMD, and functional performance as compared with the group doing home-based exercises (Watson et al. 2015). Similarly, individualized high-velocity progressive resistance training routines appear to best optimize a spectrum of musculoskeletal and functional outcomes; for full benefit, the routines should include variable moderate and load-bearing exercises as well as challenging activities for mobility and balance (Daly 2017). The ACSM (2018) highlights the frequency, intensity, types (styles), sets, repetitions, and progression recommendations as deemed appropriate given an individual's age, medical history, resistance training history, and goals (see chapter 7).

Peak bone mass is developed during childhood and adolescence, with 50% of the skeleton laid down during the teenage years (Gordon et al. 2017). Consequently, peak bone mass is a major factor associated with the risk of osteoporosis in the adult years (Mitchell et al. 2016). Bone mass is higher in physically active children than in less active children. Given that exercise-induced gains in bone mass during childhood and adolescence are maintained into adulthood, the ACSM supports the application of adult resistance training guidelines for children and adolescents who receive proper instruction and supervision (ACSM 2018). The resistance training that children and adolescents receive is to be counted toward the recommended target of 60+ min/day of MVPA.

Low back pain afflicts millions of people each year and is considered a major health issue in many countries. It is one of the top reasons people miss work and restrict their activities (Patrick, Emanski, and Knaub 2014). From 60 to 80% of adults are expected to experience low back pain at some point (Gordon and Bloxham 2016). Low back pain is also reported by adolescent athletes (Schmidt et al. 2014). Some low back problems are produced by muscular weakness or imbalance caused by a lack of physical activity (see table 1.3). For physically active people such as adolescent athletes, low back pain may be brought on by frequent bending at the waist, twisting, accommodating loads carried high on the body, heavy and repeated lifting, and holding awkward postures (Schmidt et al. 2014).

If the muscles are not strong enough to support the vertebral column in proper alignment, poor posture results and low back pain develops. Excessive weight, poor flexibility, and improper lifting habits also contribute to low back problems. By themselves, aerobic, muscle-strengthening, and flexibility programs have been shown to improve nonspecific chronic low back pain. However, research on combinations of the three exercise modalities is lacking (Gordon and Bloxham 2016).

Because the origin of low back problems is often functional rather than structural, the problem can be corrected through an exercise program that develops strength and flexibility in the appropriate muscle groups. Also, people who remain physically active throughout life retain more bone, ligament, and tendon strength, making them less prone to bone fractures and connective tissue tears (McGill 2016). Physically active people also have thicker discs between their lumbar vertebrae. This may prevent or delay the onset of degenerative disc disorders, which can also result in low back pain (Teichtahl et al. 2015).

AGING

A sedentary lifestyle and lack of adequate physical activity reduce life expectancy by predisposing the individual to aging-related diseases and by influencing the aging process itself. With aging, a progressive loss of physiological and metabolic functions occurs; however, biological aging may differ considerably among individuals because of variability in genetic and environmental factors that affect oxidative stress and inflammation. **Telomeres** are repeated DNA sequences that determine the structure and function of chromosomes. With aging and diseases associated with increased oxidative stress (e.g., CHD, diabetes mellitus, osteoporosis, and heart failure), telomere length decreases. Mechanisms underlying the relationship between physical activity and telomere length in humans are yet to be firmly established, but related work with rodent models is under way.

A study of normal, healthy twins reported that the telomere length of leukocytes is positively associated with physical activity levels during leisure time. The longer telomere length observed in more physically active individuals could not be explained by age, gender, body mass index, smoking, socioeconomic status, and physical activity at work (Cherkas et al. 2008). Similarly, postmenopausal women who engaged in a combination of aerobic and resistance exercise (≥60 min/day, 3 days/wk for >1 yr) had longer telomeres than their sedentary counterparts (Kim et al. 2012). A direct dose-response relationship between the number of movement-based behaviors engaged in and telomere length has been observed in a national sample of adults in the United States (Loprinzi, Loenneke, and Blackburn 2015). Participating in ≥300 min/wk of physical activity was positively related to longer telomere length and may protect the telomeres against shortening. Adding 1 hr/wk of vigorous LTPA seems to increase telomere length (Ogawa et al. 2017). The observations by the Loprinzi and Ogawa research groups support earlier work by Richards and associates (2008), who noted that the telomere length of leukocytes is inversely related to plasma homocysteine and C-reactive protein levels; both are known markers of inflammation and cardiovascular risk.

Although additional long-term prospective studies are needed to fully understand the antiaging effects of regular exercise, these findings suggest that exercise scientists should promote the potential benefits of leisure-time physical activity in retarding the aging process and diminishing the risk of aging-related diseases. Early indications about the relationship between telomere length and movement-based behavior counts highlight that 40 to 64 yr olds may be a very important target for physical activity promotion strategies encouraging regular participation in multiple active behaviors as they transition from middle age to older adults (Loprinzi, Loenneke, and Blackburn 2015).

Regular physical activity is believed to further promote healthy aging and longevity through **autophagy**. This process occurs within the cytosol of cells and provides a means through which damaged proteins and organelles are sequestered, reduced to usable components, and recycled (Zampieri et al. 2015). As a result, cellular components are maintained in good working order, and the cytosol is relatively free of deleterious debris (i.e., misfolded proteins, damaged mitochondria). This decreases the effects of aging on skeletal muscle (Barbieri et al. 2015) and the brain (Garatachea et al. 2015). As noted in the review by Garatachea and associates (2015), autophagy is upregulated by aerobic exercise in rodent models. Although similar research with human subjects is limited, evidence points to improved autophagy-related processes for lifelong exercisers, which, in turn, promote healthy aging.

COGNITIVE PERFORMANCE

As longevity increases, aging adults face the distinct possibility of eventually experiencing a notable decline in cognitive function. Some of the impairments affect immediate and delayed recall, visual attention, psychomotor speed, problem solving, and reasoning. Brain-training games and pastimes are growing in number and are marketed toward senior citizens, but they are typically performed in a seated and, hence, sedentary manner. Exercise and time spent being physically active may protect against cognitive decline and the onset of dementia. Likewise, higher levels of aerobic fitness help preserve or slow the rate of decline in brain and gray matter volume, which decreases age-related deterioration of key regions in the brain.

After controlling for vascular risk factors, relationships have been found between LTPA and cognitive function. Little to no LTPA is associated with diminished cognitive function and worsening scores over time (Willey et al. 2016). Northey and colleagues (2017) analyzed data from exercise-related studies conducted with adults older than 50 yr. They concluded that the cognitive function of older adults, regardless of their initial cognitive status, improved as a result of the exercise interventions. Summarily, their recommendation is that older adults engage in moderate- to vigorous-intensity exercise for no less than 45 min/day on as many days of the week as possible (Northey et al. 2017). Higher cognitive function test scores have been recorded for seniors who engage in higher levels of moderate- to vigorous-intensity physical activity (Steinberg et al. 2015). Increased sedentary time, with the exception of computer time, contributes to lower cognitive scores. From their sample of 125 adults ranging in age from 65 to 95 yr, Steinberg's team found the average sedentary time and time in MVPA were 48 hr/wk and 5 hr/wk, respectively. The latter satisfied the ACSM (2018) recommendation for MVPA per week. Results from a study investigating the postexercise effect of exercise volume on the aspect of cognitive function known as executive function (deals with problem solving, reasoning, working memory, task flexibility) also support the ACSM recommendation (Tsukamoto et al. 2017). For their sample of predominantly young male adults, the higher exercise volume based on moderate-intensity cycling improved postexercise executive function for a longer duration than did a similar exercise volume based on low-intensity cycling.

Exercise increases blood flow to the working muscles and brain in accordance with the exercise intensity. Parallels in brain blood flow, cardiac output, and oxygen consumption are known to occur. Blood flow to specific regions of the brain is believed to be associated with the areas that monitor and adjust the neural networks required to produce the appropriate level of physical work. Therefore, the mechanisms by which exercise and regular physical activity protect the cardiovascular system may be similar to those protecting the brain. For more in-depth information on this, see the review by Barnes in *Advances in Physiology Education* (2015).

There may be no one best exercise modality for preserving cognitive function as we age. Both aerobic and resistance training promote beneficial cardiorespiratory changes; intuitively, they would likewise promote beneficial changes in the brain. As reported by Northey and colleagues (2017), exercise modalities having similar efficacy in improving the cognitive function of adults ≥50 yr are tai chi, aerobic, resistance, and multicomponent training. A multimodal routine promoting variety, numerous muscle groups, challenges to balance and coordination, and intellectual stimulation may prove optimal; however, that research is sparse.

EXERCISE AS MEDICINE

As is evident in the scientific and lay literature, a physically active lifestyle that meets or exceeds the minimum recommendations established in 2008 confers numerous health-related benefits (Eijsvogels and Thompson 2015; Lundqvist et al. 2017). Even initial engagement at less than recommended levels induces health benefits (Wen et al. 2011), as does reducing the amount of time spent sitting regardless of aerobic capacity (Benatti and Ried-Larsen 2015; Bergouignan et al. 2016; Levine 2015; Same et al. 2016). Although it may not be possible to completely prevent all known chronic and noncommunicable diseases, it is certainly possible to ameliorate and delay their onset by reducing sedentary time and engaging in regular exercise and physical activity. Physical inactivity is a better predictor of mortality from all causes than are the former stalwarts of hypertension, diabetes, blood lipid levels, and smoking. Improving cardiorespiratory fitness or exercise capacity fosters biological mechanisms that favorably influence blood glucose and lipids, insulin sensitivity, body composition, inflammation, and cognitive function (Coombes et al. 2015). Likewise, sedentary behavior, defined as having an energy expenditure ≤1.5 METs, is believed to be a CVD risk factor that is independent of physical activity levels (Same et al. 2016).

A recent prospective observational investigation (Lundqvist et al. 2017) of Swedish primary care providers prescribing individualized physical activity treatment plans for inactive adult patients (27-85 yr) with at least one metabolic risk factor gives testament to the benefits of regular, individualized physical activity and exercise plans. At the 6 mo follow-up and in comparison with baseline, physical activity increased to recommended levels (30-44 min of moderate-intensity walking, 2-5 days/wk); six metabolic risk factors and health-related quality-of-life factors improved significantly, as did vitality, mental health, and social function (Lundqvist et al. 2017). The participating health care professionals received standardized training on the effects of physical activity in advance of the study, and individualized patient follow-ups (i.e., office visit, phone call) were offered. These follow-ups occurred, on average, once or twice over the course of the 6 mo period; this low frequency of provider support is indicative of the minimal impact on the primary care provider's schedule. Sadly, most medical school programs in the United States do not include training about the benefits of physical activity, basics of sound individualized exercise program prescriptions, and use of exercise as a primary prevention of many NCDs (Cardinal et al. 2015).

The ACSM created the Exercise is Medicine (EIM) initiative with a focus on getting primary care physicians and similar health care providers to include physical activity in treatment plans prescribed for their patients. Coombes and colleagues (2015) describe a six-prong approach. Generally speaking, this approach revolves around increasing awareness of the importance of a physically active lifestyle, inquiring about physical activity levels at each visit to the doctor's office, making proper referrals of patients to qualified exercise and fitness professionals, changing public and private policy to comprehensively support physically active lifestyles, alerting patients that their physical activity patterns will be discussed during office visits, and becoming role models for physically active lifestyles.

The EIM initiative (see http://exerciseismedicine.org) began in the United States and is growing as a global initiative. For information on related initiatives in participating global regions and countries, see www.exerciseismedicine.org/support_page.php/regional-updates. Opportunities abound for students and professionals in exercise science to participate in initiatives to expand public awareness and influence local public and private policy. One such opportunity is through the EIM Ambassador program (http://www.exerciseismedicine.org/support_page.php/eim-ambassadors/).

Key Points

▶ Fewer than half (49.5%) of all American adults meet the recommended amount of either the aerobic or muscle-strengthening activity needed for health benefits.

▶ The majority (79.3%) of American adults fail to meet the full set of physical activity guidelines for health.

▶ *Exercise deficit disorder* is a term describing children who do not participate in 60 min of moderate- to vigorous-intensity physical activity every day.

▶ Major chronic noncommunicable diseases associated with a lack of physical activity are CVDs, diabetes, obesity, musculoskeletal disorders, and cognitive disorders.

▶ Cardiovascular diseases are responsible for 25% of all deaths in the United States and nearly equal sex-specific percentages (36% for men, 35% for women) of all deaths before age 75 yr in Europe.

▶ The positive risk factors for CHD are age, family history, dyslipidemia, hypertension, tobacco use, prediabetes or glucose intolerance, obesity, and physical inactivity.

▶ Sedentary behavior and cardiorespiratory fitness are independent risk factors for cardiovascular and cardiometabolic disorders.

▶ The prevalence of obesity is on the rise, especially in developed countries; in the United States, 35% of adults and 30% of adolescents and children are overweight or obese.

▶ BMI is used to identify and classify individuals as overweight or obese. Cutoff values for obesity, however, vary depending on ethnicity.

▶ Individuals with three or more cardiovascular disease risk factors are said to have metabolic syndrome.

▶ Osteoporosis and low back syndrome are musculoskeletal disorders afflicting millions of people each year.

▶ FRAX is an online tool that can be used to assess your client's 10 yr risk of developing osteoporosis and experiencing a hip fracture.

▶ Moderate-intensity walking is beneficial for aerobic fitness benefits, but it may not help prevent fractures of the hip and lumbar spine.

▶ To benefit health and prevent disease, every adult should accumulate a minimum of 150 min/wk of moderate-intensity physical activity or 75 min/wk of vigorous-intensity physical activity. For additional health benefits, increase physical activity to 300 min/wk and 150 min/wk, respectively, for moderate- and vigorous-intensity exercise.

Key Terms

Learn the definition for each of the following key terms. Definitions of key terms can be found in the glossary.

angina pectoris

atherosclerosis

autophagy

body mass index (BMI)

cardiovascular disease (CVD)

cholesterol

chylomicron

coronary heart disease (CHD)

dose-response relationship

dyslipidemia

elevated blood pressure

exercise deficit disorder (EDD)

genome-wide association studies (GWAS)

HbA1c

HDL-cholesterol (HDL-C)

high-density lipoprotein (HDL)

hypercholesterolemia

hyperlipidemia

hypertension

LDL-cholesterol (LDL-C)

lipoprotein

low back pain

low-density lipoprotein (LDL)

metabolic syndrome (MetS)

myocardial infarction

myocardial ischemia

noncommunicable diseases (NCDs)

normotensive

obesity

obesity paradox

osteopenia

osteoporosis

overweight

prediabetes

sedentarism

stage 1 hypertension

stage 2 hypertension

telomeres

total cholesterol (TC)

type 1 diabetes

type 2 diabetes

very low-density lipoprotein (VLDL)

Review Questions

In addition to being able to define each of the key terms just listed, test your knowledge and understanding of the material by answering the following review questions.

1. What percentage of the American population does not get the recommended amount of physical activity for health benefits?

2. What is the recommended minimum amount of daily physical activity for health?

3. Give examples of moderate-intensity physical activity.

4. What NCDs are related to physical inactivity?

5. What percentage of Americans have some form of CVD?

6. Name four types of CVD. Which is most prevalent?

7. Explain the etiology of CHD.

8. Identify the positive and negative risk factors for CHD.

9. In terms of SBP and DBP, differentiate the elevated, stage 1 hypertension, and stage 2 hypertension categories.

10. Explain how regular physical activity affects each of the CHD risk factors as well as overall CHD risk.

11. Explain how physical inactivity differs from sedentary behavior.

12. Define obesity and overweight relative to BMI.

13. Explain the obesity paradox.

14. Define metabolic syndrome and identify its relationship to CVD.

15. Explain how regular physical activity may prevent or delay select forms of cancer and cognitive decline.

16. What types of exercise are effective for counteracting bone loss due to aging?

17. Explain how chronic adherence to moderate- to vigorous-intensity physical activity affects the aging process.

18. Explain the relationship between physical inactivity and low back pain.

CHAPTER 2

Preliminary Health Screening and Risk Classification

KEY QUESTIONS

- What are the major components of the health evaluation, and how is this information used to screen clients for exercise testing and participation?
- What factors do I need to focus on when evaluating the client's medical history and lifestyle characteristics?
- How will I know if my client is at risk for an adverse cardiovascular event during exercise or while being physically active?
- Should cardiovascular disease risk factors be identified as part of the preparticipation screening process?
- Do all clients need a physical examination and medical clearance before beginning or progressing the intensity of an exercise program?

- What are the standards for classifying blood cholesterol levels?
- How is blood pressure measured and evaluated? Are automated blood pressure devices accurate?
- How is heart rate measured? Are heart rate monitors accurate?
- What is an ECG, and does every client need to have one before or while taking an exercise test?
- Is it safe to give a graded exercise test to all clients? When does a physician need to be present?
- What are the major components of the lifestyle evaluation, and how can this information be used?
- What are the purposes of informed consent?

Before assessing your client's physical fitness profile, it is important to classify the person's health status and lifestyle. You will use information from the initial health and lifestyle evaluations to screen clients for possible adverse cardiovascular events related to exercise or physical activity. You also will use this information to identify individuals with medical contraindications to exercise, with disease symptoms and risk factors, and with special needs.

This chapter discusses the components of a comprehensive health evaluation, including a coronary risk factor profile, medical history questionnaire, lifestyle evaluation, and informed consent. It also presents guidelines and standards for classifying

blood cholesterol levels, blood pressures, and disease risk, along with techniques and procedures for measuring heart rate and blood pressure at rest and during exercise and for conducting a resting 12-lead electrocardiogram (ECG).

PRELIMINARY HEALTH EVALUATION

The purposes of the health evaluation are to detect the presence or suggestion of disease and to assess the likelihood that your client will have an unanticipated cardiovascular situation during a bout of exercise or physical activity. The components of a comprehensive health evaluation are listed in table 2.1. To evaluate the client's health status, information from questionnaires and data from clinical tests are analyzed. Minimally, for pretest health screening of clients for exercise testing and exercise program participation, you should

- administer the Physical Activity Readiness Questionnaire for Everyone (PAR-Q+),
- evaluate client participation in regular exercise in the past 3 mo,
- identify signs and symptoms of diseases,
- analyze the coronary risk factors, and
- determine if medical clearance is needed.

Step-by-step procedures for conducting a comprehensive health evaluation are listed in Procedures for Comprehensive Pretest Health Screening.

QUESTIONNAIRES AND SCREENING FORMS

Appendix A provides questionnaires and forms that may be used to obtain information for the preliminary health screening and evaluation of your clients. The client should complete the PAR-Q+, medical history questionnaire, lifestyle evaluation, and informed consent form. You will interview your client to gather information about signs and symptoms of disease, analyze your client's coronary heart disease (CHD) risk factors, and determine if it is necessary for your client to obtain a medical clearance before beginning an exercise program or progressing the existing exercise program (table 2.2).

Table 2.1 Components of a Comprehensive Health Evaluation

Component	Purpose
QUESTIONNAIRES OR SCREENING FORMS	
2018 PAR-Q+	To determine client's readiness for physical activity
Signs and symptoms of disease and medical clearance	To identify individuals in need of medical referral and to obtain evidence of physician approval for exercise testing and participation
Coronary risk factor analysis	To determine the number of coronary heart disease risk factors for client
Medical history	To review client's past and present personal and family health history, focusing on conditions requiring medical referral and clearance
Lifestyle evaluation	To obtain information about the client's living habits
Informed consent	To explain the purpose, risks, and benefits of physical fitness tests and to obtain client's consent for participation in these tests
CLINICAL TESTS	
Physical examination	To detect signs and symptoms of disease
Blood chemistry profile	To determine if client has normal values for selected blood values; values of blood cholesterol are used in the coronary risk factor analysis
Blood pressure assessment	To determine if client is hypertensive; these values are also used in the coronary risk factor analysis
12-lead electrocardiogram	To evaluate cardiac function and detect cardiac abnormalities that are contraindications to exercise
Graded exercise test	To assess functional aerobic capacity and to detect cardiac abnormalities due to exercise stress
Additional laboratory tests (e.g., angiograms, echocardiograms, pulmonary tests)	To provide a more in-depth assessment of client's health status, particularly if there is known disease

Physical Activity Readiness Questionnaire for Everyone

The PAR-Q+ (http://eparmedx.com/; see Appendix A.1) has seven general health questions that identify individuals who need medical clearance before starting an exercise program, becoming more physically active, or undergoing a fitness appraisal (see appendix A.1). If clients answer yes to any of these questions, they need to answer the follow-up questions about their medical conditions. If clients answer yes to one or more of the follow-up questions, recommend they seek additional information from a qualified professional before changing their current activity level. Also, they should complete the ePARmed-X+ (www.eparmedx.com; see appendix

A.4) on their own or with the assistance of an exercise professional. Depending on the answers to the ePARmed-X+ survey, the client will either receive clearance to participate or be offered suggestions on how to safely proceed until such clearance is attained. These suggestions include getting more information by meeting with his personal physician or a qualified exercise professional who has advanced university training. While waiting for the meeting, the client is encouraged to engage in low-intensity activities. Following the meeting, the client may receive clearance to proceed with his activity aspirations while under direct supervision of a qualified exercise professional (PAR-Q+ Collaboration 2017).

Table 2.2 ACSM Guidelines for Medical Clearance Based on Exercise History, Symptomology, and Disease Status

	Does not exercise regularly			Exercises regularly[a]		
Known disease[b]	No	Yes	Possible	No	Yes	Yes
Symptomatic[c]	No	No	Yes	No	No	Yes
Medical clearance[d]	NN	R	R	NN	NN for exercise ≤5.9 METs; R if no change in signs and symptoms in past year for exercise >6 METs	R; discontinue exercise until cleared
Exercise intensity[e]	2-5.9 METs	2-5.9 METs	2-5.9 METs	3-6+ METs	3-5.9 METs	Resume after clearance
Progression[f]	Gradually; 6+ METs OK	Gradually as tolerated	Gradually as tolerated	Gradually; 6+ METs OK	Gradually as tolerated after clearance	Gradually as tolerated

Note: Once the proper column is located from the combination of regular exercise, known disease, and symptomology, follow that column down through the rest of the table.

[a]Has performed planned, structured physical activity of moderate intensity ≥30 min on ≥3 days/wk for past 3 mo or more.

[b]Has cardiovascular (heart, peripheral vascular, or cerebrovascular), metabolic (type 1 or type 2 diabetes), or renal disease.

[c]Exhibits signs or symptoms at rest or during exertion (discomfort in cheek, jaw, neck, arms, back, and so on that may be due to ischemia; shortness of breath even when performing normal activities; dizziness or syncope; orthopnea or paroxysmal nocturnal dyspnea; edema in ankle(s); heart palpitations or tachycardia; intermittent claudication; known heart murmur; unusual fatigue).

[d]Approval from health care professional to exercise (NN = not necessary; R = recommended).

[e]2-2.9 METs (light intensity = RPE 9-11, 30%-39% HRR or $\dot{V}O_2R$; slight increase in HR and respiratory rate); 3-5.9 METs (moderate intensity = RPE 12-13, 40%-59% HRR or $\dot{V}O_2R$; noticeable increase in HR and respiratory rate); 6 METs and higher (vigorous intensity = RPE ≥14, ≥60% HRR or $\dot{V}O_2R$; substantial increase in HR and respiratory rate).

[f]In accordance with *ACSM Guidelines for Exercise Testing and Prescription, 10th Edition.*

Adapted from ACSM 2018.

PROCEDURES FOR COMPREHENSIVE PRETEST HEALTH SCREENING

Here are step-by-step procedures you should follow when conducting a comprehensive health evaluation:

- Greet the client.
- Explain the purpose of the health evaluation and lifestyle evaluation.
- Obtain the client's informed consent for health screening.
- Administer and evaluate the PAR-Q+; refer client for medical clearance if needed.
- Administer and evaluate client's medical history, focusing on signs, symptoms, and diseases; refer client for medical clearance if needed.

- Evaluate client's lifestyle profile.
- Evaluate and classify the client's cholesterol and lipoprotein levels if test results are available.
- Measure and classify the client's resting blood pressure and heart rate.
- Assess the client's coronary risk factors and current exercise participation history.
- Evaluate the client's blood chemistry profile if test results are available.

If so requested by the client's physician, you may do the following:

- Explain the purpose of and answer any questions about the 12-lead resting ECG and graded exercise test (GXT).
- Obtain the client's informed consent for these tests.
- Prepare the client and administer the 12-lead resting ECG.
- Have a physician interpret the results of the 12-lead resting ECG.

- Use the client's disease risk classification to determine whether a maximal or submaximal GXT should be administered and whether a physician needs to be present or in the immediate vicinity during this test.
- Assess the client's resting blood pressure and heart rate.
- Administer the GXT.
- Assess and classify the client's functional aerobic capacity.

Medical History Questionnaire

You should require your clients to complete a comprehensive medical history questionnaire that includes questions concerning personal and family health history (see appendix A.2). Use the questionnaire to

- examine the client's record of personal illnesses, surgeries, and hospitalizations (section A),
- assess previous medical diagnoses and signs and symptoms of disease that have occurred within the past year or are currently present (section B), and
- analyze your client's family history of diabetes, heart disease, stroke, and hypertension (section C).

Also, when reviewing the medical history, you should carefully focus on conditions that require medical referral (see Absolute and Relative Contraindications to Exercise Testing). If any of these conditions are noted, refer your client to a physician for

a physical examination and medical clearance prior to exercise testing or starting an exercise program. Some individuals have medical conditions and risk factors that outweigh the potential benefits of exercise testing. You should not administer an exercise test to individuals with absolute contraindications unless their physician orders an exercise test. Individuals with relative contraindications may be tested if the potential benefit from exercise testing outweighs the relative risk of testing. In some cases, individuals who are asymptomatic at rest can be tested using low-level endpoints. It is also important to note the types of medication being used by the client. Drugs such as digitalis, beta-blockers, bronchodilators, vasodilators, diuretics, and insulin may alter the individual's heart rate, blood pressure, ECG, and exercise capacity. If your client reports a medical condition or drug that is unfamiliar to you, be certain to consult medical references or a physician to obtain more information before conducting any exercise tests or allowing the client to participate in an exercise program.

ABSOLUTE AND RELATIVE
CONTRAINDICATIONS TO EXERCISE TESTING

Absolute Contraindications

1. Acute myocardial infarction (within 2 days)
2. Ongoing unstable angina
3. Uncontrolled cardiac arrhythmias causing symptoms or hemodynamic compromise
4. Active endocarditis
5. Symptomatic severe aortic stenosis

6. Decompensated heart failure
7. Acute pulmonary embolism, pulmonary infarction, or deep vein thrombosis
8. Acute myocarditis or pericarditis
9. Acute aortic dissection
10. Physical disability that precludes safe and adequate testing

Relative Contraindications

1. Known obstructive left main coronary artery stenosis
2. Moderate to severe aortic stenosis with uncertain relation to symptoms
3. Tachydysrhythmias with uncontrolled ventricular rates
4. Acquired advanced or complete heart attack
5. Hypertrophic obstructive cardiomyopathy with severe resting gradient

6. Recent stroke or transient ischemic attack
7. Mental impairment with limited ability to cooperate
8. Resting hypertension with systolic or diastolic blood pressure >200/110 mmHg, respectively
9. Uncorrected medical conditions, such as significant anemia, important electrolyte imbalance, and hyperthyroidism

Note: For definitions of specific medical terms, refer to the glossary.

Reprinted by permission from G.F. Fletcher, et al., "Exercise standards for testing and training: A scientific statement from the American Heart Association," *Circulation* 128 (2013): 873-934.

Signs and Symptoms of Disease and Medical Clearance

As part of the pretest health screening, you should ask your clients if they have any of the conditions or symptoms listed in appendix A.3, Risk Factors, Signs, and Symptoms of Disease. Feel free to reproduce and use this checklist.

Clients with any of the signs or symptoms on the checklist should be referred to their physician, as a signed medical clearance prior to any exercise testing or participation may be warranted. The electronic Physical Activity Readiness Medical Examination (ePARmed-X+) was designed for this purpose. The ePARmed-X+ is a physical activity–specific checklist (see appendix A.4) that is used to assess and convey medical clearance for physical activity participation or to make a referral to a medically supervised exercise program for individuals who answered yes to one of the questions in the Physical Activity Readiness Questionnaire for Everyone (PAR-Q+). For definitions of specific medical terms, refer to the glossary. The ePARmed-X+ is available electronically at www.eparmedx.com.

Coronary Risk Factor Analysis

Even though this analysis has been removed from the ACSM's (2018) health screening process for exercise preparticipation assessment, it is still important to assess your client's coronary risk profile; evaluate each item in table 2.3 carefully. If your client will not or cannot provide the information you need to in order to include or exclude a positive risk factor, then you should include it in your total risk factor count. Guidelines for classification of blood pressure and blood cholesterol levels in adults are presented in tables 2.4 and 2.5, respectively. If your client's high-density lipoprotein cholesterol (HDL-C) equals or exceeds 60 mg·dl^{-1}, subtract 1 from the total number of positive risk factors. This information is especially helpful in identifying factors related to disease prevention and management (ACSM 2018).

Table 2.3   Coronary Heart Disease Risk Factors

Positive risk factors[a]	Criteria
Age	Men: ≥45 yr, women: ≥55 yr
Family history	Myocardial infarction, coronary revascularization, or sudden death before 55 yr of age in father or other first-degree male relative (brother or son) or before 65 yr of age in mother or other first-degree female relative (sister or daughter)
Cigarette smoking	Current cigarette smoking, exposure to environmental smoke, or smoking cessation within previous 6 mo
Hypertension	Systolic BP ≥ 130 mmHg or diastolic BP ≥ 80 mmHg, measured on two separate occasions; individual is taking antihypertensive medication.
Dyslipidemia	HDL-C < 40 mg·dl⁻¹ or LDL-C ≥ 130 mg·dl⁻¹; on lipid-lowering medication; use TC ≥200 mg·dl⁻¹ if no cholesterol subfractions are available.
Diabetes	Fasting plasma glucose ≥ 126 mg·dl⁻¹ or 2 hr oral glucose tolerance test values ≥ 200 mg·dl⁻¹, measured on two separate occasions, or HbA1C ≥ 6.5%.
Obesity	Body mass index (BMI) ≥ 30 kg/m² or waist circumference > 102 cm (40 in.) for men and > 88 cm (35 in.) for women.
Physical inactivity	Not participating in ≥30 min moderate-intensity physical activity on at least 3 days/wk for at least 3 mo
Negative risk factor[b]	
High HDL-C	Serum HDL-C ≥ 60 mg·dl⁻¹.

[a]If client cannot or will not provide a risk factor value, count it as a positive risk factor except for diabetes. For diabetes, only count a missing or unknown IFG or IGT value for adults ≥45 yr with a BMI ≥25 kg/m² or for adults <45 yr with a BMI ≥25 kg/m² and additional CVD risk factors for prediabetes.

[b]If HDL-C ≥ 60 mg·dl⁻¹, subtract 1 from the sum of positive risk factors.

Data from National Cholesterol Education Program 2001; Roger et al. 2012; Whelton et al. 2017.

Table 2.4   Classification of Blood Pressure for Adults 18 yr or Older

Systolic BP (mmHg)	Category	Diastolic BP (mmHg)
<120	Normal	<80
120-129	Elevated	<80
130-139	Stage 1 hypertension	80-89
≥140	Stage 2 hypertension	≥90

Note: For individuals not taking antihypertensive medication and not acutely ill. Based on average of two or more readings on two or more occasions. When systolic and diastolic pressures fall into different categories, use the higher category for classification.

Data from Whelton et al. 2017.

Table 2.5   Classification of TC, LDL-C, Triglycerides, and HDL-C (mg·dl⁻¹)

TOTAL CHOLESTEROL, LOW-DENSITY LIPOPROTEIN CHOLESTEROL, AND TRIGLYCERIDES			
Classification	TC	LDL-C	Triglycerides
Optimal or desirable	<200	<100	<150
Near or above optimal	—	100-129	—
Borderline high	200-239	130-159	150-199
High	≥240	160-189	200-499
Very high	—	≥190	≥500
HIGH-DENSITY LIPOPROTEIN CHOLESTEROL			
Classification	HDL-C		
Low	<40	—	—
Normal	40-59	—	—
High	≥60	—	—

Data from National Cholesterol Education Program 2001.

Disease Risk Classification

The coronary risk factor analysis is no longer used to classify an individual's risk of CHD. Instead, it provides an assessment of an individual's blood chemistry values and other factors known to be associated with atherosclerotic CVD. Additionally, all but the risk factors for age and family history are considered modifiable as they are usually responsive to committed lifestyle modifications to exercise and dietary patterns. Along with your client's exercise participation habits, any signs or symptoms of cardiovascular, renal, or metabolic disease or a diagnosis of cardiovascular, renal, or metabolic disease (see appendix A.3) guides decisions regarding the need for medical clearance. Furthermore, the new ACSM (2018) screening algorithm is instrumental in determining the recommended exercise intensity.

Another tool used to estimate the 10 yr risk of a first fatal cardiovascular event due to atherosclerosis is the SCORE system (Conroy et al. 2003). The SCORE low-risk charts are used to estimate the 10 yr risk of mortality from CVD for adults from European countries with recent and substantial reductions in CV mortality risk. The high-risk chart was used to calculate the 10 yr risk of individuals from European countries not having reported such reductions. To use the chart, you must know your client's total cholesterol (mmol·L^{-1} or mg·dl^{-1}), systolic blood pressure (SBP; mmHg), age (yr), smoking status, and sex.

Since the initial publication of the SCORE system, most if not all European countries have undertaken their own investigations to determine the predictive accuracy of the original SCORE system or their own country-specific SCORE-related algorithm. By evaluating their more recent population-specific data, countries have been able to recalibrate or validate their specific SCORE-related algorithms given public health initiatives undertaken to reduce the traditional modifiable risk factors (e.g., smoking, hypertension, dyslipidemia) in the preceding decade. Among these recalibration studies, some predicted the 10 yr risk for instances of nonfatal CVD requiring hospitalization (Jørstad et al. 2017; Panagiotakos et al. 2015) as well as fatal CVD events (Jdanov et al. 2014; Rücker et al. 2016). Others (Graversen et al. 2016) evaluated the effect of adding additional variables (e.g., ECG abnormalities, high-sensitivity C-reactive protein, waist-hip ratio) to their revised algorithms. Therefore, you may want to refer to revised SCORE algorithms for the country you are interested in.

Sawano and colleagues (2016) assessed the 2003 European SCORE system for Japanese adults to determine how well it applied to a population subgroup not represented in the Conroy (2003) study. Although they did not use the SCORE system, Edwards, Addoh, and Loprinzi (2016) investigated existing equations to determine their ability to predict the 10 yr risk of a first atherosclerotic CVD event for a large sample of American adults (40 to 79 yr) free of CVD at baseline. Another tool, the Relative Risk Chart (Perk et al. 2012) may be used to educate younger people how, relative to their age group peers, their risk for an atherosclerotic event is affected by lifestyle choices (smoking) and modifiable risk factors (hypercholesterolemia, hypertension).

Lifestyle Evaluation

Planning a well-rounded physical fitness program for an individual requires that you obtain information concerning the client's living habits. The lifestyle assessment provides useful information regarding the individual's risk factor profile. Factors such as smoking, lack of physical activity, and diets high in saturated fats or cholesterol increase the risk of CHD, atherosclerosis, and hypertension. These factors can be used to pinpoint patterns and habits that need modification and to assess the likelihood of the client's adherence to the exercise program. You can obtain a lifestyle profile for your clients by using either the Lifestyle Evaluation form (appendix A.5) or the Fantastic Lifestyle Checklist (appendix A.6). The Fantastic Lifestyle Checklist is a self-administered tool for assessing a client's present health-related behaviors.

Informed Consent

Before conducting any physical fitness tests or exercise programs, you should see that each participant signs the informed consent (see appendix A.7). This form explains the purpose and nature of each physical fitness test, any inherent risks in the testing, and the expected benefits of these tests. The informed consent also assures your clients that test results will remain confidential and that their participation is strictly voluntary. If your client is underage (<18 yr), a parent or guardian must also sign the informed consent. All consent forms should be approved by your institutional review board or legal counsel.

CLINICAL TESTS

For a comprehensive health screening, you will need to evaluate information and data obtained from the physician's medical examination and clinical tests. Clinical tests provide data about your client's blood chemistry, blood pressure, cardiopulmonary function, and aerobic capacity.

Physical Examination

Your prospective exercise program participants may need to obtain a physical examination and a signed medical clearance from a physician (ePARmed-X+: www.eparmedx.com or appendix A.4) if they

- have high blood pressure or a heart condition;

- experience noticeable chest discomfort during physical activity or activities of daily living;

- have lost consciousness in the past 12 mo or were so dizzy they lost their balance;

- have been diagnosed with a chronic medical condition besides high blood pressure or heart disease;

- are taking prescribed medications for any chronic medical condition;

- have now or within the past 12 mo a bone, joint, muscle, ligament, or tendon issue that could get worse as a result of exercise or physical activity; or

- have been told by a doctor that they should perform only medically supervised activity.

The physical examination should focus on signs and symptoms of CHD and should include an evaluation of body weight, orthopedic problems, edema, acute illness, pulse rate, cardiac regularity, blood pressure (supine, sitting, and standing), and auscultation of the heart, lungs, and major arteries. The physical examination and medical history may reveal signs or symptoms of CHD, particularly if accompanied by shortness of breath, chest discomfort, leg cramps, or high blood pressure. It is recommended that clients with these symptoms obtain a signed medical clearance (see appendix A.4) prior to exercise testing or exercise participation.

Blood Chemistry Profile

Information obtained from a complete blood analysis is used to assess your client's overall health status and readiness for exercise. Table 2.6 provides normal values for selected blood variables. If any of these values fall outside of the normal range, refer your clients to their physician. Pay special attention to your client's fasting blood glucose and blood lipid values.

The National Cholesterol Education Program (NCEP) established guidelines for classifying lipoprotein levels and major risk factors that modify low-density lipoprotein cholesterol (LDL-C) treatment goals (2001). For adults 20 yr or older, the NCEP (2001) recommends that a fasting lipoprotein profile (i.e., total cholesterol, LDL-C, HDL-C, and triglycerides) be obtained every 5 yr. To classify your client's lipoprotein values, use the NCEP (2001) guidelines (see table 2.5). For nonfasting lipoprotein tests, only the total cholesterol (TC) and HDL-C values can be evaluated. If your client's TC is borderline high (200-239 mg·dl^{-1}) or high (≥240 mg·dl^{-1}), and the HDL-C level is less than 40 mg·dl^{-1}, a follow-up fasting lipoprotein test will be needed to assess LDL-C. Refer clients to their physicians for an extensive clinical evaluation and dietary therapy if they have high (160-189 mg·dl^{-1}) or very high (≥190 mg·dl^{-1}) LDL-C values. Treatment goals for lowering

Table 2.6 Normal Values for Selected Blood Variables

Variable	Ideal or typical values
Triglycerides	<150 mg·dl^{-1}
Total cholesterol	<200 mg·dl^{-1}
LDL-cholesterol	<100 mg·dl^{-1}
HDL-cholesterol	≥40 mg·dl^{-1}
TC/HDL-cholesterol	<3.5
Blood glucose	60-99 mg·dl^{-1}
Hemoglobin	13.5-17.5 g·dl^{-1} (men) 11.5-15.5 g·dl^{-1} (women)
Hemoglobin A1c	≤6%
Hematocrit	40%-52% (men) 36%-48% (women)
Potassium	3.5-5.5 meq·dl^{-1}
Blood urea nitrogen	4-24 mg·dl^{-1}
Creatinine	0.3-1.4 mg·dl^{-1}
Iron	40-190 µg·dl^{-1} (men) 35-180 µg·dl^{-1} (women)
Calcium	8.5-10.5 mg·dl^{-1}

Table 2.7 Three Risk Categories That Modify LDL-C Goals

Risk category	LDL-C goal (mg·dl⁻¹)
CHD and CHD risk equivalents[a]	<100
Multiple (2+) risk factors[b]	<130
0-1 risk factor	<160

[a]CHD risk equivalents include diabetes and atherosclerotic disease (i.e., peripheral arterial disease, abdominal aortic aneurysm, and symptomatic carotid artery disease).

[b]Risk factors include cigarette smoking, hypertension, low high-density lipoprotein cholesterol, family history of premature CHD, and age.

NCEP 2001.

LDL-C depend on the number of major risk factors (exclusive of LDL-C) the client has. To determine your client's risk factors, focus on the following in table 2.3: cigarette smoking, hypertension, low HDL-C, family history of premature CHD, and age (men ≥45 yr; women ≥55 yr). Table 2.7 is the NCEP's listing of three risk categories that modify LDL-C treatment goals.

In addition to TC and lipoproteins, you can evaluate your client's triglyceride value and the ratio of TC to HDL-C. Clients with triglyceride levels of ≥150 mg·dl⁻¹ or TC/HDL-C ratios >5.0 are at higher risk for CHD.

Resting Blood Pressure

Blood pressure (BP) is a measure of the force or pressure exerted by the blood on the arteries. The highest pressure, **systolic blood pressure (SBP)** reflects the pressure in the arteries during systole of the heart when myocardial contraction forces a large volume of blood into the arteries. Following systole, the arteries recoil and the pressure drops during diastole, or the filling phase of the heart. **Diastolic blood pressure (DBP)** is the lowest pressure in the artery during the cardiac cycle and reflects organ perfusion. The difference between the systolic and diastolic BPs is known as the **pulse pressure**. The pulse pressure creates a pulse wave that can be palpated at various sites in the body to determine pulse rate and to estimate BP.

Values used for classification of resting BP are presented in table 2.4. Normal BP (normotensive) is defined as values less than 120/80 mmHg. The elevated blood pressure category (systolic BP = 120-129 mmHg, with diastolic BP ≤80mmHg) is added to identify individuals at risk of developing hypertension. Stage 1 hypertension is defined as a resting SBP value between 130 and 139 mmHg and DBP between 80 and 89 mmHg; stage 2 hypertension blood pressure values are those equaling or exceeding 140/90 mmHg on two or more occasions (Whelton et al. 2017).

Although a blood pressure value in the elevated range does not connote a disease, it significantly increases the risk for CHD (Huang et al. 2015). Individuals with elevated blood pressures are encouraged to modify their lifestyle in order to reduce their risk of developing hypertension by

- losing body weight if overweight;
- adopting a healthy eating plan that includes a diet rich in fruits, vegetables, and low-fat dairy products but reduced in cholesterol, saturated fat, and total fat;
- restricting dietary sodium intake to no more than 2.4 g (100 mmol) per day;
- engaging in aerobic physical activities at least 150 min/wk; and
- limiting alcohol consumption to no more than 1 oz (29.6 ml) per day for men and 0.5 oz (14.8 ml) per day for women.

When lifestyle modifications are ineffective, pharmacological therapy may be required to lower BP. There are numerous drugs available to treat hypertension (see James et al. 2014), such as

- diuretics to rid the body of excess salt and fluids,
- beta-blockers to reduce heart rate and cardiac output,
- calcium channel blockers to reduce heart contractility and dilate arteries,
- direct renin inhibitors to block conversion of angiotensinogen into angiotensin-1,
- potassium channel openers to hyperpolarize vascular smooth muscles and endothelial cells,
- sympathetic nerve inhibitors to prevent constriction of arterioles,
- vasodilators to induce relaxation in smooth muscles of arterial walls, and
- angiotensin-converting enzyme inhibitors to disrupt the body's production of angiotensin, which constricts arterioles.

Additional Clinical Tests

For individuals with known or suspected CHD, additional tests may be indicated. These may include a resting 12-lead ECG, an angiogram, an echocardiogram, and a physician-monitored graded exercise test. A chest X-ray, comprehensive blood chemistry, and complete blood count may also be pertinent (ACSM 2018). For clients with known pulmonary disease, the ACSM (2018) recommends a chest X-ray, pulmonary function tests, and specialized pulmonary tests (e.g., blood gas analysis and oxygen saturation).

Graded Exercise Test

Ischemic heart disease (IHD) is often not detectable from the resting ECG, and abnormalities may not appear until the individual engages in relatively strenuous exercise. Most clinical graded exercise tests incorporate ECG monitoring and are performed in relation to the diagnosis and evaluation of IHD. It is common for clinical GXTs to be terminated at the onset of symptoms of IHD. Another reason for administering a GXT as part of the health evaluation is to assess functional aerobic capacity. A low level of functional aerobic capacity (low cardiorespiratory fitness) is now considered a strong predictor of CVD, all-cause mortality, and mortality from certain cancers. Low functional aerobic capacity may be a better predictor than are the other well-known modifiable risk factors such as type 2 diabetes, high blood pressure, smoking, and aberrant cholesterol levels (Ross et al. 2016). Healthy individuals interested in learning their cardiorespiratory fitness (CRF) levels may find graded exercise testing services available to the public through colleges and universities that have degree-granting exercise science programs; these GXTs most often are not ordered by a physician. Regardless, graded exercise tests should be administered only by trained, professionally certified personnel such as exercise scientists, physicians, and nurses.

You need to be familiar with medical conditions that are absolute and relative contraindications to exercise testing in an out-of-hospital setting (see Absolute and Relative Contraindications to Exercise Testing). Individuals with absolute contraindications should not be given a graded exercise test unless their condition has been stabilized or medically treated. In cases in which the benefits outweigh the risks, individuals with relative contraindications may perform exercise tests. These tests, however, should use low-level endpoints and be administered with caution (ACSM 2018).

As noted in statements by the American Heart Association (Myers et al. 2014), maximal exertion stress testing may be safely conducted by certified exercise specialists and allied health professionals who are well trained and experienced in screening clients prior to testing, monitoring exercise tests, and handling emergencies (ACSM 2018). To ascertain if direct supervision by a physician is needed or if the supervising physician can be nearby and immediately available while a nonphysician clinical exercise testing professional supervises the test, consult the policies of your facility and locale. The results from graded exercise tests provide a basis for prescription of exercise for healthy and coronary-prone individuals, as well as for cardiopulmonary patients.

TESTING PROCEDURES FOR BLOOD PRESSURE, HEART RATE, AND ELECTROCARDIOGRAM

One of your major responsibilities as an exercise scientist is to become proficient at measuring and monitoring BP, heart rate, and ECGs during rest and exercise. During a graded exercise test, you will be expected to obtain accurate and precise measurements of BP and heart rate while the client is exercising. Because of their importance and complexity, this section is devoted to a thorough discussion of these procedures.

MEASURING BLOOD PRESSURE

Video
2.1

Blood pressure can be measured directly or indirectly. The gold standard is the direct measurement of intra-arterial BP. This method is invasive and requires catheterization. Therefore, in clinical or field settings, BP is typically measured indirectly by auscultation or oscillometry. With advancements in technology and varying degrees of attention paid to strictly following the standard procedures for assessing blood pressure via cuff and stethoscope, automated blood pressure assessment is surpassing auscultation for resting blood pressure assessment

BLOOD PRESSURE–RELATED SMARTPHONE APPS

There are no fewer than 100 hypertension-related apps available for download (Kumar et al. 2015). Most of them allow users to track their BP, BMI, and body weight by entering the data into their smartphones. Some of these apps provide access to information about hypertension, medication adherence, and diet. Reports indicate that these tracking and educational apps include design features that make them beneficial for monitoring BP and factors related to it (e.g., body weight, stress level).

Some Android apps assess blood pressure and heart rate by using the phone's camera and microphone. These apps may provide opportunities to track blood pressure for general knowledge. It is important to understand that none of them have undergone the rigorous testing required of traditional blood pressure devices. The apps have also not been approved by the U.S. Food and Drug Administration. Therefore, health care providers should be cautious with information from these apps as provided to them by their clients.

in clinical settings. To date, unfortunately, there is no gold standard automated oscillometric device. Regardless, manual blood pressure assessment continues to be an invaluable skill; it remains the preferred method for monitoring changes in blood pressure during and after exercise (Sharman and LaGerche 2015).

For auscultation, a stethoscope and a **sphygmomanometer** consisting of a BP cuff (cloth cover and bladder) and an aneroid manometer are used. Step-by-step instructions for the auscultatory method are presented in Resting Blood Pressure Measurement Via Manual Auscultation. **Oscillometry** uses an automated electronic manometer to measure oscillations in pressure (i.e., waveforms) when the cuff is deflated. Systolic and diastolic BPs are calculated with the use of proprietary algorithms provided by each manufacturer.

Blood Pressure Measurement Techniques

Measure resting BP in the supine and exercise (sitting or standing) positions prior to testing. The client should be wearing a short-sleeved or sleeveless garment and should be seated in a quiet room. Take BP measurements rapidly, and completely deflate the cuff for at least 30 sec between consecutive readings. For more accurate results, obtain two or three determinations of pressure from each arm.

It takes a great deal of practice to become proficient at measuring BPs. When you are first learning this method, it is highly recommended that you practice with a trained BP technician, using a dual- or multiple-head stethoscope so you can listen simultaneously and compare BP readings for the same trial.

Follow the manufacturer's instructions when measuring blood pressure using an automated device.

Sources of Measurement Error

Video 2.2

Sources of error in measuring BP are numerous (adapted from Kallioinen et al. 2017, Ogedegbe and Pickering 2010; Tolonen et al. 2015) and may be related to equipment, the technician, or the client. You need to be aware of the following sources of error and do as much as possible to control them:

- Inaccurate sphygmomanometer
- Improper cuff width or length
- Cuff not centered, too loose, or over clothing
- Back, feet, or arm unsupported or elbow not at heart level
- Poor auditory acuity or reaction time of technician
- Improper rate of inflation or deflation of the cuff pressure
- Improper stethoscope placement or pressure
- Expectation bias and inexperience of the technician
- Conversation between technician and client
- Parallax error in reading the manometer
- Background noise
- Client holding onto something (e.g., cane, chair arms, treadmill handrails, or cycle ergometer handlebars)
- Client having full bladder
- Client having exercised, smoked, eaten, or consumed alcohol prior to appointment

To measure resting BP (seated position) with a manually operated aneroid or mercury device, use the following recommended procedures (adapted from Kallioinen et al. 2017; Ogedegbe and Pickering 2010; Tolonen et al. 2015):

1. Seat the client in a quiet area for at least 5 min, longer if the client is hypertensive. The client's bare arm, palm up, should be resting on a solid surface (table or desk) so that the middle of the arm is at the level of the heart. The client's back must be supported and both feet flat on the floor or other solid surface such as a step stool.

2. Select the appropriate cuff size by estimating the client's arm circumference or measuring it at the midpoint between the acromion process of the shoulder and the olecranon process of the elbow (see appendix D.4 for a description of measuring arm circumference) using an anthropometric tape measure. The bladder of the cuff should encircle 80% of an adult's arm and 100% of a child's arm.

3. Locate the brachial artery by palpating the brachial artery pulse on the anteromedial aspect of the arm below the belly of the biceps brachii and 2 to 3 cm (1 in.) above the antecubital fossa.

4. Wrap the deflated cuff snugly around the upper arm so that the midline of the cuff or artery marker is over the brachial artery pulse; if the cuff is loose, BP will be overestimated. The lower edge of the cuff should be approximately 2.5 cm (1 in.) above the antecubital fossa. Avoid placing the cuff over clothing; if the shirtsleeve is rolled up, make certain it is not occluding the circulation.

5. Position the pressure gauge so it is at your eye level and the cuff's tubing so it is not overlapping or obstructed.

6. Estimate blood pressures by locating and palpating the radial pulse (see Palpation section later in chapter for anatomical description of this site), completely closing the inflation bulb valve of the BP unit, and rapidly inflating the cuff to 70 mmHg. Slowly increase the pressure in 10 mmHg increments while palpating the radial pulse, noting when the pulse disappears (estimate of systolic BP). Partially open the valve to slowly release the pressure at a rate of 2 to 3 mmHg·sec^{-1}, noting when the radial pulse reappears (estimate of diastolic BP). Fully open the valve to completely deflate the cuff. The estimate of systolic BP from this method is used to determine how much the cuff needs to be inflated for measuring BP using the auscultatory technique. In this way, you can avoid over- or underinflating the cuff for clients with low or high BPs, respectively.

7. Position the earpieces of the stethoscope so they are aligned with the auditory canals (i.e., angled anteriorly).

8. Place the entire head of the stethoscope on the skin and over the brachial pulse (about 1 cm superior and medial to the antecubital fossa). To avoid extraneous noise, do not place any part of the head of the stethoscope underneath the cuff.

9. Close the inflation bulb valve; quickly and steadily inflate the cuff pressure to about 20 to 30 mmHg above the estimated systolic pressure previously determined by palpation.

10. Partially open the valve to slowly release the pressure at a rate of 2 to 3 mmHg·sec^{-1}. Note when you hear the first sharp thud caused by the sudden rush of blood as the artery opens. This is known as the first Korotkoff sound and corresponds to the systolic pressure (phase I).

11. Continue reducing the pressure slowly (no faster than 2 mmHg·sec^{-1}), noting when the metallic tapping sound becomes muffled (phase IV diastolic pressure) and when the sound disappears (phase V diastolic pressure). Typically, the phase V value is used as the index of diastolic pressure. However, both phase IV and V diastolic pressures should be noted. During rhythmic exercise, the phase V pressure tends to decrease because of reduction in peripheral resistance. In some cases, it may even drop to zero.

12. After noting the phase V pressure, continue deflating the cuff for at least 10 mmHg, making certain that no additional sounds are heard. Then rapidly and completely deflate the cuff.

13. Record all three BP values (phases I, IV, and V) to the nearest 2 mmHg. Wait at least 30 sec and repeat the measurement. Use the average of the two measurements for each of the three values.

The following section addresses questions about measuring BP and provides tips for taking more accurate BP measurements during rest or exercise.

Which type of sphygmomanometer provides more valid and reliable measures of resting blood pressure?

For over a century, the mercury column manometer has been considered the gold standard for indirect measurement of BP. Calibrated aneroid manometers may yield less error than automated devices when compared with mercury column manometers. As part of their systematic review of sources of inaccuracies in resting blood pressure assessment, Kallioinen and colleagues (2017) reported on the comparison of manual and automated blood pressure devices with a mercury column manometer. Of the 13 comparisons of aneroid manometers with a mercury column criterion, only one reported a significant difference, and that was for systolic blood pressure. Thirty-nine studies compared automated devices with a mercury column criterion, and significant differences were reported for systolic pressure ($n = 5$), diastolic pressure ($n = 1$), and both systolic and diastolic pressures ($n = 11$).

Although mercury column and aneroid manometers are similarly susceptible to technician error, mercury column manometers are preferred for a number of reasons. They are based on gravity, leaving little room for mechanical errors. In contrast, the aneroid manometer is a spring-based device that can fatigue with use and thereby lose its calibration more easily. It can become inaccurate without the technician's awareness, as was the case in nearly 23% of the devices checked in six accredited doctoral physical therapy programs (Arena, Simon, and Peterson 2016). Therefore, aneroid manometers must be calibrated frequently (at least every 6 mo). Often when the aneroid manometer fails the calibration test, it must be returned to the manufacturer for repair. For a complete list of recommended aneroid sphygmomanometers, see www.dableducational.org.

Unlike aneroid and mercury manometers, oscillometric devices require less calibration and maintenance; additionally, they require little technician training. Oscillometric devices are frequently used in the home setting, ambulatory blood pressure monitoring markets, and community service blood pressure screenings; they are also gaining favorability in clinical office settings. Although the common belief is that oscillometric devices may misestimate the BP of clients with irregular heart rhythms, Lakhal and associates (2015) reported similar BP values for an oscillometric device compared with intra-arterial BP measurements in a sample of arrhythmic patients ($n = 135$) and those with regular heart rhythm ($n = 136$) in three intensive care units. For a comprehensive report on the strengths and weaknesses of various oscillometric algorithms incorporated into automated blood pressure devices, see the 2015 article by Forouzanfar and colleagues.

How can I check the accuracy of an aneroid manometer?

To check the accuracy of an aneroid manometer against a mercury unit, follow the procedure adapted from Arena, Simon, and Peterson (2016) and Emmanuel (2013):

- Disconnect the bulbs of both cuffs and reconnect the bulb of the aneroid unit to the cuff of the mercury unit.
- Use a T or Y connector to reconnect the aneroid gauge being tested to the mercury unit. (*Note:* This step may be skipped if you are testing a single-tube aneroid device because the gauge is integrated into the inflation bulb handle.)
- Completely deflate the cuff being tested, and check that the aneroid gauge indicator is at zero mmHg.
- Wrap the deflated cuff around a rigid metal or plastic cylinder approximately 10 cm in diameter.
- Hold the pressure gauge of the aneroid manometer close to the mercury column and compare the two readings.
- Inflate the cuff to 250 mmHg and compare readings. Slowly deflate the cuff and compare readings at regular intervals (e.g., 200, 150, 100, and 50 mmHg).
- If the aneroid and mercury manometer pressures differ by more than 3 mmHg at any point, send the aneroid manometer to the manufacturer for adjustment.

What criteria are used to judge the accuracy of devices that measure blood pressure?

The Association for the Advancement of Medical Instrumentation (AAMI), the British Hypertension Society (BHS), the European Society of Hypertension International Protocol (ESH-IP), and the German Hypertension League (DHL) established separate criteria for judging the accuracy of BP devices. Most validation studies use one or more of these sets of criteria. For each set, measured values from the device are compared with those obtained from a mercury sphygmomanometer. To meet AAMI criteria, the measured average BP (systolic and diastolic) should not differ from the mercury standard by more than 5 mmHg, and the standard deviation should not exceed 8 mmHg. For the BHS criteria, differences in both systolic and diastolic BPs are graded as A, B, C, or D depending on the cumulative percentage of absolute individual difference scores falling within three categories: 5, 10, and 15 mmHg (see table 2.8). To be recommended, a device must achieve at least a B; A and D denote the greatest and least degree of agreement with the mercury standard.

The European Society of Hypertension (ESH) protocol, also known as the International Protocol (ESH-IP), is more complex than that of the BHS. Basically, it categorizes mean differences in BP as follows: 0 to 5 mmHg = very accurate, 6 to 10 mmHg = slightly inaccurate, 11 to 15 mmHg = moderately inaccurate, and >15 mmHg = very inaccurate. The number of comparisons cumulatively falling within 5, 10, and 15 mmHg is counted (i.e., the 5 mmHg zone represents all values falling within 0-5 mmHg; the 10 mmHg zone represents all values falling within

0-5 mmHg and 6-10 mmHg; the 15 mmHg zone represents all values falling within 0-5 mmHg, 6-10 mmHg, and 10-15 mmHg). These values are then compared against standards set for each of two phases of the validation process. Devices recommended for clinical use must pass both phases of the validation process. The 2002 ESH-IP criteria (ESH-IP1) were revised and clarified in 2010 (ESH-IP2) and made more stringent. In a retrospective investigation of validation studies, Stergiou and colleagues (2011) determined that about 33% of the BP monitors previously validated under the ESH-IP 2002 criteria failed to meet the ESH-IP 2010 requirements. For a detailed description of the ESH-IP2, see the work of O'Brien and colleagues (2010). For a detailed analysis of BP monitoring devices that passed the ESH-IP 2002 criteria yet failed the 2010 revised criteria, see the 2011 study by Stergiou and associates.

The German Hypertension League established its Quality Seal Protocol to allow evaluation of blood pressure measuring devices targeting the German market. This clinical validation protocol requires ≥96 patients in specific blood pressure and age ranges. For each patient, six standard and device-specific measurements are taken in a predefined sequence, with a 30 to 60 sec inter-assessment rest interval. Reference measurements cannot differ by more than 4 mmHg, and their averages cannot differ by more than 16 mmHg from the first to the sixth paired assessment, all completed within 40 min. Of the six paired readings, at least three qualifying readings per patient are required (288 paired readings) for subsequent analysis. Similar to the AAMI standards, the DHL Quality Seal Protocol requires that the differences between means for SBP and DBP paired readings are within 5 mmHg and standard deviations are ≤8 mmHg. Point

Table 2.8 British Hypertension Society Validation Criteria for Blood Pressure Measuring Devices

Grade[b]	CATEGORY[a]		
	≤5 mmHg	≤10 mmHg	≤15 mmHg
A	60%	85%	95%
B	50%	75%	90%
C	40%	65%	85%
D	Worse than C		

[a]Values are the cumulative percentage of absolute difference scores between the mercury standard and the test device.

[b]All three percentages must be greater than or equal to the values shown for a specific grade to be awarded.

scores are assigned based on the proximity of mean differences for both SBP and DBP pairs. A minimum 55% of the total possible score is required for earning the quality seal. For an in-depth comparison of the AAMI, BHS, ESH-IP, and DHL protocols, see the article by Beime et al. (2016).

While endorsing the need for automated BP device testing standards, Wan and colleagues (2010) highlighted the importance of reassessing device accuracy in community settings, where misestimating BP has the highest consequences. In addition to identifying eight discussion points for future consideration, Beime and colleagues (2016) highlight the typical 2-yr life cycle of a blood pressure assessment device before upgrades hit the market as a reason for short device validation protocols.

The dabl Educational Trust has a website that provides up-to-date, evidence-based information about BP measurement techniques and devices (www.dableducational.org). Here you will find tables evaluating the validity of various types of BP devices according to AAMI, BHS, and International Protocol criteria. You may also find lists of blood pressure devices validated and approved for home and clinical use on the website of the British Hypertension Society (http://bhsoc.org/bp-monitors/bp-monitors); the criteria on which they were approved are also identified.

In the future, will the mercury column manometer be banned? If so, what types of devices will replace it?

Because of the growing environmental concerns regarding the toxic effects of mercury, a global treaty was signed at the October 2013 Minamata Convention in Japan. This treaty establishes the year 2020 as the phase-out date for mercury-containing products like mercury column manometers and thermometers. As soon as 50 countries sign the treaty, it will go into effect (U.S. Environmental Protection Agency 2017). After the phase-out date, mercury-containing products cannot be manufactured, imported, or exported. Consequently, clinics and doctors' offices in many countries have been phasing out mercury manometers and thermometers. Use of automated oscillometric manometers and other devices utilizing semiconductor pressure sensors is accelerating (Asayama et al. 2016) as practitioners seek a viable replacement of the mercury column manometer.

The Scientific Committee on Emerging and Newly Identified Health Risks (SCENIHR) is on record as supporting limited use of mercury manometers but finds hybrid devices validated using ESH-IP standards to be a suitable alternative for BP assessment in a clinical setting. SCENIHR also supports the use of such hybrid devices as a criterion reference against which to validate new BP devices (Parati and Ochoa 2012). Although no health care agencies in the country forbid mercury manometers, the United States has already signed the Minamata Treaty. The National Institutes of Health (NIH) launched an initiative in 2001 to become mercury-free by replacing mercury-containing devices in its labs and facilities (National Institutes of Health 2012). None of the aneroid or nonmercury manual blood pressure sphygmomanometers for clinical use that passed AAMI, BSH, or ESH-IP1 validation criteria have received a passing score under the more conservative ESH-IP2 (dabl Educational Trust 2017); however, that may change as the website (www.dableducational.org) is updated. Alternatively, more than 40 of the automated devices on that web page have received ESH-IP2 passing scores. In assessing the accuracy of aneroid and digital manometers against the standard mercury column for the assessment of hypertensive status, Shahbabu and associates (2016) reported that the aneroid manometer was more consistently (>89%) within 5 ± 8 mmHg of the criterion than was the digital manometer (<44%).

When replacing a mercury column manometer with a mercury-free device, be sure to verify that the device has been validated using rigorous standards. It is also suggested that you conduct your own determination of equivalence between the replacement device you have chosen and your mercury column. For example, the hypertension cut-point blood pressure reading of 140/90 mmHg on the mercury column was found to be equivalent to 143/79 mmHg and 149.5/84.5 mmHg for the aneroid and digital devices, respectively, as tested by Shahbabu and colleagues (2016).

The AHA made the following recommendations for health care and fitness settings that exclusively use aneroid or automated devices (Jones et al. 2001):

- Select only devices that satisfy the validation criteria of the AAMI, BHS, or similar organizations.

- Schedule regular maintenance and calibration.
- Insist on the use of mercury manometers for calibration.
- Ensure regular training of personnel who measure BP.

Hybrid sphygmomanometers are mercury-free and combine features of both electronic and auscultatory devices. Several types of hybrid sphygmomanometers have successfully undergone clinical validation against a mercury column manometer (Stergiou et al. 2012a; Stergiou et al. 2012b). With the hybrid sphygmomanometer, the mercury column is replaced with an electronic pressure gauge. The technician uses a stethoscope to listen for the Korotkoff sounds. For older models, the technician presses a button next to the deflation knob once systolic and diastolic pressures are heard; this freezes the display showing the systolic and diastolic pressures. Newer models display both pressures after the diastolic pressure has been determined. The pressure is displayed digitally or as a simulated mercury column or aneroid display. The hybrid sphygmomanometer combines some of the best features of mercury and electronic devices and may be a good candidate to replace the mercury sphygmomanometer as the gold standard in clinical settings (Stergiou et al. 2012a).

How accurate are automated blood pressure devices?

There are many automated devices available for clinical and home use. These automated devices inflate and deflate a cuff that is placed over the brachial artery (upper arm device), radial artery (wrist device), or digital artery (finger device). The automated electronic manometer assesses oscillations in pressure while the cuff is gradually deflated. The maximum oscillation corresponds to mean arterial pressure; algorithms, which vary among manufacturers, are used to calculate systolic and diastolic pressures. An advantage of automated BP devices is that they eliminate **terminal digit bias**, the tendency of the technician to round BP values to the nearest 0 or 5 mmHg instead of reporting values rounded to the nearest even number. Factors that can affect the accuracy of automated devices include the age of mechanical components and sensors, the environment, and the provider's failure to adhere to manufacturer guidelines regarding the proper assessment procedures (Forouzanfar et al. 2015).

For a complete list of recommended, not recommended, and questionable automated upper arm, wrist, and finger blood pressure measurement devices as evaluated by AAMI, BHS, ESH-IP1, and ESH-IP2 criteria, see www.dableducational. org. Tholl and associates (2016) present the results of validations undertaken using DHL Quality Seal Protocol criteria on upper arm and wrist devices (N = 105) between 1999 and 2014.

Neuhauser and colleagues (2015) investigated the agreement in blood pressure values obtained via mercury sphygmomanometry and an oscillometric device for a sample of 65 women and 40 men. Meticulous blood pressure measurement procedures and simultaneous auscultation by two observers, blinded to each other's scores, were used in accordance with device-specific arm circumference cuff size determination guidelines. Significantly higher systolic and diastolic pressures were reported using the oscillometric device for all blood pressure categories (optimal, elevated, hypertensive). Likewise, systolic and diastolic pressures differed significantly for comparisons based on arm circumferences <28 cm and between 28 and 35 cm. Nobody in their sample had an arm circumference exceeding 36 cm. Interestingly, cuff dimensions for the oscillometric device were both wider and longer than for the mercury sphygmomanometer. Commenting on possible reasons as to why their results differed from those of other studies using the oscillometric device, Neuhauser and coauthors highlighted the changes in cuff-selection rules and cuff sizes over time, as well as their reporting of results based on stratified blood pressure and arm circumference categories. Ultimately, they have alerted clinicians to potential unintended consequences associated with the unquestioned replacement of devices and associated cuffs, as doing so may result in dramatic or attenuated differences in blood pressure values, treatment plans, and effect on comorbidities.

Generally, automated upper arm devices are more accurate than automated wrist devices for measuring resting BP. Wrist devices become inaccurate if the arm is not kept at heart level during measurement, and the position of the wrist during measurement may also influence accuracy. Tholl and colleagues (2016) reported that 11 automated wrist models in their study passed the DHL Quality Seal Protocol validation criteria. Likewise, numerous automated wrist models for home or clinical use are listed on the www.dableducational.org site and identified as passing according to at least one of the four identified protocols.

Finger devices generally are not recommended for measuring BP. Although the Finometer is listed as having satisfied the criteria of the AAMI and BHS for measuring the resting BP of black women in a clinical setting, the sample size is in question (see www.dableducational.org). As a result, finger devices should not be used for clinical measurement of BP.

Are aneroid and automated devices accurate at high altitudes?

There continue to be limited data about how non-mercury BP devices perform at higher elevations. If you consider that more than 170 million people worldwide are reported to live at or visit altitudes higher than 2,500 m (Li et al. 2012), having a valid and reliable method for assessing BP is important for monitoring the health of these people. The first study, although limited by its small sample size (N = 10), compared mercury column and aneroid BP measurements at 4,370 m (Kametas et al. 2006). Since the aneroid device fulfilled the AAMI recommendations at altitude, the authors concluded that it is a suitable alternative to mercury column manometers for adults at the altitudes similar to the Peruvian highlands. Li and colleagues (2012) reported significant differences for SBP but not DBP when comparing simultaneous BP measurements obtained with an oscillometric manometer (Omron HEM-759P) and a mercury column manometer for a sample of high-altitude (4,300 m) residents in Tibet. Another automated upper-arm oscillometric blood pressure cuff was successfully validated against a mercury column device in accordance with ESH-IP2 standards in a sample of high-altitude (3,650 m) residents (≥25 yr of age) of Tibet (Cho et al. 2013). Consequently, the Omron HEM-7201 device is suitable for use at similar altitudes. However, in their review of these two studies from the Tibetan region of China, Mingji and colleagues (2016) indicate that the extent of agreement between the two upper-arm oscillometric devices and mercury column reference measures was high for DBP whereas the agreement for SBP was inconsistent.

Can automated devices be used to measure blood pressure during exercise?

A review of the dabl Educational Trust (2017) website reveals no validation of clinical or home-use blood pressure assessment devices under exercise conditions. Therefore the lack of validity and accuracy of automated devices for measuring exercise BP as reported by Griffin, Robergs, and Heyward (1997) continues to hold true. To date, no criteria have been established to evaluate the accuracy of devices for measuring BP under stress (e.g., exercise). To assess the repeatability of automated BP measurements during exercise, a small sample of young men performed two identical maximal exertion treadmill tests; BP measurements were obtained every 4 min using a manometer that combined oscillometric and auscultatory methods (Instebo, Helgheim, and Greve 2012). Of the possible 70 pairs of SBP and DBP measurements over the two testing days, less than half of each measurement from the first day were reproducible on the second day.

The accuracy of some finger devices (i.e., Finapres and Portapres Model 2) designed for continuous and noninvasive ambulatory BP monitoring has been assessed during incremental cycle ergometer exercise (Blum et al. 1997; Eckert and Horstkotte 2002; Idema, van den Meiracker, and Imholz 1989). In these studies, the mean differences between the automated (Finapres and Portapres Model 2) and the intra-arterial measures of BP during low-intensity (~100 W) exercise ranged from 12 to 22 mmHg for systolic pressure and from −5 to −9.8 mmHg for diastolic pressure. The arm-cuff component for brachial pressure calibration with the Finapres improves its accuracy over the Portapres. Additional stabilization of the hand in the neutral position and splinting of the monitored finger to prevent grasping of the handlebars during cycling improves the peripheral pressure wave crucial for blood pressure calculation (Critoph et al. 2013). During exercise, these automated finger devices systematically underestimated and overestimated systolic and diastolic BPs, respectively, and average differences increased as exercise intensity increased. Therefore, these devices should not be used to measure BP during exercise.

Incorporating photoplethysmography, pulse wave velocity, and pulse transit time processing, alone or in combination, may improve the accuracy of these noninvasive means of blood pressure assessment in the resting state; however, published research using these devices during exercise is limited. Integrating ECG and finger plethysmography provides the means to include pulse transit time and pulse wave velocity for blood pressure determination during stationary cycling. Although the correlation between the auscultated aneroid cuff pressure and calculated systolic blood pressure was strong for the group of participants, there was a 10 to 20 mmHg difference between systolic blood pressure values (Gesche et al. 2012; Wibner et al. 2014). The differences become more pronounced as the individual mean blood pressure increases above 140 mmHg (Gesche et al. 2012).

How do body position and arm position affect blood pressure measurements?

Posture affects BP; generally, BP increases from lying (supine) to sitting to standing. Usually, resting BP is measured in the sitting position. Regardless of body position, the upper arm must be held or supported horizontally at the level of the heart (right atrium); the midsternal level most closely approximates the level of the right atrium. Raising the arm above heart level underestimates BP, and positioning the arm below heart level tends to overestimate BP. When the cuff is below the heart, there is a compounding influence of the hydrostatic pressure within the limb's vascular system, which predominantly affects SBP (Casiglia et al. 2016). Typically, the arm is supported by resting it on a table or by having the technician hold it at the elbow. Even when supine BP is measured, a pillow should be placed under the upper arm to support it at heart level.

The accuracy of automated wrist devices is greatly affected if the wrist is not held at heart level. An observational study investigated BP measurements obtained under supervision using a certified device worn at the wrist compared with measurements obtained at home without supervision after instruction at the physician's office; all participants underwent BP assessments and received training on and subsequently demonstrated the proper use of the devices and anatomical positioning (Casiglia et al. 2016). Casiglia and colleagues (2016) used a BHS-certified automated upper-arm device as their criterion, and there was no position sensor in the ESH-IP2 certified wrist cuff. In the office setting, systolic pressure was significantly lower at the wrist;

at home, significantly elevated wrist blood pressures were recorded for both SBP and DBP. Higher pressures at the wrist are associated with the wrist being below the level of the heart, and higher limb-specific hydraulic pressure is especially manifested in SBP values for those having long forearms. These differences by geographic location (office vs. home) occurred regardless of age and years of schooling (Casiglia et al. 2016); the differences highlight the importance of patient training quality in addition to the patient's ability to mimic proper procedures.

What is white coat hypertension?

In the condition known as **white coat hypertension**, individuals who have a normal BP outside of the clinical environment and are not taking any prescribed antihypertensive medications develop higher than normal values when their BP is measured by a health professional (Franklin et al. 2016; Sivén et al. 2016). To confirm this condition, BP should be measured outside of the clinical environment via self-measurement at home, 24 hr ambulatory BP monitoring, automated BP assessment in a community pharmacy, or an automated blood pressure measuring device while the client is alone in the examination room. Given the latter's more standardized and reproducible assessment of blood pressure compared with auscultation, an automated BP measurement with the client resting alone in an examination room is recommended as part of the new Canadian algorithm for determining hypertension (Cloutier et al. 2015).

Minimizing the patient-observer interaction reduces the **white coat effect,** which describes the acute elevation in blood pressure at the doctor's office, regardless of one's blood pressure at home or antihypertensive medication prescription status (Franklin et al. 2016). The likelihood of white coat hypertension is at least five times higher when a physician measures BP with the traditional manual method compared with automated BP readings taken with the client quietly resting alone in an examination room (Myers et al. 2009). In a study investigating the incidence of white coat hypertension in three different settings (home, community pharmacy, or physician's office), the same model of automated BP testing device was used in all three settings. The home and community pharmacy BP readings were similar for both SBP and DBP. The systolic and diastolic blood pressure values from both the community pharmacy and home settings were significantly lower than from the physician's office for a sample of hypertensive adults (Sendra-Lillo et al. 2011).

Studies suggest that white coat hypertension is not benign (Franklin et al. 2016; Martin and McGrath 2014; Sivén et al. 2016). A 10 yr follow-up study of 420 patients with stage 1 or 2 hypertension (of whom 18% had white coat hypertension) showed that individuals with white coat hypertension have an increased risk of CVDs (Gustavsen et al. 2003) and of developing sustained hypertension (Sivén et al. 2016) and diabetes (Martin and McGrath 2014) compared with normotensive individuals. However, awake ambulatory blood pressure is reported to more accurately predict cardiovascular events compared with BP measured in an office. Regardless of gender, DBP is higher when assessed in the doctor's office than during awake ambulatory measures after age 45 yr; SBP is also higher in the office setting, but after the age of 50 yr. Conversely, ambulatory blood pressure values are higher than those from an office setting for younger adults. Office blood pressure measurements are higher than those obtained in the home setting, but BP measurements from these two settings are more similar for elderly adults than for younger adults (Ishikawa et al. 2011). This finding suggests that health care professionals should consider white coat hypertension when evaluating cardiovascular risk factors.

What is masked hypertension?

Masked hypertension is a term coined in 2002 to describe a condition in which individuals exhibit higher than normal BP readings outside of the physician's office yet have normal BP values in the office (Sivén et al. 2016). Although white coat hypertension is more prevalent in older adults, masked hypertension occurs more frequently in younger adults (Ohkubo et al. 2005). Both, however, are harbingers for future cardiovascular events and target organ damage in comparison to normotensive individuals, even after accounting for the traditional cardiovascular risk factors (Tientcheu et al. 2015).

In their review of studies concerning the phenomenon of masked hypertension, Ogedegbe and colleagues (2010) highlighted underlying factors related to lifestyle choices and daily activities and their effect on everyday BP values. Some of the factors they cited include job stress, tobacco smoking, alcohol consumption, conflict in relationships, physical activity levels, and poor adherence with taking blood pressure medications as prescribed. They also highlighted that the risk for masked hypertension may be influenced by gender (higher for men than women) and BMI (higher for overweight and obese individuals compared with those classified as normotensive or having white coat hypertension) (Sivén et al. 2016; Ogedegbe, Agyemang, and Ravenell 2010). Regardless, if the condition is left untreated, then those with masked hypertension have a similar risk for target organ and cardiovascular damage as do those with sustained hypertension. Adults with masked hypertension have a fourfold increase in risk for developing sustained hypertension than do those with blood pressures in the normal range (Sivén et al. 2016).

What are miscuffing and cuff hypertension?

Miscuffing (i.e., undercuffing or overcuffing) is a serious source of measurement error caused by using a BP cuff with a bladder that is not appropriately scaled for the client's arm circumference. This is a potential problem regardless of whether you are using a manual or automated means of blood pressure assessment. Experts recommend using a cuff with a bladder width that is 40% of the measured upper arm circumference and a length that encircles at least 80% of the arm circumference; however, this recommendation does not guard against the risk of miscuffing. **Undercuffing** occurs when the bladder is too small for the arm circumference, leading to the overestimation of BP, known as **cuff hypertension**. Conversely, **overcuffing** underestimates BP because the bladder is too large for the arm circumference (Ringrose et al. 2015). To avoid these problems, the correct cuff and bladder size must be selected for each client. Furthermore, clients who monitor their own blood pressure with an oscillometric device at home must be made aware of the importance of purchasing a cuff that is appropriate for their own arm circumference. Many manufacturers offer devices for home and clinical use that have not undergone rigorous validation during development (Campbell et al. 2016) and ship them without offering recommendations regarding cuff size selection and its importance (Ringrose et al. 2015).

How can I determine the appropriate cuff size for my client?

To ensure accurate BP readings, you need to select a cuff size appropriate for your client's arm circumference. You should not assume that the cuff sent by the manufacturer of the in-home blood pressure measuring device is appropriate for all arms. Generally, four cuff sizes are commercially available: children, standard adult, large adult, and obese (i.e., thigh). To select the proper cuff size, measure your client's arm circumference (see appendix D.4 for a description of measuring arm circumference). For adults with larger proximal upper arm (e.g., just below the deltoid) than distal upper arm (e.g., just above the elbow) circumferences, a conical cuff may be more appropriate for BP measurements. In adults with proximal arm circumferences exceeding 32 cm, BP was significantly overestimated using a traditional rectangular-shaped cuff compared with a conical cuff. The extent of BP overestimation increased with increasing arm circumference (Palatini et al. 2012).

Similarly, you should not assume that a child's cuff is appropriate for all children. Using National Health and Nutrition Examination (NHANES) data from 2007 through 2010, Ostchega and colleagues (2014) reported that average midarm circumference for children and adolescents has increased such that approximately 53% of boys and 48% of girls aged 12 to 15 yr required a standard adult cuff; nothing smaller than a standard adult cuff was needed for 89% of boys and 57% of girls between 16 and 19 yr. A large adult cuff was required for proper cuff fit for approximately 30% and 24% of obese boys and girls, respectively. If arm circumference cannot be measured directly, you can estimate it using gender-specific prediction equations (see Ostchega et al. 2004). Table 2.9 presents recommended cuff and bladder sizes for measured or estimated arm circumferences.

How can I measure exercise blood pressure more accurately?

Measuring BP during exercise is much more difficult than doing so during rest. You should not attempt to measure exercise BP until you have demonstrated competency and have confidence in your ability to measure resting BP. It is particularly difficult to accurately measure BP when the client is running on the treadmill because of extraneous noise and arm movement during running. Sometimes you will not be able to determine diastolic BP during exercise because of the noise and vibration. Novice technicians should first practice taking BPs during cycle ergometer exercise and then try measuring BP during treadmill exercise. An expected BP response to exercise is for SBP to increase with increasing workload; usually, DBP fluctuates very little or decreases somewhat (Fletcher et al. 2013). See Tips for Measuring Exercise Blood Pressure for pointers on improving your BP measurements during exercise.

Table 2.9 Recommended Cuff and Bladder Sizes for Arm Circumferences

Client or patient	Arm circumference (cm)	Bladder width × length (cm)
Older child	NR	9 × 18
Small adult	22-26	12 × 22
Adult	27-34	16 × 30
Larger adult	35-44	16 × 36
Obese adult or high upper body muscularity (thigh cuff)	45-52	16 × 42

NR = not reported.

Data from Pickering et al. 2005.

TIPS FOR MEASURING EXERCISE BLOOD PRESSURE

Video
2.3

When measuring exercise BP, take extra precautions to ensure accurate readings, and record BP values in even numbers to the closest 2 mmHg (Sharman and LaGerche 2015).

- Instruct the client to refrain from grasping the handlebars or handrails of the exercise apparatus or your shoulder during the BP measurement.
- Position the cuff on the arm so that the tubing protruding from its bladder is superior instead of inferior. This position lessens extraneous noise caused by the tubing contacting the stethoscope during exercise.
- Stand where the client can keep the arm in the sagittal plane as much as possible. This position will distract the client less during exercise than will having the arm abducted 90°.
- Limit arm movement during the BP measurement; stabilize the client's arm with the cuff at heart level by placing and holding it firmly between your arm and trunk.
- Inflate the cuff well above the anticipated value or reading obtained during the previous stage of the graded exercise test, keeping in mind that systolic BP increases with exercise intensity.
- Position the manometer so it is no more than 3 ft (92 cm) away and is at eye level so you can read the scale easily. Errors will occur if you do not keep your eyes close to the level of the meniscus of the mercury column or perpendicular to the aneroid scale. For mercury column sphygmomanometry, use a model that is mounted on a stand with wheels so the manometer can be properly positioned during incremental stages of the exercise test. Positioning is particularly important when the client is performing graded treadmill tests that progressively increase the incline of the treadmill.

MEASURING HEART RATE

The average resting heart rate for adults is 60 to 80 beats per minute (bpm), with the average resting heart rate of women typically 7 to 10 bpm higher than that of men. Heart rates as low as 28 bpm have been reported for highly conditioned endurance athletes, whereas poorly trained sedentary individuals may have heart rates that exceed 100 bpm.

Do not use resting heart rate as a measure of cardiorespiratory fitness. There is wide variability in resting heart rate within the population, and a low resting heart rate is not always indicative of cardiorespiratory fitness level. In some cases, a low resting heart rate indicates a diseased heart or a medication that reduces heart rate. The following general guidelines may be used to classify resting heart rate:

1. <60 bpm = **bradycardia** (slow rate)
2. 60 to 100 bpm = normal rate
3. >100 bpm = **tachycardia** (fast rate)

Before you measure resting heart rate, your client should rest for 5 to 10 min in either a supine or a seated position. It is important that you measure resting heart rate carefully because this value is sometimes used in the calculation of target exercise heart rates for submaximal exercise tests, as well as for exercise prescriptions. You can measure heart rate using auscultation, palpation, heart rate monitors, or ECG recordings.

Auscultation

When measuring resting heart rate by auscultation, place the bell of the stethoscope over the third intercostal space to the left of the sternum. The sounds arising from the heart are counted for 30 or 60 sec. The 30 sec count is multiplied by 2 to convert it to beats per minute. Video 2.4

Palpation

With use of the **palpation** technique for determining heart rate, the pulse is palpated at one of the following sites:

- Brachial artery—on the anteromedial aspect of the arm below the belly of the biceps brachii, approximately 2 to 3 cm (1 in.) above the antecubital fossa
- Carotid artery—in the neck just lateral to the larynx
- Radial artery—on the anterolateral aspect of the wrist directly in line with the base of the thumb
- Temporal artery—along the hairline of the head at the temple Video 2.5

For precautions necessary for ensuring your measurement is accurate, refer to Heart Rate Determination by Palpation.

HEART RATE DETERMINATION BY PALPATION

Follow these procedures when determining heart rate by palpation:

- Use the tips of the middle and index fingers. Do not use your thumb; it has a pulse of its own and may produce an inaccurate count.

- When palpating the carotid site, do not apply heavy pressure to the area. Baroreceptors in the carotid arteries detect this pressure and cause a reflex slowing of the heart rate.

- If you start the stopwatch simultaneously with the pulse beat, count the first beat as zero. If the stopwatch is running, count the first beat as 1. Continue counting either for a set period of time (6, 10, 15, 30, or 60 sec) or for a set number of beats. When the heart rate is counted for less than 1 min, use the following multipliers to convert the count to beats per minute: 6 sec count × 10; 10 sec count × 6; 15 sec count × 4; 30 sec count × 2. Typically, shorter time intervals (i.e., 6 or 10 sec counts) are used to measure exercise and postexercise heart rates during and immediately following exercise. Because there is a rapid and immediate decline in heart rate when a person stops exercising, the 6 or 10 sec count reflects the individual's actual exercise heart rate more accurately than the longer counts do.

Heart Rate Monitors and Electrocardiogram Recordings

Video 2.6

Heart rate can also be measured using heart rate monitors or an ECG monitoring system. Generally, heart rate monitors detect either the pulse or the ECG electrical signal from the heart and provide a digital display of the heart rate. Pulse monitors use infrared sensors attached to the client's fingertip, earlobe, or wrist (i.e., heart rate watch) to detect pulsations in blood flow during the cardiac cycle. Chest-strap wire and wireless ECG-type monitors tend to be more accurate and reliable than pulse monitors, especially during vigorous exercise. However, the accuracy of wireless chest-strap monitors may be affected by electrical equipment (such as some treadmills, stair climbers, rowing machines, and video screens) generating radio or magnetic interference. Generally, heart rate monitors provide an accurate measure of ECG heart rate during rest and exercise (Vehrs et al. 2002).

Most ECG monitoring systems provide a continuous digital display of the heart rate. This value is usually recorded at the top of the ECG strip recording. If your equipment does not provide a digital readout, you can use a heart rate ruler that converts the distance of two cardiac cycles to beats per minute.

No matter which technique is used to measure heart rate, you should be aware that heart rate fluctuates easily due to temperature, anxiety, exercise, stress, eating, smoking, drinking a caffeinated beverage, time of day, body position, and some over-the-counter medications. In a supine position, the resting heart rate is lower than in either a sitting or a standing position.

TWELVE-LEAD ELECTROCARDIOGRAM

The **electrocardiogram (ECG)** is a composite record of the electrical events in the heart during the cardiac cycle. As the heart depolarizes and repolarizes during contraction, an electrical impulse spreads to the tissues surrounding the heart. Electrodes placed on opposite sides of the heart transmit the electrical potential to an ECG recorder.

In addition to providing baseline data, the resting ECG is used to detect such contraindications to exercise testing as evidence of previous myocardial infarction, ischemic ST-segment changes, conduction defects, and left ventricular hypertrophy. The reading and interpretation of ECGs require a high degree of skill and practice. As an exercise technician, you can administer the resting 12-lead ECG, but a qualified physician should interpret the results. This chapter includes only basic information about administering an ECG. You should consult other references for more detailed information concerning the reading and interpretation of ECG abnormalities (Dubin 2000; Garcia 2015; Martindale and Brown 2017; Thaler 2015).

Electrocardiogram Basics

A typical normal ECG (figure 2.1) is composed of a **P wave** that represents depolarization of the atria. The **PR interval** indicates the delay in the impulse at the atrioventricular node. Electrical currents generated during ventricular depolarization and contraction produce the **QRS complex**. The **T wave** and **ST segment** correspond to ventricular repolarization.

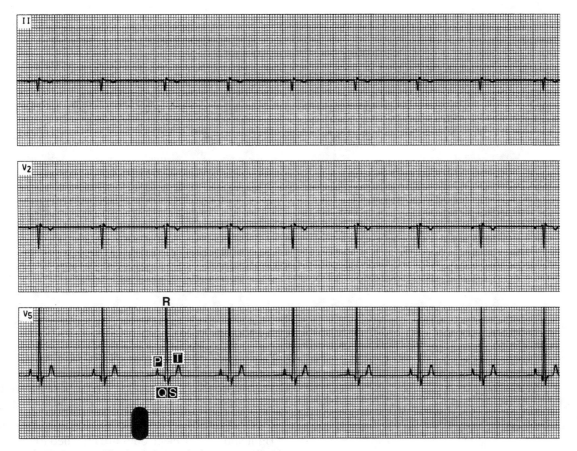

FIGURE 2.1 Typical normal electrocardiogram.

A lead is a pair of electrodes placed on the body and connected to an ECG recorder. An axis is an imaginary line connecting the two electrodes. A standard 12-lead ECG consists of three **limb leads**, three **augmented unipolar leads**, and six **chest leads**. Each of the 12 ECG leads records a different view of the heart's electrical activity. Thus, the tracings from the various leads differ from one another.

Resting 12-Lead Electrocardiogram Procedures

To create the 12 leads, 10 electrodes are used. The electrodes for the three limb leads (I, II, and III) are placed on the right arm, left arm, and left leg. A ground electrode is placed on the right leg. This is electronically equivalent to placing the electrodes at the shoulders and the symphysis pubis. Limb lead I measures the voltage differential between the left and right arm electrodes. Limb leads II and III measure the voltage between the left leg and right (lead II) and left (lead III) arms. Figure 2.2 shows the

three limb leads and three augmented unipolar leads.

The three augmented unipolar leads are aVF (feet), aVL (left), and aVR (right). The augmented unipolar lead compares the voltage across one of the limb electrodes with the average voltage across the two opposite electrodes. Lead aVL, for example, records the voltage across an electrode placed on the left arm and the average voltage across the other two limb electrodes (see figure 2.2).

The six chest leads (V_1 to V_6) measure the voltage across a specific area of the chest, with the average voltage across the other three limb leads. Figure 2.3 illustrates electrode placement for the chest leads, V_1 through V_6.

During the resting ECG, the client should lie quietly in a supine position on a table. The electrode sites should be shaved if hair is present and should be cleaned with alcohol. Remove the superficial layer of skin at each site by rubbing it with fine-grain emery paper or a gauze pad. Disposable electrodes contain electrode gel and adhesive discs. After applying the electrode, tap it firmly to test for noisy leads. You should always calibrate the ECG recorder prior to

Video 2.7

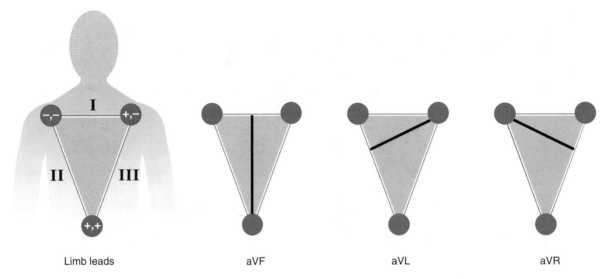

FIGURE 2.2 Three limb leads and three augmented unipolar leads.

use by recording the standard 1 mV deflection per centimeter. Also, to standardize the time base for the ECG, set the paper speed to 25 mm·sec^{-1}.

ANATOMICAL LOCATIONS FOR CHEST ELECTRODES

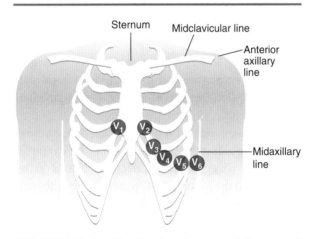

FIGURE 2.3 Electrode placement for chest leads, V1 to V6.

V_1—fourth intercostal space to the right of the sternal border

V_2—fourth intercostal space to the left of the sternal border

V_3—at the midpoint of a straight line between V_2 and V_4

V_4—fifth intercostal space along the midclavicular line

V_5—horizontal to V_4 on the anterior axillary line

V_6—horizontal to V_4 and V_5 on the midaxillary line

The 12-Lead Exercise ECG

To avoid poor ECG tracings caused by moving limbs during exercise, the electrode configuration is modified slightly for an exercise 12-lead ECG (see figure 2.4). The right and left arm electrodes are placed below the right and left clavicles, respectively. The right and left leg electrodes are attached to the right and left sides of the trunk, below the rib cage on the anterior axillary line. The six chest electrodes are positioned as previously described.

Video 2.8

Video 2.9

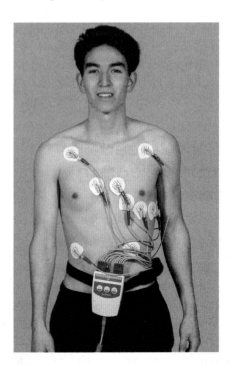

FIGURE 2.4 Electrode placement for 12-lead exercise electrocardiogram.

Key Points

▶ The purpose of the health evaluation is to detect disease and to assess disease risk.

▶ Important components of the health evaluation are a medical history, CHD risk factor analysis, physical examination, clinical tests, and medical clearance.

▶ The lifestyle evaluation includes information about the diet, tobacco and alcohol use, physical activity, and psychological stress levels of the individual.

▶ All clients are required to sign an informed consent prior to taking any physical fitness tests or participating in an exercise program.

▶ The resting evaluation of cardiorespiratory function includes heart rate, BP, and a 12-lead ECG that is interpreted by a qualified physician.

▶ Resting BP can be assessed using auscultation or automated BP devices.

▶ Appropriate blood pressure cuff size for the client's arm is critical for accurate BP assessment.

▶ Heart rate may be taken using auscultation, palpation, heart rate monitors, or ECG recordings.

▶ The 12-lead ECG includes three limb leads (I, II, III), three augmented unipolar leads (aVF, aVR, aVL), and six chest leads (V_1 through V_6).

▶ A graded maximal exercise test is the best way to assess functional aerobic capacity, but submaximal exercise tests can be used to estimate a client's maximal functional aerobic capacity.

Key Terms

Learn the definition for each of the following key terms. Definitions of key terms can be found in the glossary.

augmented unipolar leads
auscultation
bradycardia
chest leads
cuff hypertension
diastolic blood pressure (DBP)
electrocardiogram (ECG)
elevated blood pressure
limb leads
masked hypertension
miscuffing
normotensive
oscillometry
overcuffing
palpation

PR interval
pulse pressure
P wave
QRS complex
sphygmomanometer
stage 1 hypertension
stage 2 hypertension
ST segment
systolic blood pressure (SBP)
tachycardia
terminal digit bias
T wave
undercuffing
white coat effect
white coat hypertension

Review Questions

In addition to being able to define each of the key terms, test your knowledge and understanding of the material by answering the following review questions.

1. Identify the purpose of each component of the comprehensive health evaluation.

2. At minimum, a pretest health screening should include four items. Name these.

3. Identify cardiovascular, pulmonary, metabolic, and musculoskeletal diseases or disorders that may limit exercise performance (name three signs or symptoms for each category).

4. Identify the positive and negative risk factors for CHD. Specify the criteria for each of these risk factors.

5. Identify the cutoff values for classifying resting BPs.

6. Identify the cutoff values for classifying TC, LDL-C, HDL-C, and triglycerides.

7. Explain the importance of BP cuff size selection.

8. Name three methods for measuring BP. Which one is considered the gold standard? Is each method accurate at high altitude?

9. Describe the proper positioning of the wrist for assessing resting blood pressure with a wrist cuff.

10. Name three sources of error in measurement of BP.

11. Identify two BP devices that are best suited for assessing BP during exercise.

12. Describe three things you should do to ensure accurate BP readings during exercise.

13. Describe the effects of miscuffing on BP readings.

14. What effect do arm position and body posture have on BP readings?

15. Name three methods for measuring heart rate.

16. Identify the component parts of a typical normal ECG tracing. What does each component represent relative to the cardiac cycle?

17. Describe the anatomical locations for placement of the 10 electrodes used to obtain a 12-lead ECG recording.

18. Name three absolute and three relative contraindications to exercise testing.

CHAPTER 3

Principles of Assessment, Prescription, and Exercise Program Adherence

KEY QUESTIONS

▶ What are the essential components of a physical fitness profile?

▶ What are the purposes of physical fitness tests and how can I use the results?

▶ Several physical fitness tests are available; how do I select the best test for my client?

▶ Are field tests as good as laboratory tests for measuring physical fitness?

▶ What is the best way to interpret test results for my client?

▶ What are the essential elements of an exercise prescription?

▶ Is one type of exercise better than others for improving each component of physical fitness?

▶ Does high-intensity exercise improve physical fitness faster than low-intensity exercise?

▶ Is it safe to exercise every day?

▶ When should I increase the frequency, intensity, and duration in an exercise prescription? Can these elements be increased simultaneously?

▶ Do older people benefit as much from exercise as younger people?

▶ How can I get my clients to stick with their exercise programs?

▶ How can technology be used to promote physical activity?

Health and fitness professionals need to master the basic principles of physical fitness assessment and exercise prescription. You must know how to use the results of physical fitness tests to plan scientifically sound exercise programs that are individualized to meet your clients' needs, interests, and abilities. With your knowledge, leadership, and guidance, your clients can reduce their risk of disease and improve their health and physical fitness levels safely and effectively.

As an exercise specialist, you will have diverse responsibilities, such as

- educating clients about the positive benefits of regular physical activity;

- conducting pretest health evaluations to screen clients for exercise participation (see chapter 2);

- selecting, administering, and interpreting tests designed to assess each component of physical fitness;

- designing individualized exercise programs;

- leading exercise classes;

- analyzing your clients' exercise performance and correcting performance errors;

- educating your clients about the dos and don'ts of exercise; and

- motivating your clients to improve their adherence to exercise.

Exercise specialists play many roles: educator, leader, technician, and artist. To be effective in these roles, you must integrate knowledge from many disciplines such as anatomy, physiology, chemistry, nutrition, education, and psychology, as well as refine your exercise testing, prescription, and leadership skills.

This chapter presents principles of exercise testing and prescription, along with information about exercise program adherence and the use of technology to promote physical activity.

PHYSICAL FITNESS TESTING

In order to plan and administer physical fitness tests, you must understand the following:

- The components of physical fitness to be tested
- Purposes of physical fitness testing
- Testing order and the testing environment
- Test validity, reliability, and objectivity
- Prediction equation evaluation
- Test administration and interpretation

COMPONENTS OF PHYSICAL FITNESS

Physical fitness is the ability to perform occupational, recreational, and daily activities without becoming unduly fatigued. As an exercise specialist, one of your primary responsibilities is to assess each of the following physical fitness components:

1. *Cardiorespiratory endurance.* **Cardiorespiratory endurance** is the ability of the heart, lungs, and circulatory system to supply oxygen and nutrients efficiently to working muscles. Exercise physiologists measure the **maximum oxygen consumption ($\dot{V}O_2max$)**, or the rate of oxygen utilization of the muscles during aerobic exercise, in order to assess cardiorespiratory endurance and maximal functional aerobic capacity. Physical fitness evaluations should include a test of cardiorespiratory function during rest and exercise. Graded exercise tests (GXTs) are used for this purpose. Improved cardiorespiratory endurance is one of the most important benefits of aerobic exercise training programs. Chapters 4 and 5 present detailed information about graded exercise testing and aerobic exercise programs.

2. *Musculoskeletal fitness.* **Musculoskeletal fitness** refers to the ability of the skeletal and muscular systems to perform work. This requires muscular strength, muscular endurance, muscular power, and bone strength. **Muscular strength** is the maximal force or tension level that can be produced by a muscle group, **muscular endurance** is the ability of a muscle to maintain submaximal force levels for extended periods, **muscular power** refers to the rate of force development, and **bone strength** is related to the risk of bone fracture and is a function of the mineral content and density of the bone tissue. Resistance training is one of the most effective ways to improve the strength of muscles and bones and to develop muscular endurance. Plyometrics and explosive free weight lifts are effective means of developing muscular power. Chapters 6 and 7 provide detailed information about assessing musculoskeletal fitness and designing resistance training programs.

3. *Body weight and body composition.* **Body weight (BW)** refers to the size or mass of the individual. **Body composition** refers to body weight in terms of the absolute and relative amounts of muscle, bone, and fat tissues. Aerobic exercise and resistance training are effective in altering body weight and composition. Chapters 8 and 9 discuss body composition assessment techniques and exercise programs for weight management.

4. *Flexibility.* **Flexibility** is the ability to move a joint or series of joints fluidly through the complete range of motion. Flexibility is limited by factors such as bony structure of the joint and the size and strength of muscles, ligaments, and other connective tissues. Daily stretching can greatly improve flexibility. Chapters 10 and 11 give more information about assessing flexibility and designing stretching programs.

5. *Balance.* **Balance** is the ability to keep the body's center of gravity within the base of support when maintaining a static position, performing voluntary movements, or reacting to external disturbances. **Functional balance** refers to the ability to perform daily movement tasks requiring balance such as picking up an object from the floor, dressing, and turning to look at something behind you. Tai chi and yoga are two examples of activities that can be used to improve balance. Chapter 12 addresses the assessment of balance and design of programs for improving balance.

PURPOSES OF PHYSICAL FITNESS TESTING

As mentioned in chapter 2, it is imperative that you carefully screen your clients prior to exercise testing, identify any contraindications to exercise testing, determine if medical clearance is recommended prior to initiating an exercise program, and obtain each client's informed consent before conducting any physical fitness tests. You can use laboratory and field tests to assess each component of physical fitness and to develop physical fitness profiles for your clients. Results from these tests enable you to identify strengths and weaknesses and to set realistic and attainable goals for your clients. Data from specific tests (e.g., heart rates from a GXT) will help you make accurate and precise exercise prescriptions for each client. Also, you can use baseline and follow-up data to evaluate the progress of exercise program participants.

TESTING ORDER AND THE TESTING ENVIRONMENT

When you administer a complete battery of physical fitness tests in a single session, use the following test sequence to minimize the effects of previous tests on subsequent test performance:

- Resting blood pressure and heart rate
- Body composition and balance
- Cardiorespiratory endurance
- Muscular fitness
- Flexibility

Often, clients are apprehensive about taking physical fitness tests. Test anxiety may affect the validity and reliability of test results. Therefore, you should put your clients at ease by establishing good rapport, projecting a sense of relaxed confidence, and creating a testing environment that is friendly, quiet, private, safe, and comfortable. Room temperature should be maintained at 70 to 74 °F (21-23 °C), and the relative humidity should be controlled whenever possible. For pretest health screening and interpretation of the client's test results, the room should have comfortable chairs and a table for completing questionnaires and paperwork, as well as an examination table or bed for the resting evaluation of heart rate, blood pressure, and the 12-lead electrocardiogram. All equipment used for physical testing should be carefully calibrated and prepared before your clients arrive for testing. This will ensure valid test data and efficient use of time.

TEST VALIDITY, RELIABILITY, AND OBJECTIVITY

To accurately assess your clients' physical fitness status, you must select tests that are valid, reliable, and objective. It is necessary to understand these basic concepts fully in order to evaluate the relative worth of specific physical fitness tests and prediction equations.

Test Validity

With regard to physical fitness testing, test **validity** is the ability of a test to *measure accurately*, with minimal error, a specific physical fitness component. **Reference** (or **criterion**) **methods** are used to obtain *direct* measures of physical fitness components. However, some physical fitness components cannot always be measured directly, requiring the use of *indirect* measures for estimation of the value of the reference measure. For example, exercise physiologists consider the direct measurement of $\dot{V}O_2max$ (i.e., collection and analysis of expired gas samples) during maximal exercise to be the criterion measure of cardiorespiratory fitness. Direct measurement of $\dot{V}O_2max$, however, requires expensive equipment, considerable technical expertise, and very high levels of client motivation. Therefore in the laboratory setting, $\dot{V}O_2max$ is usually estimated using formulas to convert the amount of work output during a GXT to oxygen consumption (see chapter 4). In field settings, prediction equations are used to estimate $\dot{V}O_2max$ from a combination of physiological, demographic, and performance predictor variables.

One way in which researchers quantify the validity of physical fitness tests is by calculating the relationship between predicted scores (y') and the criterion scores (y) using correlation coefficients ($r_{y,y'}$). This value, $r_{y,y'}$, is known as the **validity coefficient**. The magnitude of the validity coefficient cannot exceed 1.0. The closer the value is to 1.0, the stronger the validity of the test. Valid physical fitness field tests and prediction equations typically have validity coefficients in excess of $r_{y,y'} = .80$.

Because field tests indirectly estimate a physical fitness component, there will be a difference between the measured (reference) and predicted values for that component. This difference $(y - y')$ is called the **residual score**. The **standard error of estimate** (*SEE*) is a measure of prediction error and is used to quantify the accuracy of the prediction equation and the validity of the field test. The magnitude of the *SEE* depends on the size of the residual scores and reflects the average degree of deviation of individual data points around the **line of best fit** (or **regression line**) depicting the linear relationship between the measured and the predicted scores. When individual data points fall close to the regression line, the *SEE* is small (see figure 3.1). A valid field test has a high validity coefficient and a small prediction error.

In addition to test validity, test sensitivity and specificity are often reported. **Sensitivity** refers to the probability of correctly identifying individuals who have risk factors for a specific disease or syndrome. An example is the probability of correctly identifying individuals with risk factors for CVD (cardiovascular disease) using body mass index (BMI) and waist circumference cutoff values. **Specificity** is a measure of the ability to correctly identify individuals with no risk factors. Given that the sensitivity and specificity of tests are typically

less than 1.00 (i.e., <100% correct), some individuals will be identified as having risk factors even though they have none (**false positive**), and some will be identified as having no risk factors when they do have some (**false negative**).

Test Reliability

Reliability is the ability of a test to yield *consistent* and *stable* scores across trials and over time. For example, the skinfold test is considered to be reliable because a trained skinfold technician obtains similar skinfold values when taking duplicate measurements on the same person. Researchers quantify reliability by calculating the relationship between trial 1 and trial 2 test scores or day 1 and day 2 test scores. This value, $r_{x1,x2}$, is known as the **reliability coefficient**. The magnitude of the reliability coefficient cannot exceed 1.0. In general, physical fitness tests have high reliability coefficients, typically exceeding $r_{x1,x2} = .90$.

It is important to know that test reliability affects test validity. Tests with poor reliability also have poor validity because unreliable tests fail to produce consistent test scores. It is possible, however, for a test to have excellent reliability ($r_{x1,x2} > .90$) but poor validity. Even when a test yields stable and precise values across trials or between days, it may not validly measure a specific physical fitness component. For example, researchers reported high test-retest reliability ($r_{x1,x2} = .99$) for the sit-and-reach test but also noted that this test has poor validity ($r_{y,y'} = .12$) as a measure of low back flexibility in women (Jackson and Langford 1989).

Test Objectivity

Objectivity is also known as intertester reliability. Objective tests yield similar test scores for a given individual when the same test is administered by different technicians. Objectivity is quantified by calculating the correlation between pairs of test scores measured on the same individuals by two different technicians. This value, $r_{1,2}$, is known as the **objectivity coefficient**. As with validity and reliability coefficients, the magnitude of the objectivity coefficient cannot exceed 1.0. Most physical fitness tests have high objectivity coefficients ($r_{1,2} > .90$), especially when highly trained technicians practice together and carefully follow standardized testing procedures.

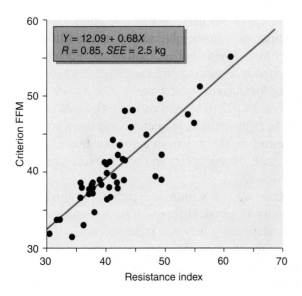

FIGURE 3.1 Line of best fit and SEE (prediction error).

PREDICTION EQUATION EVALUATION

Although reference measures obtained in the laboratory setting provide the most valid assessment of each physical fitness component, these tests are expensive and time consuming and require considerable technical expertise. In field and clinical settings, you can obtain estimates of these reference measures by selecting valid field tests and prediction equations that have good predictive accuracy. Table 3.1 provides an overview of the types of tests used in laboratory and field settings to assess each physical fitness component.

To select the most appropriate tests for measuring your clients' physical fitness, it is important to evaluate the relative worth of the fitness tests and their prediction equations. To do this, you should ask the following questions:

What reference measure was used to develop the prediction equation?

As mentioned earlier, the reference or criterion measure of a specific physical fitness component is obtained by directly measuring the component. Reference measures are used as a gold standard for validating field tests and developing prediction equations that accurately estimate the reference measure. For example, skinfold prediction equations are developed and cross-validated through comparison of the estimated body density (calculated from the skinfold equation) against the reference measure of body density typically obtained from hydrodensitometry (underwater weighing). Similarly, the validity of the sit-and-reach test for measuring low back flexibility was tested by comparing sit-and-reach scores with range of motion values (reference measure) directly measured by X-ray or goniometric methods. Table 3.1 describes reference measures

Table 3.1 Direct (Reference) and Indirect (Field) Measures of Physical Fitness Components

Physical fitness component	Reference measure	Laboratory or reference method	Indirect measures or field tests	Group prediction error (*SEE* and *TE*)	Individual prediction error*	Chapter
Cardiorespiratory endurance	Direct measurement of $\dot{V}O_2$max ($ml\cdot kg^{-1}\cdot min^{-1}$)	Maximal GXT	Submaximal GXT, distance run/walk tests, step tests	$<5.0\ ml\cdot kg^{-1}\cdot min^{-1}$	$\pm10\ ml\cdot kg^{-1}\cdot min^{-1}$	4
Muscular strength	Maximal force (kg) or torque (Nm)	Isokinetic or 1-RM tests	Submaximal tests (2-RM to 10-RM value)	<2.0 kg	±4 kg	6
Body composition	Db ($g\cdot cc^{-1}$), FFM (kg), or %BF	Hydrodensitometry or dual-energy X-ray absorptiometry	Bioimpedance, skinfolds, anthropometry	$<0.0080\ g\cdot cc^{-1}$ <3.5 kg FFM (men) <2.8 kg FFM (women) $<3.5\%$ BF	±6.0 kg ±5.0 kg $\pm7.0\%$	8
Bone strength	Bone mineral content and bone density	Dual-energy X-ray absorptiometry	Anthropometric measures of bony width	NR	NR	8
Flexibility	ROM at joint (degrees)	X-ray or goniometry	Linear measures of ROM	$<6°$	$\pm12°$	10
Balance	None	Computerized balance assessment	Timed performance on balance tasks; distance reached	NR	NR	12

Db = total body density; FFM = fat-free mass; %BF = relative body fat; *SEE* = standard error of estimate; *TE* = total error; GXT = graded exercise test; ROM = range of motion; RM = repetition maximum; NR = not reported; Nm = newton-meter.

*95% limits of agreement.

that experts commonly use to assess each physical fitness component. Field tests and prediction equations developed using indirect methods instead of reference methods as the criterion have questionable validity.

How large was the sample used to develop the prediction equation?

Large randomly selected samples (N = 100-400 subjects) are generally needed to ensure the data are representative of the population for whom the prediction equation was developed. Also, equations based on large samples tend to have more stable regression weights for each predictor variable in the equation.

What is the ratio of sample size to the number of predictor variables in the equation?

In multiple regression, the correlation between the reference measure of the physical fitness component and the predictors in the equation is represented by the **multiple correlation coefficient (R_{mc})**. The larger the R_{mc} (up to maximum value of 1.00), the stronger the relationship. The size of R_{mc} will be artificially inflated if there are too many predictors in the equation compared with the total number of subjects. Statisticians recommend a minimum of 20 subjects per predictor variable. For example, if a skinfold (SKF) prediction equation has three predictors (e.g., triceps SKF, calf SKF, and age), then the minimum sample size needs to be 60 subjects. Prediction equations that are based on small samples or that have a poor subject-to-predictor ratio are suspect and should not be used.

What were the sizes of the R_{mc} and the standard error of estimate for the prediction equation?

In general, the R_{mc} for equations predicting physical fitness components exceeds .80. This means that at least 64% [R^2 = .80^2 × 100] of variance in the reference measure can be accounted for by the predictors in the equation. As you can easily see, the larger the R_{mc}, the greater the amount of shared variance between the reference measure and predictor variables. When you evaluate the relative worth of a prediction equation, it is more important to focus on the size of the prediction error (SEE) than on the R_{mc} because the magnitude of R_{mc} is greatly affected by sample size and variability of the data. Keep in mind that SEE reflects the degree of deviation of individual data points (participants' scores) around the line of best fit through the entire sample's data points. In multiple regression, the line of best fit is the regression line that depicts the linear relationship between the reference measure and all the predictor variables in the equation. Table 3.1 presents standard values for evaluating prediction errors of physical fitness prediction equations.

To whom is the prediction equation applicable?

To answer this question, you need to pay close attention to the physical characteristics of the sample used to derive the equation. Factors such as age, gender, race, fitness level, and body fatness need to be examined carefully. Prediction equations are either population specific or generalized. **Population-specific equations** are intended only for individuals from a specific homogeneous group. For example, separate skinfold equations have been developed for boys and girls 6 to 17 years of age (see table 8.3). Population-specific equations are likely to systematically over- or underestimate the physical fitness component if they are applied to individuals who do not belong to that population subgroup. On the other hand, there are **generalized prediction equations** that can be applied to individuals who differ greatly in physical characteristics. Generalized equations are developed using diverse, heterogeneous samples, and they account for differences in physical characteristics by including these variables as predictors in the equation. For example, the prediction equation for the Rockport walking test (see chapter 4) is generalized because gender and age are predictors in this equation.

How were the variables measured by the researchers who developed the prediction equation?

It is important to know not only which variables are included in a prediction equation but also how each one of these predictors was measured by the researchers developing the equation. Although it is highly recommended that standardized procedures be used for all physical fitness testing, this is not always done. For example, the suprailiac skinfold used in the skinfold equations developed by Jackson, Pollock, and Ward (1980) is measured above the iliac crest at the anterior axillary line. In contrast, the *Anthropometric Standardization Reference Manual* (Lohman, Roche, and Martorell 1988) recommends that the suprailiac skinfold be measured above the iliac crest at the midaxillary line. For most individuals, there will be a difference between skinfold thicknesses measured at these two sites. Thus, larger-than-expected prediction errors may result if physical fitness variables are not measured according to the descriptions provided by the researchers who developed the equation.

Was the prediction equation cross-validated on another sample from the population?

An equation must be tested on other samples from the population before its validity or predictive accuracy can be determined. For example, the Rockport 1.0 mi (1.6 km) walking test was originally developed to assess the cardiorespiratory fitness of women and men aged 20 to 69 (Kline et al. 1987). Other researchers cross-validated this equation to establish its predictive accuracy for women 65 yr of age or older (Fenstermaker, Plowman, and Looney 1992) and for male officers and enlisted men (19 to 44 yr) of the U.S. Air Force (Weiglein et al. 2011). In general, prediction equations that have not been cross-validated on the original study sample or on additional samples in other studies should not be used.

What were the sizes of the validity coefficient ($r_{y,y''}$) and the prediction errors when this equation was applied to the cross-validation sample (i.e., what is the group predictive accuracy of the equation)?

An equation with good predictive accuracy has a moderately high validity coefficient ($r_{y,y''} > .80$) and an acceptable prediction error (see the group prediction error column in table 3.1). In cross-validation studies, the accuracy of an equation for estimating the reference values of a group is assessed by analyzing two types of prediction error: the *SEE* and the total error (*TE*). As mentioned, the *SEE* reflects the average deviation of individual data points from the regression line, or line of best fit (see figure 3.1). The **total error** (*TE*) is the average degree of deviation of individual data points from the line of identity (see figure 3.2). The **line of identity** has a slope of 1.0 and a y-intercept equal to 0. When an equation closely predicts the actual or measured scores of the cross-validation sample, individual data points fall close to the line of identity (i.e., *TE* is small). Acceptable values for evaluating group prediction errors (*SEE* and *TE*) are presented in table 3.1.

Was the average predicted score similar to the average reference score for the cross-validation sample?

The prediction equation should yield similar mean values for the actual (measured or reference) and

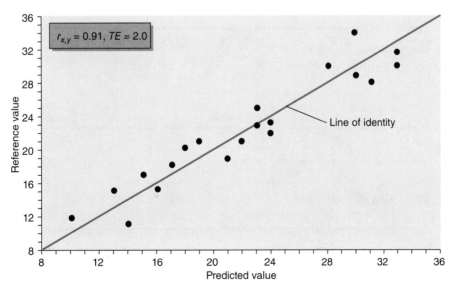

FIGURE 3.2 Line of identity and total error (prediction error).

predicted scores of the cross-validation sample. The **constant error (CE)** is the difference between the actual and predicted means. The means are compared using a paired *t*-test, and they should not differ significantly from each other. A large significant difference indicates a **bias** or systematic difference (i.e., over- or underestimation) between the original validation sample and the cross-validation sample. This difference is caused by technical error or biological variability between the samples.

How good is the prediction equation for estimating reference values of individual clients (i.e., what is the individual predictive accuracy of the equation)?

Although a prediction equation may accurately estimate the average reference score for a specific group, it may not necessarily give accurate estimates for all individuals comprising that group. To evaluate how well a prediction equation works for individuals, researchers use the **Bland and Altman method** (1986), which sets **limits of agreement** around the average difference $(\bar{d})$ between the actual and predicted scores for the sample. With this method, difference scores (actual − predicted values) and average scores [(actual + predicted values) / 2] are calculated for each individual in the sample and are plotted on a graph (see figure 3.3). When the difference scores are normally distributed, 95% lie within ±2 standard deviations from the overall mean

difference $(\bar{d})$ for the group. In this case, the standard deviation of the difference scores (S_d) is used to set the upper $(+2S_d)$ and lower $(-2S_d)$ limits of agreement. Smaller 95% limits of agreement indicate that the equation has a better individual predictive accuracy. The limits of agreement estimate how well you will be able to predict your clients' actual value when using the equation. In the example in figure 3.3, the predictive accuracy of the equation for estimating the actual relative body fat (%BF) of individual clients is approximately ±6% BF (note the upper and lower limits of agreement on the *y*-axis of the graph).

In summary, you should apply all of the following evaluation criteria when selecting field tests and prediction equations that indirectly assess the physical fitness of your clients:

- An acceptable method is used to derive reference measures of the physical fitness component.

- A large sample (N = 100-400) and 20 to 40 subjects per predictor variable are used to develop the equation.

- The sizes of the multiple correlation and validity coefficients exceed .80.

- The group prediction errors (*SEE* and *TE*) are acceptable (see table 3.1).

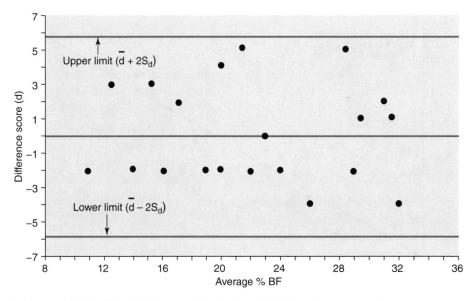

FIGURE 3.3 Bland-Altman plot with 95% limits of agreement.

- Demographic characteristics (e.g., age, gender, race, fitness status) of the validation and cross-validation samples are described.

- The prediction equation is cross-validated in the original study or on independent samples from other studies.

- The constant error (bias), or difference between the measured and predicted means for the cross-validation sample, is not statistically significant.

- The 95% limits of agreement are acceptable (see table 3.1).

PHYSICAL FITNESS TESTS: ADMINISTRATION AND INTERPRETATION

To obtain good test results, it is important to prepare your clients for physical fitness testing by giving them appropriate instructions at least 1 day before the scheduled exercise tests.

Pretest Instructions

Give the client directions to the testing facility and make special arrangements if the facility requires a parking pass. Make sure the client has the following instructions in preparation for the test:

- Wear comfortable clothing, socks, and athletic shoes, if available.

- Drink plenty of fluids during the 24 hr period before the test.

- Refrain from eating, smoking, and drinking alcohol or caffeine for 3 hr prior to the test.

- Do not engage in strenuous physical activity the day of the test.

- Get adequate sleep (6-8 hr) the night before the test.

Test Administration

Later chapters give detailed procedures for administering laboratory and field tests for each physical fitness component. Your technical skills and expertise in administering these tests are directly related to your mastery of standardized testing procedures and the amount of time you spend practicing testing techniques. For example, to become a proficient skinfold technician, you should practice on at least 50 people (Jackson and Pollock 1985). You also need a great deal of practice in order to measure exercise blood pressures and heart rates accurately and to coordinate the timing of these measurements during a GXT on the treadmill or cycle ergometer. Remember that you cannot obtain valid test scores if you do not follow the standardized testing procedures.

Test Interpretation

After collecting the test data, you must analyze and interpret the results for each client. Computer software programs are available that display and compare the client's test results against normative data. Some graphs display the individual's physical fitness profile so you and your client can easily pinpoint strengths as well as physical fitness components in need of improvement.

To classify your clients' physical fitness status, you should compare test scores against established norms. For this purpose, age-gender norms are provided for many of the cardiorespiratory fitness, muscular fitness, body composition, flexibility, and balance tests included in this book. For some tests, percentile rankings are used to classify a client's performance. To illustrate the interpretation of a percentile ranking, let's use the example of a 35 yr old male client whose sit-and-reach score ranks in the 60th percentile. This ranking means his score is better than 60% of the scores of all males the same age taking this test.

When interpreting results for clients, use lay language, rather than highly technical terms and jargon, to explain their test scores. Whenever possible, try to phrase poor results in positive terms. For example, if a female client's body fat level is classified as obese, do not embarrass and alarm her by saying something like this: "Your underwater weighing test indicates you are obese and need to lose at least 20 pounds to achieve a healthy body fat level in order to reduce your risk of diseases linked to obesity. You need to decrease your caloric intake and increase your caloric expenditure by dieting and exercising. The sooner you start a weight management program, the better."

Instead, you should use a more positive and less intimidating approach when interpreting this result. The following approach is more appropriate, especially for clients with low **self-efficacy** or motivation to initiate and adhere to an exercise program: "Women with more than 35% body fat are at risk for disease. If you wish, I will evaluate your daily calorie intake and suggest healthy foods you like to eat that are low in fat. Also, we can discuss ways to increase your physical activity level. I think we can find some activities you will enjoy and have time for, so that you'll burn more calories each day. With these changes, you should be able to lower your body fat to a healthy level in a reasonable amount of time."

BASIC PRINCIPLES FOR EXERCISE PROGRAM DESIGN

A number of basic training principles apply to all types of exercise programs, whether they improve cardiorespiratory fitness, musculoskeletal fitness, body composition, or flexibility.

- *Specificity-of-training principle.* The **specificity principle** states that the body's physiological and metabolic responses and adaptations to exercise training are specific to the type of exercise and the muscle groups involved. For example, physical activities requiring continuous, dynamic, and rhythmic contractions of large muscle groups are best suited for stimulating improvements in cardiorespiratory endurance; stretching exercises develop range of joint motion and flexibility; and resistance exercises are effective for improving muscular strength and muscular endurance. Furthermore, the gains in muscular fitness are specific to the exercised muscle groups, type and speed of contraction, and training intensity.

- *Overload training principle.* To promote improvements in physical fitness components, the physiological systems of the body must be taxed using loads that are greater (**overload principle**) than those to which the individual is accustomed. Overload can be achieved through increases in the frequency, intensity, and duration of aerobic exercise. Muscle groups can be effectively overloaded through increases in the number of repetitions, sets, or exercises in programs that improve muscular fitness and flexibility.

- *Principle of progression.* Throughout the training program, you must progressively increase the training volume, or overload, to stimulate further improvements (i.e., **progression principle**). The progression needs to be gradual because doing too much, too soon may cause musculoskeletal injuries. This is a major reason why some individuals drop out of exercise programs.

- *Principle of initial values.* Individuals with low initial physical fitness levels will show greater relative (%) gains and a faster rate of improvement in response to exercise training than individuals with average or high fitness levels (**initial values principle**). For example, during the first month of an aerobic exercise program, the $\dot{V}O_2$max of a client with poor cardiorespiratory endurance capacity may improve 12% or more, whereas a highly trained endurance athlete may improve only 1% or less.

- *Principle of interindividual variability.* Individual responses to a training stimulus are quite variable and depend on a number of factors such as age, initial fitness level, and health status (i.e., **interindividual variability principle**). You therefore must design exercise programs with the specific needs, interests, and abilities of each client in mind and develop personalized exercise prescriptions that take into account individual differences and preferences.

- *Principle of diminishing returns.* Each person has a genetic ceiling that limits the extent of improvement that is possible from exercise training. As individuals approach their genetic ceiling, the rate of improvement in physical fitness slows and eventually levels off (i.e., **diminishing returns principle**).

- *Principle of reversibility.* The positive physiological effects and health benefits of regular physical activity and exercise are reversible. When individuals discontinue their exercise programs (detraining), exercise capacity diminishes quickly. Within a few months, most of the training improvements are lost (i.e., **reversibility principle**).

THE ART AND SCIENCE OF EXERCISE PRESCRIPTION

Traditionally, some exercise specialists have focused on rigidly applying scientific principles of exercise prescription and have devoted little or no attention to the *art* of exercise prescription. As an exercise programming artist, you need to be creative and flexible, able to modify the exercise prescription based on your clients' goals, behaviors, and responses to the exercise. Using both a scientific and an artistic approach will enable you to personalize the exercise prescription, increasing the probability your clients will make long-term commitments to include physical activity and exercise as an indispensable part of their lifestyles.

BASIC ELEMENTS OF THE EXERCISE PRESCRIPTION

Although prescriptions are individualized for each client, basic elements are common to all exercise prescriptions. These include mode, intensity, duration, frequency, and progression.

Mode

As mentioned earlier, the specificity-of-training principle implies that certain types of exercise training are better suited than others for developing specific components of physical fitness. Table 3.2 presents types of training and examples of exercise modes that optimize improvements for each physical fitness component.

To promote changes in body composition and bone strength, many experts recommend using more than one type of exercise training. For body composition changes, you should prescribe a combination of aerobic exercise to reduce body fat and resistance exercise to build muscle and bone. Similarly, high-intensity weight-bearing activities, plyometrics, and resistance training are all effective for building bone mass for improved bone health.

Intensity

Exercise intensity dictates the specific physiological and metabolic changes in the body during exercise training. As mentioned previously, the initial exercise intensity in the exercise prescription depends on the client's program goals, age, capabilities, preferences, and fitness level. This intensity should stress, but not overtax, the cardiopulmonary and musculoskeletal systems. Later chapters provide detailed information and guidelines on selecting exercise intensities for the development of each physical fitness component as well as for the progression of exercise intensity.

Duration

Duration and intensity of exercise are inversely related: The higher the intensity, the shorter the duration of the exercise. Exercise duration depends not only on the intensity of exercise but also on the client's health status, initial fitness level, functional capability, and program goals. For improved health benefits, the American College of Sports Medicine

Table 3.2   Types of Training and Exercise Modes for Improving Physical Fitness Components

Physical fitness component	Type of training	Exercise modes
Cardiorespiratory endurance	Aerobic exercise	Walking, jogging, cycling, rowing, swimming, stair climbing, simulated cross-country skiing, aerobic dance, step aerobics, elliptical activity
Muscular strength and muscular endurance	Resistance exercise	Free weights, exercise machines, body weight exercises, exercise bands
Bone strength	Weight-bearing high-impact aerobic exercise and resistance exercise	Load-bearing calisthenics, high-intensity cardio, plyometrics, free weights, body weight exercises, exercise machines, whole-body vibration, walking for femoral neck strength
Body composition	Aerobic exercise and resistance exercise	Same modes as listed for cardiorespiratory endurance and muscular strength
Flexibility	Stretching exercise	Static stretches, PNF stretches, yoga, tai chi, Pilates
Balance	Balance training	Tai chi, yoga, Pilates, balance exercises

PNF = proprioceptive neuromuscular facilitation.

(ACSM) and the Centers for Disease Control and Prevention (CDC) recommend that every individual should accumulate at least 150 min/wk of moderate-intensity or 75 min/wk of vigorous-intensity aerobic exercise or a weekly combination of moderate- and vigorous-intensity aerobic exercise. This amount of physical activity can be achieved in either daily continuous bouts (e.g., 30 min moderate-intensity exertion 5 days/wk) or multiple bouts of shorter duration throughout the day (e.g., multiple bouts of 10 min or more in a day), depending on the client's functional capacity and time constraints.

As the client adapts to the exercise training, the duration of exercise may be slowly increased (e.g., by 5-10 min per session) about every 1 to 2 wk for at least the first month. For older and less fit individuals, the ACSM (2018) recommends increasing exercise duration, rather than intensity, in the initial stages of the exercise program; however, gradually moving the client toward the minimum threshold requirement of both duration and intensity is important in terms of maximizing the benefits of the program. For most clients, the duration of aerobic, resistance, and flexibility exercise workouts should not exceed 60 min. This will lessen the chance of overuse injuries and exercise burnout.

Frequency

Frequency typically refers to the total number of weekly exercise sessions. Research shows that exercising 3 days/wk on alternate days is sufficient to improve various components of physical fitness. However, frequency is related to the duration and intensity of exercise and varies depending on the client's program goals and preferences, time constraints, and functional capacity. Sedentary clients with poor initial fitness levels may exercise more than once a day, and clients with diabetes should exercise daily or miss no more than 2 consecutive days in a week. When improved health is the primary goal of the exercise program, the ACSM and CDC recommend either 3 days/wk of vigorous-intensity exercise or 5 days/wk of moderate-intensity exercise or 3 to 5 days/wk of a combination of moderate- and vigorous-intensity exercise. If you prescribe daily physical activity for an apparently healthy client, it is important to vary the type of exercise (i.e., aerobic, resistance, flexibility, and balance exercises) or exercise mode (e.g., walking, cycling, and weightlifting) to lessen the risk of overuse injuries to the bones, joints, and muscles.

Progression of Exercise

Throughout the exercise program, physiological and metabolic changes enable the individual to perform more work. For continued improvements, the cardiopulmonary and musculoskeletal systems must be progressively overloaded through periodic increases in the frequency, intensity, and duration of the exercise.

When applying the principle of progression to an exercise prescription, increase the frequency, intensity, and duration gradually, and do so one element at a time. A simultaneous increase in frequency, intensity, and duration, or in any combination of these elements, may overtax the individual's physiological systems, thereby increasing the risk of exercise-related injuries and exercise burnout. Generally, for older and less fit clients, it is better to increase exercise duration, instead of exercise intensity, especially during the initial stage of their exercise prescriptions. Using subjective ratings of perceived exertion is more beneficial than metabolic equivalent (MET) levels when progressing the exercise prescription of an older adult. On a 10-point scale, a 5 or 6 is representative of moderate intensity (noticeably increased heart rate, or HR, and breathing rate) while a 7 or 8 represents vigorous intensity (substantial increases in HR and breathing rate) (ACSM 2018).

STAGES OF PROGRESSION IN THE EXERCISE PROGRAM

Most individualized exercise programs include initial conditioning, improvement, and maintenance stages. The **initial conditioning stage** typically lasts 1 to 6 wk and serves as a primer to familiarize the client with exercise training. During this stage, you should prescribe stretching exercises, light calisthenics, and low-intensity aerobic or resistance exercises. Have your clients progress slowly by increasing exercise duration first, followed by small increases in exercise intensity. The initial stage of the exercise program may be skipped for some physically active individuals provided their initial fitness level is good to excellent and they are accustomed to the exercise modes prescribed for their programs.

The **improvement stage** of the exercise program typically lasts 4 to 8 mo, and the rate of progression is more rapid than in the initial conditioning stage. During this stage, the frequency, intensity, and duration are systematically and slowly advanced, one element at a time, until the client's fitness goal is reached.

The **maintenance stage** of the exercise program helps clients preserve the level of fitness they achieved by the end of the improvement stage. This stage should continue on a regular, long-term basis. The amount of exercise required to maintain the client's physical fitness level is less than that needed to improve specific fitness components. Thus, the frequency of a specific mode of exercise used to develop any given fitness component can be decreased and that mode replaced with other types of physical activities. By the end of the improvement stage, for example, a client may be jogging 5 days/wk. For maintenance, jogging may be reduced to 2 or 3 days/wk, and different aerobic activities (e.g., swimming, rowing, cycling, stair climbing) or other types of exercise and sport activities (e.g., weightlifting, hiking, tennis) may be substituted the other 3 days. Including a variety of enjoyable physical activities during this stage helps clients counteract boredom and maintain their interest level.

EXERCISE PROGRAM ADHERENCE

Exercise professionals face the challenge of convincing individuals to start exercising and to make a lifelong commitment to a physically active lifestyle. Approximately 8 out of every 10 adults (78.5%) in the United States do not get the recommended amount of physical activity (Centers for Disease Control and Prevention 2015b). Exercise specialists play an important role in educating the public about why regular physical activity is absolutely essential for good health and on how to exercise safely and effectively.

Of those individuals starting an exercise program, almost 50% will drop out within 1 yr (Dishman, Sallis, and Orenstein 1985). A newer survey indicates there is a 3.7% probability (i.e., very small) that a new member will maintain active membership beyond 1 yr. It is anticipated that 37% will quit by the third month (Sperandei, Vieira, and Reis 2016). As an exercise specialist, you must help your clients develop a positive attitude toward physical activity and make a firm commitment to the exercise program. To increase adherence, you need to be aware of factors related to exercise attrition.

Many factors influence regular participation in physical activity and adherence to an exercise program (see table 3.3). Although every individual is unique, terminating a fitness center membership may not mean the client stopped participating in regular physical activity. Statistical predictors of continued fitness center membership are associated with initial physical activity level, body mass index, and age at enrollment. The key motivating factors are health, aesthetics, hypertrophy, and weight loss (Sperandei, Vieira, and Reis 2016). Knowing the factors associated with continued participation in physical activity will direct your approach and the steps you take to facilitate your clients' adherence to their exercise programs. Focus on factors that are potentially modifiable, such as exercise facilities, program variables (e.g., exercise intensity and perceived exertion), enjoyable scenery while exercising, and support from their spouse, family, friends, and peers.

As an exercise specialist, you also need to understand and implement psychological models related to successful behavior change. For an excellent overview of behavior change theories and discussion of strategies you can use to help your clients adopt and maintain a physically active lifestyle, see Napolitano and colleagues (2010). Models that may be useful for encouraging exercise and improving adherence to exercise include the following:

- Behavior modification model
- Health belief model
- Social cognitive model
- Transtheoretical model of health behavior change (stages of motivational readiness for change)
- Decision-making theory
- Model of reasoned action and theory of planned behavior
- Self-determination theory

With the **behavior modification model**, clients become actively involved in the change process by

Table 3.3 Select Factors Related to Physical Activity Participation and Exercise Program Adherence

Category	Positive factors	Negative factors
Demographic and biological	Education Gender[a] Socioeconomic status	Age Race[b] Overweight or obesity
Psychological, cognitive, emotional	Enjoyment of exercise Expected benefits of exercise Perceived health and fitness Self-efficacy Self-motivation	Barriers to exercise Mood disturbance
Behavioral	Activity history during adulthood Healthy dietary habits	Smoking
Social-cultural	Physician influence Support from spouse, family, friends, or peers	Social isolation
Environmental	Access to exercise facilities Satisfaction with exercise facility Exercise equipment at home Enjoyable scenery Observing others exercising Neighborhood safety	Climate or season Urban location
Program	Exercise leadership and supervision Variety of exercise modes and activities	Initial exercise intensity Perceived effort

[a]Males are more likely to be physically active than females.

[b]Whites are more physically active than non-whites.

Data from Sallis and Owen 1999; Trost et al. 2002.

setting realistic short- and long-term goals, developing a plan to achieve these goals, and signing a contract that describes each goal and how it may be achieved. Throughout the exercise program, you should provide your clients with feedback and revise the plan as needed. You can help your clients adopt physical activity into their lifestyle, develop a social support system, and implement behavior counseling strategies such as keeping a diary of their physical activity. Sometimes it can be effective to give rewards such as T-shirts, certificates, emblems, and pins to recognize the attainment of specific goals, such as walking a total of 50 mi (80.5 km) in 1 mo. Help your clients set both short-term and long-term goals that are attainable. For this purpose, you can periodically reevaluate your clients' fitness levels to assess improvement. You can state goals in performance or physiological terms. An example of a short-term performance goal is to complete a 3 mi (4.8 km) fun run in less than 33 min. A long-term physiological goal might be to increase maximum

oxygen uptake ($\dot{V}O_2max$) by 15% in 4 mo. As the exercise specialist, you must help each individual set realistic goals.

The **health belief model** is based on the assumption that individuals will engage in exercise on a regular basis because they perceive the threat of disease and believe this threat is severe and they are susceptible to disease. When the benefits outweigh the barriers, individuals will take action and adopt exercise into their lifestyle. Self-efficacy and cues to action are important components of this model (ACSM 2018).

The **social cognitive model**, developed by Bandura (1982), is based on the concepts of self-efficacy and outcome expectation. The likelihood that people will engage in a specific behavior, like exercising regularly, depends on their self-efficacy or perception of their ability to perform the task, as well as their confidence in making the behavioral change (Grembowski et al. 1993). To assess self-efficacy, have your clients rate, on a scale of 0% to 100%, their confidence in making the specific behavior change. Individuals with high self-efficacy ratings (≥70%) believe they have the knowledge and skill to exercise successfully. As a result, they are more likely to succeed in making a long-term behavior change. To increase self-efficacy, educate your clients so they fully understand their beliefs, and help them identify specific barriers to engaging in physical activity. Techniques for improving your clients' exercise self-efficacy include performance mastery (e.g., teach your clients scientifically sound and safe exercise principles and techniques, and allow them to practice these techniques); modeling (e.g., give clients an opportunity to observe role models who are performing the exercise successfully); positive reinforcement (e.g., compliment clients when they perform activities correctly or improve a specific physical fitness component); and emotional arousal (e.g., educate clients about the health benefits of physical activity and exercise). Ashford, Edmunds, and French (2010) provide a detailed review and analysis of studies designed to change self-efficacy for the promotion of lifestyle and recreational physical activity.

The **transtheoretical model** describes the process clients go through when adopting a change in health behavior (e.g., exercising). The basic concepts of this model are as follows:

- Clients progress through five stages of changes at different rates.
- In this process, clients may move back and forth through the stages of change.
- Clients use different cognitive and behavioral strategies in this process.
- Clients weigh the costs and benefits of the health behavior change.

To effectively apply this model, the exercise specialist needs to be aware of the client's stage of readiness for participating in exercise. The **stages of motivational readiness for change model** is based on the premise that individuals move through a series of stages as they adopt and maintain a new habit (Prochaska and DiClemente 1982). This model has been used to facilitate long-term changes in health behaviors such as smoking (Gökbayrak et al. 2015), weight management (da Silva et al. 2015), dietary modification (Knight et al. 2015), and stress management (Jones et al. 2017) as well as in physical activity behaviors (Dishman, Jackson, and Bray 2014). A client's ability to make a long-term commitment to an exercise program or to daily physical activity is based on the individual's motivational readiness for change. The following example illustrates the five stages of motivational readiness in terms of changing exercise behavior:

1. Precontemplation: Client does not exercise and does not intend to start exercising.
2. Contemplation: Client is not exercising but intends to start.
3. Preparation: Client is exercising but is not meeting the recommended amount of physical activity.
4. Action: Client has been performing the recommended amount of exercise regularly for less than 6 mo.
5. Maintenance: Client has been exercising regularly at the recommended amount for 6 mo or longer.

Individuals are at different stages of readiness for change; therefore, you need to match intervention strategies to the client's stage and tailor your approach to meet the individual's needs, interests, and concerns. Detailed descriptions of how to plan and deliver physical activity intervention strategies specific to the stages of change are available (see ACSM 2018; de Vries et al. 2016; Hebden et al. 2013; Partridge et al. 2015; Pekmezi, Barbera, and Marcus 2010).

The **decision-making theory** proposes that individuals decide whether or not to engage in a behavior by weighing the perceived benefits and costs of that behavior. Clients are more likely to exercise when they perceive that the benefits outweigh the costs (e.g., "I feel better about myself when I exercise even though it takes time from my busy schedule"). Clients in early stages of motivational change (e.g., precontemplation stage) tend to perceive more disadvantages compared with clients in later stages (e.g., action stage) of change (Pekmezi, Barbera, and Marcus 2010). To assess your clients' motivational readiness and decisional balance for exercise, you may use a 16-item self-report tool (see Marcus, Rakowski, and Rossi 1992).

The **theory of reasoned action** proposes a way to understand and predict an individual's behavior. According to this theory, intention is the most important determinant of behavior; intention is highly influenced by the individual's attitudes and subjective behavioral norms. For example, believing that exercise results in positive outcomes leads to a favorable attitude about engaging in physical activity and the intention to do so. Subjective behavioral norms, or perceptions about what others think or believe about exercise, may also influence a client's intention (Downs 2006). The **theory of planned behavior** extends the theory of reasoned action by taking into consideration the client's perception of behavioral control (i.e., perceived power and control). This theory proposes that individuals intend to perform a specific behavior (e.g., exercising) if they evaluate it positively (e.g., attitude), believe others think it is important (subjective norms), and perceive the behavior to be under their control (e.g., power). Although this theory provides useful information behind the formulation of intention for adopting exercise behavior, intention alone is insufficient for predicting whether or not your clients will adopt a physically active lifestyle (Napolitano et al. 2010). A client's perception of control influences his intention and behavior toward becoming physically active. You can bolster your clients' belief in control through strategies to reduce barriers, increase opportunities, and increase access to resources for participation (Motalebi et al 2014).

In helping your clients adopt and maintain a physically active lifestyle, it is also important to understand their motivation or degree of determination for changing or avoiding this behavior. Motivation is a complex construct; it may be described as falling along a continuum, ranging from no motivation (i.e., amotivation) to intrinsic motivation. The schematic (Teixeira et al. 2012) of the **self-determination theory** (Deci and Ryan 2000) depicts mediating mechanisms that may influence specific psychological needs (i.e., autonomy, competence, and relatedness). These needs ultimately lead through a continuum of motivation and on toward adoption and maintenance of exercise behavior. The self-determination theory identifies four levels of motivation (Mears and Kilpatrick 2008):

1. Amotivation: The individual has no intention or desire to engage in exercise.

2. Other-determined motivation: The individual is motivated to exercise by outside factors such as rewards, guilt, fear, or pressure; long-term adherence is unlikely. Possible motives for exercising may be "I exercise to lose weight" or "My partner thinks I should exercise more."

3. Self-determined extrinsic motivation: The individual values exercise, is motivated by extrinsic factors like improved health or gains in fitness, and freely chooses (i.e., autonomy) to exercise without a sense of outside pressure. A possible motive for exercising may be "I exercise because it is an important part of my healthy lifestyle."

4. Intrinsic motivation: The individual engages in exercise for the sheer enjoyment and satisfaction it brings to sense of well-being; enjoying exercise for its own sake leads to adherence. The probable motive for exercising is "I am a physically active person, and I exercise because I like doing it."

The ultimate goal of this approach is to get clients to value physical activity and to think of themselves as exercisers rather than to use exercise to attain an external goal like weight loss. Some individuals may never reach the point of exercising for sheer enjoyment of the activity; however, valuing exercise may be enough to get clients to adhere to their exercise regimens (Rodgers and Loitz 2009). Much more research, including longitudinal research, is needed to better understand why people do or do not adopt a physically active lifestyle. Analyzing results by gender may reveal information that is lost when looking at the data of men and women together (Teixeira et al. 2012).

Questionnaires have been developed to assess your clients' exercise motivation. The Behavioral Regulation in Exercise Questionnaire measures your clients' level of motivation on a continuum, ranging from amotivation to intrinsic motivation (Markland and Tobin 2004). The Exercise Motivation Inventory (Markland and Ingledew 1997) measures specific motives (i.e., guilt, enjoyment, fitness) for engaging in exercise; Egli and colleagues (2011) identified differences in exercise motivation by age, race, and sex with this questionnaire. You can use questionnaire results to help your clients understand their level of motivation and to develop ways to improve their exercise motivation. Rodgers and Loitz (2009) offer suggestions and steps you can take to understand and improve your clients' motivation to exercise (see Tips to Enhance Exercise Motivation).

As an exercise specialist, you need to integrate principles from each of these models and implement

TIPS TO ENHANCE EXERCISE MOTIVATION

Try to understand why the client is there:

- Is the motive external? Try to move the client's focus to a value motive.
- Focus on integrating the exercise with the client's sense of self.

Create opportunities to experience competence:

- Put clients in a position where they can easily see and hear you and receive direction from you.
- Celebrate meaningful successes; don't over-emphasize trivial accomplishments.
- Use clear, appropriate communication strategies; avoid jargon.
- Be respectful of your client's efforts.

Create opportunities for autonomy:

- Give choices and options.
- Relate the exercises to your client's goals.
- Avoid coercive and controlling encouragement.

Create opportunities for relatedness:

- Introduce the client to other participants.
- Give tips and instructions on the expected behavior, including proper etiquette.
- Communicate understanding of your client's perspective.

Bottom line:

- Pay attention to factors that create opportunities for your clients to feel competent, related, and autonomous.
- Encourage value motives for exercising; downplay external reasons for exercising.

Based on Rodgers and Loitz 2009.

STRATEGIES TO INCREASE EXERCISE PROGRAM ADHERENCE

- Recruit physician support of the exercise program.
- Prescribe moderate-intensity exercise to minimize injury and complications.
- Advocate exercising with others.
- Offer a variety of enjoyable exercise and fitness activities.
- Provide positive reinforcement through periodic testing.

- Recruit support for the program from clients' families and friends. Add optional recreational games to the conditioning program.
- Use progress charts to record exercise achievements.
- Establish a reward system to recognize participant accomplishments.
- Provide qualified exercise professionals who are well trained, innovative, and enthusiastic.

strategies to improve your clients' exercise program adherence. The ACSM (2018) recommends program modifications and motivational strategies to increase long-term adherence to an exercise program (see Strategies to Increase Exercise Program Adherence). The key to increasing exercise program adherence lies in the leadership, education, and motivation that you provide. First, you must be a positive role model. You also must be knowledgeable and able to educate clients about exercise and fitness, provide motivation, and encourage social support. The mediators most likely to help clients become more physically active include self-regulation, self-efficacy, and autonomous motivation (Teixeira et al. 2015).

USING TECHNOLOGY TO PROMOTE PHYSICAL ACTIVITY

Technology is a double-edged sword. Computers, for example, contribute to sedentary leisure-time behaviors (e.g., playing seated computer games, surfing the web). On the other hand, technology is being used to promote physical activity and change exercise behavior. For years, **wearable technology** such as pedometers, accelerometers, and heart rate monitors have been used as motivational tools. Integration of these older tools with newer technologies (e.g., smartphones, apps) has expanded the potential for technology to provide nearly instantaneous feedback, monitoring, and promotion of physical activity by the individual and by one's social network. Clinicians, trainers, and health promotion experts are using physical activity interventions that incorporate technology to encourage and change exercise behavior. Such interventions are more effective if they incorporate behavior change theory, especially planned behavior theory, include multiple behavior change techniques, and utilize multiple methods (e.g., text messaging, social media posts) for interacting with clients (Webb et al. 2010). Efforts are under way to identify the most synergistic combination of behavior change techniques and tools with the greatest likelihood of increasing physical activity behaviors, regardless of how the behavioral change message is delivered (van Genugten et al. 2016). In this section, questions addressing the use of various technologies for promoting exercise program adherence are addressed.

How are pedometers used to promote physical activity?

Video 3.1

Pedometers count and track the number of steps taken over the course of a day. Most pedometers provide a fairly accurate count of steps taken while walking, jogging, and running. Clients can track and monitor their progress in meeting exercise program goals. Pedometers are fairly simple, low-cost devices. They are sometimes given away as incentives for participating in an activity-related initiative such as health fairs, community-based programs, or employee wellness programs. Pedom-

eter-based walking programs are associated with significant decreases in BMI, body weight, waist circumference, systolic blood pressure, and CVD risk factors. Improvements in quality of life and HDL-C values have also been reported (Cayir, Menekse, and Akturk 2015; Guglani, Shenoy, and Singh 2014; Miyazaki et al. 2015).

Do pedometers have to be positioned at the waist to ensure accuracy?

To provide accurate step counts, older, simpler pedometer models need to be attached in an upright position to a firm waistband or the shank of the lower leg. However, newer pedometers with piezo-electric sensors are position-independent and can be worn anywhere on the body (Lee et al. 2015; Liu et al. 2015). Studies revealed that the accuracy of pedometer step counts is related to the combination of walking speed and where the pedometer is worn (Ehrler, Weber, and Lovis 2016; Femina et al. 2016; Lee et al. 2015). For people who walk at a slow pace, have difficulty walking, or shuffle their feet, a wrist-worn pedometer is more accurate than one at the hip. For those capable of moving at faster speeds, a waist-worn pedometer is more accurate than pedometers worn elsewhere (Ehrler, Weber, and Lovis 2016; Lee et al. 2015).

What is the recommended number of steps per day for health benefits?

Tracking progress toward an age-appropriate goal for steps taken in a day is key as a person moves from being irregularly active to being more consistently active. For adults, accumulating 10,000 steps per day (see table 3.4) is a recommended goal. Accumulating 8,000 to 9,000 steps per day at a rate of 100 steps·min^{-1} or more is equivalent to 30 min of adult moderate-intensity physical activity, the health benefit

Table 3.4 Classification of Pedometer-Based Activity for Adults and Children

Classification*	Adults	Girls (6-12 yr)	Boys (6-12 yr)
Sedentary	<5,000	<7,000	<10,000
Low active	5,000-7,499	7,000-9,499	10,000-12,499
Somewhat active	7,500-9,999	9,500-11,999	12,500-14,999
Active	10,000-12,499	12,000-14,499	15,000-17,499
Highly active	≥12,500	≥14,500	≥17,500

*These descriptors are used for adults; for children, the following descriptors are used: copper, bronze, silver, gold, and platinum (copper and platinum representing the lowest and highest levels of activity, respectively).

threshold. For adult weight loss, accumulating 11,000 to 13,000 steps·day^{-1} is recommended. For children, researchers recommend a higher step count goal: 12,000 steps·day^{-1} for girls and 15,000 steps·day^{-1} for boys (Katanista et al. 2015; Tudor-Locke et al. 2004).

What additional information can be tracked using a pedometer?

Some newer pedometers can estimate how far the wearer has traveled, the total time spent walking or jogging at a moderate intensity, and how many 10-min bouts of moderate-intensity activity were performed. Although some pedometers provide an estimate of the calories expended during physical activity, these results generally underestimate the reference values. Additional information about the validity and accuracy of pedometers is available (Femina et al. 2016; Lee et al. 2015; Tudor-Locke et al. 2011).

Are accelerometers better than pedometers for monitoring activity?

Accelerometers record acceleration of the body or body segments moment by moment. Consequently, they may provide more detailed information about the frequency, duration, intensity, and patterns of movement than do traditional pedometers. Some accelerometers can identify body position (e.g., seated, standing) and estimate daily energy expenditure. Like pedometers, however, accelerometers do not provide accurate estimates of energy expenditure and should not be worn at the hip during slow walking. Accelerometers provide an objective measure of the wearer's compliance with an aerobic exercise prescription or the recommended physical activity guidelines for cardiorespiratory health (see chapter 1). Since the data storage capacity of accelerometers is larger than that of pedometers, your clients can store weeks' worth of their activity data.

Accelerometer technology is now integrated into some of the newer types of pedometers. As a result, some pedometers may be capable of providing several of the same features and functions as an accelerometer.

Do accelerometers need to be placed at a specific location on the body to ensure accuracy?

The internal workings of accelerometers (piezoelectric sensors plus miniaturized gyroscopes, inclinometers, magnetometers, and so on) make them location-independent. This means they can be worn anywhere on the body. Keep in mind that accelerometers require body segment motion in order to track activities; so, for example, the counts will be inaccurate if an accelerometer is worn at the wrist during cycling.

What type of device should my clients use to track and monitor HR during exercise?

Heart rate monitors can be used to measure HR during rest and exercise and to monitor exercise intensity. Typically, these monitors use a simple strap worn next to the skin just below the pectoral muscles. The strap continuously transmits the HR data to a nearby device (e.g., a watch-style receiver or your smartphone) and displays the HR in bpm. Because HR is linearly related to oxygen uptake, it can be used to estimate exercise energy expenditure. However, remember that HR may be affected by factors such as temperature, humidity, hydration, and emotional stress as well as some medications and dietary supplements. Any one of these factors may affect the accuracy of the estimated energy expenditure.

There are numerous watch-style heart rate monitors that do not require a chest strap. These monitors vary in price and features, so tell your clients to do their research before investing in one. For example, if a client wants to monitor HR while swimming or playing water polo, the monitor needs to be waterproof. Some wrist-worn monitors track heart rate in a continuous fashion. Others need to be touched in order to display the HR. The latter could present some challenges in tracking HR while cycling or skiing. Not all watch-style HR monitors have been properly validated; clients should determine whether the device has been tested by unbiased, reputable, independent sources.

Do smartphone cameras accurately measure HR?

Smartphone cameras measure HR by sending a light beam through the skin and monitoring how the light is reflected as the blood flows rhythmically through the capillaries. This technology is known as **photoplethysmography (PPG)**. It takes a few moments for the proprietary algorithm in the smartphone app to measure the pulsatile fluctuations before converting them into bpm. The quality of contact between the user's finger and the camera lens can greatly influence the results. Thus, exercise

HR may actually be a few beats higher than what is displayed. The algorithms differ among devices and apps depending on the manufacturers. Consequently, these devices may yield inaccurate or different results. Smartphone apps that have not been approved by the U.S. Food and Drug Administration should not be used to medically monitor HR.

My client likes to hike and run in the mountains. Is there some type of technology that would help him track these activities?

Global positioning system (GPS) technology may meet your client's needs. GPS technology uses a combination of satellites and ground stations to calculate geographic locations. This means there is a line-of-sight requirement between the user and the satellites; without it (e.g., when spelunking or when indoors), the user cannot count on GPS being able to compute location at that moment (Cho, Rodriguez, and Evenson 2011). GPS units that can be worn on the wrist, hip, or upper arm are commercially available and provide information about altitude, distance, travel time, and average velocity while hiking. When used in conjunction with accelerometry, GPS-enabled devices can assess and monitor the intensity of physical activity and estimate calories expended (Rodriguez, Brown, and Troped 2005; Schutz and Herren 2000; Troped et al. 2008). The ability of the GPS to accurately calculate location depends on the GPS unit and the environment in which it is used. The projected location may be single to double digits (in meters) away from the actual location. As a result, calculations of the distance between two geographic locations, the elapsed time to travel that distance, and the average velocity of travel may also be affected (Jankowska, Schipperijn, and Kerr 2015).

My client's smartphone has a GPS and accelerometer. Will this work to track her outdoor activities?

This is an ongoing area for research. One study reported that the combination of smartphones, Bluetooth, GPS, and accelerometry is a cost-effective method of monitoring the details (time and space) of day-to-day movements both indoors and out (Schenk et al. 2011). As the technology develops, GPS in combination with the global telecommunications networks may become more widely used to assess and promote physical activity worldwide. However, intra- and interunit validity and reliability need to be established as part of any future research project incorporating GPS technology (Abraham et al. 2012).

Should I encourage children to play some of the active video games?

Active video games (AVGs) provide an enjoyable way to be physically active (Bailey and McInnis 2011; Maddison et al. 2011; Zhu 2008). Therefore, this style of activity may be a good way to show children that exercise can be fun. These games can be played alone or with others and provide an alternative to exercising outdoors during inclement weather. AVGs may also serve as a transition to participation in sports and physical activities (Chamberlin and Gallagher 2008).

When the AVG requires the players to actively move, then this style of game play is known as **exergaming**. Although there is little research about the effects of exergaming, reductions in waist circumference, blood pressure, and weight gain have been noted for overweight children who participate (Maddison et al. 2011; Murphy et al. 2009). One study reported that MET levels for exergaming range from moderate to vigorous intensity; Wii boxing is at the low end of moderate intensity, but Sportwall and Xavix are vigorous-intensity exergames (Bailey and McInnis 2011).

What types of active video games are available?

Games that can be played at multiple skill levels are good choices since they provide a form of progression. Dance Dance Revolution (DDR) in its various renditions is a fun way to promote physical activity and weight loss in obese children and adults (Epstein et al. 2007; Zhu 2008). It is available for home use on Wii and Xbox. The number of calories burned while playing appears to be directly related to experience level; inexperienced players burn fewer calories than do experienced players (Sell, Lillie, and Taylor 2008). Overall, DDR games can provide a moderate-intensity workout (Bailey and McInnis 2011). Bronner, Pinkser, and Noah (2015) reported that the freeware version of DDR, StepMania Endless, requires a level of energy expenditure that equates to vigorous intensity (9.2 ± 2.0 METs).

Wii Sports is a home video game that uses body motions to mimic sport activities such as tennis, golf, bowling, baseball, and boxing. Although playing Wii Sports will not burn as many calories as actually playing the sport, children playing Wii bowling, tennis, golf, and boxing games burn 2% more calories than do children playing sedentary computer games (Graves et al. 2007). Wii boxing, preferred more by boys than girls, can be played at varying levels of difficulty—all of which provide moderate-intensity MET level exertion. Miyachi and colleagues (2010) quantified the MET levels for Wii Sports games for adults. They reported that the average MET level of all Wii Sports games for adults is only 3.0, which places this activity at the low end of moderate-intensity exercise.

What are the potential health benefits gained from playing active video games?

There are several documented benefits associated with playing AVGs. These include improved cognitive processes in children (Best 2011) and older adults (Bleakley et al. 2015). Increased energy expenditure (Warburton et al. 2009) and improved range of motion (Barry et al. 2016; Parry et al. 2014; Staiano and Flynn 2014) were also reported. Balance, mental health, and timed walking along a narrow path improved for senior citizens who finished a 3 mo video dancing intervention (30 min per session, twice weekly) (Studenski et al. 2010). Active video game play holds promise for promoting functional independence, improving balance, preventing falls, reducing premature disability, and maintaining health by increasing the physical activity levels of adults and seniors (deJong 2010). Adults at least 6 mo past their stroke event successfully played Wii tennis and boxing at a moderate intensity level while standing (Hurkmans et al. 2011). Consequently, playing AVGs can be beneficial in helping children and adults of all ages reap the benefits of physical activity regardless of their ability to stand and walk.

Do Wii Fit videos provide a good training workout?

Wii Fit Plus offers more than 60 training activities. These activities are categorized into four areas: aerobics (e.g., hula hoops and running), strength training (e.g., lunges and leg extensions), yoga, and balance training. Each category is made up of multiple types of exercises and activities. This exercise modality uses the handheld Wii remote controller and a balance board peripheral for some of the activities (e.g., running in place and yoga poses). At the beginner level, only the resistance and aerobic training activities provide moderate-intensity MET levels.

How may virtual reality technology be used to promote physical activity?

Virtual reality, or simulation technology, is an exciting advancement of the human-computer interface. It certainly has the potential to gain ground in the interactive healthy behaviors domain. There are two styles of virtual reality. Immersive virtual reality uses head-mounted displays, body-motion sensors, real-time graphics, and very high-tech interface devices (e.g., specialized helmets) to provide an individualized experience in a simulated environment (Rizzo et al. 2011). Nonimmersive virtual reality uses current flat-screen (e.g., television or computer screens) and traditional interface devices, such as keyboards, game pads, and joysticks. Although this technology is still evolving, the Xbox Kinect system uses a special camera and reflective adhesive markers to capture full-body movement. Since the user's body is the interface device, the user can move more naturally. With further interdisciplinary research and development, this style of interactive exergaming may offer full body–interaction gaming that further promotes physically active lifestyles (Rizzo et al. 2011).

How can persuasive technology be used to promote exercise program adherence?

Persuasive technology is defined as a computer system, device, or application that intentionally changes a person's attitude or behavior (Fogg 2003). This technology uses tools (e.g., pedometer or balance board), media (e.g., video and audio), and social interaction (e.g., playing with another person or networking) to persuade individuals to adopt the behavior without their conscious knowledge. Although DDR was not developed specifically to promote physical activity, it has changed exercise attitudes and behavior among children and youth by incorporating principles of persuasive technology. DDR uses video, music, and a dance platform to capture interest and engage children in the activity without making them fully aware that they are exercising. The emerging field of persuasive technology has enormous potential for promoting physical activity and healthy behaviors (Fogg and Eckles 2007; Zhu 2008).

Are social networks useful for promoting exercise program adherence?

With the explosion of social networking (e.g., Facebook, Twitter, Instagram, and YouTube), exercise professionals and fitness consumers have innumerable opportunities for nearly instantaneous sharing and accessing of information. This information exchange is facilitated through mobile technologies and the Internet. Unprecedented opportunities now exist for directly accessing social networks to deliver health behavior change interventions. Although social media and apps have a greater capacity to infiltrate social networks and create a contagion, they are challenging to develop, and the user must formally consent (e.g., subscribe, download). Conversely, online pages and groups offer low barriers to social networking (Cobb and Graham 2012). Facebook is a feasible platform for delivering social support interventions for physical activity among young college-age women (Cavallo et al. 2012). Websites and mass-reach broadcast media are two of the delivery mechanisms underlying social marketing strategies (Peterson, Chandlee, and Abraham 2008). These media are now accessible to everyone with smartphone technology. To best leverage social media technology to educate and interact with clients, health behavior and fitness professionals are encouraged to consider the POST (people, objectives, strategies, technology) approach as discussed by Torgan and Cousineau (2012).

Key Points

- The essential components of physical fitness are cardiorespiratory endurance, musculoskeletal fitness, body composition, and flexibility.

- Valid, reliable, and objective laboratory and field tests have been developed to assess each fitness component.

- Test validity refers to the ability of a physical fitness test to accurately measure a specific fitness component.

- Test reliability is the ability of a test to yield consistent and stable scores across trials and over time.

- Objective tests give similar test scores when different technicians administer the test to the same client.

- All physical fitness prediction equations need to be validated and cross-validated to determine their applicability and suitability for use in the field.

- The line of best fit is a regression line depicting a linear relationship between a reference measure and all the predictor variables in the regression equation.

- The *SEE* is a type of prediction error that reflects the degree of deviation of individual data points around the line of best fit or regression line.

- The *TE* is a type of prediction error that reflects the degree of deviation of individual data points around the line of identity.

- Sensitivity and specificity are measures of the ability of a test to correctly identify individuals with and without risk factors for diseases.

- Use standard evaluation criteria to judge the relative worth of newly developed physical fitness tests and prediction equations.

- The Bland and Altman method evaluates how well a prediction equation works for estimating a physical fitness component of an individual within a group.

- To obtain valid and reliable test results, clinicians must follow standardized testing procedures and have technical skills.

- Established norms for most tests are available and are used to classify physical fitness status based on the client's test scores.

- When explaining test results to clients, clinicians need to be positive and to use simple, nontechnical terms.

- To design an effective exercise program, it is necessary to understand and apply training principles. These principles include specificity, overload, progression, initial values, interindividual variability, diminishing returns, and reversibility.

▶ The basic elements of an exercise prescription are mode, intensity, duration, frequency, and progression.

▶ The exercise prescription should be individualized to meet the needs, interests, and abilities of the client.

▶ The three stages of an exercise program are initial conditioning, improvement, and maintenance.

▶ Throughout the improvement stage of an exercise program, the frequency, intensity, and duration of exercise are increased, one at a time.

▶ Physical activity participation and exercise adherence are related to demographic, biological, psychological, cognitive, emotional, behavioral, social, cultural, and environmental factors.

▶ When developing strategies for increasing exercise program adherence, it is important to integrate principles and concepts from psychological models and theories related to successful behavior change.

▶ To promote physical activity participation and adherence, pedometers, accelerometers, HR monitors, GPS units, active video gaming, social networking, and smartphone apps can be used.

▶ Persuasive technology uses tools, media, and social interaction to promote physical activity and healthy behaviors.

Key Terms

Learn the definition of each of the following key terms. Definitions of terms can be found in the glossary.

accelerometer

balance

behavior modification model

bias

Bland and Altman method

body composition

body weight (BW)

bone strength

cardiorespiratory endurance

constant error (CE)

criterion method

decision-making theory

diminishing returns principle

exergaming

false negative

false positive

flexibility

functional balance

generalized prediction equations

global positioning system (GPS)

health belief model

heart rate monitor

improvement stage

initial conditioning stage

initial values principle

interindividual variability principle

limits of agreement

line of best fit

line of identity

maintenance stage

maximum oxygen consumption ($\dot{V}O_2$max)

multiple correlation coefficient (R_{mc})

muscular endurance

muscular power

muscular strength

musculoskeletal fitness

objectivity

objectivity coefficient

overload principle

pedometer

persuasive technology

photoplethysmography (PPG)

physical fitness

population-specific equations

progression principle

reference method

regression line

reliability

reliability coefficient

residual score

reversibility principle

self-determination theory

self-efficacy	theory of planned behavior
sensitivity	theory of reasoned action
social cognitive model	total error (*TE*)
specificity	transtheoretical model
specificity principle	validity
stages of motivational readiness for change model	validity coefficient
standard error of estimate (*SEE*)	wearable technology

Review Questions

In addition to being able to define each of the key terms, test your knowledge and understanding of the material by answering the following review questions.

1. Define physical fitness. Name and define the four components of physical fitness.

2. What is the recommended sequence of testing for administering a complete physical fitness test battery?

3. Identify the reference (criterion) method for each of the four components of physical fitness.

4. Which is more important: test validity or test reliability? Explain your choice.

5. Select one physical fitness component and explain how you can determine the relative worth or predictive accuracy of a field test developed to assess this component.

6. Select one physical fitness component and give an example of how each of the seven training principles can be applied to it.

7. Identify exercise modes suitable to develop each of the four components of fitness.

8. Identify the three elements of an exercise prescription. For older or less fit clients, which of the elements should be increased first during the initial stage of their exercise programs?

9. Name the three stages of an exercise program. On average, how long should each stage last?

10. Identify three positively related and three negatively related factors associated with physical activity participation.

11. Choose one of the psychological models related to successful behavior change and give specific examples of how this model could be applied to a client undertaking a resistance training program to develop muscular fitness.

12. Explain why pedometers and accelerometers worn at the hip occasionally give different counts than one worn at the wrist.

13. Elaborate on factors relating to activity tracker accuracy during walking, running, and cycling.

14. How does GPS technology contribute to understanding environmental influences on exercise and physical activity?

15. Explain how you would select an app for your client.

16. What is persuasive technology, and how can it be used to promote physical activity?

CHAPTER 4

Assessing Cardiorespiratory Fitness

KEY QUESTIONS

▶ How is cardiorespiratory fitness ($\dot{V}O_2max$) assessed?

▶ What is a graded exercise test?

▶ How is $\dot{V}O_2max$ estimated from a graded exercise test and field test data?

▶ Should all clients be given a maximal graded exercise test? What factors should I consider in determining whether to give my client a maximal or submaximal exercise test?

▶ How accurate are submaximal exercise tests and field tests in assessing cardiorespiratory fitness?

▶ What exercise modes are suitable for graded exercise testing?

▶ What are the standardized testing procedures for graded exercise testing?

▶ What are the criteria for terminating a graded exercise test?

▶ Is it safe to give children and older adults a graded exercise test?

One of the most important components of physical fitness is cardiorespiratory endurance. Cardiorespiratory endurance is the ability to perform dynamic exercise involving large muscle groups at moderate to high intensity for prolonged periods (American College of Sports Medicine 2018). Every physical fitness evaluation should include an assessment of cardiorespiratory function during both rest and exercise.

This chapter presents guidelines for graded exercise testing as well as maximal and submaximal exercise test protocols and procedures. Although many of the graded exercise test (GXT) protocols presented in this chapter were developed years ago, these classic protocols are still widely used in research and clinical settings. In addition, each of these protocols meets the ACSM (2018) guidelines for graded exercise tests. The chapter also addresses graded exercise testing for children and older adults and includes a discussion of cardiorespiratory field tests. All of the test protocols included in this chapter are summarized in appendix B.1, Summary of Graded Exercise Test and Cardiorespiratory Field Test Protocols.

DEFINITION OF TERMS

Exercise physiologists consider directly measured **maximum oxygen uptake ($\dot{V}O_2max$)** the most valid measure of functional capacity of the cardiorespiratory system. The $\dot{V}O_2max$, or rate of oxygen uptake during maximal exercise, reflects the capacity of the heart, lungs, and blood to deliver oxygen to the working muscles during dynamic exercise involving large muscle mass. The $\dot{V}O_2max$ is widely accepted as the criterion measure of cardiorespiratory fitness.

Traditionally, a plateau in oxygen consumption despite an increase in workload is the criterion used to determine the attainment of a true $\dot{V}O_2max$ during a maximum exercise tolerance test. Evidence suggests, however, that the incidence of a $\dot{V}O_2$ plateau during incremental exercise testing is highly variable, ranging from 16% to 94% (Day et al. 2003; Edvardsen, Hem, and Anderssen 2014; Magnan et al. 2013; Mier, Alexander, and Mageean 2012; Yoon, Kravitz, and Robergs 2007). In fact, studies have established that a plateau phenomenon is not

Video 4.1

a prerequisite for identifying a true $\dot{V}O_2$max in the majority of individuals (Noakes 2008; Poole and Jones 2017). Some researchers now suggest that a **verification bout** of constant load exertion (~10% higher than the highest workload achieved in a ramp trial) is more appropriate for determining $\dot{V}O_2$max (Poole and Jones 2017). According to Magnan and colleagues (2013), the incidence of a plateau for inactive people is related to body mass index (BMI), waist-to-hip ratio, sense of self-efficacy, gender, and method for determining the plateau. However, when participants attain similar $\dot{V}O_2$max values without consistently attaining a plateau with four different maximal exertion treadmill protocols, then the impact of protocol selection and day-to-day biologic variability cannot be overlooked (Beltz et al. 2016).

$\dot{V}O_2$ **peak** is the highest rate of oxygen consumption measured during the exercise test, regardless of whether or not a $\dot{V}O_2$ plateau is reached. $\dot{V}O_2$ peak may be higher than, lower than, or equal to $\dot{V}O_2$max. For many individuals who do not reach an actual $\dot{V}O_2$ plateau, the $\dot{V}O_2$ peak attained during a maximum-effort incremental test to the limit of tolerance is a valid index of $\dot{V}O_2$ max (Day et al. 2003; Hawkins et al. 2007; Howley 2007).

Maximal and submaximal $\dot{V}O_2$ are expressed in absolute or relative terms. **Absolute $\dot{V}O_2$** is measured in liters per minute (L·min^{-1}) or milliliters per minute (ml·min^{-1}) and provides a measure of energy cost for non-weight-bearing activities such as leg or arm cycle ergometry. Absolute $\dot{V}O_2$ is directly related to body size; thus, men typically have a larger absolute $\dot{V}O_2$ max than women.

Because absolute $\dot{V}O_2$ depends on body size, $\dot{V}O_2$ is typically expressed relative to body weight (i.e., in ml·kg^{-1}·min^{-1}). **Relative $\dot{V}O_2$max** is used to classify an individual's cardiorespiratory (CR) fitness level or to compare fitness levels of individuals differing in body size. Relative $\dot{V}O_2$ can also be used to estimate the energy cost of weight-bearing activities such as walking, running, and stair climbing. However, although the relationship between absolute $\dot{V}O_2$max and body mass is strong ($r = .86$), it is not perfect ($r = 1.00$). Therefore, when $\dot{V}O_2$max is expressed simply as a linear function of body mass, CR fitness levels of heavier (>75.4 kg) and lighter (<67.7 kg) individuals may be under- or overclassified, respectively (Heil 1997). Some experts propose scaling exercise capacity (i.e., $\dot{V}O_2$, 6 min walk test distance) to an exponential function of body mass (Buresh and Berg 2002; Dourado and McBurnie 2012; Heil 1997). A current limitation of doing so is that the norms used to classify CR fitness levels were established for relative $\dot{V}O_2$ max values expressed as ml·min^{-1}·kg^{-1} and not as ml·min^{-1}·kg$^{0.67}$ or ml·min^{-1}·kg$^{0.75}$, where the exponents are suggested to correct relative oxygen consumption for body mass. Carrick-Ranson and colleagues (2012) suggested that scaling relative to fat-free mass (FFM; see chapter 8), the most metabolically active tissue, is more appropriate than is allometric scaling. They used scaling relative to FFM to demonstrate that a decrease in maximal heart rate, not maximal stroke volume and total blood volume, is the likely source of the age-related decline in $\dot{V}O_2$ for both men and women.

Expressing $\dot{V}O_2$ relative to the individual's FFM (i.e., as ml·kgFFM^{-1}·min^{-1}) provides you with an estimate of cardiorespiratory endurance that is independent of changes in body weight. For example, your client's improvement in relative $\dot{V}O_2$ max following a 16 wk aerobic exercise program may reflect both improved capacity of the cardiorespiratory system (increase in absolute $\dot{V}O_2$ max) and weight loss (increase in relative $\dot{V}O_2$ expressed as ml·kg^{-1}·min^{-1} due to a decrease in body weight). Thus, expressing $\dot{V}O_2$ max relative to FFM, instead of body weight, reflects the oxygen consumption of the tissues most active during exercise and physical activity.

The rate of oxygen consumption can also be expressed as a gross $\dot{V}O_2$ or net $\dot{V}O_2$. **Gross $\dot{V}O_2$** is the total rate of oxygen consumption and reflects the caloric costs of both rest and exercise (gross $\dot{V}O_2$ = resting $\dot{V}O_2$ + exercise $\dot{V}O_2$). On the other hand, **net $\dot{V}O_2$** represents the rate of oxygen consumption in excess of the resting $\dot{V}O_2$ and is used to describe the caloric cost of the exercise. Both gross and net $\dot{V}O_2$ can be expressed in either absolute (e.g., L·min^{-1}) or relative (ml·kg^{-1}·min^{-1}) terms. Unless specified as a net $\dot{V}O_2$, the $\dot{V}O_2$ values reported throughout this book refer to gross $\dot{V}O_2$.

GRADED EXERCISE TESTING: GUIDELINES AND PROCEDURES

Exercise scientists and physicians use exercise tests to evaluate functional cardiorespiratory capacity

($\dot{V}O_2$ max) objectively. The $\dot{V}O_2$ max, determined from graded maximal or submaximal exercise tests, is used to classify the cardiorespiratory fitness levels of your clients (see table 4.1). You can use baseline and follow-up data to evaluate the progress of exercise program participants and to set realistic goals for your clients. You can use the heart rate (HR) and oxygen uptake data obtained during the graded exercise test to make accurate, precise exercise prescriptions.

As discussed in chapter 2, an individual's exercise history, disease status (i.e., known versus nonexistent cardiovascular, metabolic, or renal disease), and positive symptomology, or lack thereof, for those same three diseases now drive the preparticipation screening process. As the preparticipation screening algorithm indicates (see table 2.2), the recommended initial exercise program intensity is dependent on the individual's exercise history, disease status, symptomology, and requirement for medical clearance. The ACSM (2018) no longer recommends a graded **maximal exercise test** before engaging in an exercise program. However, one may be included as part of the medical clearance process. For medical conditions that constitute absolute and relative contraindications to exercise testing, see chapter 2. For risk stratification of patients in medical fitness and cardiac rehabilitation facilities, the American

Association of Cardiovascular and Pulmonary Rehabilitation (AACVPR) has a more thorough set of risk stratification procedures you need to follow (Williams 2001).

GENERAL GUIDELINES FOR EXERCISE TESTING

You may use a maximal or submaximal graded exercise test (GXT) to assess the cardiorespiratory fitness of the individual. The selection of a maximal or submaximal GXT depends on

- your client's habitual exercise patterns, risk factors, and diagnosis or symptomology of cardiovascular, metabolic, or renal disease;
- your reasons for administering the test (physical fitness testing or clinical testing); and
- the availability of appropriate equipment and qualified personnel.

In clinical and research settings, $\dot{V}O_2$ max is typically measured directly, which requires expensive equipment and experienced personnel. Although $\dot{V}O_2$ max can be predicted from maximal exercise intensity with a fair degree of accuracy, **submaximal exercise tests** also provide a reasonable estimate of cardiorespiratory fitness level. They are less costly,

Table 4.1 Cardiorespiratory Fitness Classifications: $\dot{V}O_2$max (ml·kg^{-1}·min^{-1})

Age (yr)	Poor	Fair	Good	Excellent	Superior
WOMEN					
20-29	≤33	34-39	40-45	46-51	52+
30-39	≤27	28-31	32-36	37-40	41+
40-49	≤24	25-28	29-32	33-38	39+
50-59	≤21	22-24	25-28	29-32	33+
60-69	≤18	19-21	22-24	25-27	28+
MEN					
20-29	≤44	45-49	50-56	57-62	63+
30-39	≤39	40-44	45-49	50-57	58+
40-49	≤35	36-39	40-45	46-52	53+
50-59	≤30	31-34	35-40	41-46	47+
60-69	≤26	27-29	30-35	36-40	41+

Note: Graded treadmill test data with metabolic gas collection

Adapted from L.A. Kaminsky, R. Arena, and J. Myers, "Reference Standards for Cardiorespiratory Fitness Measured With Cardiopulmonary Exercise Testing: Data From the Fitness Registry and the Importance of Exercise National Database," *Mayo Clinic Proceedings* 90 no. 11 (2015): 1515-1523.

less time consuming, and not as risky. Submaximal exercise testing, however, is considered less sensitive as a diagnostic tool for coronary heart disease (CHD).

In either case, the exercise test should be a multistage graded test. This means the individual exercises at gradually increasing submaximal workloads. Many commonly used exercise test protocols require that each workload be performed for 3 min. The GXT protocol is the means through which maximum functional capacity ($\dot{V}O_2$max) is determined. When direct measures are being used, a combination of specific criteria is applied to confirm that the individual being tested gave a maximal effort. One of those criteria requires that oxygen uptake plateaus and does not increase by more than 150 ml·min^{-1} with a further increase in workload. Poole and Jones (2017) recommend confirming maximal effort by utilizing a constant supramaximal load verification bout instead of relying on a plateau or secondary criteria. Historically, however, combinations of the following secondary criteria have been used to confirm that an individual who did not attain a $\dot{V}O_2$ plateau gave a maximal effort and, hence, attained a true $\dot{V}O_2$max:

- Failure of the HR to increase with increases in exercise intensity
- Venous lactate concentration exceeding 8 mmol·L^{-1}
- **Respiratory exchange ratio (RER)** greater than 1.15
- **Rating of perceived exertion (RPE)** greater than 17 using the original Borg scale (6-20)

It should be noted that one's ability to satisfy one or more of these secondary criteria has been shown to be related to age and sex (Edvardsen, Hem, and Anderssen 2014). If the test is terminated before the person reaches a plateau in $\dot{V}O_2$ and an RER greater than 1.15, the GXT is considered to be a measure of $\dot{V}O_2$peak rather than $\dot{V}O_2$max. Children, older adults, sedentary individuals, and clients with known disease are more likely than other groups to attain a $\dot{V}O_2$peak rather than a $\dot{V}O_2$max. For CHD screening and classification purposes, bringing a person to at least 85% of the age-predicted maximal HR is desirable because some electrocardiogram (ECG) abnormalities do not appear until the HR reaches this level of intensity.

Evidence suggests that maximal exercise tests are no more dangerous than submaximal tests provided you carefully follow guidelines for exercise tolerance testing and continuously monitor the physiological responses of the exercise participant. Eight nonfatal and no fatal events were identified in a retrospective study of 5,060 symptom-limited exercise tests (adverse event rate of 0.16%) performed on clients with various underlying high-risk cardiac diagnoses (Skalski, Allison, and Miller 2012). For clinical testing, the risk of an exercise test being fatal is no greater than 0.4 to 0.5 per 10,000 tests (Atterhog, Jonsson, and Samuelsson 1979; Goodman, Thomas, and Burr 2011; Rochmis and Blackburn 1971; Skalski, Allison, and Miller 2012), although the risk of myocardial infarction has been estimated to be 4 per 10,000 tests (Thompson 1993). Based on a review of studies including clients with and without CVD, Goodman and colleagues (2011) identified the average risk of an adverse event during exercise testing as being less than 2.9 nonfatal and 0.3 fatal events per 10,000 tests. The risk for apparently healthy individuals (without known disease or symptomology) is very low, with no complications occurring in 380,000 exercise tests done on young individuals (Levine, Zuckerman, and Cole 1998). Similarly, there were no complications reported in the 700,000-plus exercise tests performed on sports-persons and athletes in the studies reviewed by Goodman and colleagues (2011). As a result, Goodman and colleagues concluded that the risks of maximal exertion exercise testing reflect a fatal-event incidence of 0.2 to 0.8 per 10,000 tests and a nonfatal-event incidence of 1.4 per 100,000 tests.

Nonphysicians may safely supervise exercise tests as long as they have demonstrated the competencies required to do so. Individual competencies, training, support, and certifications recommended for the continued safe monitoring of exercise tests by nonphysicians are identified in the 2014 scientific statement from the AHA (Myers et al. 2014). This statement also lists medical conditions for which a physician should be present in the room during exercise testing.

GENERAL PROCEDURES FOR CARDIORESPIRATORY FITNESS TESTING

At least 1 day before the exercise test, you should give your client pretest instructions (see chapter 3).

Prior to graded exercise testing, the client should read and sign the informed consent and complete the 2018 PAR-Q+; see appendix A.1, Physical Activity Readiness Questionnaire for Everyone (PAR-Q+). Step-by-step instructions are listed in Procedures for Administering a Graded Exercise Test.

Pretest, exercise, and recovery HRs can be measured using the palpation or auscultation technique (see chapter 2) if a HR monitor or ECG recorder is unavailable. Because of extraneous noise and vibration during exercise, it may be difficult to obtain accurate measurements of BP, especially when your client is running on the treadmill. To become proficient at taking exercise BP, you need to practice as much as possible.

For years, the Borg scales have been used to obtain ratings of perceived exertion (RPEs) during exercise testing. The original scale (6-20) and the revised scale (0-10) allow clients to rate their degree of exertion subjectively during exercise; the two scales are highly related to exercise HRs and $\dot{V}O_2$. Both RPE scales take into account the linear rise in HR and $\dot{V}O_2$ during exercise. The revised scale also reflects nonlinear changes in blood lactate and ventilation during exercise. Ratings of 6 on the original scale and 0 on the revised scale correspond to no exertion at all; ratings of 10 on the revised scale and 19 on the original scale usually correspond with the maximal level of exercise (Borg 1998). Moderate-intensity exercise is rated between 12 and 14 on the original scale and rated 5 or 6 on the revised scale. Ratings of perceived exertion are useful in determining the endpoints of the GXT, particularly for patients who are taking beta-blockers or other medications that may alter the HR response to exercise. You can teach your clients how to use the RPE scales to monitor relative intensities during aerobic exercise programs.

Alternatively, you may use OMNI scales to obtain a client's RPE for various modes of exercise testing. The OMNI scales can be used to measure RPE for the overall body, the limbs, and the chest. These scales were originally developed for children and adolescents and used a picture system to illustrate intensity (0 = extremely easy to 10 = extremely hard) of effort during exercise. Later the scales were modified for use with adults engaging in cycle ergometer, treadmill, stepping, elliptical, and resistance exercises. As part of the validation testing for the cycling, stepping, elliptical, and treadmill ergometry scales, the OMNI RPE values have been correlated with HR and $\dot{V}O_2$ data. Concurrent validity coefficients ranged from .82 to .95 for HR and OMNI RPE; likewise, the validity coefficients ranged between .88 and .96 for $\dot{V}O_2$ and OMNI RPE (Guidetti et al. 2011; Krause et al. 2012; Mays et al. 2010; Robertson 2004). For resistance exercise, RPE values from the OMNI scale were correlated with weight lifted, yielding validity coefficients ranging from .72 to .91 (Robertson 2004; Robertson et al. 2005). A derivation of the OMNI 0 to 10 RPE scale uses sketches of simple facial expressions (e.g., smiling, frowning, neutral expression) and a numeric scale (Chen, Chiou, et al. 2017). The correlations of RPE with stationary cycling workload and with heart rate for young adults ($r > .97$) were nearly identical for the Borg 10-point and facial expression scales. For children, the two scales were perceived similarly for RPE and workload ($r > .97$). The facial expression scale ($r > .90$) was more closely related to heart rate than was the Borg scale ($r > .49$).

Appendix B.4 contains sample instructions, procedures, and OMNI pictorial scales for boys, girls, and adults engaging in cycling, treadmill walking or running, stepping, and resistance exercise. Like the Borg scales, the OMNI scales can be used by your clients to monitor the intensity of their workouts during aerobic and resistance exercise training. For a detailed discussion of how to use these scales, refer to the work of Chen, Chiou, and colleagues (2017); Guidetti and colleagues (2011); Robertson (2004); Krause and colleagues (2012); and Mays and colleagues (2010). Table 4.2 summarizes the verbal cues corresponding to the numerical values of the OMNI RPE scales.

Table 4.2 Verbal Cues for OMNI RPE Scales

Adults	Children
Extremely easy = 0	Not tired at all = 0
Easy = 2	A little tired = 2
Somewhat easy = 4	Getting more tired = 4
Somewhat hard = 6	Tired = 6
Hard = 8	Really tired = 8
Extremely hard = 10	Very, very tired = 10

Procedures for Administering a Graded Exercise Test

Video 4.2

- Measure the client's resting HR and blood pressure (BP) in the exercise posture (see chapter 2 for these procedures).

- Begin the GXT with a 2 to 3 min warm-up to familiarize the client with the exercise equipment and prepare him for the first stage of the exercise test.

- During the test, monitor HR, BP, and ratings of perceived exertion (RPEs) at regular intervals. Measure HR at least two times during each stage, near the end of the second and third minutes of each stage. A steady-state HR (two HR measurements within ±5 bpm) should be reached for each stage of the test. Do not increase the workload until a steady-state HR is reached.

- Blood pressure should be measured during the last minute of each stage of the test and repeated if a hypotensive or hypertensive response is observed.

- Rating of perceived exertion should be assessed near the end of the last minute of each exercise stage using either the Borg or OMNI scales.

- Throughout the exercise test, continuously monitor the client's physical appearance and symptoms.

- Discontinue the GXT when the test termination criteria are reached (e.g., 70% HRR or 85% HRmax, if the client requests stopping the test, or if any of the indications for stopping an exercise test are apparent [see General Indications for Termination of a Graded Exercise Test]).

- Have the client cool down by exercising at a low work rate that does not exceed the intensity of the first stage of the exercise test (e.g., walking on the treadmill at 2 mph [53.6 m·min^{-1}] and 0% grade, or cycling on the cycle ergometer at 50 to 60 revolutions per minute [rpm] and zero resistance). Active recovery reduces the risk of hypotension from venous pooling in the extremities.

- During recovery, continue measuring postexercise HR and BP for at least 5 min. If an abnormal response occurs, extend the recovery period. The HR and BP during active recovery should be stable but may be higher than preexercise levels. Continue monitoring the client's physical appearance during recovery.

- If your client has signs of discomfort or if an emergency occurs during the test, use a passive cooldown with the client in a sitting or supine position.

Based on ACSM 2018.

TEST TERMINATION

In a maximal or submaximal GXT, the exercise usually continues until the client voluntarily terminates the test or a predetermined endpoint is reached. As an exercise technician, however, you must be acutely aware of all indicators for stopping a test. If you notice any of the signs or symptoms listed in General Indications for Termination of a Graded Exercise Test, you should stop the exercise test prior to the client's reaching $\dot{V}O_2$max (for a maximal GXT) or the predetermined endpoint (for a submaximal GXT).

MAXIMAL EXERCISE TEST PROTOCOLS

Many maximal exercise test protocols have been devised to assess cardiorespiratory capacity. As

the exercise technician, you must be able to select an exercise mode and test protocol that are suitable for your clients given their age, gender, and health and fitness status. Commonly used modes of exercise are treadmill walking or running and stationary cycling. Arm ergometry is useful for persons with paraplegia and clients who have limited use of the lower extremities. Also, combined leg and arm ergometry and total body recumbent stepper exercise tests may be suitable alternatives to treadmill testing for assessing the cardiorespiratory fitness of older persons with balance deficits, gait impairments, and decreased coordination (Billinger, Loudon, and Gajewski 2008; Loudon et al. 1998). Bench stepping is not highly recommended but could be useful in field situations when large groups need to be tested. Whichever mode of exercise you choose, be sure to adhere to

GENERAL INDICATIONS FOR TERMINATION OF A GRADED EXERCISE TEST

1. Onset of angina or angina-like symptoms
2. Drop in systolic BP of >10 mmHg from baseline BP despite an increase in workload
3. Excessive rise in BP: systolic pressure >250 mmHg or diastolic pressure >115 mmHg
4. Shortness of breath, wheezing, leg cramps, or claudication
5. Signs of poor perfusion (e.g., ataxia, dizziness, pallor, cyanosis, cold or clammy skin, or nausea)
6. Failure of HR to rise with increased exercise intensity
7. Noticeable change in heart rhythm
8. Client's request to stop
9. Physical or verbal manifestations of severe fatigue
10. Failure of the testing equipment

Note: For definitions of specific terms, refer to the glossary.

Adapted from American College of Sports Medicine, *ACSM's Guidelines for Exercise Testing and Prescription,* 10th ed. (Philadelphia: Lippincott Williams & Wilkins, 2018), 84, with permission of Wolters Kluwer.

the principles explained in General Principles of Exercise Testing.

The exercise test may be continuous or discontinuous. A **continuous exercise test** is performed with no rest between work increments. Continuous exercise tests can vary in the duration of each exercise stage and the magnitude of the increment in exercise intensity between stages. Researchers recommend a total test duration between 8 and 12 min to increase the probability of moderately and highly trained individuals reaching $\dot{V}O_2$ max (Fletcher et al. 2013; Gibbons et al. 2002). A slightly longer, hence less aggressive, test may be better suited for less fit individuals (Beltz et al. 2016). Midgley and colleagues (2008) challenged the 8 to 12 min recommendation (American College of Sports Medicine 2014; Fletcher et al. 2013; Gibbons et al. 2002) based on an extensive review of studies dealing with this topic. They concluded that the duration of cycle ergometer tests should be between 7 and 26 min and that treadmill tests should be between 5 and 26 min to yield a valid determination of $\dot{V}O_2$ max. This recommendation assumes that an adequate warm-up precedes the shorter-duration tests and that the treadmill grade does not exceed 15% during the protocol. For most continuous exercise test protocols, the exercise intensity is increased gradually (2 to 3 METs for low-risk individuals) throughout the test, and the duration of each stage is usually 2 or 3 min, allowing most individuals to reach a steady-state $\dot{V}O_2$ during each stage. Across the stages of this type of GXT, the workload may increase linearly or nonlinearly. Each increment in workload is dictated by the specific protocol and does not vary among individuals. Although this type of GXT is widely used in research and clinical settings, it may not be optimal for assessing the functional capacity of all individuals, especially those with low exercise tolerance.

Continuous ramp-type tests are widely used because they can be individualized for the client's estimated exercise tolerance. For example, increments in work rate during a ramp protocol are much higher for endurance-trained athletes than for sedentary individuals (e.g., 30 W·min^{-1} vs. 10 W·min^{-1}). Also, each exercise stage for ramp protocols is much shorter (e.g., 20 sec) than that of the traditional continuous GXT protocols (2-3 min). **Ramp protocols** provide continuous and frequent increments in work rate throughout the test so that the $\dot{V}O_2$ increases linearly; they are designed to bring individuals to their limit of exercise tolerance in approximately 10 min. In a study comparing four ramp protocol durations (5, 8, 12, and 16 min) during incremental cycling exercise, Yoon and colleagues (2007) reported that the optimal protocol duration to elicit $\dot{V}O_2$ max of healthy, moderately to highly trained men and women is between 8 and 10 min.

Because of the frequent (e.g., every 10 or 20 sec) increases in work rate with ramp protocols, $\dot{V}O_2$ plateaus are rarely observed. Regardless, when *plateau* is defined as a change in $\dot{V}O_2$ ·min^{-1} <0.5

General Principles of Exercise Testing

1. Typically, you will use either a treadmill or stationary cycle ergometer for graded exercise testing. All equipment should be calibrated before use.

2. Begin the GXT with a 2 to 3 min warm-up to orient the client to the equipment and prepare her for the first stage of the GXT.

3. The initial exercise intensity should be considerably lower than the anticipated maximal capacity.

4. Exercise intensity should be increased gradually throughout the stages of the test. Work increments may be 2 METs or greater for apparently healthy individuals and as small as 0.5 MET for patients with disease.

5. Closely observe contraindications for testing and indications for stopping the exercise test. When in any doubt about the safety or benefits of testing, do not perform the test at that time.

6. Monitor the HR at least two times, but preferably each minute, during each stage of the GXT. Heart rate measurements should be taken near the end of each minute. If the HR is higher than 110 bpm and does not reach steady state (two HRs within ±5 or 6 bpm), extend the work stage an additional minute or until the HR stabilizes.

7. Measure BP and RPE once during each stage of the GXT, in the later portion of the stage. Repeat BP if the value indicates a hypertensive or hypotensive response.

8. Continuously monitor client appearance and symptoms.

9. For submaximal GXTs, terminate the test when the client's HR reaches 70% HRR (heart rate reserve) or 85% HRmax (maximal heart rate), unless the protocol specifies a different termination criterion. Also, stop the test immediately if there is an emergency situation, if the client fails to conform to the exercise protocol, or if the client experiences signs of discomfort.

10. The test should include a cool-down period of at least 5 min, or longer if abnormal HR and BP responses are observed. During recovery, HR and BP should be monitored each minute. For active recovery, the workload should be no more than that used during the first stage of the GXT. A passive recovery is used in emergency situations and when clients experience signs of discomfort and cannot perform an active cool-down.

11. Exercise tolerance in METs should be estimated for the treadmill or ergometer protocol used, or directly assessed if oxygen uptake is measured during the GXT.

12. The testing area should be quiet and private. The room temperature should be 21 to 23 °C (70-72 °F) or less and the humidity 60% or less if possible.

Note: Medical clearance recommended for individuals having known cardiovascular, renal, and metabolic disease or symptomology thereof.

L·min^{-1} during the final 30 sec of a cycling protocol (Yoon, Kravitz, and Robergs 2007), plateaus are observable for moderately and highly trained adults. However, as previously mentioned, the $\dot{V}O_2$ peak from ramp-type protocols appears to be a valid index of $\dot{V}O_2$max even without a plateau in $\dot{V}O_2$ (Day et al. 2003). The ramp approach potentially improves the prediction of $\dot{V}O_2$max given that $\dot{V}O_2$ increases linearly across work rates. Ramp protocols allow some individuals to reach a higher exercise tolerance compared with traditional GXT protocols. However,

there are disadvantages. To design an individualized ramp protocol, the maximum work rate for each client must be predetermined or accurately estimated from training records or questionnaires so you can select a work rate that allows the client to reach peak exercise tolerance in approximately 10 min. Also, ramp protocols increase work rate frequently (e.g., 25-30 stages in a 10 min test), requiring more expensive electromagnetically braked cycle ergometers and programmable treadmills that make rapid and smooth transitions between the stages of the exercise test. Finally, inexperienced technicians may have difficulty measuring exercise BP during each minute of the ramp protocol.

For **discontinuous exercise tests**, the client rests 5 to 10 min between workloads. The workload is progressively increased until the client reaches maximum exercise tolerance (exhaustion). Typically, each stage of the discontinuous protocol lasts 5 or 6 min, allowing $\dot{V}O_2$ to reach a steady state. On average, discontinuous tests take five times longer to administer than do continuous tests. Similar $\dot{V}O_2$max values are attained using discontinuous and continuous (increasing workload every 2-3 min) protocols (Maksud and Coutts 1971); therefore, continuous tests are preferable in most research and clinical settings.

McArdle, Katch, and Pechar (1973) compared the $\dot{V}O_2$max scores as measured by six commonly used continuous and discontinuous treadmill and cycle ergometer tests. They noted that the $\dot{V}O_2$max scores for the cycle ergometer tests were approximately 6% to 11% lower than for the treadmill tests. Many subjects identified local discomfort and fatigue in the thigh muscles as the major factors limiting further work on both the continuous and discontinuous cycle ergometer tests. For the treadmill tests, subjects indicated windedness and general fatigue as the limiting factors and complained of localized fatigue and discomfort in the calf muscles and lower back. Lambrick and associates (2017) compared continuous and discontinuous treadmill protocols for healthy children. Although the duration of the discontinuous protocol was longer, this type of protocol elicited similar values for $\dot{V}O_2$ peak and maximal HR. However, peak running speed was faster and RER lower for the discontinuous protocol.

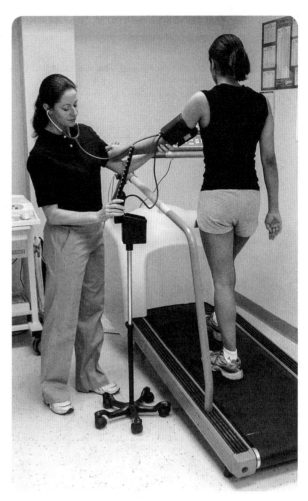

FIGURE 4.1 Treadmill.

TREADMILL MAXIMAL EXERCISE TESTS

Video 4.3

Generally, the treadmill is the preferred exercise test modality in the United States (Balady et al. 2010). For treadmill maximal exercise tests, the exercise is performed on a motor-driven treadmill with variable speed and incline (see figure 4.1). Speed varies up to 25 mph (40 km·hr⁻¹), and the incline is measured in units of elevation per 100 horizontal units and is expressed as a percentage. The workload on the treadmill is raised through increases in the speed or incline or both. Workload is usually expressed in miles per hour and percent grade.

It is difficult and expensive to measure oxygen consumption during exercise. Therefore, ACSM (2018) equations (table 4.3) to estimate the metabolic cost of exercise ($\dot{V}O_2$) may be used. These equations provide a valid estimate of $\dot{V}O_2$ for steady-state exercise only. When used to estimate the maximum rate of energy expenditure ($\dot{V}O_2$max), the measured $\dot{V}O_2$ will be less than the estimated $\dot{V}O_2$ if steady state is not reached. Also, because maximal exercise involves both aerobic and anaerobic components, the $\dot{V}O_2$max will be overestimated since the contribution of the anaerobic component is not known.

Before using any of the ACSM metabolic equations to estimate $\dot{V}O_2$, make certain that all units of measure match those in the equation (see Converting Units of Measure).

The ACSM metabolic equations in table 4.3 are useful in clinical settings for estimating the total

Table 4.3   Metabolic Equations for Estimating Gross $\dot{V}O_2$

Exercise mode gross $\dot{V}O_2$ (ml·kg^{-1}·min^{-1})	Resting $\dot{V}O_2$ (ml·kg^{-1}·min^{-1})	Comments
Walking $\dot{V}O_2 = S^a \times 0.1 + S \times G^b \times 1.8$	+3.5	1. For speeds of 50-100 m·min^{-1} (1.9-3.7 mph) 2. 0.1 ml·kg^{-1}·m^{-1} = O_2 cost of walking horizontally 3. 1.8 ml·kg^{-1}·m^{-1} = O_2 cost of walking on incline (% grade of treadmill)
Running $\dot{V}O_2 = S^a \times 0.2 + S \times G^b \times 0.9$	+3.5	1. For speeds >134 m·min^{-1} (>5.0 mph) 2. If truly jogging (not walking), this equation can also be used for speeds of 80-134 m·min^{-1} (3-5 mph) 3. 0.2 ml·kg^{-1}·m^{-1} = O_2 cost of running horizontally 4. 0.9 ml·kg^{-1}·m^{-1} = O_2 cost of running on incline (% grade of treadmill)
Leg ergometry $\dot{V}O_2 = W^c / M^d \times 1.8 + 3.5$	+3.5	1. For work rates between 50 and 200 W (300-1,200 kgm·min^{-1}) 2. kgm·min^{-1} = kg × m·rev^{-1} × rev·min^{-1} 3. Monark and Bodyguard = 6 m·rev^{-1}; Tunturi = 3 m·rev^{-1} 4. 1.8 ml·kg^{-1}·min^{-1} = O_2 cost of cycling against external load (resistance) 5. 3.5 ml·kg^{-1}·min^{-1} = O_2 cost of cycling with zero load
Arm ergometry $\dot{V}O_2 = W^c / M^d \times 3.0 +$ none	+3.5	1. For work rates between 25 and 125 W (150-750 kgm·min^{-1}) 2. kgm·min^{-1} = kg × m·rev^{-1} × rev·min^{-1}; m·rev^{-1} for Monark arm ergometer = 2.4 m 3. 3.0 ml·kg^{-1}·min^{-1} = O_2 cost of cycling against external load (resistance) 4. None = due to small mass of arm musculature, no special term for unloaded (zero load) cycling needed
Stepping $\dot{V}O_2 = F^e \times 0.2 + F \times ht^f \times 1.8 \times 1.33$	+3.5	1. Appropriate for stepping rates between 12 and 30 steps·min^{-1} and step heights between 0.04 m (1.6 in.) and 0.40 m (15.7 in.) 2. 0.2 ml·kg^{-1}·m^{-1} = O_2 cost of moving horizontally 3. 1.8 ml·kg^{-1}·m^{-1} = O_2 cost of stepping up (bench height) 4. 1.33 includes positive component of stepping up (1.0) + negative component of stepping down (0.33)

[a]S = speed of treadmill in m·min^{-1}; 1 mph = 26.8 m·min^{-1}.

[b]G = grade (% incline) of treadmill in decimal form (e.g., 10% = 0.10).

[c]W = work rate in kgm·min^{-1}; 1 Watt = 6.12 kgm·min^{-1}.

[d]M = body mass in kilograms; 1 kg = 2.2 lb.

[e]F = frequency of stepping in steps per minute.

[f]ht = bench height in meters; 1 in. = 0.0254 m.

ACSM 2018.

rate of energy expenditure (gross $\dot{V}O_2$) during steady-state treadmill walking or running. The total energy expenditure, in ml·kg^{-1}·min^{-1}, is a function of three components: speed, grade, and resting energy expenditures. For treadmill walking, the oxygen cost of raising one's body mass against gravity (vertical work) is approximately 1.8 ml·kg^{-1}·m^{-1}, and 0.1 ml·kg^{-1}·m^{-1} of oxygen is needed to move the body horizontally. For treadmill running, the oxygen cost for vertical work is one-half that for treadmill walking (0.9 ml·kg^{-1}·m^{-1}), whereas the energy expenditure for running on the treadmill (0.2 ml·kg^{-1}·m^{-1}) is twice that for walking. See ACSM Walking Equation for an example of how to take these three factors into account when figuring $\dot{V}O_2$.

The $\dot{V}O_2$ estimated from the ACSM walking equation (see table 4.3) is reasonably accurate for walking speeds between 50 and 100 m·min^{-1} (1.9-3.7 mph). However, since the equation is more accurate for walking up a grade than on the level, $\dot{V}O_2$ may

Converting Units of Measure

- Convert body mass (M) in pounds to kilograms (1 kg = 2.2 lb). For example, 170 lb / 2.2 = 77.3 kg.
- Convert treadmill speed (S) in miles per hour to meters per minute (1 mph = 26.8 m·min⁻¹). For example, 5.0 mph × 26.8 = 134.0 m·min⁻¹.
- Convert treadmill grade (G) from percent to decimal form by dividing by 100. For example, 12% / 100 = 0.12.

- Convert METs to ml·kg⁻¹·min⁻¹ by multiplying (1 MET = 3.5 ml·kg⁻¹·min⁻¹). For example, 6 METs × 3.5 = 21.0 ml·kg⁻¹·min⁻¹.
- Convert kgm·min⁻¹ to watts (W) (1 W ≈ 6 kgm·min⁻¹) by dividing. For example, 900 kgm·min⁻¹ / 6 = 150 W.
- Convert step height in inches to meters (1 in. = 0.0254 m) by multiplying. For example, 8 in. × 0.0254 = 0.2032 m.

ACSM Walking Equation

To calculate the gross $\dot{V}O_2$ for a 70 kg (154 lb) subject who is walking on the treadmill at a speed of 3.5 mph and a grade of 10%, follow these steps:

$$\dot{V}O_2 = \text{speed} + (\text{grade} \times \text{speed}) + \text{resting } \dot{V}O_2 \text{ (ml·kg}^{-1}\text{·min}^{-1})$$

$$= [\text{speed (m·min}^{-1}) \times 0.1] + [\text{grade (decimal)} \times \text{speed (m·min}^{-1}) \times 1.8] + 3.5$$

1. Convert the speed in mph to m·min⁻¹; 1 mph = 26.8 m·min⁻¹.

$$3.5 \text{ mph} \times 26.8 = 93.8 \text{ m·min}^{-1}$$

2. Calculate the speed component (S).

$$S = \text{speed (m·min}^{-1}) \times 0.1$$

$$= 93.8 \text{ m·min}^{-1} \times 0.1$$

$$= 9.38 \text{ ml·kg}^{-1}\text{·min}^{-1}$$

3. Calculate the grade × speed component (G × S). Convert % grade into a decimal by dividing by 100.

$$G \times S = \text{grade (decimal)} \times \text{speed} \times 1.8$$

$$= 0.10 \times (93.8 \text{ m·min}^{-1}) \times 1.8$$

$$= 16.88 \text{ ml·kg}^{-1}\text{·min}^{-1}$$

4. Calculate the total gross $\dot{V}O_2$ in ml·kg⁻¹·min⁻¹ by adding the speed, grade × speed, and resting $\dot{V}O_2$ (R).

$$\dot{V}O_2 = S + (S \times G) + R$$

$$= (9.38 + 16.88 + 3.5) \text{ ml·kg}^{-1}\text{·min}^{-1}$$

$$= 29.76 \text{ ml·kg}^{-1}\text{·min}^{-1}$$

be underestimated as much as 20% during walking on the level. For the ACSM running or jogging equations, the $\dot{V}O_2$ estimates are relatively accurate for speeds exceeding 134 m·min⁻¹ (5 mph) and speeds as low as 80 m·min⁻¹ (3 mph) provided that the client is jogging and not walking (American College of Sports Medicine 2014). When HRs fall between 110 bpm and 85% of age-predicted maximum HR, the ACSM running equation provides a reasonably good (*SEE* [standard error of estimate] = 4.2 to 4.35 ml·kg⁻¹·min⁻¹) estimation of maximal aerobic capacity (Marsh 2012).

Figure 4.2 illustrates commonly used treadmill exercise test protocols. These protocols conform to the general guidelines for maximal exercise testing. Some of the protocols are designed for a specific population, such as well-conditioned athletes or high-risk cardiac patients. The exercise intensity for each stage of the various treadmill test protocols can be expressed in METs. The MET estimations for each stage of some commonly used treadmill protocols are listed in table 4.4.

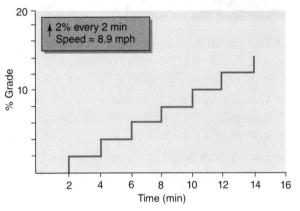

Costill and Fox (1969)
For: highly trained
Warm-up: 10-min walk or run
Initial workload: 8.9 mph, 0%, 2 min

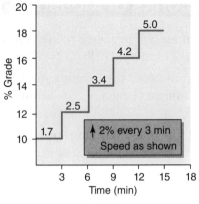

Bruce et al. (1973)
For: normal and high risk
Initial workload: 1.7 mph, 10%, 3 min = normal
                 1.7 mph, 0-5%, 3 min = high risk

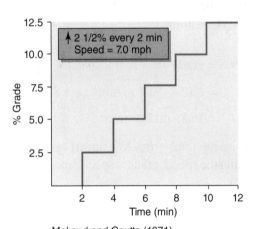

Maksud and Coutts (1971)
For: highly trained
Warm-up: 10-min walking, 3.5 mph, 0%
Initial workload: 7 mph, 0%, 2 min

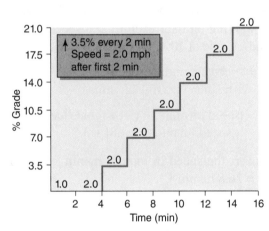

Naughton et al. (1964)
For: cardiac and high risk
Initial workload: 1.0 mph, 0%, 2 min

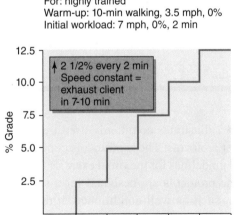

Modified Åstrand (Pollock et al. 1978)
For: highly trained
Warm-up: 5-min walk or jog
Initial workload: 5-8 mph, 0%, 3 min

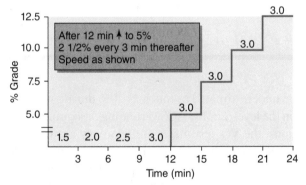

Wilson et al. (1978)
For: cardiac and high risk
Initial workload: 1.5 mph, 0%, 3 min

FIGURE 4.2 Treadmill exercise test protocols.

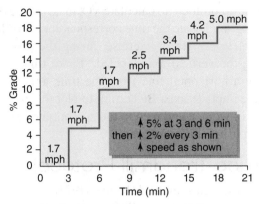

Modified Bruce (Lerman et al. 1976)
For: normal and high risk
Initial workload: 1.7 mph, 0%, 3 min

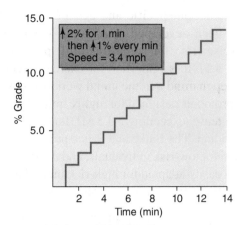

Balke and Ware (1959)
For: normal risk
Initial workload: 3.4 mph, 0%, 1 min

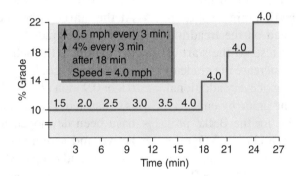

Kattus (1968)
For: cardiac and high risk
Initial workload: 1.5 mph, 10%, 3 min

FIGURE 4.2 *(continued)*

Table 4.4   **MET Estimations for Each Stage of Commonly Used Treadmill Protocols**

Stage[a]	Bruce	Modified Bruce[b]	Balke	Naughton
1	4.6	2.3	3.6	1.8
2	7.0	3.5	4.5	3.5
3	10.2	4.6	5.0	4.5
4	12.1	7.0	5.5	5.4
5	14.9	10.2	5.9	6.4
6	17.0	12.1	6.4	7.4
7	19.3	14.9	6.9	8.3

[a]Percent grade and speed for each stage are illustrated in figure 4.2.

[b]Stage 1 = 0% grade, 1.7 mph; Stage 2 = 5% grade, 1.7 mph.

Population-specific and generalized equations have been developed to estimate $\dot{V}O_2$ max from exercise time for some treadmill protocols (see table 4.5). It is important for exercise technicians to keep in mind that the initial workload in some of the protocols designed for highly trained athletes is too intense (exceeding 2-3.5 METs) for the average individual. The Balke and Bruce protocols are well suited for low-risk individuals, and the Bruce protocol is easily adapted for high-risk individuals using an initial workload of 1.7 mph at 0% to 5% grade.

Balke Treadmill Protocol

To administer the Balke and Ware (1959) exercise test protocol (see figure 4.2), set the treadmill speed at 3.4 mph (91.1 m·min⁻¹) and the initial grade of the treadmill at 0% during the first minute of exercise. Maintain a constant speed on the treadmill throughout the entire exercise test. At the start of the second minute of exercise, increase the grade to 2%. Thereafter, at the beginning of every additional minute of exercise, increase the grade by only 1%.

Use the prediction equation for the Balke protocol in table 4.5 to estimate a client's $\dot{V}O_2$ max from exercise time. Alternatively, you can use a nomogram (see figure 4.3) developed for the Balke treadmill protocol to calculate $\dot{V}O_2$ max. To use this nomogram, locate the time corresponding to the last complete minute of exercise during the protocol along the vertical axis labeled "Balke time," and draw a horizontal line from the time axis to the oxygen uptake axis. Be certain to plot the exercise time of women and men in the appropriate column when using this nomogram.

Bruce Treadmill Protocol

The Bruce, Kusumi, and Hosmer (1973) exercise test is a multistaged treadmill protocol (see figure 4.3). The protocol increases the workload by changing both the treadmill speed and percent grade. During the first stage (minutes 1-3) of the test, the normal individual walks at a 1.7 mph pace at 10% grade. At the start of the second stage (minutes 4-6), increase the grade by 2% and the speed to 2.5 mph (67 m·min⁻¹). In each subsequent stage of the test, increase the grade by 2% and the speed by either 0.8 or 0.9 mph (21.4 or 24.1 m·min⁻¹) until the client is exhausted. Prediction equations for this protocol have been developed to estimate the $\dot{V}O_2$ max of active and sedentary women and men, cardiac patients, and people who are elderly (see table 4.5). As an alternative, you may use the nomogram (see

Table 4.5 Population-Specific and Generalized Equations for Treadmill Protocols

Protocol	Population	Reference	Equation
Balke	Active and sedentary men	Pollock et al. (1976)	$\dot{V}O_2$max = 1.444(time) + 14.99 r = .92, SEE = 2.50 (ml·kg⁻¹·min⁻¹)
	Active and sedentary women[a]	Pollock et al. (1982)	$\dot{V}O_2$max = 1.38(time) + 5.22 r = .94, SEE = 2.20 (ml·kg⁻¹·min⁻¹)
Bruce[b]	Active and sedentary men	Foster et al. (1984)	$\dot{V}O_2$max = 14.76 − 1.379(time) + 0.451(time²) − 0.012(time³) r = .98, SEE = 3.35 (ml·kg⁻¹·min⁻¹)
	Active and sedentary women	Pollock et al. (1982)	$\dot{V}O_2$max = 4.38(time) − 3.90 r = .91, SEE = 2.7 (ml·kg⁻¹·min⁻¹)
	Cardiac patients and elderly persons[c]	McConnell and Clark (1987)	$\dot{V}O_2$max = 2.282(time) + 8.545 r = .82, SEE = 4.9 (ml·kg⁻¹·min⁻¹)
Naughton	Male cardiac patients	Foster et al. (1983)	$\dot{V}O_2$max = 1.61(time) + 3.60 r = .97, SEE = 2.60 (ml·kg⁻¹·min⁻¹)

SEE = standard error of estimate.

[a]For women, the Balke protocol was modified: speed 3.0 mph; initial workload 0% grade for 3 min, increasing 2.5% every 3 min thereafter.

[b]For use with the standard Bruce protocol; cannot be used with modified Bruce protocol.

[c]This equation is used only for treadmill walking while holding the handrails.

figure 4.4) developed for the Bruce protocol. Plot the client's exercise time for this protocol along the vertical axis labeled "Bruce time," and draw a horizontal line from the time axis to the oxygen uptake. Again, be certain to use the appropriate column for men and women.

Modified Bruce Protocol

The modified Bruce protocol (see figure 4.2) is more suitable than the Bruce protocol for high-risk and elderly individuals. However, with the exception of the first two stages, this protocol is similar to the standard Bruce protocol. Stage 1 starts at 0% grade and a 1.7 mph walking pace. For stage 2, the % grade is increased to 5%. McInnis and Balady (1994) compared physiological responses to the stan-

dard and modified Bruce protocols in patients with CHD and reported similar HR and BP responses at matched exercise stages despite the additional 6 min of low-intensity exercise performed using the modified Bruce protocol.

Note that the prediction equations for the Bruce protocol (see table 4.5) can be used for only the standard, not the modified, Bruce protocol. To estimate $\dot{V}O_2$ for the modified Bruce protocol, use the ACSM metabolic equation for walking (see table 4.3).

Self-Paced Protocols

Self-paced protocols are designed to be somewhat free-form in that the individual adjusts the treadmill speed and incline or cycling workload to his liking with the understanding that he needs to reach the

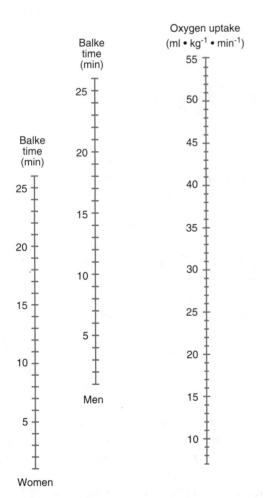

FIGURE 4.3 Nomogram for Balke graded exercise test.

Reprinted by permission from N.K. Ng, *METCALC Software: Metabolic Calculations in Exercise and Fitness* (Champaign, IL: Human Kinetics, 1995), 30.

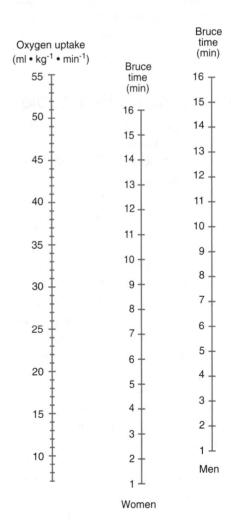

FIGURE 4.4 Nomogram for standard Bruce graded exercise test.

Reprinted by permission from N.K. Ng, *METCALC Software: Metabolic Calculations in Exercise and Fitness* (Champaign, IL: Human Kinetics, 1995), 32.

point of exhaustion within 8 to 12 min. In most situations, speed and incline can only be adjusted upward. Periodic data collection is required, just as it is with standard GXTs. Also, when metabolic gas analysis collection is used with this style of ramp protocol, a specific time increment (e.g., every 30 sec) is identified; HR and RPE are obtained and expired gas values during that increment are averaged for further analysis. In this example, $\dot{V}O_2$ max may then be identified as the highest 30 sec average. Comparison of these incremental averages from the last minute or two of the protocol may reveal the attainment of a $\dot{V}O_2$ plateau (e.g., <2 ml·kg^{-1}·min^{-1} increase; Nieman 2003).

Sperlich and colleagues (2015) compared self-paced, standard GXT, and ramped maximal exertion treadmill protocols. Their results indicate that a self-paced protocol can be completed, on average, within 10 min and produce RPE, blood lactate, HR, and RER values that satisfy the secondary criteria for determining maximal exertion. The lowest $\dot{V}O_2$ max occurred with the standard GXT protocol.

Treadmill Ramp Protocols

Kaminsky and Whaley (1998) developed a standardized ramp protocol (i.e., BSU/Bruce ramp protocol) for assessing the functional cardiorespiratory capacity of symptomatic, sedentary, and apparently healthy individuals. For this protocol, the treadmill speed increases gradually (in 0.1-0.4 mph, or 2.68-10.72 m·min^{-1}, increments) every minute. The minimum speed is 1.0 mph (26.8 m·min^{-1}); the maximum speed is 5.8 mph (155 m·min^{-1}). The treadmill grade also increases gradually (by 0%-5%) every minute. The minimum grade is 0%; the maximum grade is 20%. Every 3 min during this ramp protocol, the work rates (i.e., speed and grade) equal those of the traditional Bruce protocol (see table 4.6). For example, during the sixth minute of exercise, the treadmill speed (2.5 mph, or 53.6 m·min^{-1}) and grade (12%) are the same, allowing comparisons between the two types of protocols. The ramp approach has the advantage of avoiding large, unequal increments in workload. Also, it results in uniform increases in hemodynamic and physiological responses to incremental exercise and more accurately estimates exercise capacity and ventilatory threshold.

Porszasz and colleagues (2003) devised a ramp protocol that increases work rate linearly so that the individual walking on a treadmill reaches

Table 4.6 Comparison of Work Rates for the Standard Bruce Protocol and the Bruce Ramp Protocol

Minute[a]	SPEED (MPH)[b]		GRADE (%)	
	SB	BR	SB	BR
1	1.7	1.0	10	0
2	1.7	1.3	10	5
3	*1.7*	*1.7*	*10*	*10*
4	2.5	2.1	12	10
5	2.5	2.3	12	11
6	*2.5*	*2.5*	*12*	*12*
7	3.4	2.8	14	12
8	3.4	3.1	14	13
9	*3.4*	*3.4*	*14*	*14*
10	4.2	3.8	16	14
11	4.2	4.1	16	15
12	*4.2*	*4.2*	*16*	*16*
13	5.0	4.5	18	16
14	5.0	4.8	18	17
15	*5.0*	*5.0*	*18*	*18*
16	5.5	5.3	20	18
17	5.5	5.6	20	19
18	5.5	5.8	20	20

SB = standard Bruce protocol; BR = Bruce ramp protocol.

[a]Boldfaced italics identify the times during the two protocols when the work rates are equivalent.

[b]To convert mph to m·min^{-1}, multiply by 26.8.

exhaustion in approximately 10 min. To linearly increase work rate over time, it is necessary to couple linear increases in walking speed with curvilinear increases in treadmill grade. Because this protocol starts with slow walking (i.e., 0.5-1.0 mph, or 13.4-26.8 m·min^{-1}), it is suitable for individuals with low exercise tolerance as well as for sedentary individuals with a range of exercise tolerances. As with all types of ramp protocols, this protocol is individualized. The peak work rate, a comfortable range of walking speeds, and the increments in treadmill incline or grade are determined for each client.

This protocol compares favorably to cycle ergometer ramp protocols that increase work rate linearly so that maximum exercise tolerance is reached in ~10 min. The slope of the relationship between $\dot{V}O_2$ and work rate, however, is consistently steeper on the treadmill than on the cycle ergometer (Porszasz et al. 2003). This steeper slope reflects additional use of the limbs (i.e., swinging the arms and legs) and frictional force as treadmill speed increases. For each individual, the time course for the grade increments needed to elicit a linear increase in work rate can be calculated with a prediction equation based on the client's body weight, desired initial and final walking speeds, initial grade, and estimated peak work rate (see Porszasz et al. 2003). These individual variables, along with the prediction equation for increasing grade, can be programmed into the computer of a contemporary treadmill. Thus, each individualized ramp protocol is controlled by the computer so that the frequent increases in speed and grade are smooth and rapid.

Video 4.4

CYCLE ERGOMETER MAXIMAL EXERCISE TESTS

The cycle ergometer is a widely used instrument for assessing cardiorespiratory fitness and is the preferred modality for exercise tests conducted on individuals with conditions affecting their ability to safely walk or jog on a treadmill (Balady et al. 2010). On a friction-type cycle ergometer (see figure 4.5), resistance is applied against the flywheel using a belt and weighted pendulums. The hand wheel adjusts the workload by tightening or loosening the brake belt. The workload on the cycle ergometer is raised through increases in the resistance on the flywheel. The power output is usually expressed in kilogram-meters per minute (kgm·min^{-1}) or watts (1 W ≈ 6 kgm·min^{-1}) and is easily measured using the equation

$$power = force \times distance / time$$

where force equals the resistance or tension setting on the ergometer (kilograms) and distance is the distance traveled by the flywheel rim for each revolution of the pedal multiplied by the number of revolutions per minute. On the Monark and Bodyguard cycle ergometers, the flywheel travels 6 m per pedal revolution. Therefore, if a resistance of 2 kg is applied and the pedaling rate is 60 rpm, then

$$power = 2 \text{ kg} \times 6 \text{ m} \times 60 \text{ rpm} = 720 \text{ kgm·min}^{-1}$$
$$or\ 120\ W.$$

To calculate the distance traveled by the flywheel of cycle ergometers with varying-sized flywheels,

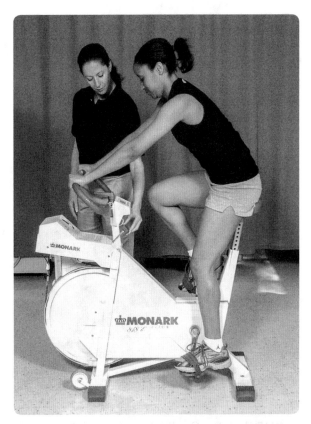

FIGURE 4.5 Cycle ergometer (mechanically braked).

measure the circumference (in meters) of the resistance track on the flywheel and multiply the circumference by the number of flywheel revolutions during one complete revolution (360°) of the pedal (Gledhill and Jamnik 1995).

When you are standardizing the work performed on a friction-type cycle ergometer, the client should maintain a constant pedaling rate. Some cycle ergometers have a speedometer that displays the individual's pedaling rate. Check this dial frequently to make certain your client is maintaining a constant pedaling frequency throughout the test. If a speedometer is not available, use a metronome to establish your client's pedaling cadence. Controlling the pedaling rate on an electrically braked cycle ergometer (figure 4.6) is unnecessary. An electromagnetic braking force adjusts the resistance for slower or faster pedaling rates, thereby keeping the power output constant. This type of cycle ergometer, however, is difficult to calibrate.

Most cycle ergometer test protocols for untrained cyclists use a pedaling rate of 50 or 60 rpm, and

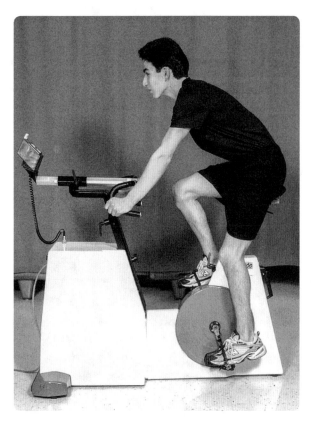

FIGURE 4.6 Cycle ergometer (electrically braked).

power outputs are increased by 150 to 300 kgm·min^{-1} (25-50 W) in each stage of the test. However, you can use higher pedaling rates (≥80 rpm) for trained cyclists. A pedaling rate of 60 rpm produces the highest $\dot{V}O_2$max when compared with rates of 50, 70, or 80 rpm (Hermansen and Saltin 1969). Figure 4.7 illustrates some widely used discontinuous and continuous maximal exercise test protocols for the cycle ergometer. Guidelines for use of cycle ergometers are presented in Testing With Cycle Ergometers.

To calculate the energy expenditure for cycle ergometer exercise, use the ACSM equations provided in table 4.3. The total energy expenditure or gross $\dot{V}O_2$, in ml·kg^{-1}·min^{-1}, is a function of the oxygen cost of pedaling against resistance (power output in watts), the oxygen cost of unloaded cycling (approximately 3.5 ml·kg^{-1}·min^{-1} at 50-60 rpm with zero resistance), and the resting oxygen consumption. The cost of cycling against an external load or resistance is approximately 1.8 ml·kg^{-1}·m^{-1}. For a sample calculation, see ACSM Leg Ergometry Equation.

Keep in mind that the leg and arm ergometry equations are accurate in estimating $\dot{V}O_2$ only if the client attains a steady state during the maximal GXT. If, for example, the client is able to complete only 1 min of exercise during the last stage of the maximal test protocol, the power output from the previous stage (in which the client reached steady state) should be used to estimate $\dot{V}O_2$max rather than the power output corresponding to the last stage.

Testing With Cycle Ergometers

The following guidelines are suggested for the use of cycle ergometers:

1. Calibrate the cycle ergometer often by hanging known weights from the belt of the flywheel and reading the dial on the hand wheel.

2. Always release the tension on the belt between tests.

3. Establish pedaling frequency before setting the workload.

4. Check the load setting frequently during the test because it may change as the belt warms up.

5. Set the metronome so that one revolution is completed for every two beats (e.g., set the metronome at 120 for a test requiring a pedaling frequency of 60 rpm).

6. Adjust the height of the seat so the knee is slightly flexed (about 25°) at maximal leg extension with the ball of the foot on the pedal.

7. Have the client assume an upright seated posture, with hands properly positioned on the handlebars.

Åstrand (1965)
Type: continuous
For: normal risk
Initial workload: 600 kgm (100 W) (men)
                       300 kgm (50 W) (women)

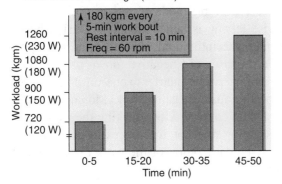

Fox (1973)
Type: discontinuous
For: normal risk
Initial workload: 750-900 kgm (125-150 W) (men)
                       450-600 kgm (75-100 W) (women)

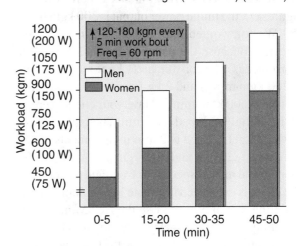

Åstrand (1956)
Type: discontinuous
For: normal risk
Initial workload: 720 kgm (100 W)

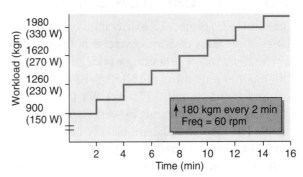

McArdle et al. (1973)
Type: continuous
For: normal risk
Initial workload: 900 kgm (150 W)

FIGURE 4.7   Cycle ergometer exercise test protocols.

ACSM Leg Ergometry Equation

To calculate the energy expenditure of a 62 kg (136 lb) woman cycling at a work rate or power output of 360 kgm·min⁻¹, follow these steps:

1. Calculate the energy cost of cycling at the specified power output.

   $\dot{V}O_2$ = work rate[a] (W) / body mass (M) × 1.8

   = 360 kgm·min⁻¹ / 62 kg × 1.8

   = 10.45 ml·kg⁻¹·min⁻¹

2. Add the estimated cost of cycling at zero load (i.e., 3.5 ml·kg⁻¹·min⁻¹).

   $\dot{V}O_2$ = 10.45 ml·kg⁻¹·min⁻¹ + 3.5 ml·kg⁻¹·min⁻¹

   = 13.95 ml·kg⁻¹·min⁻¹

3. Add the estimated resting energy expenditure (3.5 ml·kg⁻¹·min⁻¹).

   $\dot{V}O_2$ = 13.95 ml·kg⁻¹·min⁻¹ + 3.5 ml·kg⁻¹·min⁻¹

   = 17.45 ml·kg⁻¹·min⁻¹

[a]Work rate is in kgm·min⁻¹.

Video
4.5

Åstrand Cycle Ergometer Maximal Test Protocol

For the Åstrand (1965) continuous test protocol (see figure 4.7), the initial power output is 300 kgm·min^{-1} (50 W) for women and 600 kgm·min^{-1} (100 W) for men. Because the pedaling rate is 50 rpm, the resistance is 1 kg for women (1 kg × 6 m × 50 rpm = 300 kgm·min^{-1}) and 2 kg for men (2 kg × 6 m × 50 rpm = 600 kgm·min^{-1}). Have your client exercise at this initial workload for 2 min. Then increase the power output every 2 to 3 min in increments of 150 kgm·min^{-1} (25 W) and 300 kgm·min^{-1} (50 W) for women and men, respectively. Continue the test until the client is exhausted or can no longer maintain the pedaling rate of 50 rpm. Use the ACSM metabolic equation for leg ergometry to estimate $\dot{V}O_2$ from your client's power output during the last steady-state stage of the GXT.

Fox Cycle Ergometer Maximal Test Protocol

The Fox (1973) protocol is a discontinuous test consisting of a series of 5 min exercise bouts with 10 min rest intervals. The starting workload is between 750 and 900 kgm·min^{-1} (125-150 W) for men and 450 and 600 kgm·min^{-1} (75-100 W) for women. The progressive increments in work depend on the client's HR response and are usually between 120 and 180 kgm·min^{-1} (20-30 W). The client exercises until exhausted or until no longer able to pedal for at least 3 min at a power output that is 60 to 90 kgm·min^{-1} (10-15 W) higher than the previous workload. You can use the metabolic equations to convert the power output from the last steady-state stage of this protocol to $\dot{V}O_2$max.

Self-Paced Cycle Ergometer Maximal Test Protocol

For self-paced cycle ergometer protocols, the client adjusts the pedaling cadence and flywheel resistance throughout the test protocol. Mauger and Sculthorpe (2012) designed a self-paced, maximal exertion 10-min protocol. This protocol requires the rider to select workloads for five 2 min stages. For each stage, there is a target RPE, also known as a stage "clamp", culminating in an RPE of 20 on the Borg scale for the last stage. Compared with the traditional cycling protocol, the self-paced **RPE-clamped protocol** results in a $\dot{V}O_2$max value that is approximately 8% higher and a peak power output that is 35 W higher, on average. Conversely, other researchers report no difference in maximal values for self-paced RPE-clamped protocols compared with more traditional ones using the same modality (Chidnok et al. 2013; Evans, Parfitt, and Eston 2014). The self-paced protocol is perceived as being preferred over the traditional ramp protocol (Evans, Parfitt, and Eston 2014). The clamping technique produces similar maximal results in comparison to standardized protocols, regardless of the modality; therefore, it is a viable alternative for maximal exertion testing.

BENCH STEPPING MAXIMAL EXERCISE TESTS

The least desirable mode of exercise for maximum exercise testing is bench stepping. During bench stepping, the individual is performing both positive (up phase) and negative (down phase) work. Approximately one-quarter to one-third less energy is expended during negative work (Morehouse 1972). This factor, coupled with adjusting the step height and stepping rate for differences in body weight, makes standardization of the work extremely difficult.

General Procedures

Most step test protocols increase the intensity of the work by gradually increasing the height of the bench or stepping rate. The work (W) performed can be calculated using the equation W = F × D, where F is body weight in kilograms and D is bench height multiplied by number of steps per minute. For example, a 50 kg (110 lb) woman stepping at a rate of 22 steps·min^{-1} on a 30 cm (0.30 m) bench is performing 330 kgm·min^{-1} of work (50 kg × 0.30 m × 22 steps·min^{-1}).

The following equations can be used to adjust the step height and stepping rate for differences in body weight to achieve a given work rate (Morehouse 1972):

$$\text{step height (cm)} = \text{work (kgcm·min}^{-1})$$
$$/ \text{body weight (kg)}$$
$$\times \text{stepping rate}$$

$$\text{stepping rate (steps·min}^{-1}) = \text{work (kgcm·min}^{-1})$$
$$/ \text{body weight (kg)}$$
$$\times \text{step height (cm)}$$

For example, if you devise a graded step test protocol that requires a client weighing 60 kg (132 lb) to exercise at a work rate of 300 kgm·min^{-1}, and the stepping rate is set at 18 steps·min^{-1}, you need to determine the step height that corresponds to the work rate:

$$\text{step height} = 300 \text{ kgm·min}^{-1} / (60 \text{ kg} \times 18$$
$$\text{steps·min}^{-1})$$

$$= 0.28 \text{ m, or 28 cm}$$

Alternatively, you may choose to keep the step height constant and vary the stepping cadence for each stage of the GXT. For example, if the step height is set at 30 cm (0.30 m), and the protocol requires that a client weighing 60 kg (132 lb) exercise at a work rate of 450 kgm·min^{-1}, you need to calculate the corresponding stepping rate for this client:

$$\text{stepping rate} = 450 \text{ kgm·min}^{-1} / (60 \text{ kg} \times 0.30 \text{ m})$$

$$= 25 \text{ steps·min}^{-1}$$

You can calculate the energy expenditure in METs using the ACSM metabolic equation for stepping exercise (see table 4.3). The total gross $\dot{V}O_2$ is a function of step frequency, step height, and the resting energy expenditure. The oxygen cost of the horizontal movement is approximately 0.2 ml·kg^{-1}·m^{-1} for each four-count stepping cycle. The oxygen demand for stepping up is 1.8 ml·kg^{-1}·m^{-1}; approximately one-third more must be added (i.e., constant of 1.33 in equation) to account for the oxygen cost of stepping down. For an example of such calculations, see ACSM Stepping Equation.

Nagle, Balke, and Naughton Maximal Step Test Protocol

Nagle, Balke, and Naughton (1965) devised a graded step test for assessing work capacity. Have your client step at a rate of 30 steps·min^{-1} on an automatically adjustable bench (2-50 cm). Set the initial bench height at 2 cm and increase the height 2 cm every minute of exercise. Use a metronome to

ACSM Stepping Equation

To calculate the energy expenditure for bench stepping using a 16 in. (about 40 cm) step height at a cadence of 24 steps·min^{-1}, use the following procedure:

$$\dot{V}O_2 \text{ in ml·kg}^{-1}·\text{min}^{-1} = [\text{frequency (F) in} \text{ steps·min}^{-1}$$
$$\times 0.2] + (\text{step height in m·step}^{-1}$$
$$\times \text{F in steps·min}^{-1} \times 1.33$$
$$\times 1.8) + \text{resting } \dot{V}O_2$$

1. Calculate the $\dot{V}O_2$ for the stepping frequency (F).

$$\dot{V}O_2 = \text{stepping frequency (F)} \times 0.20$$
$$= 24 \text{ steps·min}^{-1} \times 0.20$$
$$= 4.8 \text{ ml·kg}^{-1}·\text{min}^{-1}$$

2. Convert the bench height to meters (1 in. = 2.54 cm or 0.0254 m).

$$\text{ht} = 16 \text{ in.} \times 0.0254 \text{ m}$$
$$= 0.4064 \text{ m}$$

3. Calculate the $\dot{V}O_2$ for the vertical work performed during stepping.

$$\dot{V}O_2 = \text{bench ht} \times \text{stepping rate} \times 1.33 \times 1.8$$
$$= 0.4064 \text{ m} \times 24 \text{ steps·min}^{-1} \times 1.33 \times 1.8$$
$$= 23.35 \text{ ml·kg}^{-1}·\text{min}^{-1}$$

4. Add resting $\dot{V}O_2$ to the calculated $\dot{V}O_2$ from steps 1 and 3.

$$\dot{V}O_2 = 4.8 \text{ ml·kg}^{-1}·\text{min}^{-1} + 23.35 \text{ ml·kg}^{-1}·\text{min}^{-1}$$
$$+ 3.5 \text{ ml·kg}^{-1}·\text{min}^{-1}$$
$$= 31.65 \text{ ml·kg}^{-1}·\text{min}^{-1}$$

establish the stepping cadence (four beats per stepping cycle). To establish a cadence of 30 steps·min^{-1}, set the metronome at 120 (30 × 4). Terminate the test when the subject is fatigued or can no longer maintain the stepping cadence. Use the ACSM metabolic equation for stepping exercise to calculate the energy expenditure ($\dot{V}O_2$max) corresponding to the step height and stepping cadence during the last work stage of this protocol.

RECUMBENT STEPPER MAXIMAL EXERCISE TEST

Billinger and colleagues (2008) developed a maximum exercise test using a total body recumbent stepper (NuStep TRS 4000). The protocol begins with a 2 min warm-up at load setting 1 (50 W). Immediately after the warm-up, the initial workload is set to 4 (75 W). The resistance is increased progressively until the participant reaches test termination criteria. A constant cadence (115 steps·min^{-1}) is used throughout the exercise protocol. Compared with treadmill testing (Bruce protocol), the recumbent stepper test elicits a lower HRmax (181 vs. 188 bpm) and $\dot{V}O_2$ (3.13 vs. 3.67 L·min^{-1}) on average. These differences are expected given the seated posture during the recumbent stepper exercise test. The correlation coefficients for $\dot{V}O_2$max ($r = .92$) and HRmax ($r = .96$) indicate a strong relationship between the Bruce protocol and the recumbent stepper protocol.

This test modality may be especially useful for assessing the cardiorespiratory fitness of individuals with neuromuscular disorders that impair gait, coordination, and balance. Seated steppers are now widely used as a training modality in rehabilitation centers, fitness centers, and retirement communities.

SUBMAXIMAL EXERCISE TEST PROTOCOLS

It is desirable to directly determine the functional cardiorespiratory capacity of the individual for classifying the aerobic fitness level and prescribing an aerobic exercise program. However, this is not always practical to do. The actual measurement of $\dot{V}O_2$max requires expensive laboratory equipment,

a considerable amount of time to administer, and a high level of motivation on the part of the client.

Alternatively, you can use submaximal exercise tests to predict or estimate the $\dot{V}O_2$max of the individual. Many of these tests are similar to the maximal exercise tests described previously but differ in that they are terminated at some predetermined HR intensity. You will monitor the HR, BP, and RPE during the submaximal exercise test. The treadmill, cycle ergometer, and bench stepping exercises are commonly used for submaximal exercise testing.

ASSUMPTIONS OF SUBMAXIMAL EXERCISE TESTS

Submaximal exercise tests assume that a *steady-state HR* is achieved and is consistent for each exercise work rate. Steady-state HR is usually achieved in 3 to 4 min at a constant submaximal work rate. Also, it is assumed that a *linear relationship exists between $\dot{V}O_2$ and HR* within the range of 110 to 150 bpm. The HR and work rate from two submaximal work outputs can be plotted (i.e., HR-$\dot{V}O_2$ relationship) and extrapolated to HRmax to estimate $\dot{V}O_2$max from submaximal data (see figure 4.10). Although the linear relationship between HR and $\dot{V}O_2$ holds for light to moderate workloads, the relationship between oxygen uptake and work rate becomes curvilinear at heavier workloads. If your clients are taking medications that alter HR, you should not use submaximal HR data to estimate their $\dot{V}O_2$max.

Another assumption of submaximal testing is that the *mechanical efficiency during cycling or treadmill exercise is constant for all individuals.* However, a client with poor mechanical efficiency while cycling has a higher submaximal HR at a given workload, and the actual $\dot{V}O_2$max is underestimated because of this inefficiency. As a result, $\dot{V}O_2$max predicted by submaximal exercise tests tends to be overestimated for highly trained individuals and underestimated for untrained, sedentary individuals.

Submaximal tests also assume that the *HRmax for clients of a given age is similar.* However, it has been shown to vary as much as ±11 bpm, even after controlling for variability due to age and training status (Londeree and Moeschberger 1984). Also, for submaximal tests, the HRmax is estimated from age. The equation HRmax = 220 − age is widely used. The HRmax of approximately 5% to 7% of men and women is more than 15 bpm less than their age-predicted values. On the other hand, 9% to 13% exceed their age-predicted HRmax by more than 15 bpm (Whaley et al. 1992). Because of interindividual variability in HRmax and the potential inaccuracy with use of age-predicted values, there may be considerable error (±10%-15%) in estimating your clients' $\dot{V}O_2$ max, especially when submaximal data are extrapolated to an age-predicted HRmax.

In addition, Tanaka, Monahan, and Seals (2001) noted that the traditional age-predicted equation (220 − age) overestimates the measured HRmax of younger individuals and increasingly underestimates the actual HRmax of individuals older than 40 yr. After reviewing numerous studies of healthy adults (18-81 yr), the authors reported that age singly accounts for 80% of the variance in HRmax and is independent of gender and physical activity status. They derived an equation to predict HRmax from age: HRmax = 208 − (0.7 × age). Estimates from this equation differ from those of the traditional one, particularly in older (>40 yr) adults. For example, the age-predicted HRmax for a 60 yr old client is 166 bpm for the revised equation (208 − [0.7 × 60] = 166 bpm) and 160 bpm for the traditional equation (220 − 60 = 160 bpm).

Gellish and colleagues (2007) modeled the relationship between HRmax and age as individuals grow older. Their data yielded a prediction equation (HRmax = 207 − [0.7 × age]) that is similar to the equation derived by Tanaka and colleagues (2001). The confidence interval (CI) for predicting HRmax of adults 30 to 75 yr was ±5 to 8 bpm. Additionally, Gellish and colleagues developed a quadratic equation, HRmax = 192 − (0.007 × age^2). Although this quadratic equation improves the prediction error (95% CI = ±2-5 bpm), it is not practical to use.

After determining there was no difference in HRmax compared to that obtained through treadmill testing, Cleary and colleagues (2011) suggested that the highest HR from two 200 m maximal exertion sprints is a suitable alternative to the age-related HRmax prediction equations for adults (18-33 yr). Of interest, they found that the Gellish quadratic equation and the gender-specific equations of Fairbarn and colleagues (1994) (women: [HRmax = 201 − (0.63 × age)]; men: HRmax = [208 − (0.80

× age)]) produced estimations similar to that from the 200 m sprint.

Because of interindividual variability in HRmax and the potential inaccuracy of age-predicted equations, the actual HRmax should be measured directly (by ECG or HR monitor) whenever possible. An accurate HRmax is particularly important in situations in which

- the exercise test is terminated at a predetermined percentage of either HRmax (%HRmax method) or heart rate reserve (HRR = % [HRmax − HRrest] + HRrest),
- the client's $\dot{V}O_2$ max is estimated from submaximal exercise test data that are extrapolated to an age-predicted HRmax,
- or HRmax is used to determine target exercise HRs for aerobic exercise prescriptions (see chapter 5).

TREADMILL SUBMAXIMAL EXERCISE TESTS

Video 4.6

Treadmill submaximal tests provide an estimate of functional cardiorespiratory capacity ($\dot{V}O_2$ max) and assume a linear increase in HR with successive increments in workload. Compared to clients with low cardiorespiratory fitness levels, the well-conditioned individual presumably is able to perform a greater quantity of work at a given submaximal HR.

A **perceptually regulated exercise test (PRET)** offers an alternative to estimating $\dot{V}O_2$ peak using HR. These tests are performed on cycle ergometers and treadmills. PRETs require that the workload be adjusted so that the individual exercises in a graded format (3 min stages) at intensities associated with four different RPE values (9, 11, 13, 15). Metabolic gas data collected during the last 30 sec of each stage are averaged and plotted against the corresponding RPE; the linear regression technique is used to extrapolate to an RPE of 19 or 20 for the estimation of $\dot{V}O_2$ peak.

Eston and colleagues (2012) validated a PRET for treadmill testing for a mixed group of active and sedentary adults (18-72 yr). They concluded that extrapolating to an RPE of 19 is valid for estimating $\dot{V}O_2$ peak for sedentary and active adults. Evans and colleagues (2015) included PRET protocols in their review of submaximal treadmill tests for estimating $\dot{V}O_2$peak. They discussed the importance of familiarizing individuals with the Borg 6 to 20 RPE scale before the test begins. Additionally, Evans and colleagues (2015) commented on the benefit of using self-identified workloads at each of the RPEs instead of using an age-predicted maximal HR.

You can also use treadmill maximal test protocols (figure 4.2) to identify the slope of an individual's HR response to exercise. The $\dot{V}O_2$max can be predicted from either one (single-stage model) or two (multistage model) submaximal HRs. The accuracy of the single-stage model is similar to that of the multistage model.

Multistage Model

To estimate $\dot{V}O_2$max with the multistage model, use the HR and workload data from two or more submaximal stages of the treadmill test. Be sure your client reaches steady-state HRs between 115 and 150 bpm (Golding 2000). Determine the slope (b)

by calculating the ratio of the difference between the two submaximal (SM) workloads (expressed as $\dot{V}O_2$) and the corresponding change in submaximal HRs:

$$b = (SM_2 - SM_1) / (HR_2 - HR_1)$$

Calculate the $\dot{V}O_2$ for each workload using the ACSM metabolic equation (table 4.3), and use the following equation to predict $\dot{V}O_2$max:

$$\dot{V}O_2max = SM_2 + b(HRmax - HR_2)$$

If the actual maximal HR is not known, estimate it using one of the age-predicted HRmax equations previously mentioned. See Multistage Model for Estimating $\dot{V}O_2$max for an example that illustrates how $\dot{V}O_2$max is estimated from submaximal treadmill test data for a 38 yr old male. In this example, the Bruce protocol was administered to the client. Please note that this model may be used for any multistage GXT test.

MULTISTAGE MODEL FOR ESTIMATING $\dot{V}O_2$MAX

Submaximal Data From Bruce Protocol

Stage 2[a]

$\dot{V}O_2$[b] = 24.5 ml·kg^{-1}·min^{-1} (SM$_2$)

HR = 145 bpm (HR$_2$)

Stage 1[a]

$\dot{V}O_2$ = 16.1 ml·kg^{-1}·min^{-1} (SM$_1$)

HR = 130 bpm (HR$_1$)

Maximal HR: 220 – age = 182 bpm

Slope (b) = (SM$_2$ – SM$_1$) / (HR$_2$ – HR$_1$)

$\quad$ b = (24.5 – 16.1) / (145 – 130)

$\quad$ b = 8.4 / 15

$\quad$ b = 0.56

$\dot{V}O_2$max: = SM$_2$ + b(HRmax – HR$_2$)

$\quad$ = 24.5 + 0.56(182 – 145)

$\quad$ = 24.5 + 20.72

$\dot{V}O_2$max = 45.22 ml·kg^{-1}·min^{-1}

[a]Stages 1 and 2 refer to the last two stages of the GXT completed by the client, and not the first and second stage of the test protocol. For example, if the client completes three stages of the submaximal exercise test protocol, data from stage 2 and stage 3 are used to estimate $\dot{V}O_2$.

[b]$\dot{V}O_2$ is calculated using ACSM metabolic equations (see table 4.3). $\dot{V}O_2$ can be expressed in L·min^{-1}, ml·kg^{-1}·min^{-1}, or METs.

Single-Stage Model

To estimate $\dot{V}O_2$ max with the single-stage model, use one submaximal HR and one workload. The steady-state submaximal HR during a single-stage GXT should reach 130 to 150 bpm. Formulas for Men and Women shows formulas that have been developed (Shephard 1972).

FORMULAS FOR MEN AND WOMEN

Men

$$\dot{V}O_2\text{max} = SM_{\dot{V}O_2} \times [(HR_{max} - 61) / (HR_{SM} - 61)]$$

Women

$$\dot{V}O_2\text{max} = SM_{\dot{V}O_2} \times [(HR_{max} - 72) / (HR_{SM} - 72)]$$

$SM_{\dot{V}O_2}$ is calculated using the ACSM metabolic equations (see table 4.3). Estimate HRmax (if not known) using one of the age-predicted HRmax formulas; HRsubmax is the submaximal HR.

Single-Stage Model for Estimating $\dot{V}O_2$ max provides an example to illustrate how this model is used to predict $\dot{V}O_2$ max from submaximal treadmill data for a 45 yr old female. In this example, the Balke protocol was administered. Please note that this model may be used for any GXT protocol.

Single-Stage Treadmill Walking Test

Ebbeling and colleagues (1991) developed a single-stage treadmill walking test suitable for estimating $\dot{V}O_2$ max of healthy, low-risk adults 20 to 59 yr. The Ebbeling treadmill test also produced high test-retest reliability and validity with $\dot{V}O_2$ max for a sample of middle-aged (45-65 yr) women (Mitros et al. 2011). For this protocol, walking speed is individualized and ranges from 2.0 to 4.5 mph (53.6-120.6 m·min^{-1}) depending on your client's age, gender, and fitness level. Establish a walking pace during a 4 min warm-up at 0% grade. The warm-up work bout should produce a HR within 50% to 70% of the individual's age-predicted HRmax. The test consists of brisk walking at the selected pace for an additional 4 min at 5% grade. Record the steady-state HR at this workload, and use

SINGLE-STAGE MODEL FOR ESTIMATING $\dot{V}O_2$ MAX

Submaximal Data From Balke Protocol: Stage 3

$$\dot{V}O_2 = 5.0 \text{ METs } (SM_{\dot{V}O_2})$$
$$HR = 148 \text{ bpm } (HR_{SM})$$

Maximal HR: 220 – age = 175 bpm

$$\dot{V}O_2\text{max}: = SM_{\dot{V}O_2} \times [(HR_{max} - 72)$$
$$/ (HR\text{submax} - 72)]$$
$$= 5 \times [(175 - 72) / (148 - 72)]$$
$$= 5 \times (103 / 76)$$
$$= 6.8 \text{ METs}$$

it in the following equation to estimate $\dot{V}O_2$ max:

$\dot{V}O_2$ max = 15.1 + 21.8(speed in mph) (ml·kg^{-1}·min^{-1})

– 0.327(HR in bpm)

– 0.263(speed × age in years)

+ 0.00504(HR × age)

+ 5.48(gender: female = 0; male = 1)

Single-Stage Treadmill Jogging Test

You can estimate the $\dot{V}O_2$ max of younger adults (18-28 yr) using a single-stage treadmill jogging test (George et al. 1993). For this test, select a comfortable jogging pace ranging from 4.3 to 7.5 mph (115.2-201 m·min^{-1}), but not more than 6.5 mph (174.2 m·min^{-1}) for women and 7.5 mph (201 m·min^{-1}) for men. Have the client jog at a constant speed for about 3 min. The steady-state exercise HR should not exceed 180 bpm. Estimate $\dot{V}O_2$ max using the following equation:

$\dot{V}O_2$ max = 54.07 – 0.1938(body weight in kg (ml·kg^{-1}·min^{-1})

+ 4.47(speed in mph)

– 0.1453(HR in bpm)

+ 7.062(gender: female = 0; male = 1)

Video
4.7

CYCLE ERGOMETER SUBMAXIMAL EXERCISE TESTS

Cycle ergometer multistage submaximal tests can be used to predict $\dot{V}O_2$ max. These tests are either continuous or discontinuous and are based on the assumption that HR and oxygen uptake are linear functions of work rate. The HR response to submaximal workloads is used to predict $\dot{V}O_2$ max.

Alternatively, PRETs may be used if metabolic gases are collected during the submaximal cycling test. Instruct your client to pedal for 3 min each at an RPE of 9, 11, 13, and 15. Plot the average $\dot{V}O_2$ from the last 30 sec of each stage against the respective RPE value. Extrapolate the regression line to an RPE of 20 to estimate $\dot{V}O_2$ peak. PRETs remove errors associated with using an equation to calculate an age-predicted maximal heart rate (Coquart et al. 2016; Evans et al. 2015).

Åstrand-Ryhming Cycle Ergometer Submaximal Exercise Test Protocol

The Åstrand-Ryhming protocol (1954) is a single-stage test that uses a nomogram to predict $\dot{V}O_2$ max from HR response to one 6 min submaximal workload. A power output is selected that produces a HR between 125 and 170 bpm. The initial workload is usually 450 to 600 kgm·min⁻¹ (75-100 W) for trained, physically active women and 600 to 900 kgm·min⁻¹ (100-150 W) for trained, physically active men. An initial workload of 300 kgm·min⁻¹ (50 W) may be used for unconditioned or older individuals.

During the test, measure the HR every minute and record the average HR during the fifth and sixth minutes. If the difference between these two HRs exceeds 5 or 6 bpm, extend the work bout until a steady-state HR is achieved. If the HR is less than 130 bpm at the end of the exercise bout, increase the workload by 300 kgm·min⁻¹ (50 W) and have the client exercise an additional 6 min.

To estimate $\dot{V}O_2$ max for this protocol, use the modified Åstrand-Ryhming nomogram (see figure 4.8). This nomogram estimates $\dot{V}O_2$ max (in L·min⁻¹) from submaximal treadmill, cycle ergometer, and step test data. For each test mode, the submaximal HR is plotted with either oxygen cost for treadmill

exercise ($\dot{V}O_2$ in L·min⁻¹), power output (kgm·min⁻¹) for cycle ergometer exercise, or body weight (kg) for stepping exercise. For the cycle ergometer test, plot the client's power output (kgm·min⁻¹) and the steady-state exercise HR in the corresponding columns of the Åstrand-Ryhming nomogram (see figure 4.8). Connect these points with a ruler, and read the estimated $\dot{V}O_2$ max at the point where the line intersects the $\dot{V}O_2$ max column.

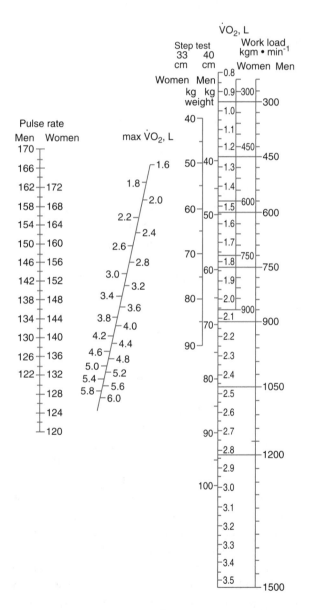

FIGURE 4.8 Modified Åstrand-Ryhming nomogram.

From "Aerobic Capacity in Men and Women with Special Reference to Age," by I. Åstrand, 1960. *Acta Physiologica Scandinavica* 49 (Suppl. 169), p. 51. Copyright 1960 by *Acta Physiologica Scandinavica*. Reprinted by permission.

The correlation between measured $\dot{V}O_2$ max and the $\dot{V}O_2$ max estimated from this nomogram is $r = .74$. The prediction error is ±10% and ±15%, respectively, for well-trained and untrained individuals (Åstrand and Rodahl 1977). A cross-validation study of this protocol and nomogram yielded a validity coefficient of .82 and a prediction error of 5.1 ml·kg^{-1}·min^{-1} for estimating the $\dot{V}O_2$ max of adults 18 to 44 yr (Swain et al. 2004).

For clients younger or older than 25 yr, you must use the following age-correction factors to adjust the $\dot{V}O_2$ max predicted from the nomogram for the effect of age. For example, if the estimated $\dot{V}O_2$ max from the nomogram is 3.2 L·min^{-1} for a 45 yr old client, the adjusted $\dot{V}O_2$ max is 2.5 L·min^{-1} (3.2 × 0.78 = 2.5 L·min^{-1}).

YMCA Cycle Ergometer Submaximal Exercise Test Protocol

The YMCA protocol (Golding 2000) is a cycle ergometer submaximal test for women and men. This protocol uses three or four consecutive 3 min workloads on the cycle ergometer designed to raise the HR to between 110 bpm and 85% of the age-predicted HRmax for at least two consecutive workloads. The pedal rate is 50 rpm, and the initial workload is 150 kgm·min^{-1} (25 W). Using a friction-type cycle ergometer, set the resistance to 0.5 kg (0.5 kg × 50 rpm × 6 m = 150 kgm·min^{-1}). To

achieve this work rate using a plate-loaded cycle ergometer, use one weight plate (1.0 kg) and reduce the pedaling frequency to 25 rpm (1.0 kg × 25 rpm × 6 m = 150 kgm·min^{-1}). Use the HR during the last minute of the initial workload to determine subsequent workloads (see figure 4.9). If the HR is less than 86 bpm, set the second workload at 600 kgm·min^{-1}. If HR is 86 to 100, the workload is 450 kgm·min^{-1} for the second stage of the protocol. If the HR at the end of the first workload exceeds 100 bpm, set the second workload at 300 kgm·min^{-1}.

Set the third and fourth workloads accordingly (see figure 4.9). Measure the HR during the last 30 sec of minutes 2 and 3 at each workload. If these HRs differ by more than 5 or 6 bpm, extend the workload an additional minute until the HR stabilizes. If the client's steady-state HR reaches or exceeds 85% of the age-predicted HRmax during the third workload, terminate the test.

Calculate the energy expenditure ($\dot{V}O_2$) for the last two workloads using the ACSM metabolic equations (see table 4.3). To estimate $\dot{V}O_2$ max from these data, use the equations for the multistage model to calculate the slope of the line depicting the HR response to the last two workloads. Alternatively, you can graph these data to estimate $\dot{V}O_2$ max (see figure 4.10). To do this, plot the $\dot{V}O_2$ for each workload and corresponding HRs. Connect these two data points with a straight edge, extending the line so that it intersects the predicted maximal HR line. To extrapolate $\dot{V}O_2$ max, drop a perpendicular line from the point of intersection to the x-axis of the graph. If this is done carefully, the graphing method and multistage method will yield similar estimates of $\dot{V}O_2$ max.

AGE-CORRECTION FACTORS FOR ÅSTRAND-RYHMING NOMOGRAM

Age	Correction factor
15	1.10
25	1.00
35	0.87
40	0.83
45	0.78
50	0.75
55	0.71
60	0.68
65	0.65

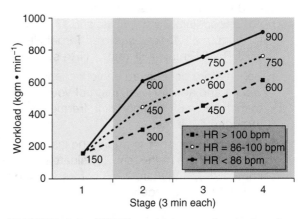

FIGURE 4.9 YMCA cycle ergometer protocol.

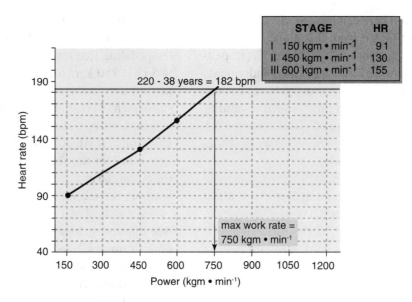

STAGE		HR
I	150 kgm • min^{-1}	91
II	450 kgm • min^{-1}	130
III	600 kgm • min^{-1}	155

220 - 38 years = 182 bpm

max work rate = 750 kgm • min^{-1}

FIGURE 4.10 Plotting heart rate versus submaximal work rates to estimate maximal work capacity and $\dot{V}O_2$max.

PRELIMINARY PROCEDURES AND GENERAL INSTRUCTIONS FOR SWAIN PROTOCOL

To select the protocol, follow these steps:

1. Measure the body weight and record your client's age.

2. Classify your client's activity level as either *active* (>90 min/wk of vigorous activity or >120 min/wk of moderate-intensity exercise) or *inactive* (<90 min/wk of vigorous activity or <120 min/wk of moderate-intensity exercise). Vigorous activities include running, vigorous cycling, or any equivalent; moderate-intensity activities include brisk walking, moderate cycling, or any equivalent.

3. Estimate your client's age-predicted HRmax (220 – age). Calculate the target exercise HRs corresponding to 45%, 55%, and 75% HRR (see figure 5.3 for an example). Target HR = %HRR × (HRmax – HRrest) + HRrest.

4. Select a protocol based on your client's body weight and activity level. Instruct your client to maintain a 60 rpm pedaling frequency throughout the test.

5. Measure exercise HRs during the last 15 sec of each minute of the test. Terminate the test immediately if the target HR corresponding to 75% HRR is exceeded.

To estimate maximum workload and the corresponding $\dot{V}O_2$max from the final 6 min stage of this test, use the following steps:

1. Calculate the power in watts (W) for the final 6 min workload. Power$_{6 min}$ (W) = resistance (kg) × 60 rpm × 9.81 m·sec^{-2}.

2. Average the fifth- and sixth-minute HRs from the final stage (HR$_{6 min}$), and calculate the client's age-predicted HRmax using 220 – age.

3. Calculate the client's %HRR for the final stage: %HRR = (HR$_{6 min}$ – HRrest) / (HRmax – HRrest).

4. Estimate the client's maximum workload or power in watts (W) by dividing the power of the final stage, calculated in step 1, by the %HRR calculated in step 3: power$_{max}$ (W) = power$_{6 min}$ / %HRR.

5. Use the ACSM metabolic equation for cycle ergometry to convert maximum power to an estimated $\dot{V}O_2$max: $\dot{V}O_2$max = 7 + [10.8 × power$_{max}$ (W) / body mass in kg].

Based on Swain et al. 2004.

Swain Cycle Ergometer Submaximal Exercise Test Protocol

Swain and colleagues (2004) devised a submaximal cycle ergometry protocol for estimating $\dot{V}O_2$max based on the relationship between heart rate reserve (HRR) and $\dot{V}O_2$reserve ($\dot{V}O_2$R) rather than on the HR-$\dot{V}O_2$ relationship. This protocol gradually approaches a target HR of 65% to 75% HRR in 1 min stages. This target HR zone is equivalent to 65% to 75% $\dot{V}O_2$R. When the client reaches her target HR, she continues to exercise at that workload for an additional 5 min. The initial work rate and incre-

ments in work rate differ depending on the client's body mass and activity level (see figure 4.11). The predictive validity of this test was good ($r = .89$; *SEE* = 4.0 ml·kg⁻¹·min⁻¹) for estimating the $\dot{V}O_2$max of adults ages 18 to 44 yr. However, more cross-validation studies are needed to determine this test's applicability to older or high-risk clients.

Figure 4.11 illustrates the Swain test protocols for active and inactive clients who weigh <90 kg or ≥90 kg (198 lb). To select the appropriate protocol and to calculate your client's estimated $\dot{V}O_2$max, follow the instructions in Preliminary Procedures and General Instructions for Swain Protocol.

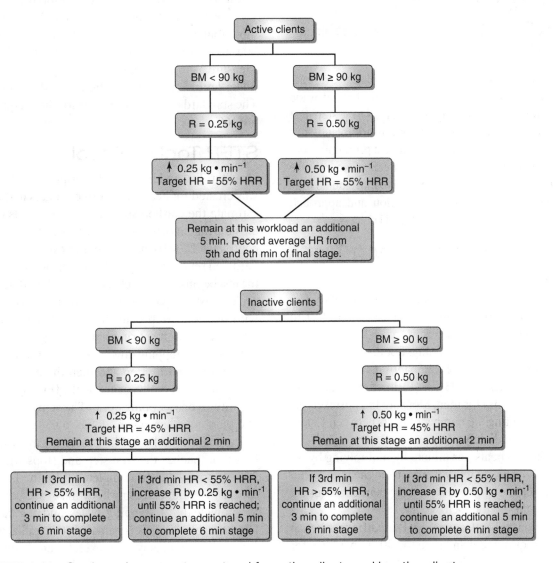

FIGURE 4.11   Swain cycle ergometer protocol for active clients and inactive clients.

Fox Single-Stage Cycle Ergometer Test Protocol

You can modify the maximal exercise test protocol (see figure 4.7) designed by Fox (1973) to predict $\dot{V}O_2$max (ml·min^{-1}). Have your client perform a single workload (i.e., 900 kgm·min^{-1} or 150 W) for 5 min. The standard error of estimate for this test is ±246 ml·min^{-1}, and the standard error of prediction is ±7.8%. The correlation between actual and predicted $\dot{V}O_2$ max is $r = .76$. To estimate $\dot{V}O_2$ max, measure the HR at the end of the fifth minute of exercise (HR$_5$) and use the following equation:

$$\dot{V}O_2 \max (\text{ml·min}^{-1}) = 6,300 - 19.26(\text{HR}_5)$$

BENCH STEPPING SUBMAXIMAL EXERCISE TESTS

There are many step tests available to evaluate cardiorespiratory fitness; however, few provide equations for predicting $\dot{V}O_2$ max. Only step test protocols with prediction equations are included in this section. Although these step test protocols were designed to be submaximal, the energy expenditure required of obese, short, or inactive individuals may exceed moderate-intensity exertion and approach $\dot{V}O_2$ max levels (Hansen et al. 2011).

Åstrand-Ryhming Step Test Protocol

As mentioned previously, you can use the Åstrand-Ryhming nomogram (see figure 4.8) to predict $\dot{V}O_2$ max from postexercise HR and body weight during bench stepping. For this protocol, the client steps at a rate of 22.5 steps·min^{-1} for 5 min. The bench height is 33 cm (13 in.) for women and 40 cm (15.75 in.) for men. Measure the postexercise HR by counting the number of beats between 15 and 30 sec immediately after exercise (convert this 15 sec count to beats per minute by multiplying by 4). Correct the predicted $\dot{V}O_2$ max from the nomogram if your client is older or younger than 25 yr (using the age-correction factors).

Hansen and colleagues (2011) modified the bench height requirement and used the 40 cm platform for the middle-aged (45 ± 13 yr) participants at least 170 cm tall. A 33 cm platform was used for those shorter than 170 cm. Not everyone was able to complete the 5 min exercise period. Given the level of exertion required for stepping (from 75% to over 95% $\dot{V}O_2$max), Hansen and colleagues suggested that medical supervision of fixed-rate stepping tests may be required.

Queens College Step Test Protocol

In a step test to predict $\dot{V}O_2$ max devised by McArdle and colleagues (1972), the client steps at a rate of 22 steps·min^{-1} (females) or 24 steps·min^{-1} (males) for 3 min. The bench height is 16.25 in. (41.3 cm). Have your client remain standing after the exercise. Wait 5 sec and then take a 15 sec HR count. Convert the count to beats per minute by multiplying by 4. If you are administering this test simultaneously to more than one client, you should teach your clients how to measure their own pulse rates (see How to Measure Your Pulse Rate). To estimate $\dot{V}O_2$ max in ml·kg^{-1}·min^{-1}, use the equations listed in table 4.7. The standard error of prediction for these equations is ±16%.

STEP Tool Protocol

The Step Test and Exercise Prescription (STEP) tool was created for health care professionals to quickly estimate the cardiorespiratory fitness levels of clients during an office visit. For this test, your client completes 20 self-paced stepping cycles on a standardized set of two steps (20 cm step height). Before the test begins, let your client practice for 10 stepping cycles. Instruct your client to step onto the first step with one foot, step onto the second step with the other foot, and then bring both feet together on the second step. Stepping down is done similarly—first one foot down one step and then the other foot to the floor. When both feet are on the floor again, that constitutes one stepping cycle. The stepping pattern is up, up, together, down, down, together (Knight, Stuckey, and Petrella 2014). Timing begins when the first foot touches the first step and stops when the 20th stepping cycle is completed. Maximal aerobic capacity is estimated using body mass, age, sex, time to complete the 20 stepping cycles, and postexercise HR (see table 4.7). HR is palpated at the radial artery for 6 sec immediately after exercise and multiplied by 10 to get beats per minute. This equation was independently validated using several adult popula-

Table 4.7 Prediction Equations for Cardiorespiratory Field Tests

Field test	Equation[a]	Source
DISTANCE RUN/WALK		
1.0 mi steady-state jog	$\dot{V}O_2max = 100.5 - 0.1636(BW, kg) - 1.438(time, min) - 0.1928(HR, bpm) + 8.344(gender)^b$	George et al. (1993)
1.0 mi run/walk (8-17 yr)	$\dot{V}O_2max = 108.94 - 8.41(time, min) + 0.34(time, min)^2 + 0.21(age \times gender)^b - 0.84(BMI)^c$	Cureton et al. (1995)
1.0 mi run/walk (13-16 yr)	$\dot{V}O_2peak = 7.34 \times speed, m \cdot sec^{-1} + 0.23(age, yr \times gender^b) + 17.75$	Burns et al. (2016)
1.5 mi run/walk	$\dot{V}O_2max = 88.02 - 0.1656(BW, kg) - 2.76(time, min) + 3.716(gender)^b$	George et al. (1993)
1.5 mi run/walk	$\dot{V}O_2max = 100.16 + 7.30(gender)^b - 0.164(BW, kg) - 1.273(time, min) - 0.1563(HR, bpm)$	Larsen et al. (2002)
12 min run	$\dot{V}O_2max = 0.0268(distance, m) - 11.3$	Cooper (1968)
15 min run	$\dot{V}O_2max = 0.0178(distance, m) + 9.6$	Balke (1963)
1.0 mi walk	$\dot{V}O_2max = 132.853 - 0.0769(BW, lb) - 0.3877(age, years) + 6.315(gender)^b - 3.2649(time, min) - 0.1565(HR, bpm)$	Kline et al. (1987)
STEP TESTS		
Åstrand	Men: $\dot{V}O_2max (L \cdot min^{-1}) = 3.744 [(BW + 5) / (HR - 62)]$ Women: $\dot{V}O_2max (L \cdot min^{-1}) = 3.750 [(BW - 3) / (HR - 65)]$	Marley and Linnerud (1976)
Queens College	Men: $\dot{V}O_2max = 111.33 - (0.42 HR, bpm)$ Women: $\dot{V}O_2max = 65.81 - (0.1847 HR, bpm)$	McArdle et al. (1972)
STEP tool	$\dot{V}O_2max (L \cdot min^{-1}) = 3.9 + (1511 / time^d) \times [(weight, kg / HR, bpm) \times 0.124] - (age, yr \times 0.032) - (gender^e \times 0.633)$	Knight, Stuckey, and Petrella (2014)
Individualized	$\dot{V}O_2max (ml \cdot kg^{-1} \cdot min^{-1}) = 45.938 + 0.253(gender)^b - 0.140(weight, kg) + 0.670(PFA) + 0.429(FSR) - 0.149(45sRHR)$	Webb et al. (2014)
Self-paced (≥65 yr)	Men: $\dot{V}O_2max (ml \cdot kg^{-1} \cdot min^{-1}) = 129.6 - (3.82 O_2 pulse) - (5.32 time to completion, s) - (0.22 age, yr) - (0.24 BMI^c) - (0.12 HR, bpm)$ Women: $\dot{V}O_2max (ml \cdot kg^{-1} \cdot min^{-1}) = 116.4 - (5.10 O_2 pulse) - (2.81 time to completion, s) - (0.24 age, yr) - (0.24 BMI^c) - (0.14 HR, bpm)$	Petrella et al. (2001)

HR = heart rate; m = meters; PFA = perceived functional ability score; FSR = final step rate, steps·min⁻¹; 45sRHR = HR at 45 sec after test termination; O₂ pulse = step test $\dot{V}O_2$ cost / HR.

[a]All equations estimate $\dot{V}O_2max$ in $ml \cdot kg^{-1} \cdot min^{-1}$ unless otherwise specified.

[b]For gender, substitute 1 for males and 0 for females.

[c]BMI = body mass index, or body weight (BW, in kg) / ht² (in meters).

[d]Time is in seconds

[e]For gender, substitute 1 for males and 2 for females

tions, ranging in age from 18 to 85 yr, but may not be suitable for people using medications to control their HR. Knight, Stuckey, and Petrella (2014) assessed the predictive accuracy of the equation against the Bruce treadmill protocol. There was a moderately strong relationship ($r = .79$) between the $\dot{V}O_2$ estimated from the STEP and the average $\dot{V}O_2$ during the last 30 sec of the treadmill test. However, the STEP tool systematically overpredicted $\dot{V}O_2$ max by 6.4 ml·kg⁻¹·min⁻¹. The 95% confidence interval was 4.1 to 8.7 ml·kg⁻¹·min⁻¹.

Webb Step Test Protocol

The Webb protocol was developed for college-age adults and uses the client's perceived functional ability (PFA) as determined by questionnaire (George, Stone, and Burkett 1997). Step height is calculated using your client's height (step height = 0.19 × height in cm), and termination HR is 75% of your client's age-predicted HRmax (207 − [0.7 × age]). Instruct your client to wear a heart rate monitor. The initial stepping cadence depends on your client's PFA (see Webb et al. 2014). Use a metronome to help your client maintain the proper stepping cadence (steps·min^{-1}) in an up, up, down, down fashion. A brief familiarization with the stepping cadence is recommended. Your client steps at the initial cadence for 2 min. Record the HR and RPE in the last 30 sec of each stage. At the end of each 2 min stage, increase the stepping cadence by 5 steps·min^{-1}, but do not change the step height. Continue this pattern until the termination HR is attained. Have your client finish this stage and immediately sit down; record the HR immediately and again every 15 sec for 1 min. To estimate $\dot{V}O_2$ max (see table 4.7), use the final stepping rate (cadence, FSR) and posttest HR at the 45 sec interval.

ADDITIONAL MODES FOR SUBMAXIMAL EXERCISE TESTING

If you are working at a health or fitness club, you may have access to stair climbers, recumbent steppers, and rowing ergometers. You can use some of these exercise machines for submaximal exercise testing of your clients.

Stair Climbing Submaximal Test Protocols

In light of the popularity of and continued interest in step aerobic training, you may choose to use a simulated stair climbing machine to estimate the aerobic fitness of some clients. The StairMaster 4000 PT and 6000 PT are two step ergometers commonly used in health and fitness settings. The StairMaster 4000 PT has step pedals that go up and down, whereas the 6000 PT model has a revolving staircase. Howley, Colacino, and Swensen (1992) reported that the HR response to increasing submaximal workloads (4.7 and 10 METs) on the StairMaster 4000 PT step ergometer was linear. Also, compared against values with treadmill exercise, the HRs measured during stepping were systematically higher (7-11 bpm) at each submaximal intensity. However, the MET values read from the step ergometer were about 20% higher than the measured MET values. To obtain more accurate MET values for each submaximal intensity, use the following equation:

$$\text{actual METs} = 0.556 + 0.745 \, (\text{StairMaster 4000 PT MET value})$$

The StairMaster 4000 PT test protocol, developed by the manufacturer, provides a relatively more accurate estimate of $\dot{V}O_2$max for young women (20-25 yr) who use this device for aerobic training ($r = .57$; $SEE = 5.3$ ml·kg^{-1}·min^{-1}; $CE = 1.0$ ml·kg^{-1}·min^{-1}) as compared with estimates for their untrained counterparts ($r = .00$; $SEE = 6.7$ ml·kg^{-1}·min^{-1}; $CE = 6.9$ ml·kg^{-1}·min^{-1}) (Roy et al. 2004). This finding illustrates that the exercise testing mode should match the exercise training mode (i.e., application of the specificity principle).

To estimate $\dot{V}O_2$max, measure the steady-state HR and calculate the corrected MET value for each

How to Measure Your Pulse Rate

1. Use your middle and index fingers to locate the radial pulse on the outside of your wrist just below the base of your thumb. Do not use your thumb to feel the pulse because it has a pulse of its own and may produce an inaccurate count.

2. If you cannot feel the radial pulse, try locating the carotid pulse by placing your fingers lightly on the front of your neck, just to the side of your voice box. Do not apply heavy pressure because this will cause your HR to slow down.

3. Use a stopwatch or the second hand of your wristwatch and count the number of pulse beats for a 6, 10, or 15 sec period.

4. Convert the pulse count to beats per minute using the following multipliers: 6 sec count × 10; 10 sec count × 6; and 15 sec count × 4.

5. Remember this value and record it on your scorecard.

of two submaximal exercise intensities (e.g., 4 and 7 METs). Each stage of the test should last 3 to 6 min in order to produce steady state. Then use either the multistage model formulas (see Multistage Model for Estimating $\dot{V}O_2$max) or the graphing method (see figure 4.10) to predict $\dot{V}O_2$max.

During the test, clients may hold the handrail lightly for balance but should not support their body weight. If they support their body weight, $\dot{V}O_2$max will be overestimated (Howley et al. 1992). Also, compared against the value with treadmill testing, your clients' estimated $\dot{V}O_2$max may be lower because stair climbing produces systematically higher HRs at any given submaximal exercise intensity.

Recumbent Stepper Submaximal Test Protocol

The YMCA submaximal cycling protocol has been adapted for use with the NuStep T5xr recumbent stepper and can be used to estimate the $\dot{V}O_2$ peak (r = .91; SEE = 4.09 ml·kg^{-1}·min^{-1}; TE = 4.11 ml·kg^{-1}·min^{-1}) of your clients, 20-60 yr (Billinger et al. 2012). The Billinger equation may also be used for older adults, 60-80 yr (r = .87; SEE = 4.2 ml·kg^{-1}·min^{-1}) (Herda et al. 2013).

The client must maintain a stepping rate between 90 and 100 steps·min^{-1} throughout the protocol. Similar to the YMCA cycling protocol, the stage change is dependent on the client's having attained a steady-state HR. The initial workload is 30 W, and workload is increased every 3 min in accordance with the HR-derived protocol track. Use the HR during the last 10 sec of the second and third minutes of each stage to determine if steady-state HR has been attained (within ± 5 bpm). If the HR at the end of the initial stage is less than 80 bpm, set the second workload at 125 W. If HR is 80 to 89 bpm, the workload is 100 W for the second stage of the protocol. If the initial stage HR is 90 to 100 bpm, the second-stage workload is 75 W. If the HR at the end of the first workload exceeds 100 bpm, set the second workload at 50 W. Subsequent workloads increase 25 W every third minute thereafter, assuming a steady-state HR was achieved in the previous stage. The protocol terminates when the client reaches 85% of the age-predicted HRmax or volitional exhaustion. Estimate $\dot{V}O_2$ peak (ml·kg^{-1}·min^{-1}) using the following equation:

$$\dot{V}O_2 \text{ peak} = 125.707 - (0.476 \times \text{age, yr})$$
$$+ (7.686 \times \text{sex}) - (0.451 \times \text{wt, kg})$$
$$+ (0.179 \times W_{end\_submax})$$
$$- (0.415 \times HR_{end\_submax})$$

Note: For sex, 0 = female and 1 = male.
W_{end_submax} = watts equivalent to final workload.
HR_{end_submax} = HR at test termination.

Rowing Ergometer Submaximal Test Protocols

Submaximal exercise protocols have been developed for the Concept II rowing ergometer and can be used to estimate your clients' $\dot{V}O_2$ max. The Hagerman (1993) protocol is designed for noncompetitive or unskilled rowers. Before beginning the test, set the fan blades in the fully closed position and select the small axle sprocket. For this test, select a submaximal exercise intensity (the HR should not exceed 170 bpm) that the client can sustain for 5 to 10 min. Measure the exercise HR at the end of each minute. Continue the rowing exercise until the client achieves a steady-state HR. Use the Hagerman (1993) nomogram (see figure 4.12) to estimate $\dot{V}O_2$max from the submaximal power output (watts) and the steady-state HR during the last minute of exercise.

ELLIPTICAL CROSS-TRAINER SUBMAXIMAL TEST PROTOCOL

Dalleck, Kravitz, and Roberts (2006) developed an equation to predict $\dot{V}O_2$ max from submaximal testing using an elliptical cross-trainer. Their participants performed three 5 min stages. Cadence and HR were recorded for the second stage. Compared with $\dot{V}O_2$ max from an elliptical test to exhaustion, the prediction equation

$$\dot{V}O_2 \text{ max} = 73.676 + 7.383(\text{gender})$$
$$- 0.317(\text{weight, kg})$$
$$+ 0.003957(\text{age} \times \text{cadence})$$
$$- 0.006452(\text{age} \times \text{heart rate at stage 2})$$

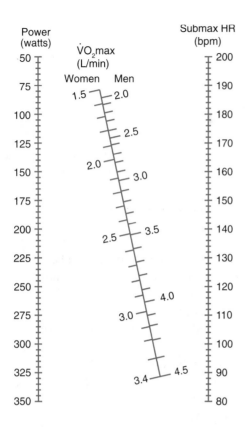

FIGURE 4.12 Concept II nomogram for estimating $\dot{V}O_2$max in noncompetitive and unskilled male and female rowers.

From *Concept II Rowing Ergometer Nomogram for Prediction of Maximal Oxygen Consumption* by Dr. Fritz Hagerman, Ohio University, Athens, OH. The nomogram is not appropriate for use with non-Concept II ergometers and is designed to be used by noncompetitive or unskilled rowers participating in aerobic conditioning programs. Adapted by permission of Concept II, Inc., 105 Industrial Park Drive, Morrisville, VT 05661 (800) 245-5676.

estimated $\dot{V}O_2$ max well ($r = .86$; *SEE* = 3.91 ml·kg^{-1}·min^{-1}). Furthermore, the actual and predicted $\dot{V}O_2$ max values were similar for the sample of healthy young adults (29.5 ± 7.1 yr). For details about the testing protocol, see Dalleck, Kravitz, and Robergs (2006).

Newer models of elliptical cross-trainers display a value for METs. Mays and associates (2016) used both steady-state and non-steady-state HRs recorded over the course of submaximal trials. These HR values were used to estimate $\dot{V}O_2$peak. The $\dot{V}O_2$peak predicted from the MET levels as derived from the device's proprietary equations was lower than that derived from the two (steady state and combined steady state and non-steady state) HR-based prediction equations. The displayed MET levels may be inaccurate across the spectrum of exercise intensities. The authors cautioned trainers about designing

exercise programs based on $\dot{V}O_2$ peak values derived from these displayed MET values.

FIELD TESTS FOR ASSESSING AEROBIC FITNESS

The maximal and submaximal exercise tests using a treadmill or a cycle, rowing, arm-crank, or elliptical ergometer are not well suited for measuring the cardiorespiratory fitness of large groups in a field situation. Thus, a number of performance tests such as distance runs have been devised to predict $\dot{V}O_2$ max (see table 4.7). These tests are practical, inexpensive, less time consuming than the treadmill or cycle ergometer tests, easy to administer to large groups, and suitable for personal training settings; they can be used to classify the cardiorespiratory fitness levels of healthy men (≤45 yr) and women (≤55 yr). You cannot use field tests to detect CHD because HR, ECG, and BP are usually not monitored during the performance. Most field tests used to assess cardiorespiratory endurance involve walking, running, swimming, cycling, or bench stepping; they require that clients be able to accurately measure their postexercise HR. Pollock, Broida, and Kendrick (1972) found that with practice, men could learn to measure their own pulse rates accurately. The correlation between manual and electronic measurements of pulse rate ranged between $r = .91$ and .94. Similar results ($r = .95$) were reported for college women for pulse rates measured manually and electronically (Witten 1973). Prior to administering field tests that require the measurement of HR, you should teach your clients how to measure their pulse rates using the palpation technique described in How to Measure Your Pulse Rate.

DISTANCE RUN TESTS

The most commonly used distance runs involve distances of 1.0 or 1.5 mi (1,600 or 2,400 m) to evaluate aerobic fitness. Distance run tests are based on the assumption that the fitter individual will be able to run a given distance in less time or to run a greater distance in a given period of time. Using factor analysis, Disch, Frankiewicz, and Jackson (1975) noted that runs greater than 1.0 mi tended to load exclusively on the endurance factor rather than the speed factor.

You should be aware that the relationship between distance runs and $\dot{V}O_2$max has not been firmly established. Although performance on a distance run can be accurately measured, it may not be an accurate index of $\dot{V}O_2$max or a substitute for the direct measurement of $\dot{V}O_2$max. Endurance running performance may be influenced by other factors such as motivation; percent fat (Cureton et al. 1978; Katch et al. 1973); running efficiency (pacing ability); lactate threshold (Costill and Fox 1969; Costill, Thomason, and Roberts 1973); and storage and reuse of elastic energy, lower leg architecture, and body weight (Lacour and Bourdin 2015).

The correlations between distance run tests and $\dot{V}O_2$ max tend to vary considerably ($r = .29$-$.97$) depending on the client's age, sex, and training status. Sample size, test distance, and testing procedures may also affect this relationship (Mayorga-Vega et al. 2016). Generally, the longer the run, the higher the correlation with $\dot{V}O_2$max. On the basis of this observation, it is recommended that you select a test with a distance of at least 1.0 mi (1,600 m) or duration of at least 9 min.

The most widely used distance run tests are the 9 and 12 min runs and the 1.0 and 1.5 mi runs. Some physical fitness test batteries for children and adolescents recommend using either the 9 min or 1.0 mi run test.

9 or 12 Min Run Test

To administer the 9 or 12 min run test, use a 400 m track or flat course with measured distances so the number of laps completed can be easily counted and multiplied by the course distance. Place markers to divide the course into quarters or eighths of a mile so you can quickly determine the exact distance covered in 9 or 12 min. Instruct your clients to run as far as possible. Walking is allowed, but the objective of these tests is to cover as much distance as possible in either 9 or 12 min. At the end of the test, calculate the total distance covered in meters and use the appropriate equation in table 4.7 to estimate the client's $\dot{V}O_2$ max.

1.5 Mile Run/Walk Test

The 1.5 mi (2.4 km) run/walk test is conducted on a 400 m track or flat measured area. To measure the course, use an odometer or measuring wheel. For the 1.5 mi run, instruct your clients to cover the specified distance in the fastest possible time. Walking is allowed, but the objective is to cover the distance in the shortest possible time while maintaining a steady exercise pace. Call out the elapsed time (in minutes and seconds) as each client crosses the finish line. You can use a HR monitor to ensure that participants maintain a steady exercise pace during this test. Instruct your clients to keep their target HR between 60% and 90% HRmax. The exercise HR at the end of the test, along with gender, body mass, and elapsed exercise time, can be substituted into the Larsen equation (see table 4.7) to estimate the $\dot{V}O_2$ max of young (18-29 yr) adults (Larsen et al. 2002). Cross-validation of this equation yielded a high validity coefficient ($r = .89$) and small prediction errors ($SEE = 2.5$ ml·kg^{-1}·min^{-1}; $TE = 2.68$ ml·kg^{-1}·min^{-1}) for a sample of young military personnel (Taylor et al. 2002).

To use the $\dot{V}O_2$max prediction equations for the 1.5 mi run/walk test (see table 4.7), convert the seconds to minutes by dividing the seconds by 60. For example, if a client's time for the test is 12:30, the exercise time is converted to 12.5 min (30 / 60 sec = 0.5 min).

1.0-Mile Jogging Test

One limitation of distance run tests is that individuals are encouraged to run as fast as possible and give a maximal effort, thereby increasing the risk of cardiovascular and orthopedic injuries. The potential risk is even greater for untrained individuals who do not run or jog regularly and have difficulty selecting a proper jogging pace. To address this problem, George and colleagues (1993) developed a submaximal 1 mi (1.6 km) track jogging test for 18 to 29 yr old women and men that requires only moderate steady-state exertion.

For this test, instruct your clients to select a comfortable, moderate jogging pace and to measure their postexercise HR immediately following the test. The elapsed time for 1 mi should be at least 8 min for males and 9 min for females, and the postexercise HR (15 sec count × 4) should not exceed 180 bpm. To help establish a suitable pace, precede the timed 1 mi test with a 2 to 3 min warm-up. Use either an indoor or outdoor track for this test. Record the time, in minutes, required to jog 1 mi, and have your clients measure their postexercise HRs using the palpation technique (radial or carotid sites). Estimate the client's $\dot{V}O_2$ max using the prediction equation for the 1.0 mi steady-state jog test (see table 4.7).

20 m Shuttle Run Test

Video 4.8

A field test used to estimate $\dot{V}O_2$ max, the 20 m shuttle run is also known by other names such as the beep test and the PACER. There are several derivations of the protocol and equations used to predict $\dot{V}O_2$ max (see Mayorga-Vega, Aguilar-Soto, and Viciana 2015). This test is performed by having individuals (adults and children) run back and forth between markers (e.g., cones, lines taped or painted on the floor) that are 20 m apart. A prerecorded soundtrack establishes the speed needed to cover the distance between markers. The test begins with a sound, and the 20 m distance must be covered before the next sound is heard. When that sound is heard, the runner turns around and returns to the original marker. This pattern continues as the time between sounds decreases incrementally. The test ends when the runner cannot cover the 20 m distance before the sound.

Permutations of this test are based on starting speed (i.e., 7.5 to 8.5 km·h⁻¹) and increases in speed (i.e., 0.5 to 1.0 km·h⁻¹) each minute (Mayorga-Vega, Aguilar-Soto, and Viciana 2015). A review of the studies validating the 20 m shuttle run for estimating $\dot{V}O_2$ max indicates a moderate to high criterion-related validity ($r = .66-.84$) for the performance scores alone. The validity improves ($r = .78-.95$) when participant-specific demographics (e.g., body mass, sex, age) are included in the prediction equation (Mayorga-Vega, Aguilar-Soto, and Viciana 2015). The authors concluded that the 20 m shuttle run is a viable option for estimating cardiorespiratory fitness of adults (Mayorga-Vega, Aguilar-Soto, and Viciana 2015) and should be used instead of other traditional walk/run protocols (Mayorga-Vega et al. 2016).

Walking Test

The Rockport Walking Institute (1986) has developed a walking test to assess cardiorespiratory fitness for men and women ages 20 to 69 yr. Because this test requires only fast walking, it is useful for testing older or sedentary individuals (Fenstermaker, Plowman, and Looney 1992). The test was developed and validated for a large heterogeneous sample of

86 women and 83 men (Kline et al. 1987). The cross-validation analysis resulted in a high validity coefficient and small standard error of estimate (*SEE*), indicating that the 1.0 mi walking test yields a valid submaximal assessment of estimated $\dot{V}O_2$ max. Other researchers have substantiated the predictive accuracy of this equation for women 65 yr of age and older (Fenstermaker, Plowman, and Looney 1992), military men (18-44 yr) (Weiglein et al. 2011), and adults (19-44 yr) (Seneli et al. 2013). Testing on a nonmotorized treadmill did not alter the walking time, but the postexercise HR was increased. Consequently, $\dot{V}O_2$ max is significantly underestimated when using a nonmotorized treadmill for this 1.0 mi walking test (Seneli et al. 2013).

To administer this test as originally designed, instruct your clients to walk 1.0 mi as quickly as possible and to take their HR immediately at the end of the test by counting the pulse for 15 sec. It is important that clients know how to take their pulse accurately. The walking course should be a measured mile that is flat and uninterrupted, preferably a 400 m track. Clients should warm up for 5 to 10 min before the test and wear good walking shoes and loose-fitting clothes.

To estimate a client's $\dot{V}O_2$ max, use the generalized equation for the 1.0 mi walking test (see table 4.7). Alternatively, you can use the Rockport relative fitness charts (appendix B.2) or the sex-specific equations (see Kline et al. 1987) to classify your client's cardiorespiratory fitness level. Locate the walking time and corresponding postexercise HR (bpm) on the appropriate chart for the individual's age and gender. These charts are based on body weights of 125 lb for women and 170 lb for men. If the client weighs substantially more than this, the cardiorespiratory fitness level will be overestimated.

STEP TESTS

The major advantage of using step tests to assess cardiorespiratory fitness is that they can be administered to large groups in a field situation without requiring expensive equipment or highly trained personnel. Most of these step tests use postexercise and recovery HRs to evaluate aerobic fitness, but they do not provide an estimate of the individual's $\dot{V}O_2$ max. Step test protocols and scoring procedures are described in appendix B.3, Step Test Protocols.

MONITORING HRS DURING FIELD TESTS

If you monitor field test HRs with a technological device (i.e., heart rate monitor, accelerometer, pulse oximeter, smart watch, or smartphone app) instead of palpating postexercise HR, you are advised to record the HR displayed at the postexercise time interval specified by the protocol when it was created and validated (e.g., 15 sec postexercise for the 1 mi walk and 1 mi jogging tests). Using a HR captured for a different time interval may introduce additional error in the estimation of $\dot{V}O_2$max.

Many smart devices detect HR noninvasively by using light to detect changes in microvascular blood volume or blood flow at the wrist or in the nail bed. This light-based technique is known as photoplethysmography (PPG). Proprietary algorithms within the device and app convert the fluctuations in blood flow and blood volume into HRs. Therefore, the quality of the algorithms and the integrity of the blood-sensor interface are important for the accuracy of devices relying on PPG. Increasing exercise intensities, alterations in wrist position, tattoos, and skin pigmentation patterns may compromise the integrity of the blood-sensor interface (Spierer et al. 2015). If you plan on using a smart device to measure HR, look for one that has been successfully validated against an ECG reference (i.e., no significant differences between device and ECG means, small *SEEs*, correlations ≥.80). Errors in the calculation of HR lead to errors in the estimation of $\dot{V}O_2$max. See the research of El-Amrawy, Pharm, and Nounou (2015) and LeBoeuf and colleagues (2014) for their assessments of PPG technology for accurate monitoring of HR.

The validity of step tests is highly dependent on the accurate measurement of pulse rate. Step tests that use recovery HR tend to have lower validity than those using the time required for the HR to reach a specified level during performance of a standardized workload (Baumgartner and Jackson 1975). The correlation coefficients between step test performance and $\dot{V}O_2$ max range between $r = .32$ and .77 (Cureton and Sterling 1964; deVries and Klafs 1965; McArdle et al. 1972).

ADDITIONAL FIELD TESTS

In addition to running, walking, and step tests, cycling and swimming tests have been devised for use in field situations (Cooper 1977). The 12 min cycling test, using a bike with no more than three speeds, is conducted on a hard, flat surface when the wind velocity is less than 10 mph (268 m·min⁻¹). These conditions limit the effect of outside influences on the rider's performance. Five- and 10-speed bikes are not employed unless use of the lower gears can be restricted. Use an odometer to measure the distance traveled in 12 min. In the 12 min swimming test, the client may use any stroke and rest as needed. Norms for the 12 min cycling test and 12 min swimming test are available (Cooper 1977).

Of these two tests, the swimming test is the less preferred because the outcome is highly skill dependent. For example, a skilled swimmer with an average cardiorespiratory fitness level will probably be able to swim farther in 12 min than a poorly skilled swimmer with an above-average cardiorespiratory fitness level. In fact, Conley and colleagues (1991, 1992) reported that the 12 min swim has low validity ($r = .34$-.42) as a cardiorespiratory field test for male and female recreational swimmers. Whenever possible, select an alternative field test and avoid using the 12 min swim test.

EXERCISE TESTING FOR CHILDREN AND OLDER ADULTS

You may need to modify the generic guidelines for exercise testing (see General Principles of Exercise Testing earlier in the chapter) of low-risk adults when you are assessing cardiorespiratory fitness of children and older adults. You must take into account growth, maturation, and aging when selecting exercise testing modes and protocols for these groups.

ASSESSING CARDIORESPIRATORY FITNESS OF CHILDREN

In the laboratory setting, you can assess the cardiorespiratory fitness of children using either the treadmill

WORKING WITH GPS-CAPABLE DEVICES

Most smart devices that have integrated GPS capabilities require line of sight with the satellites used for triangulating location (Hillsdon et al. 2015). This makes it challenging to rely on GPS for accurate calculation of distances if the activities are performed indoors or in a high-density urban environment (Jankowska, Schipperijn, and Kerr 2015). Newer receivers that have a SiRFstarIII GPS chip are reported to work indoors, which should reduce the amount of missing data (McGrath, Hopkins, and Hinckson 2015). Two commercially available GPS units were compared against the time it took research subjects to cover the reference distance of 2.4 km while jogging at two speeds and walking on an outdoor 400 m track (Benson, Bruce, and Gordon 2015). Significant differences in time to completion and distance covered were found. Precise spatial accuracy is required when using GPS features to set distance. Otherwise, spatial inaccuracies will influence the time to completion of field tests. Therefore, at this point, it is not recommended that you use the GPS features of smart devices for distance and time to completion when conducting a field test to estimate $\dot{V}O_2$max.

---

or cycle ergometer. Treadmill testing is usually preferable, especially for younger children, because their shortened attention span may not allow them to maintain a constant pedaling rate during a cycle ergometer test. Also, children younger than 8 yr or shorter than 50 in. (127 cm) may not be tall enough to use a standard cycle ergometer. To accommodate children, modify the seat height, pedal crank length, and handlebar position.

For treadmill testing, you may choose to use the modified Balke protocol (see table 4.8) because the speed is constant and the means of increasing intensity is to change the grade. Either the modified Balke protocol or the modified Bruce protocol (i.e., 2 min instead of 3 min stages) may be used when assessing the cardiorespiratory fitness levels of children. Age and gender endurance-time norms for children (4-18 yr) for the modified Bruce protocol are available elsewhere (Wessel, Strasburger, and Mitchell 2001).

For cycle ergometer testing, you can use the McMaster protocol (see table 4.8). For this protocol, the pedaling frequency is 50 rpm, and increments in work rate are based on the child's height. As an alternative, a new **steep ramp cycling protocol (SRP)** has demonstrated both high reliability and validity for accurately assessing $\dot{V}O_2$ peak of children and adolescents (Bongers et al. 2013). After a 3 min warm-up at a power output of 25 W, the ramp trial begins with workload increments of either 10, 15, or 20 W per 10 sec; the increments are determined by participant height (<120 cm, 120-150 cm, and >150 cm, respectively). The ramp protocol continues until the pedaling cadence falls below 60 rpm

and the participant exhibits other signs of maximal exertion. The SRP was validated against a separate maximal exertion cycling protocol with metabolic gas collection; the following equation was derived:

$$\dot{V}O_2 \text{peak (ml·min}^{-1}) = 8.262 \times W_{SRP} + 177.096 \ (R^2 = .917; \ SEE = 237.4 \text{ ml·min}^{-1}).$$

The mean difference between predicted and measured $\dot{V}O_2$ peak was 0.3 ml·min^{-1}, and no systematic bias was noted in the Bland and Altman analysis (1986). Test-retest comparison of the SRP indicated high reproducibility of peak power output ($ICC = .986$).

Children, like adults, may not exhibit a plateau in oxygen consumption during ramp protocol testing. Only 34% of the children undergoing metabolic gas analysis in the study by Bongers and colleagues (2013) demonstrated a plateau in $\dot{V}O_2$. Barker and colleagues (2011) confirmed that children exert their maximal effort during a ramp cycling protocol. This confirmation was made by having the children rest 15 min and then perform a supramaximal cycling trial at 105% of the peak power output attained during the ramp protocol. Subsequent analysis revealed similar $\dot{V}O_2$ peak values between the two cycling protocols. In addition to noting a low incidence of a plateau during the ramp cycling trial, Barker and colleagues (2011) commented that had they relied on the other secondary indicators of maximal exertion (i.e., RER and HR), they would have underestimated $\dot{V}O_2$ max by 10% to 20%, on average, in their sample of healthy 9 and 10 yr olds.

Field tests, such as the 1.0 mi (1.6 km) run/walk, are widely used to assess the cardiorespiratory fit-

Table 4.8 Graded Exercise Test Protocols for Children (Skinner 1993)

MODIFIED BALKE TREADMILL PROTOCOL				
Activity classification	Speed (mph)	Initial grade (%)	Increment (%)	Duration (min)
Poorly fit	3.0	6	2	2
Sedentary	3.25	6	2	2
Active	5.0	0	2.5	2
Athletes	5.25	0	2.5	2

MCMASTER CYCLE ERGOMETER PROTOCOL			
Height (cm)	Initial work rate: kgm·min^{-1} (watts)	Increments: kgm·min^{-1} (watts)	Duration (min)
120	75 (12.5)	75 (12.5)	2
120-139.9	75 (12.5)	150 (25)	2
140-159.9	150 (25)	150 (25)	2
≥160	150 (25)	300 (50) for boys 150 (25) for girls	2

ness of children 5 to 17 yr of age. These tests are part of the Physical Best Program (American Alliance for Health, Physical Education, Recreation and Dance 1988), Fitnessgram (Cooper Institute for Aerobics Research 1994), and the President's Challenge Test (President's Council on Physical Fitness and Sports 1997), as well as national physical fitness surveys of children and youth (Ross and Pate 1987). To estimate $\dot{V}O_2$ peak of 8 to 17 yr olds for the 1.0 mi run/walk test, you can use a generalized prediction equation (see table 4.7) (Cureton et al. 1995). You can also use a BMI-independent prediction equation for adolescents 13 to 16 yr to estimate $\dot{V}O_2$ peak (Burns et al. 2016). For younger children (5-7 yr), the 0.5 mi (0.8 km) run/walk test is recommended (Rikli, Petray, and Baumgartner 1992). Criterion-referenced standards for the 1.0 mi test are available elsewhere (American Alliance for Health, Physical Education, Recreation and Dance 1988; Cooper Institute for Aerobics Research 1994). A review of literature and in-depth analysis of equations designed to estimate $\dot{V}O_2$ max for young people (<18 yr) is available (Ferrar et al. 2014).

In Canada and Europe, the multistage 20 m shuttle run test, developed by Leger and colleagues (1988), is a popular alternative to distance running/walking field tests to estimate the aerobic fitness of children (8-19 yr) in educational settings. This test has been cross-validated using other samples of European, Canadian, and American children (Anderson 1992; Mahar et al. 2011; van Mechelen, Holbil, and Kemper 1986).

For this test, children run back and forth continuously on a 20 m (indoor or outdoor) course. The running speed is set using a sound signal emitted from a prerecorded tape. The starting pace is 8.5 km·hr^{-1}, and the speed is increased 0.5 km·hr^{-1} each minute until they can no longer maintain the pace. The maximal aerobic speed at this stage is used, in combination with age, in the original equation to estimate $\dot{V}O_2$ max (ml·kg^{-1}·min^{-1}) as follows:

$$\dot{V}O_2 \text{ max} = 31.025 + 3.238(\text{speed, km·hr}^{-1})$$
$$- 3.248(\text{age, yr})$$
$$+ 0.1536(\text{age} \times \text{speed})$$

Mahar and colleagues (2011) evaluated this and several other equations for a sample of schoolchildren. In an attempt to improve the fitness category classification resulting from these equations, they devised and cross-validated quadratic and linear equations that improve both the prediction of $\dot{V}O_2$ max and the fitness level categorization of children aged 10 to 16 yr.

$$\dot{V}O_2 \text{ max} = 41.76799 + (0.49261 \times \text{laps}) - (0.00290 \times \text{laps}^2) - (0.61613 \times \text{BMI}) + (0.34787 \times \text{gender} \times \text{age}),$$ where boys = 1 and girls = 0; $R = .75$, $R^2 = .56$, $SEE = 6.17$ ml·kg^{-1}·min^{-1}

$$\dot{V}O_2 \, max = 40.34533 + (0.21426 \times laps) - (0.79472 \times BMI) + (4.27293 \times gender) + (0.79444 \times age); R = .74, R^2 = .54, SEE = 6.29 \, ml \cdot kg^{-1} \cdot min^{-1}$$

Two other incremental running tests have been validated against a graded treadmill test and shown reliable in terms of test-retest determination of maximal heart rate. Bendiksen and colleagues (2012) investigated the suitability of the modified Yo-Yo Intermittent Recovery Level 1 test (YYIR1C) and the Anderson test (1992) for assessing the cardiorespiratory health of children aged 6 to 10 yr. The criterion measure was the maximal heart rate attained during an incremental treadmill test. Both tests require the children to run back and forth between two cones (or lines). The maximal heart rate and number of laps completed are recorded and used for interpretation. The YYIR1C uses a distance of 16 m. After returning to the starting point, the child engages in a 10 sec active recovery by jogging around a third cone located 4 m behind the starting location. The speed at which the child needs to complete the 16 m laps up and back is controlled by the prerecorded YYIR1 disc. The 16 m running pace becomes progressively faster, while the active recovery period remains at 10 sec. The child runs until failing twice to complete the 16 m distance within the designated time increment.

Similarly, in the Anderson test, children run between two cones (or lines) 20 m apart. However, the children run as fast as possible and take one step beyond each demarcation before turning and running back. The children run in this manner for 15 sec, at which time a whistle is blown and the children stop as quickly as possible (within two steps) to rest for 15 sec. The last 3 sec of the rest period are counted off (e.g., "3, 2, 1, run"). According to protocol, this pattern continues for 10 min. The average maximal heart rates from the YYIR1C and Anderson tests were similar, at 207 and 206 bpm, respectively, and slightly higher than that from the incremental treadmill test (203 bpm). Consequently, Bendiksen and colleagues (2012) reported that these two field tests are sensitive enough to detect fitness-based differences in this age group.

A stepping protocol that uses postexercise HR to identify a child's cardiorespiratory fitness level was investigated by Jankowski and colleagues (2015). Polish schoolchildren (6 to 12 yr) performed the 3 min Kasch Pulse Recovery Test (KPR Test).

Using a bench that was 30.5 cm (12 in.) in height, the children stepped up and down to the pace of a metronome set to 24 steps·min⁻¹. The children sat immediately after the test ended so the 1 min recovery HRs could be determined; the average of electronically collected recovery HRs was computed. Age and gender criterion tables were developed to classify a child's fitness level based on the percentile associated with postexercise HR. The authors commented that this simple protocol requires minimal equipment and is suitable for screening large numbers of children for the purpose of establishing their cardiorespiratory fitness levels. However, the HR categories have not yet been validated against gold standard reference values of aerobic capacity. The details of the gender- and age-specific criterion HRs are available elsewhere (Jankowski et al. 2015).

ASSESSING CARDIORESPIRATORY FITNESS OF OLDER ADULTS

Smith and colleagues (2016) reviewed and evaluated 13 submaximal exercise equations to estimate $\dot{V}O_2 max$ of apparently healthy older adults (mean age ≥65 yr). Modalities included treadmills, recumbent steppers, and stationary stepping. Although they reported that walking and running modalities are preferred, the most accurate (no significant differences between measured and estimated $\dot{V}O_2 \, max$, r^2 = .90) estimation of aerobic capacity was produced using the self-paced stepping protocol developed by Petrella et al. (2001).

To assess the cardiorespiratory fitness of elderly clients, you can also use modified versions of treadmill and cycle ergometer protocols. The following modifications for standard GXT protocols are recommended:

- Extend the warm-up to more than 3 min.

- Set an initial exercise intensity of 2 to 3 METs; work increments should be 0.5 to 1.0 MET (e.g., Naughton treadmill protocol; see table 4.4).

- Reduce the treadmill speed to the walking ability of your client when needed.

- Extend the duration of each work stage (at least 3 min), allowing enough time for the client to attain steady state.

- Select a protocol likely to produce a total test time of 8 to 12 min.

Select treadmill protocols that increase grade instead of speed, especially for older clients with poor ambulation. You can modify the standard Balke protocol (see figure 4.2) by having the client walk at 0% grade and 3.0 mph (4.8 km·hr^{-1}) or slower initially and by increasing the duration of each stage to at least 3 min. If elderly clients are more comfortable holding on to the handrails during a treadmill test, you can use the standard Bruce protocol and the McConnell and Clark (1987) prediction equation to estimate their $\dot{V}O_2$ max (see table 4.5). Alternatively, you could use cycle ergometer GXTs for older individuals with poor balance, poor neuromuscular coordination, or impaired vision. You can also use field tests to estimate the cardiorespiratory fitness of your older (60-94 yr) clients. The Senior Fitness Test battery (Rikli and Jones 2013) includes two measures of aerobic endurance: the 6 min walking test and the 2 min step test.

Self-Paced Step Test (Petrella et al. 2001)

Purpose: Quick assessment of the aerobic capacity of older adults in an office setting.

Application: Monitor functional aerobic capacity within the time constraints of a doctor's appointment.

Equipment: You will need a stopwatch, a valid HR monitor, and two contiguous steps, 20 cm each.

Test procedures: Instruct your client to fast for 2 hr or more before the test. Record your client's height and weight and convert those into a BMI value. A single stepping cycle is completed by following the pattern of stepping up with one foot, up to the next step with the other foot, together with both feet on the second step, down one step with one foot, down to the floor with the other foot, together with both feet on the floor. After the familiarization period (see the safety tips), let the client rest 5 min before completing 20 steps at his normal stair climbing pace. Time (in sec) how long it takes the client to complete the 20 steps. Record the HR immediately after completion of the 20th stepping cycle.

Scoring: See table 4.7 for the gender-specific equations using normal stepping pace for predicting $\dot{V}O_2$ max for this protocol. To compute the oxygen cost of stepping, use the equation

O_2 cost = [(F × step ht × 1.78 × 1.30 + 1/3F]

where F equals the stepping frequency.

Safety tips: Clinically screen the client to rule out known or possible silent ischemic heart disease, unstable metabolic disease, orthopedic issues that may affect stepping, unstable pulmonary disease, or medications that alter heart rate. Familiarize your client to the step height and stepping procedure by having him climb up and down the steps 10 times at a self-described slow pace while following the stepping pattern. Stand close by to steady the client and prevent any falls as necessary.

Validity and reliability: There were strong correlations ($r \geq .90$) between self-paced stepping estimations and measured $\dot{V}O_2$ max (ml·kg^{-1}·min^{-1}; Balke ramp treadmill protocol) for both men and women. No differences between predicted and measured $\dot{V}O_2$ max values were found 2 to 4 wk after baseline assessment. Test-retest results 52 wk later produced strong correlations for $\dot{V}O_2$ max ($r \geq .97$), heart rate ($r \geq .92$), and stepping time ($r \geq .90$) for both sexes.

6 Min Walking Test

Video 4.9

Purpose: Assess aerobic endurance.

Application: Measure ability to perform activities of daily living such as walking, stair climbing, shopping, and sightseeing.

Equipment: You will need a 5 × 20 yd (4.6 × 18.3 m) rectangular walking area, a measuring tape, a stopwatch, four cones, masking tape, index cards, and chairs.

Test procedures: Use masking tape or chalk to mark 5 yd (4.6 m) lines on a flat, rectangular course. Place cones on the inside corners of the rectangle. Instruct participants to walk (not jog) as fast as possible around the course for 6 min. Partners can keep track of the total number of laps and distance covered by marking the index card each time a lap is completed. Administer one trial; measure total distance to the nearest 5 yd. Test two or more people at a time for motivation.

Scoring: Calculate the total distance covered in 6 min. Each mark on the index card represents 50 yd (45.6 m). Use table 4.9 to determine a client's percentile ranking.

Safety tips: Place chairs around the outside of the walking course in case a client needs to sit and rest during the test. Select a level, well-lit walking area with a nonslip surface. Discontinue the test if the client shows signs of overexertion. Have the client cool down by stepping in place for 1 min.

Validity and reliability: The 6 min walking distance was positively related ($r = .78$) to submaximal treadmill walking time (Bruce protocol, time to reach 85% HRmax). This walking test detects the expected performance declines across age groups and discriminates between individuals with high and low physical activity levels and functional ability test scores. The test-retest reliability was $r = .94$.

Casanova and colleagues (2011) followed standard procedure to evaluate the 6 min walking test performance of 444 adults (40-80 yr) from seven countries. The effect of age on distance walked was significant for ages ≥60 yr, regardless of gender. They found no difference in distance walked based on self-reported activity levels (sedentary vs. physically active). Casanova and associates reported geographic variations in the distance walked that could not be explained by anthropometric variables. Consequently, they urge caution when using existing predictive equations and standard curves when interpreting results of the 6 min walking test.

Table 4.9 6 Min Walking Test Norms for Older Adults

	60-64 YR		65-69 YR		70-74 YR		75-79 YR		80-84 YR		85-89 YR		90-94 YR	
Percentile rank	**F**	**M**	**F**	**M**	**F**	**M**	**F**	**M**	**F**	**M**	**F**	**M**	**F**	**M**
95	741	825	734	800	709	779	696	762	654	721	638	710	564	646
90	711	792	697	763	673	743	655	716	612	678	591	659	518	592
85	690	770	673	738	650	718	628	686	584	649	560	625	488	557
80	674	751	653	718	630	698	605	661	560	625	534	596	463	527
75	659	736	636	700	614	680	585	639	540	604	512	572	441	502
70	647	722	621	685	599	665	568	621	523	586	493	551	423	480
65	636	710	607	671	586	652	553	604	508	571	476	532	406	461
60	624	697	593	657	572	638	538	586	491	554	458	512	388	440
55	614	686	581	644	561	625	524	571	477	540	443	495	373	422
50	603	674	568	631	548	612	509	555	462	524	426	477	357	403
45	592	662	555	618	535	599	494	539	447	508	409	459	341	384
40	582	651	543	605	524	586	480	524	433	494	394	442	326	366
35	570	638	529	591	510	572	465	506	416	477	376	422	308	345
30	559	626	515	577	497	559	450	489	401	462	359	403	291	326
25	547	612	500	562	482	544	433	471	384	444	340	382	273	304
20	532	597	483	544	466	526	413	449	364	423	318	358	251	279
15	516	578	463	524	446	506	390	424	340	399	292	329	226	249
10	495	556	439	499	423	481	363	394	312	370	261	295	196	214
5	465	523	402	462	387	445	322	348	270	327	214	244	150	160

F = females; M = males.

Note: Values represent distance in yards; to convert yards to meters, multiply by 0.91.

Adapted by permission from R. Rikli and C. Jones, *Senior Fitness Test Manual*, 2nd ed. (Champaign, IL: Human Kinetics, 2013), 156.

2 Min Step Test

Purpose: Alternative test of aerobic endurance when time, space, or weather prohibits administering the 6 min walking test.

Application: Measure ability to perform activities of daily living such as walking, stair climbing, shopping, and sightseeing.

Equipment: You will need a stopwatch, a tape measure, masking tape, and a tally counter to count steps.

Test procedures: Determine the minimum knee-stepping height of the client by identifying the midpoint between the kneecap (midpatellar level) and iliac crest. Mark this point on the anterior aspect of the client's thigh and on a nearby wall or chair. These marks are used to monitor knee height during the test. Ask the client to step in place for 2 min, lifting the right knee as high as the target level marked on the wall. Use the tally counter to count the number of times the right knee reaches the target level. If the proper knee height cannot be maintained, ask the client to slow down or stop until she can execute proper form; keep the stopwatch running. Administer one trial.

Scoring: Count the number of times the right knee reaches the target level in 2 min. Use table 4.10 to determine your client's percentile ranking.

Safety tips: Clients with poor balance should stand close to a wall, doorway, or chair for support in case they lose their balance during the test. Spot each client carefully. Have the client cool down after the test by walking slowly for 1 min. Discontinue the test if your client shows signs of overexertion.

Validity and reliability: The 2 min step test scores were moderately correlated ($r = .73$-$.74$) with

Table 4.10 2 Min Step Test Norms for Older Adults

Percentile rank	60-64 YR F	60-64 YR M	65-69 YR F	65-69 YR M	70-74 YR F	70-74 YR M	75-79 YR F	75-79 YR M	80-84 YR F	80-84 YR M	85-89 YR F	85-89 YR M	90-94 YR F	90-94 YR M
95	130	135	133	139	125	133	123	135	113	126	106	114	92	112
90	122	128	123	130	116	124	115	126	104	118	98	106	85	102
85	116	123	117	125	110	119	109	119	99	112	93	100	80	96
80	111	119	112	120	105	114	104	114	94	107	88	95	76	91
75	107	115	107	116	101	110	100	109	90	103	85	91	72	86
70	103	112	104	113	97	107	96	105	87	99	81	87	69	83
65	100	109	100	110	94	104	93	102	84	96	79	84	66	79
60	97	106	96	107	90	101	90	98	81	93	76	81	63	76
55	94	104	93	104	87	98	87	95	78	90	73	78	61	72
50	91	101	90	101	84	95	84	91	75	87	70	75	58	69
45	88	98	87	98	81	92	81	87	72	84	67	72	55	66
40	85	96	84	95	78	89	78	84	69	81	64	69	53	62
35	82	93	80	92	74	86	75	80	66	78	61	66	50	59
30	79	90	76	89	71	83	72	77	63	75	59	63	47	55
25	75	87	73	86	68	80	68	73	60	71	55	59	44	52
20	71	83	68	82	63	76	64	68	56	67	52	55	40	47
15	66	79	63	77	58	71	59	63	51	62	47	50	36	42
10	60	74	57	72	52	66	53	56	46	56	42	44	31	36
5	52	67	47	67	43	67	45	47	37	48	39	36	24	26

F = females; M = males.

Note: Values represent number of times right knee reaches target level.

Adapted by permission from R. Rikli and C. Jones, *Senior Fitness Test Manual*, 2nd ed. (Champaign, IL: Human Kinetics, 2013), 157.

Rockport 1 mi walking scores and treadmill walking (Bruce protocol, time to reach 85% HRmax) in older adults. This step test detected expected performance declines across age groups and discriminated between exercisers and nonexercisers. The test-retest reliability was $r = .90$.

Key Points

▶ The best way to assess cardiorespiratory capacity (cardiorespiratory fitness) is through a GXT in which the functional $\dot{V}O_2$max is measured.

▶ Unless contraindications to exercise are observed or medical clearance is not granted, it is advised that you administer a valid functional aerobic capacity test for your client before creating an exercise program.

▶ Before, during, and after a maximal or submaximal exercise test, closely monitor the HR, BP, and RPE.

▶ Treadmill, cycle ergometer, and bench stepping are the most commonly used modes of exercise for exercise testing.

▶ The choice of exercise mode and exercise test protocol depends on the purpose of the test and on the age, gender, and health and fitness status of the individual.

▶ Verification of maximal exercise effort is attained with short bouts of supramaximal exercise on the same modality.

▶ Self-paced protocols allow the individual to adjust workloads during graded maximal and submaximal tests.

▶ Clamping stages of an exercise test by RPE values provides the individual with a stage-specific target during a self-paced protocol.

▶ Submaximal exercise tests are used to estimate the functional cardiorespiratory capacity by predicting the $\dot{V}O_2$max of the individual. Failure to meet the assumptions underlying submaximal exercise tests produces a ±10% to 20% error in the prediction of $\dot{V}O_2$max from submaximal HR data.

▶ Field tests are the least desirable way of assessing aerobic fitness and should not be used for diagnostic purposes. However, field tests are useful for assessing the cardiorespiratory fitness of large groups.

▶ Commonly used field tests include distance runs, walking tests, step tests, and shuttle runs.

▶ Distance runs should last at least 9 min to assess aerobic function. Distance runs usually range between 1 and 2 mi (1,600 and 3,200 m) or 9 and 12 min.

▶ The validity of step tests for assessing cardiorespiratory fitness is highly dependent on obesity, height, fitness level, and the accurate measurement of HR; step test validity is usually somewhat lower than the validity of distance run tests.

▶ For children and older adults, select a treadmill protocol that increases grade rather than speed.

▶ The 6 min walking test or step tests can be used to assess cardiorespiratory fitness of older adults in field settings.

Key Terms

Learn the definition for each of the following key terms. Definitions of key terms can be found in the glossary.

absolute $\dot{V}O_2$

continuous exercise test

discontinuous exercise test

graded exercise test (GXT)

gross $\dot{V}O_2$

maximal exercise test

maximum oxygen uptake ($\dot{V}O_2$max)

net $\dot{V}O_2$

perceptually regulated exercise test (PRET)

ramp protocols

rating of perceived exertion (RPE)

relative $\dot{V}O_2$max

respiratory exchange ratio (RER)

RPE-clamped protocol

self-paced protocol

steep ramp cycling protocol (SRP)

submaximal exercise test

verification bout

$\dot{V}O_2$max

$\dot{V}O_2$peak

Review Questions

In addition to being able to define each of the key terms listed, test your knowledge and understanding of the material by answering the following review questions.

1. What is the most valid and direct measure of functional cardiorespiratory capacity?

2. What is the difference between absolute and relative $\dot{V}O_2$?

3. What is the difference between gross and net $\dot{V}O_2$?

4. What is the difference between $\dot{V}O_2$max and $\dot{V}O_2$peak?

5. What factors should you consider when choosing a maximal or submaximal exercise test protocol for your client?

6. Identify the ACSM criteria for attainment of $\dot{V}O_2$max during a GXT.

7. Explain the pros and cons of requiring a plateau in $\dot{V}O_2$ consumption to call a test "maximal."

8. How do you perform a verification bout to confirm whether the client gave maximal effort? Describe the similarities and differences between self-paced and RPE-clamped protocols.

9. During a GXT, what three variables are monitored at regular intervals?

10. List three reasons for stopping a GXT.

11. What is active recovery, and why is it recommended for graded exercise testing?

12. How do the continuous, discontinuous, and ramp exercise testing protocols differ?

13. Calculate the gross $\dot{V}O_2$ for a 60 kg woman running on a treadmill at a speed of 6.0 mph and a grade of 10%.

14. Calculate the gross $\dot{V}O_2$ for an 80 kg man cycling on a Monark cycle ergometer at a pedaling frequency of 70 rpm and a resistance of 3.5 kg.

15. Calculate the energy expenditure for bench stepping using an 8 in. step and a cadence of 30 steps·min^{-1}.

16. Name three types of field tests for estimating aerobic capacity.

17. Which type of testing, treadmill or cycle ergometer, should be used for assessing the cardiorespiratory fitness of children?

18. How should standard GXT protocols be modified for testing older adults?

19. For whom is a GXT on an elliptical cross-trainer appropriate and why?

CHAPTER 5

Designing Cardiorespiratory Exercise Programs

KEY QUESTIONS

▶ What are the basic components of an aerobic exercise prescription?

▶ How is the aerobic exercise prescription individualized to meet each client's goals and interests?

▶ What methods are used to prescribe and monitor exercise intensity?

▶ Which exercise modes are best suited for an aerobic exercise prescription?

▶ How often does a client need to exercise to improve and maintain aerobic fitness?

▶ How long does a client need to exercise to improve aerobic fitness?

▶ Is discontinuous aerobic training as effective as continuous training?

▶ How effective are multimodal cross-training programs?

▶ What are the physiological benefits of aerobic exercise training?

Once you have assessed an individual's cardiorespiratory fitness status, you are responsible for planning an aerobic exercise program to develop and maintain the cardiorespiratory endurance of that program participant—a program that will meet the individual's needs and interests, taking into account age, gender, physical fitness level, and exercise habits. Appendix A.5, Lifestyle Evaluation, provides forms that will help you determine your clients' exercise patterns and preferences.

In designing the exercise prescription, keep in mind that some people engage in aerobic exercise to improve their health status or reduce their disease risk, while others are primarily interested in enhancing their physical fitness ($\dot{V}O_2$max) levels or physical appearance. Given that the quantity of exercise needed to promote health is less than that needed to develop and maintain higher levels of physical fitness, you must adjust the exercise prescription according to your client's primary goal.

This chapter provides guidelines for writing individualized exercise prescriptions that promote health status as well as develop and maintain cardiorespiratory fitness. It compares various training methods and aerobic exercise modes and presents examples of individualized exercise programs.

THE EXERCISE PRESCRIPTION

It is important to consider each client's goals and purposes for engaging in an exercise program. The primary goal for exercising may affect the mode, intensity, frequency, duration, and progression of the exercise prescription. For example, the quantity of physical activity needed to achieve health benefits or reduce one's risk of illness and death is less than the amount of activity typically prescribed when the client's goal is to make substantial improvements in cardiorespiratory fitness. When the primary goal for the exercise prescription is improved health, refer to

Guidelines for Exercise Prescription for Improved Health.

On the other hand, when the primary goal for the exercise prescription is to improve cardiorespiratory fitness, refer to ACSM (2018) Guidelines for Exercise Prescription for Improved Health and Cardiorespiratory Fitness.

ELEMENTS OF A CARDIORESPIRATORY EXERCISE WORKOUT

Each exercise workout of the aerobic exercise prescription and program should include the following phases:

- Warm-up (5-10 min)
- Endurance conditioning (20-60 min)
- Cool-down (5-10 min)
- Stretching (≥10 min)

The purpose of the warm-up is to increase blood flow to the working cardiac and skeletal muscles, increase body temperature, decrease the chance of muscle and joint injury, and lessen the chance of abnormal cardiac rhythms. During the warm-up, the tempo of the exercise is gradually increased to prepare the body for a higher intensity of exercise performed during the conditioning phase. The warm-up starts with 5 to 10 min of low-intensity (<40% $\dot{V}O_2$ reserve [$\dot{V}O_2R$]) to moderate-intensity (40%-60% $\dot{V}O_2R$) aerobic activity (e.g., brisk walking for clients who jog or slow jogging for clients who run during their endurance conditioning phase).

During the endurance conditioning phase of the workout, aerobic exercise is performed according to the exercise prescription following the **FITT-VP principle** (i.e., F = frequency; I = intensity; T = time, duration; T = type, mode of activity; V = volume, quantity; P = progression) (ACSM 2018). This phase usually lasts 20 to 60 min, depending on the exercise intensity. Bouts of 10 min are acceptable as long as the client accumulates at least 30 min of moderate-intensity or 20 min of vigorous-intensity exercise that day. The conditioning phase is followed immediately by the cool-down phase.

A cool-down phase immediately after endurance exercise is needed to reduce the risk of cardiovascular complications caused by stopping exercise suddenly. During cool-down, the individual continues exercising (e.g., walking, jogging, or cycling) at a low intensity for 5 to 10 min. This light activity allows the heart rate (HR) and blood pressure (BP) to return to near baseline levels, prevents the pooling of blood in the extremities, and reduces the possibility of dizziness and fainting. The continued pumping action of the muscles increases the venous return and speeds up the recovery process.

The stretching phase usually lasts at least 10 min and is performed after the warm-up or cool-down phase. Static stretching exercises for the legs, lower back, abdomen, hips, groin, and shoulders are usually included (for specific flexibility exercises, see appendix F.1). Stretching exercises after the cool-down phase may help reduce the chance of muscle cramps or muscle soreness.

TYPES (MODES) OF EXERCISE

If the primary goal of the exercise program is to develop and maintain cardiorespiratory fitness, pre-

Guidelines for Exercise Prescription for Improved Health

The following aerobic exercise guidelines are from the U.S. Department of Health and Human Services (2015).

1. **Mode:** Select endurance-type physical activities.
2. **Intensity:** Prescribe at least moderate-intensity physical activities (3 to 6 METs [metabolic equivalents of task]).
3. **Frequency and duration:** Schedule at least 150 to 300 min/wk (e.g., 30 min, 5 days/wk or 60 min, 3 days/wk). Duration varies according to the type and intensity of activity (see Examples of Moderate-Intensity and Vigorous-Intensity Aerobic Activities, chapter 1).

ACSM Guidelines for Exercise Prescription for Improved Health and Cardiorespiratory Fitness (FITT-VP)

1. **Frequency:** Schedule moderate-intensity exercise at least 5 days/wk, vigorous-intensity exercise at least 3 days/wk, or a combination of moderate- and vigorous-intensity exercise 3 to 5 days/wk.

2. **Intensity:** Prescribe moderate-intensity (3.0-6.0 METs or 40%-<60% $\dot{V}O_2R$ or HRR) or vigorous-intensity (>6.0 METs or ≥60%-89% $\dot{V}O_2R$ or HRR) or a combination of moderate- and vigorous-intensity exercise. Intensity varies depending on the client's cardiorespiratory fitness classification.

3. **Progression:** Gradually adjust the exercise prescription for each client in accordance with the conditioning effect, participant characteristics, new exercise test results, or performance during the exercise sessions. The rate of progression depends on the individual's age, functional capacity, health status, and goals. For apparently healthy adults, a reasonable progression increases duration by 5 to 10 min every 1 to 2 wk for the first 4 to 6 wk of their exercise program. Typically, the aerobic exercise prescription consists of three stages: initial conditioning, improvement, and maintenance.

4. **Time (duration):** Schedule 30 to 60 min of moderate-intensity exercise (≥150 min/wk), 20 to 60 min of vigorous-intensity exercise (≥75 min/wk), or a combination of moderate- and vigorous-intensity exercise to attain recommended targeted volumes of exercise. Continuous exercise bouts of 10 min or more may be accumulated throughout the day.

5. **Type (mode):** Select rhythmic aerobic activities that can be maintained continuously and that involve large muscle groups and require little skill to perform (see Classification of Aerobic Exercise Modalities). Introduce other aerobic activities requiring more stamina or skill later in the program.

6. **Volume (quantity):** For most adults, target approximately 1,000 kcal·wk^{-1} moderate-intensity exercise or physical activity (150 min/wk at 3.0-6.0 METs or 40%-<60% $\dot{V}O_2R$). When combined with the recommended duration, daily pedometer step counts (≥5,400 to 7,900 steps·day^{-1}) fulfill this category. More steps per day are required for weight loss and subsequent weight maintenance. An energy expenditure between 500 and 1,000 MET·min·wk^{-1} is the recommended quantity of exercise or physical activity for most adults. To compute **MET·min·wk^{-1}**, multiply the MET value of an activity by the number of minutes it is performed in the week.

Based on ACSM (2018).

scribe aerobic activities using large muscle groups in a continuous, rhythmic fashion. In the initial and improvement stages of the exercise program, it is important to closely monitor the exercise intensity. Therefore, you should select modes of exercise that allow the individual to maintain a constant exercise intensity and that are not highly dependent on the participant's skill. **Type A activities** require minimal skill or physical fitness to perform. Activities such as walking, cycling, and aqua-aerobics are best suited for this purpose. **Type B activities** are vigorous-intensity exercises that require minimal skill but average physical fitness. Jogging and Spinning are examples of type B activities. You may prescribe type B activities in the initial and improvement stages for individuals who exercise regularly. **Type C activities** include endurance activities that require both skill and average physical fitness levels. Swimming, skating, and cross-country skiing should be prescribed only for individuals who have acquired these skills or who possess adequate physical fitness levels to learn these skills. **Type D activities** are recreational sports that may improve physical fitness. These should be performed in addition to the person's regular aerobic exercise program. Examples of type D activities are racket sports, hiking, soccer, basketball, and downhill skiing. You should consider using type C and D activities to add variety in the later stages (maintenance stage) of your clients' exercise programs.

In addition to walking, jogging, and cycling, other exercise modalities provide a sufficient cardiorespiratory demand for improving aerobic fitness. Exercise modalities such as machine-based stair climbing, elliptical training, and rowing offer your exercise program participants a variety of options for their exercise prescription. Many individuals prefer to cross-train to add variety and enjoyment to their aerobic workouts. But are these exercise modes just as effective as traditional type A and B activities (walking, jogging, and cycling)? The answer to this question is not simple, and it depends on the method (%$\dot{V}O_2$ max or perceived exertion) used to equate different exercise modalities.

During exercise at a prescribed percentage of $\dot{V}O_2$max, Thomas and colleagues (1995) noted that six different aerobic exercise modes (treadmill jogging, Nordic skiing, shuffle skiing, stepping, cycling, and rowing) produced relatively similar cardiovascular responses (see figure 5.1), but that

cycling resulted in a significantly higher rate of perceived exertion (RPE) compared with the other modes. Likewise, other researchers have reported that the relationship between HR and $\dot{V}O_2$ at constant submaximal intensities was similar for treadmill jogging, in-line skating (Wallick et al. 1995), and aerobic dancing with arms used extensively above the head or kept below the shoulders (Berry et al. 1992). In contrast, Parker and colleagues (1989) reported that the average steady-state HR during 20 min of aerobic dancing was significantly higher than that for treadmill jogging when the subjects exercised at the same relative intensity (60% $\dot{V}O_2$max). Likewise, Howley, Colacino, and Swensen (1992) noted that HR response during electronic step ergometer exercise was systematically higher than that from treadmill exercise at the same submaximal $\dot{V}O_2$. Also, supporting the body weight during step ergometer exercise significantly reduces the HR and oxygen consumption compared with lightly holding on to the handrails for balance.

When exercise modes are equated using subjective RPEs, research suggests that treadmill jogging may be superior to other aerobic exercise modes

CLASSIFICATION OF AEROBIC EXERCISE MODALITIES

These lists contain examples of moderate amounts of physical activity. More vigorous activities, such as stair walking and running, require less time (15 min). On the other hand, less vigorous activities like washing and waxing the car require more time (45-60 min).

Type A Activities	Type B Activities	Type C Activities	Type D Activities
Cycling (indoors)	Jogging and running	Aerobic dancing	Basketball
Walking	Rowing*	In-line skating	Downhill skiing
Aqua-aerobics	Stair climbing*	Nordic skiing (outdoors)	Handball
Slow dancing	Simulated climbing*	Rope skipping	Racket sports
	Nordic skiing*	Swimming	Hiking
	Elliptical training*		
	Spinning		
	Fast dancing		

Note: Type A activities require minimal skill and physical fitness; type B activities require average physical fitness but minimal skill; type C activities require both skill and average physical fitness levels; and type D activities are recreational sports that should be prescribed only in addition to a regular, aerobic exercise program.

*Machine-based activities.

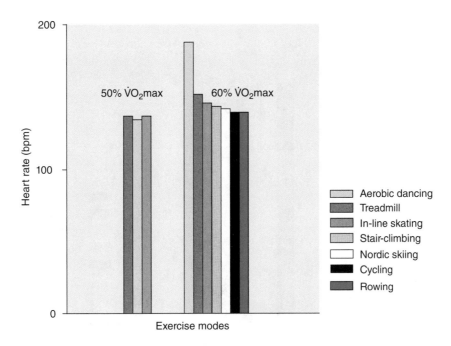

FIGURE 5.1 Comparison of steady-state heart rate response at submaximal exercise intensities for various aerobic exercise modes.

in terms of total oxygen consumption and rate of energy expenditure (Hulsey et al. 2012; Kravitz, Robergs, and Heyward 1996; Kravitz et al. 1997b; Zeni, Hoffman, and Clifford 1996). Subjects exercising on seven different modalities at a somewhat hard (RPE = 13 or 14) intensity for 15 to 20 min experienced a greater total oxygen consumption for treadmill jogging compared with stepping, rowing, Nordic skiing, cycling, and shuffle skiing (Kravitz et al. 1997b; Thomas et al. 1995). Also, the rate of energy expenditure during treadmill exercise was 20% to 40% greater than during stationary cycling (Kravitz et al. 1997b; Zeni, Hoffman, and Clifford 1996) and 42% higher than arm crank exercise (Schrieks, Barnes, and Hodges 2011). Hulsey and colleagues (2012) reported that kettlebell swinging intervals require 25% to 39% less energy than does treadmill exercise at the same RPE. In addition, steady-state exercise HRs were higher (see figure 5.2) for treadmill jogging compared with cycling and aerobic riding (Kravitz et al. 1996; Kravitz et al. 1997b; Zeni, Hoffman, and Clifford 1996). Similarly, HR and RPE were higher during kettlebell swings and sumo deadlifts compared with treadmill walking at the same $\dot{V}O_2$ (Thomas et al. 2014). The average net energy expenditure of young adults (18-28 yr; 29.1-55.2 ml·kg^{-1}·min^{-1}) was 5.56 kcal·min^{-1} higher over 1,600 m when running (160 m·min^{-1}) compared with walking (86 m·min^{-1}) on a treadmill (Wilkin, Cheryl, and Haddock 2012).

When selecting aerobic exercise modes for a client's exercise prescription, you should consider how easily the exercise intensity can be graded and adjusted in order to overload the cardiorespiratory system throughout the improvement stage. For aerobic dance, work rates can be progressively increased by means of quicker cadences and upper body exercise using light (1-4 lb [0.45-1.8 kg]) hand-held weights (Kravitz et al. 1997a). The intensity of in-line skating can be effectively graded by increasing the skating velocity (Wallick et al. 1995). The intensity of rowing, stair climbing, and simulated whole-body climbing exercise can be incremented progressively using a variety of exercise machine settings (Brahler and Blank 1995; Howley, Colacino, and Swensen 1992).

Prescribe rope-skipping activities with caution; the exercise intensity for skipping 60 to 80 skips·min^{-1} is approximately 9 METs. This value exceeds the maximum MET capacity of most sedentary individuals. Also, the exercise intensity is not easily graded because doubling the rate of skipping

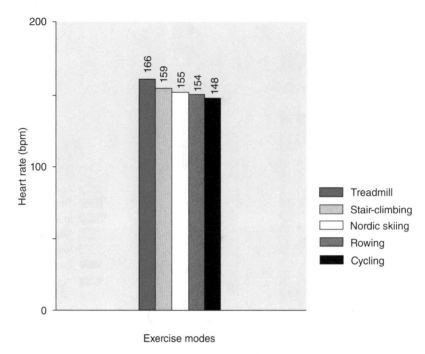

FIGURE 5.2 Comparison of steady-state heart rate response at somewhat hard intensity (rating of perceived exertion = 13 or 14) for various aerobic exercise modes.

increases the energy requirement by only 2 or 3 METs. Town, Sol, and Sinning (1980) reported an average energy expenditure of 11.7 to 12.5 METs for skipping at rates of 125, 135, and 145 skips·min⁻¹. They concluded that rope skipping is a strenuous exercise that may not serve well as a form of graded aerobic exercise.

When selecting exercise modes for your older clients, you need to consider their functional aerobic capacity, musculoskeletal problems, and neuromuscular coordination (impaired vision or balance). Select activities that are enjoyable and convenient. For many older adults, walking is an excellent mode. Stationary cycling and aquatic exercise can be used for individuals with impaired vision or balance. Research reviewed by Jahnke and colleagues (2010) suggests that tai chi and qigong demonstrate similar health benefits pertaining to balance improvement and fall prevention, cardiorespiratory fitness, physical function, and quality of life in older adults.

INTENSITY OF EXERCISE

Exercise intensity is a key factor in determining physiological adaptations to the exercise stimulus (Wolpern et al. 2015). Traditionally, exercise inten-

sity has been expressed as a straight percentage of the individual's maximal aerobic capacity ($\dot{V}O_2$max), peak oxygen consumption ($\dot{V}O_2$peak), or heart rate reserve (HRR). However, research has suggested that the %$\dot{V}O_2$ max is not equivalent (1:1 ratio) to the %HRR for cycling and treadmill exercise (Morán-Navarro et al. 2016; Swain and Leutholtz 1997; Swain et al. 1998). The ACSM changed its recommendation regarding the method used to calculate exercise intensity for aerobic exercise prescriptions. Instead of expressing relative intensity as a straight percentage of $\dot{V}O_2$ max (%$\dot{V}O_2$ max) or HRmax (%HRmax), the ACSM (2018) recommends using the **percent $\dot{V}O_2$ reserve (%$\dot{V}O_2$R)**. The $\dot{V}O_2$R is the difference between the $\dot{V}O_2$ max and resting oxygen consumption ($\dot{V}O_2$ rest). With this modification, percent values for the %$\dot{V}O_2$R and %HRR methods for prescribing exercise intensity are approximately equal, thereby improving the accuracy of calculating a target $\dot{V}O_2$, particularly for clients who are engaging in low-intensity aerobic exercise (Swain 1999). There is individual variability in resting oxygen consumption; this introduces questions regarding the assumed constant (1 MET = 3.5 ml·kg⁻¹·min⁻¹) ascribed to $\dot{V}O_2$ rest (Mansoubi et al. 2015). Consequently, when it is available, the actual

$\dot{V}O_2$ rest should be used when determining $\dot{V}O_2R$.

Regardless of the method used, intensity and duration of exercise are indirectly related. In other words, the higher the exercise intensity, the shorter the duration of exercise required and vice versa. Before prescribing the exercise intensity for aerobic exercise, carefully evaluate the individual's initial cardiorespiratory fitness classification, goals for the program, exercise preferences, and injury risks. Your client can improve cardiorespiratory fitness with either lower-intensity, longer-duration exercise or higher-intensity, shorter-duration exercise. Historically, low to moderate intensities of longer duration were recommended for most individuals. Higher-intensity exercise may increase the risk of orthopedic injury and, consequently, discourage continued participation in the exercise program. Regardless, high-intensity interval training (HIT) is receiving interest as an increasingly popular and time-efficient rival of endurance training for improving cardiorespiratory fitness. In a detailed analysis and evaluation of studies comparing traditional endurance training with HIT, the mean effect between the two training styles is small. Nevertheless, HIT's influence on $\dot{V}O_2$ max is greater than is that of endurance training (Milanović, Sporiš, and Weston 2015).

Part of the art of exercise prescription is being able to select an exercise intensity that is adequate to stress the cardiovascular system without overtaxing it. According to the ACSM (2018), the initial exercise intensity for apparently healthy adults is 40% to <90% $\dot{V}O_2R$ or HRR, depending on their initial physical fitness classification (i.e., fair to excellent cardiorespiratory fitness level). Lower-intensity exercise (30%-59% $\dot{V}O_2R$ or HRR) may be sufficient to provide important health benefits for sedentary clients or older individuals with poor initial cardiorespiratory fitness levels. For most individuals, intensities of 55% to 80% $\dot{V}O_2R$ are sufficient to improve cardiorespiratory fitness. As a general rule, the more fit the individual, the higher the exercise intensity needs to be to produce further improvement in cardiorespiratory fitness. In fact, Morán-Navarro and colleagues (2016) reported that the thresholds denoting the switch from aerobic to anaerobic metabolism for highly trained male cyclists (20.5 ± 7.5 yr) occurred between 62% and 89% HRR. This finding suggests that highly fit individuals may require a higher exercise intensity than what is generally prescribed for the average adult. Exercise intensity can be prescribed using the $\dot{V}O_2$ reserve, HR, RPE, or talk test method.

$\dot{V}O_2$ Reserve (MET) Method

First, measure the client's functional aerobic capacity ($\dot{V}O_2$ max or $\dot{V}O_2$ peak) using a graded exercise test (see chapter 4). Express the client's $\dot{V}O_2$ max in relative terms: $ml \cdot kg^{-1} \cdot min^{-1}$ or METs (metabolic equivalents of task). The $\dot{V}O_2R$ calculations presented here assume that 1 MET is approximately equal to $3.5\ ml \cdot kg^{-1} \cdot min^{-1}$. Therefore, given a $\dot{V}O_2$ max of 35 $ml \cdot kg^{-1} \cdot min^{-1}$, for example, the metabolic equivalent would be 10 METs (35 / 3.5 = 10 METs).

Next determine the $\dot{V}O_2$ reserve ($\dot{V}O_2R$). As mentioned previously, the $\dot{V}O_2R$ is the difference between $\dot{V}O_2$ max and $\dot{V}O_2$ rest ($\dot{V}O_2R = \dot{V}O_2$ max − $\dot{V}O_2$ rest). The percentage of $\dot{V}O_2R$ depends on the initial cardiorespiratory fitness level of the client. To calculate the target $\dot{V}O_2$ (in METs) based on the $\dot{V}O_2R$, use the following equation:

$$\text{target } \dot{V}O_2 = [\text{relative exercise intensity (\%)} \times \dot{V}O_2 R] + \dot{V}O_2 \text{ rest}$$

For example, the target $\dot{V}O_2$ corresponding to 50% $\dot{V}O_2R$ for a client with a $\dot{V}O_2$ max of 10 METs is calculated as follows:

$$\text{target } \dot{V}O_2 = [0.50 \times (10 - 1 \text{ MET})] + 1 \text{ MET}$$

$$= (0.50 \times 9 \text{ METs}) + 1 \text{ MET}$$

$$= 4.5 + 1.0 \text{ METs, or } 5.5 \text{ METs}$$

The exercise intensity (METs) for walking, jogging, running, cycling, and bench-stepping activities is directly related to the speed of movement, power output, or mass lifted. Use the ACSM equations (table 4.3) to calculate the speed or work rates corresponding to a specific MET intensity for the exercise prescription. For example, to estimate how fast a woman should jog on a level course to be exercising at an intensity of 8 METs, follow these steps:

1. Convert the METs to $ml \cdot kg^{-1} \cdot min^{-1}$.

$$\dot{V}O_2 = 8 \text{ METs} \times 3.5\ ml \cdot kg^{-1} \cdot min^{-1}$$

$$= 28\ ml \cdot kg^{-1} \cdot min^{-1}$$

2. Substitute known values into the ACSM running equation and solve for speed.

$$28 \text{ ml·kg}^{-1}\text{·min}^{-1} = [\text{speed (m·min}^{-1}) \times 0.2]$$
$$+ 3.5 \text{ ml·kg}^{-1}\text{·min}^{-1}$$

$$28.0 \text{ ml·kg}^{-1}\text{·min}^{-1} - 3.5 = \text{speed (m·min}^{-1}) \times 0.2$$
$$122.5 \text{ m·min}^{-1} = \text{speed}$$

3. Convert speed to mph.

$$1 \text{ mph} = 26.8 \text{ m·min}^{-1}$$

$$122.5 \text{ m·min}^{-1} / 26.8 \text{ m·min}^{-1} = 4.57 \text{ mph}$$

4. Convert mph to minute per mile pace.

$$\text{pace} = 60 \text{ min/hr} / \text{mph}$$

$$= 60 \text{ min/hr} / 4.57 \text{ mph}$$

$$= 13.1 \text{ min·mi}^{-1} \text{ (or } 8.1 \text{ min·km}^{-1})$$

Average MET values for selected conditioning exercises, sports, and recreational activities are presented in appendix E.3, Gross Energy Expenditure for Conditioning Exercises, Sports, and Recreational Activities. When estimating MET values for children and adolescents, use the compendium of energy expenditures (MET values) developed for youth (see McMurray et al. 2015; Ridley, Ainsworth, and Olds 2008). Prescribing exercise intensity using only MET values has certain limitations. The caloric costs (i.e., average MET values) of conditioning exercises are only estimates of energy expenditure. The caloric costs of activities, particularly type C activities, vary greatly with the individual's skill level. Although these MET estimates provide a starting point for prescribing exercise intensity, environmental factors such as heat, humidity, altitude, and pollution may alter the HR and RPE responses to exercise. Therefore, you should use the HR or RPE method along with the MET method to ensure that the exercise intensity does not exceed safe limits.

Heart Rate Methods

There are three ways to prescribe exercise intensity for your clients using HR data. Each of these approaches is based on the assumption that HR is a linear function of exercise intensity (i.e., the higher the exercise intensity, the higher the HR).

Heart Rate Versus MET Graphing Method

When a submaximal or maximal graded exercise test (GXT) is administered, the client's steady-state HR response to each stage of the exercise test can be plotted (see figure 5.3). The HRmax is the HR observed at the highest exercise intensity during

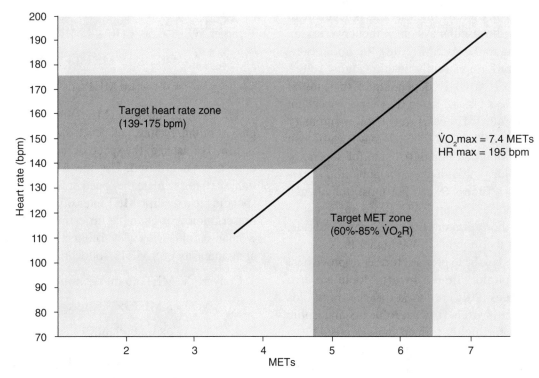

FIGURE 5.3 Plotting target heart rate zone using graded exercise test data (heart rate vs. METs). HRmax = maximal heart rate; $\dot{V}O_2R$ = oxygen reserve.

a maximal GXT. For submaximal GXTs, you can estimate a client's HRmax using one of the age-predicted HRmax formulas (e.g., 220 − age). From this graph, you can obtain HRs corresponding to given percentages of the estimated functional capacity or $\dot{V}O_2$max. In our example, the functional capacity of the individual is 7.4 METs, and the HRmax is 195 bpm. The HRs corresponding to exercise intensities of 4.8 and 6.4 METs (60%-85% $\dot{V}O_2$R) are 139 and 175 bpm, respectively. During exercise workouts, the individual should measure the HR using an HR monitor or palpation to verify that the appropriate exercise intensity is reached.

It is important to note that the HR response to graded exercise is dependent to some extent on the mode of exercise testing. For example, compared with treadmill testing, exercising on an electronic step ergometer elicits higher HRs, and stationary cycling typically results in somewhat lower HRs at the same relative exercise intensities. When using this method to obtain HRs for an exercise prescription, be sure to match the exercise testing and training modes by selecting a testing mode that elicits HR responses that are similar to those obtained for the training mode (see figure 5.1). For example, if your client chooses skating as a training mode and you do not have a skating treadmill, you should administer an incremental slide board GXT, given that the relationship between HR, $\dot{V}O_2$, %$\dot{V}O_2$max, and ventilation at submaximal exercise intensities is similar for these two exercise modes (Piucco et al. 2017).

Heart Rate Reserve Method

When HR data from a GXT are not available, you can use the **Karvonen method**, or **percent heart rate reserve (%HRR) method**, to determine target HRs for a client's exercise prescription. The **heart rate reserve (HRR) method** takes into account the resting HR and maximal HR. The HRR is the difference between the maximal HR and resting HR. A percentage of HRR is added to the client's resting HR to determine the target exercise HR:

$$\text{target HR} = [\% \text{ exercise intensity} \times (\text{HRmax} - \text{HRrest})] + \text{HRrest}$$

As previously mentioned, the percent values for the HRR method closely approximate the percent values for the $\dot{V}O_2$R method (Azevedo et al. 2011; Lounana et al. 2007; Swain and Leutholtz 1997). The ACSM (2018) recommends using 40% to <90% HRR for most adults. Deconditioned individuals may need to start at 30% HRR. For example, if

$$\text{maximal HR} = 178 \text{ bpm,}$$

$$\text{resting HR} = 68 \text{ bpm, and}$$

$$\text{exercise intensity} = 60\% \text{ HRR, then}$$

$$\text{target exercise HR} = 0.60(178 - 68) + 68$$
$$\text{or } 134 \text{ bpm.}$$

Percentage of Maximal Heart Rate Method

You also can use a straight percentage of maximal HR (**percent heart rate maximum, %HRmax**) to estimate exercise intensity and determine target exercise HR. This method is based on the fact that the %HRmax is related to %$\dot{V}O_2$R and %HRR. In table 5.1, you can see that 67% and 94% HRmax correspond to exercise intensities of 45% and 85% $\dot{V}O_2$R or HRR. Using this method, you will typically prescribe target HRs between 64% and 96% HRmax depending on the fitness level of your client.

With use of this technique, the actual maximal HR must be known or must be predicted either from the HR response to submaximal workloads or from the HRmax prediction equations, such as

Table 5.1 Comparison of Methods for Prescribing Exercise Intensity for Healthy Adults

CR fitness classification	%HRR or %$\dot{V}O_2$R	%HRmax	RPE
Poor	30-45	57-67	Light-moderate
Fair	40-55	64-74	Light-moderate
Average	55-70	74-84	Moderate-hard
Good	65-80	80-91	Moderate-hard
Excellent	70-<90	84-96	Somewhat hard-hard

HRR = heart rate reserve; RPE = rating of perceived exertion.

220 − age or 206.9 − (0.67 × age). For example, if the age-predicted maximal HR is 180 bpm and the exercise intensity is set at 70% HRmax, the target exercise HR is equal to 126 bpm.

$$\%HRmax \times HRmax = target\ HR$$

$$0.70 \times 180\ bpm = 126\ bpm$$

Compared with the Karvonen (%HRR) method, the %HRmax method tends to give a lower value when the same relative intensity is used. If in our example the client's resting HR is 80 bpm, the target HR using the Karvonen method is 150 bpm [0.70 × (180 − 80) + 80 bpm] compared with 126 bpm for the %HRmax method.

Limitations of Heart Rate Methods

Exclusive use of HR to develop intensity recommendations for your clients' exercise prescriptions may lead to large errors in estimating relative exercise intensities ($\%\dot{V}O_2R$) for some individuals. This is especially true when HRmax is predicted from age (220 − age) instead of being directly measured. In about 30% of the population, an age-predicted prescription of 60% HRR may be as low as 70% or as high as 80% of the actual HRmax (Dishman 1994). Measured HRmax varies with exercise mode. Therefore, your clients' perceived effort may differ among exercise modes even during exercise at the same submaximal HR. Also, medications, emotional states, and environmental factors (e.g., temperature, humidity, and air pollution) can affect your clients' exercise training HRs. You should consider using RPEs to adjust the exercise intensity in such situations.

Rating of Perceived Exertion Method

In light of the limitations associated with using HR for setting exercise intensity, consider using a combination of HR and RPE in developing prescriptions for your clients. You can use RPEs to prescribe and monitor exercise intensity for healthy and clinical clientele (Reed and Pipe 2016; Tang et al. 2016). The ACSM (2018) recommends using RPE values (10-point scale) to prescribe exercise intensity for older adults (moderate intensity: 5 to 6; vigorous intensity: 7 to 8). The RPE scales (see table 4.2 and appendix B.4) are valid and reliable tools for assess-

ing the level of physical exertion during continuous aerobic exercise (Guidetti et al. 2011; Krause et al. 2012; Mays et al. 2010; Reed and Pipe 2016; Scherr et al. 2013; Tang et al. 2016).

During the GXT, the client rates the intensity of each stage of the test using an RPE scale. You can use the intensities (METs) corresponding to somewhat hard (6 on OMNI scale or 12 on Borg RPE scale) to hard (8 on OMNI scale or 16 on Borg RPE scale) to set the minimum and maximum training intensities for the exercise prescription. Compared with the %HRR method, RPEs between 12 and 16 closely approximate 40% and 84% HRR, respectively (Pollock et al. 1998). Strong correlations between the OMNI-RPE and $\dot{V}O_2$ (r = .93-.96) as well as HR (r = .96-.97) and the Borg RPE scale (r = .96-.98) were reported (Mays et al. 2010). Similarly, Scherr and colleagues (2013) reported a correlation between RPE (6-20 scale) and blood lactate (r = .84 for a quadratic regression) that was higher than that between RPE and HR (r = .74 for a linear regression); their sample consisted of 2,560 Caucasians (13-83 yr) who were classified as either sedentary (failed to meet the ACSM's recommended guidelines for physical activity) or athletic (performed at least 10 hr of exercise weekly or were members of a national team). As reported by Scherr and colleagues (2013), the relationships between RPE and associated exercise intensity variables (HR or blood lactate) were strong and independent of gender, medical history, age, level of physical activity, and testing modality (treadmill or stationary cycle).

With practice, an individual can learn to associate RPE with a specific target exercise HR, especially at higher exercise intensities (Smutok, Skrinar, and Pandolf 1980). Thus, the RPE can be used instead of HR, or in combination with HR, to monitor training intensity and to adjust the exercise prescription for conditioning effects. Parfitt, Evans, and Eston (2012) reported that sedentary clients are able to successfully use RPE to monitor their exercise intensity. Those who exercised 3 days/wk at an RPE of 13 (somewhat hard) on the Borg 6-20 scale improved their aerobic capacity by 17% in 8 wk. Moreover, the majority of the exercise intervention group perceived their exercise sessions as being pleasant and reported that their selected exercise intensity felt good (Parfitt, Evans, and Eston 2012). Interestingly, Scherr and colleagues (2013) confirmed that an RPE in the range of 11 to 13 is appropriate for untrained or less fit individuals, while those with higher levels of fitness would benefit from aerobic training in the RPE range of 13 to 15. Compared with men, women are more likely to overestimate RPE, especially if the women are infrequent exercisers. In contrast, men and regular exercisers tend to underestimate their level of physical activity compared with accelerometry data (Skatrud-Mickelson et al. 2011). Consequently, as an exercise professional, you must remain aware that some of your clients may likely misestimate their level of exertion.

One advantage of RPE as a method of monitoring exercise intensity is that your clients do not need to stop exercising in order to check their HRs. Unfortunately, exercising at a given RPE value produces very different metabolic responses when performing kettlebell swings (34.1 ml·kg^{-1}·min^{-1}) compared with treadmill running (46.7 ml·kg^{-1}·min^{-1}) (Hulsey et al. 2012). For an extensive review of research pertaining to the use of perceived exertion for prescribing exercise intensity, see the studies of Dishman (1994) and Robertson (2004). Parfitt and colleagues (2012) describe how allowing clients to select their exercise intensity based on RPE theoretically supports the sense of self-determination and perception of exercise autonomy, both of which may improve client adherence to an exercise prescription.

Monitoring Exercise Intensity

Throughout the aerobic exercise program, carefully monitor exercise intensity in order to ensure your clients' safety and to confirm that your clients are exercising at or near the prescribed intensity. The HR and RPE methods can be used for this purpose. Teach your clients how to monitor exercise intensity using HR palpation techniques (see chapter 2), HR monitors, and the RPE scales (see table 4.2).

Research assessing the validity and reliability of using motion and physiological response monitors to track exercise intensity for a variety of exercise modalities is ongoing. Some exercise modalities are more suitable than others when monitoring HR via technology. In addition to working well for land-based exercise, some HR monitors work well in fresh water (e.g., swimming pools) but must be waterproofed for use in salt water (i.e., swimming in the ocean). Raffaelli and colleagues (2012) reported that monitoring intensity during water aerobics is

better done by HR palpation than accelerometry.

Some clients prefer using a talk test to monitor their exertion. The **talk test** is a measure of the ability to converse comfortably while exercising, and it is based on the relationship between exercise intensity and pulmonary ventilation. **Pulmonary ventilation**, or the movement of air into and out of the lungs, increases linearly with exercise intensity ($\dot{V}O_2$) up to a point. At the breaking point, known as the **ventilatory threshold (VT)**, pulmonary ventilation increases exponentially relative to the exercise intensity and rate of oxygen consumed. At the ventilatory threshold, it becomes difficult to speak during exercise. However, Quinn and Coons (2011) found that the talk test was more strongly associated with **lactate threshold** (exercise intensity at which blood lactate value increases by at least 1 mmol·L^{-1} compared with the previous blood sample) and RPE than with the VT in young men.

Studies of college-age students (Persinger et al. 2004), clinically stable cardiac patients (Reed and Pipe 2014), and athletes (Jeans et al. 2011; Recalde et al. 2002) showed that individuals who pass the talk test are exercising at intensities within the accepted guidelines for the exercise prescription. Those failing the talk test are exercising at intensities that exceed the prescribed level but that may be appropriate for high-intensity intervals. In a group of competitive male cyclists (21-37 yr), Gillespie's research team (2015) found that the point of failure on the talk test (definitely unable to speak comfortably) equated to their cyclists' ventilatory thresholds. The talk test provides a fairly precise and consistent method for monitoring exercise during stationary cycling and treadmill exercise (Persinger et al. 2004). The accuracy of the talk test to predict VT is improved by using speech passages that are ≥93 words in length (Schroeder et al. 2017).

Similarly, the **counting talk test (CTT)** is an objective method for monitoring exercise intensity (Loose et al. 2012). The counting talk test is normalized relative to how far one can count during rest; following a maximal inhalation, one begins counting at a comfortable pace (i.e., one one-thousand, two one-thousand, and so on). The highest digit counted prior to a second inhalation is the number (CTT_{rest}) used for future exercise intensity determinations. During exercise, the counting procedure is repeated, with the highest number spoken before breathing again divided by the baseline value to derive a %CTT$_{rest}$. Exercising at 30% to 40% CTT$_{rest}$ or 40% to 50% CTT$_{rest}$ is equivalent to being in the moderate- to vigorous-intensity range for those with a CTT$_{rest}$ of at least 25 or <25, respectively. The CTT is reliable as well as significantly and inversely related to %HRR and RPE (r = −.64 to −.77) for walking, stationary cycling, elliptical training, and stair stepping (Loose et al. 2012).

FREQUENCY OF EXERCISE

The frequency of the exercise sessions depends on the client's caloric goals, health and fitness level, preferences, time constraints, and targeted exercise intensity. Health and fitness benefits result from moderate-intensity aerobic exercise performed at least 5 days/wk. Vigorous-intensity aerobic exercise performed more than 5 days/wk may result in overuse injuries for individuals lacking moderate to high levels of aerobic fitness and variety in exercise modalities. A combination of moderate- and vigorous-intensity aerobic exercise performed 3 to 5 days/wk is recommended (ACSM 2018) for attaining and retaining health and fitness benefits. Exercising fewer than three times per week is not recommended even though some health and fitness benefits may be realized by doing so. Individuals with poor cardiorespiratory fitness levels should exercise at light to moderate intensities a minimum of 5 days/wk. Multiple daily exercise bouts of at least 10 min duration each may be prescribed for sedentary clients having poor aerobic fitness.

In terms of improving $\dot{V}O_2$max, the sequence of exercise sessions seems to be less important than the total work (volume) performed during the training. Similar improvements were noted for individuals who trained every other day (M-W-F) and three consecutive days (M-T-W) (Moffatt, Stamford, and Neill 1977).

TIME (DURATION) OF EXERCISE

As an exercise specialist, you must prescribe an appropriate combination of exercise intensity and duration so that the individual adequately stresses the cardiorespiratory system without overexertion. As mentioned earlier, the intensity and duration of exercise are inversely related (the lower the exercise intensity, the longer the duration of the exercise). The ACSM (2018) recommends 20 to 60 min of continuous or intermittent activity per day. Healthy asymptomatic individuals can usually sustain exercise intensities of 60% to <90% $\dot{V}O_2R$ for 20 to 30 min. To improve cardiorespiratory fitness levels, aerobic exercise of moderate intensity and duration (30-60 min) is recommended for most adults (ACSM 2018). During the initial 4 to 6 wk of an aerobic exercise program, session duration can be increased by 5 to 10 min every other week until the desired number of minutes per week are attained (ACSM 2018). Poorly conditioned and older individuals may be able to exercise continuously at a low intensity (<40% $\dot{V}O_2R$) for only 5 to 10 min. They may need to perform multiple sessions (e.g., three 10 min exercise bouts) in a given day to accumulate 30 min of aerobic exercise.

An alternative way of estimating the duration of exercise is to use the caloric cost of the exercise. To achieve health benefits, ACSM (2018) recommends a minimum of 150 min/wk of moderate-intensity exercise or at least 75 min/wk of vigorous-intensity exercise or a combination thereof that results in the desired volume of exercise. Exercising at these combinations of minimum duration and intensity is equivalent to a minimal weekly caloric threshold of 1,000 kcal from physical activity or exercise. Consequently, you may target **caloric thresholds** of 150 to 400 kcal·day^{-1}; however, be aware that the ACSM (2018) cautions against using absolute exercise intensities (e.g., kcal·min^{-1}) since they do not account for individual differences in body weight, fitness level, or gender.

During the initial stage of the exercise program, however, weekly exercise caloric expenditure may be considerably lower (200-600 kcal·wk^{-1}). To attain 300 min/wk of moderate-intensity exercise in the improvement stage, your client's caloric expenditure must increase from 1,000 to 2,000 kcal·wk^{-1}. This can be accomplished by gradually increasing the frequency, intensity, and duration of the exercise. For example, in order for a 60 kg (132 lb) woman who is exercising at an intensity of 7 METs five times per week to reach a weekly net caloric threshold of 1,500 kcal·wk^{-1}, she needs to expend 300 kcal per exercise session (1,500 kcal / 5 = 300 kcal). You can estimate the gross caloric cost of her exercise (kcal·min^{-1}) using the following formula:

gross caloric cost (kcal·min^{-1}) = METs × 3.5
× body mass
in kg / 200

To calculate the net caloric expenditure from her activity, subtract the resting oxygen consumption (1 MET) from the gross $\dot{V}O_2$ ($\dot{V}O_2$ cost of exercise + $\dot{V}O_2$ rest) and substitute this value (7 − 1 = 6 METs) into the equation:

net caloric cost = 6 METs × 3.5 × 60 kg / 200

= 6.3 kcal·min^{-1}

Therefore, she needs to exercise approximately 48 min (300 kcal / 6.3 kcal·min^{-1}) five times per week in order to achieve her weekly net caloric expenditure goal of 1,500 kcal.

Santos and colleagues (2012) investigated the influence of body mass (60-100 kg) and fitness levels (16.4-61.2 ml·kg^{-1}·min^{-1}) on the energy expenditure and exercise program recommendations endorsed by the ACSM. They derived equations for estimating individualized training intensity (%$\dot{V}O_2$R), duration (min/wk), frequency (days/wk), and weekly energy expenditure (kcal·wk^{-1}) to account for individual variability in a given exercise session. The energy expenditure equation suggested by the ACSM (2018) overestimated energy expenditure for individuals with low aerobic fitness levels while underestimating energy expenditure for everyone else. For additional information about their suggested adjustments to the ACSM equations and how these adjustments were derived, see Santos and colleagues (2012).

VOLUME OF EXERCISE

The frequency, intensity, and duration of exercise determine the quantity or **volume of exercise**. The **MET·min** is an index of energy expenditure and is calculated by multiplying the MET value of activities by the number of minutes the activity is performed per week (e.g., 6 METS × 150 min = 900 MET·min·wk^{-1}). Using this measure of exercise volume, the total amount of physical activity can be standardized across individuals and types of activities (ACSM 2018). The ACSM (2018) recommends ≥500-1,000 MET·min·wk^{-1} as a target volume of exercise for adults. This volume is equivalent to moderate-intensity exercise (3 to 6 METs) for about 150 min/wk.

In addition, pedometers (see chapter 3) can be used to quantify the amount of exercise. Total step counts of 5,400 to 7,900 steps·day^{-1} meet the physical activity recommendations (≥500 to 1,000 MET·min·wk^{-1}) for most adults. Walking 1 mi at a moderate intensity (100 steps·min^{-1}) yields about 3,000 to 4,000 steps on average. It is best to use pedometer counts in combination with recommended time and duration of exercise (e.g., 100 steps·min^{-1}) for 30 min and 150 min/wk.

PROGRESSION OF EXERCISE

Physiological changes associated with aerobic endurance training (see Physiological Changes Induced by Cardiorespiratory Endurance Training) enable the individual to increase the total work performed. The greatest conditioning effects occur during the first 6 to 8 wk of the exercise program. Aerobic endurance may improve as much as 3% per week during the first month, 2% per week for the second month, and 1% per week or less thereafter. For continued improvements, the cardiorespiratory system must be overloaded through adjustments in the intensity and duration of the exercise to the new level of fitness. The degree and rate of improvement depend on the age, health status, and initial fitness level of the participant. For the average person, aerobic training programs generally produce a 5% to 20% increase in $\dot{V}O_2$max (Pollock 1973). Sedentary, inactive persons may improve as much as 40% in aerobic fitness, while elite athletes may improve only 5% because they begin at a level much closer to their genetic limits. Do not expect older individuals entering the exercise program to improve as quickly as younger individuals even when the initial fitness levels are the same.

STAGES OF PROGRESSION

As discussed in chapter 3, the three stages of progression for cardiorespiratory exercise programs are the initial conditioning, improvement, and maintenance stages.

Initial Conditioning

The initial conditioning stage may last 1 to 6 wk, depending on the client's rate of adaptation to the exercise program. In this stage, each exercise session should include a warm-up, moderate-intensity aerobic activity (3-6 METs), low-intensity muscular fitness exercises, and a cool-down that emphasizes stretching exercises (ACSM 2006). Clients starting a moderate-intensity aerobic conditioning program should exercise a minimum of 3 days/wk. The duration of the aerobic exercise should be at least 20 min and progress to 30 min. After clients are able to sustain aerobic activity at 55% to 60% HRR for 30 min, they progress to the improvement stage.

Improvement

The improvement stage usually lasts 4 to 8 mo. During this stage, the rate of progression is more rapid. Intensity, duration, and frequency of exercise should always be increased independently. Either duration or frequency should be increased before intensity is increased. Increase the duration no more than 10 min per session every week or two in the first month until your clients are able to sustain moderate to vigorous exercise for 20 to 60 min. Frequency should progress from 3 to 5 days/wk. Once the desired duration and frequency are reached, the exercise intensity may be increased gradually to reduce the likelihood of injury, soreness, and overtraining (ACSM 2018).

Rate of progression during this stage depends on a number of factors. Cardiac patients, older adults, and less fit individuals may need more time for the

PHYSIOLOGICAL CHANGES INDUCED BY CARDIORESPIRATORY ENDURANCE TRAINING

Cardiorespiratory System

Increases	Decreases
Heart size and volume	Resting heart rate
Blood volume and total hemoglobin	Submaximal exercise heart rate
Stroke volume—rest and exercise	Blood pressure (if high)
Cardiac output—maximum	
$\dot{V}O_2max$	
Oxygen extraction from blood	
Lung volume	

Musculoskeletal System

Increases
Mitochondria—number and size
Myoglobin stores
Triglyceride stores
Oxidative phosphorylation

Other Systems

Increases	Decreases
Strength of connective tissues	Body weight (if overweight)
Heat acclimatization	Body fat
High-density lipoprotein cholesterol	Total cholesterol
Mood	Low-density lipoprotein cholesterol
Cognitive function	Depression
Telomere length	Incidence of Alzheimer's disease

body to adapt to a higher conditioning intensity. Ultimately, older or less fit adults should strive to achieve 30 to 60 min/day of moderate-intensity activity (5 or 6 on a 10-point RPE scale) or 20 to 30 min/day of vigorous-intensity activity (>6 on a 10-point RPE scale) or any equal combination thereof.

Maintenance

After achieving the desired level of cardiorespiratory fitness, an individual enters the maintenance stage of the exercise program. This stage continues on a regular, long-term basis if the individual has made a lifetime commitment to exercise.

The goal of this stage is to maintain the cardiorespiratory fitness level and the weekly exercise caloric expenditure achieved during the improvement stage. Have your clients accomplish this goal by engaging in aerobic activities 3 to 5 days/wk at the intensity and duration that were reached at the end of the improvement stage. Reducing the training frequency from 5 to 3 days/wk does not adversely affect $\dot{V}O_2$max as long as the training intensity remains the same. However, clients should participate in other activities an additional 2 or 3 days/wk. To this end, a variety of enjoyable activities from the type C and D classifications may be selected to counteract boredom and to maintain the interest level of the participant. For example, an individual who was running 5 days/wk at the end of the improvement stage may choose to run only 3 days/wk and substitute Zumba, in-line skating, racquetball, or high-intensity circuit resistance training using body weight on the other 2 days.

AEROBIC TRAINING METHODS AND MODES

Either continuous or discontinuous training methods can improve cardiorespiratory endurance. **Continuous training** involves one continuous aerobic exercise bout performed at low to moderate intensities without rest intervals. **Discontinuous training** consists of several intermittent low- to high-intensity exercise bouts interspersed with rest periods. Both training methods produce significant improvements in $\dot{V}O_2$max (Landram et al 2016; Milanović, Sporiš, and Weston 2015). Results from research comparing improvements in $\dot{V}O_2$max resulting from high-in-

tensity interval (discontinuous) training versus continuous endurance training are mixed. However, a recent literature review and detailed analysis on the topic indicate that high-intensity interval training is only slightly better than continuous endurance training for improving $\dot{V}O_2$max (Milanović, Sporiš, and Weston 2015). One concern about high-intensity intermittent training is the possibility of exercise burnout. Pollock and colleagues (1977) reported that the dropout rate of adults in a high-intensity interval (discontinuous) training program was twice that of those in a continuous jogging program. Thus, for the typical client, **high-intensity interval training** may be better suited for stimulating short-term (e.g., 4 wk) improvements in cardiorespiratory fitness and for adding variety to the exercise program. More research addressing the long-term health benefits of interval training and its effects on exercise adherence for the general population is warranted.

CONTINUOUS TRAINING

All the exercise modes listed as type A or B activities (see Classification of Aerobic Exercise Modalities earlier in this chapter) are suitable for continuous training. One advantage of continuous training is that the prescribed exercise intensity (e.g., 75% HRR) is maintained fairly consistently throughout the duration of the steady-paced exercise. Generally, continuous exercise at low to moderate intensities is safer, more comfortable, and better suited for individuals initiating an aerobic exercise program.

Walking, Jogging, and Cycling

The most popular modes of continuous training are walking, jogging or running, and cycling. Exercise programs using walking, jogging, and cycling provide similar cardiorespiratory benefits (Pollock, Cureton, and Greninger 1969; Pollock, Dimmick, et al. 1971; Pollock et al. 1975; Wilmore et al. 1980). Improvements in $\dot{V}O_2$max are comparable for most commonly used exercise modes. Pollock, Dimmick, and colleagues (1975) compared running, walking, and cycling exercise programs of middle-aged men who trained at 85% to 90% HRmax. All three groups showed significant improvements in $\dot{V}O_2$max. These results indicate that improvement in $\dot{V}O_2$max is independent of the mode of training when frequency, intensity, and duration of exercise are held constant and are prescribed in accordance with sound, scientific principles.

Aerobic Dance

For nearly 50 yr, aerobic dance has been a popular mode of exercise for improving and maintaining cardiorespiratory fitness. A typical aerobic dance workout begins with a low-intensity warm-up (approximately 5 min) of the major muscle groups. This is followed by 20 to 30 min of either high- or low-impact (both feet simultaneously leaving the floor or one foot always on the floor, respectively) aerobic dancing. The music and speed of movement increase until the age-appropriate target training intensity is reached. A cool-down that includes stretching concludes the session and typically lasts 5 min. Handheld weights (1-4 lb [0.5-2 kg]) can also be used to increase exercise intensity. Heart rates should be monitored frequently during exercise to ensure they stay within the target zone.

Zumba is a highly popular style of exercise that typically blends large muscle group movements of the upper and lower body with Latin-style music (Domene et al. 2016). It can be performed on land or in a swimming pool. Single-session energy expenditure is reported to exceed the current recommendations (ACSM 2018) for improving and maintaining cardiorespiratory fitness, making Zumba a moderate- to vigorous-intensity exercise enjoyed by young, middle-aged, and older adults alike (Dalleck et al. 2015; Domene et al. 2016; Luettengen et al. 2012). The average MET levels (4.3 ± 0.4 and 6.2 ± 0.3, respectively) in the studies by Dalleck and colleagues (2015) and Domene and colleagues (2016) exceed that corresponding to treadmill walking at 3.5 mph with no incline (3.8 METs). After a 16 wk Zumba intervention (3 days/wk, 60 min/session), the estimated $\dot{V}O_2$max values of the participating sedentary and overweight or obese women had improved significantly as did numerous other physiological variables associated with improved health (Krishnan et al. 2015).

Step Ergometry and Stair Climbing

Step ergometry (machine-based stair climbing) is a popular exercise modality in health and fitness clubs.

Research shows a linear HR response to graded submaximal exercise performed on stair climbing ergometers. However, the MET levels displayed on the StairMaster 4000 PT overestimate the actual MET intensity of the exercise (Howley, Colacino, and Swensen 1992). When prescribing exercise intensity using this type of stair climber, be certain to adjust the machine's estimates for each MET level using the following equation:

$$\text{actual METs} = 0.556 + 0.745 \\ (\text{StairMaster MET setting})$$

MET level and %HRR estimations attained while ascending 100 steps or 17.3 m (17.3 cm steps; 20 steps per floor) within 2 min indicate that stair climbing demands an effort increasing from moderate (3.5 METs; 56%-61% HRR) to vigorous (7.6 METs; 69%-80% HRR) intensity during ascent for both men and women, respectively. Descending the same stairs requires approximately 3 METs of effort (Al Kandari et al. 2016). Consequently, your clients may be able to introduce short bouts of moderate- to vigorous-intensity exercise wherever an accessible stairwell is available. To estimate the $\dot{V}O_2$ requirement of stair climbing at a given cadence (number of steps / time to complete) and step height, see table 4.3. Should climbing multiple flights of stairs initially prove too difficult for unfit clients, Takaishi and associates (2014) recommend they perform multiple repetitions of ascending and descending fewer flights of stairs. This will allow clients to accumulate the necessary 30 min of moderate-intensity exercise without the physiological stress of climbing continuously. Acute, intense bouts of stair climbing produce similar physiologic results as equivalent bouts (3 × 20 sec) of all-out cycling and, therefore, are suitable as a sprint interval modality (Allison et al. 2017).

Elliptical Training

Elliptical training machines are popular in the fitness industry. Elliptical trainers are designed for either upper body, lower body, or combined upper and lower body exercise. The lower body motion during exercise on an elliptical trainer is a cross between the actions performed with machine-based stair climbing and upright stationary cycling. With elliptical trainers, the feet move in an egg-shaped, or elliptical, pattern, and the feet stay in contact with the footpads of the device throughout the exercise.

Unlike running or jogging, this form of exercise may provide a high-intensity workout with low-impact forces comparable to those for walking (Klein, White, and Rana 2016; Lu, Chien, and Chen 2007).

Kravitz and colleagues (1998) reported that the average energy expenditure during forward-backward exercise with no resistance and against resistance for 5 min (125 strides·min^{-1}) was, respectively, 8.1 and 10.7 kcal·min^{-1}. Exercise intensities ranged between 72.5% and 83.5% HRmax (age predicted). Compared against treadmill exercise, upper body elliptical training at self-selected intensities produced similar $\dot{V}O_2$, HR, and RPE responses (Crommett et al. 1999). Although there was no difference in $\dot{V}O_2$ between combined upper and lower body elliptical training and treadmill exercise, upper and lower body elliptical training produced a significantly higher HR and RPE (Crommett et al. 1999). Compared with steady-state treadmill exercise at self-identified training velocity (no incline), the RPE response focusing on legs only was higher for traditional elliptical training (150-160 strides·min^{-1} at steady-state HR from prior treadmill bout). There were no differences by modality for upper body or whole-body RPEs. When matched for whole-body RPE from the treadmill exercise, results regarding differences in HR responses, by modality, are equivocal (Brown et al. 2010; Green et al. 2004). Mier and Feito (2006) reported significantly different $\dot{V}O_2$, ventilation, and RPE values when comparing traditional elliptical exercise performed using legs only ($\dot{V}O_2$: 18.7 ± 3.0 ml·kg^{-1}·min^{-1}; V_E: 38.9 ± 3.0 L·min^{-1}; RPE: 10.9 ± 1.9) with elliptical training using both arms and legs combined ($\dot{V}O_2$: 19.2 ± 3.0 ml·kg^{-1}·min^{-1}; V_E: 37.7 ± 8.3 L·min^{-1}; RPE: 10.3 ± 1.9). Additionally, they commented on the large interindividual variability in $\dot{V}O_2$ at each stage of exercise, possibly related to the gender, body composition, and elliptical training experience of the exerciser.

Traditional elliptical training is a viable substitute for treadmill and stair climbing exercise (Brown et al. 2010; Green et al. 2004). Egaña and Donne (2004) reported similar and significant increases in $\dot{V}O_2$max values following a 12 wk intervention (30-40 min·day^{-1}; 3 days/wk; 70%-90% HRmax) of traditional elliptical training as compared against treadmill running and stair climbing.

Outdoor elliptical bicycles (ebikes) are a cross between traditional elliptical trainers and bicycles.

As described by Klein, White, and Rana (2016), the pedal angle of the two styles of elliptical trainers is different, with the ebike allowing for leg movement patterns more reflective of running than cycling. Results from their crossover study comparing 4 wk of ebike training against run-only training with experienced runners indicate similar significant increases in VT compared with baseline for both modalities (Klein, White, and Rana 2016). No differences were found between modalities for any of the performance variables of interest. Ebike training provides a no-impact alternative to running that induces similar physiological responses.

Water-Based Exercise

Water-based exercise, such as water aerobics or walking in waist-deep water, has been promoted as an effective way to increase the cardiorespiratory fitness of young, middle-aged, and older adults. Improvements in muscular strength may also be realized because of resistance provided by the water as body segments move through it. This exercise is especially popular among individuals who are older, overweight, or afflicted with orthopedic disabilities. Bergamin and associates (2012) provide a comprehensive analysis of the effect of water-based training on the physical fitness of elderly adults.

Although this will vary based on the style of water-based exercise, a typical exercise session includes the following phases:

- Warm-up—5 to 10 min of stretching before entering the pool, followed by walking slowly in the water

- Endurance phase—20 to 30 min of continuous walking, jogging, kicking, arm swinging, and dancing in the water

- Resistance phase—10 min of resistance exercises performed underwater with foam noodles, dumbbells, barbell-like devices, and leg pads

- Cool-down—5 to 10 min of stretching

In older women (60-75 yr) participating in water-based exercise training 3 days/wk for 12 wk, $\dot{V}O_2$peak increased by 12% while total cholesterol and low-density lipoprotein cholesterol decreased by 11% and 17%, respectively. Also, muscle strength and arm and leg power increased significantly in response to exercising the limbs against the resistance of water (Takeshima et al. 2002). For a thorough review of the influences of environmental conditions on physiological responses during water-based exercise (with the head out and body submerged), see the review by Barbosa and associates (2009).

Innovative Aerobic Exercise Modes

New and innovative modes of aerobic exercise are introduced every year by the fitness industry in order to stimulate and maintain exercise participation of clients. Many of these new programs combine traditional exercise modes (e.g., stationary cycling, stepping, tai chi, and martial arts) with music. Fitness centers throughout the United States now offer group exercise classes using programs such as BodyCombat, RPM, BodyJam, BodyPump, BodyStep, and Tae Bo. BodyCombat is an aerobic workout that combines movements from karate, boxing, taekwondo, and tai chi with fast-paced music. RPM is an indoor cycling workout to music that includes warm-up, pace, hill, mixed terrain, interval, free spin, mountain climb, and stretch segments. BodyJam integrates current dance styles with trending music genres popular with young adults. BodyPump is a conditioning class of low-weight, high-repetition workouts choreographed to music. Tae Bo is an aerobic exercise routine that combines music with elements of taekwondo and kick boxing to promote aerobic fitness.

Rixon and colleagues (2006) compared exercise HRs and estimates of energy expenditure for BodyCombat (73% HRmax; 9.7 kcal·min^{-1}), RPM (74.3% HRmax; 9.9 kcal·min^{-1}), BodyStep (72.4% HRmax; 9.6 kcal·min^{-1}), and BodyPump (60.2% HRmax; 8.0 kcal·min^{-1}) routines. With the exception of BodyPump, the intensity and duration of these exercise routines appear to be sufficient to meet physical activity recommendations for improving health and for weight management. Eight inactive women (BMI: 29.9 ± 2.3 kg/m^2) participated in an 8 wk RPM studio cycling program (3 days/wk), increasing in session duration from 20 min to 50 min by week 3 (Faulkner et al. 2015). The program was a mix of low-, moderate-, and high-intensity cycling, and the average training intensity (83% HRmax) met the ACSM (2018) criteria for vigorous intensity. Faulkner's research team found that the studio cycling program was an effective means for significantly improving maximal aerobic capacity (11.8%), body fat levels (–13.6%), and blood lipid profile (LDL: –23%; total cholesterol: –13%). Although the group exercise classes described by Rixon and colleagues are taught in thousands of fitness clubs internationally, further research is needed to determine the health benefits and effects of these exercise programs on aerobic fitness.

Kettlebell exercise is a popular whole-body, aerobic training modality. It involves the rhythmic swinging and ballistic lifting of nonsymmetrical hand weights. The available research on this modality is sparse and equivocal. Farrar, Mayhew, and Koch (2010) found that kettlebell swinging is suitable for improving aerobic fitness. As expected, the average %HRmax during kettlebell exercise (87% HRmax) was higher than the corresponding average %$\dot{V}O_2$max (65.3% $\dot{V}O_2$max) (Farrar, Mayhew, and Koch 2010). Thomas and colleagues (2014) compared a 30 min kettlebell routine against 30 min of moderate-intensity treadmill walking (with incline) at the $\dot{V}O_2$ of the kettlebell routine. They reported that their kettlebell routine required similar aerobic effort even though the HR and RPE were consistently higher for the kettlebell routine. Jay and colleagues (2011) reported no significant improvements in aerobic capacity following an 8 wk kettlebell training intervention for a predominantly (85%) female sample of adults (44 yr and 23 kg·m^{-2} on average). Conversely, a 6% improvement in maximal aerobic capacity was reported for a group of top-tier female collegiate soccer players who performed high-intensity kettlebell snatches at a 1:1 work-to-rest ratio for 20 min three times a week for 4 wk (Falatic et al. 2015). Beltz and colleagues (2013) reported a 13% increase in aerobic capacity for young adults completing kettlebell classes (two classes a week for 8 wk) in a university setting.

DISCONTINUOUS TRAINING

As mentioned previously, discontinuous training involves a series of low- to high-intensity exercise bouts interspersed with rest or relief periods. All of the exercise modes listed as type A and type B activities (see Classification of Aerobic Exercise Modalities earlier in this chapter) are suitable for discontinuous training. Because of the intermittent nature of this form of training, the exercise intensity and total amount of work performed can be greater than with continuous training, making discontinuous training a versatile method that is widely used by athletes, as well as individuals with low cardiorespiratory fitness. In fact, the ACSM (2018) recommends the use of discontinuous (intermittent) training for symptomatic individuals who are able to tolerate only low-intensity exercise for short periods of time (3-5 min). Interval training, treading, Spinning, and circuit resistance training are examples of intermittent, or discontinuous, training.

Interval Training

Interval training involves a repeated series of exercise work bouts interspersed with rest or relief periods. This method is popular among athletes because it allows them to exercise at higher relative intensities during the work interval than are possible with longer-duration continuous training. Interval training programs can also be modified to improve speed and anaerobic endurance, as well as aerobic endurance, simply by changing the exercise intensity and length of the work and relief intervals.

An example of interval training is work intervals run at a pace such that a distance of 1,100 yd (1,005 m) is covered in 3 to 4 min. Each work interval is then followed by a rest-relief interval of 1.5 to 2 min. This sequence is repeated three times. During the rest-relief interval, the individual may walk or jog while recovering from the work bout. For aerobic interval training, the ratio of work to rest-relief is usually 1:1 or 1:0.5. Each work interval is 3 to 5 min and is repeated three to seven times. The exercise intensity usually ranges between 70% and 85% $\dot{V}O_2$ max. The overload principle is applied by increasing the exercise intensity or length of the work interval, decreasing the length of the rest-relief interval, or increasing the number of work intervals per exercise session. For a discussion of interval training and sample programs, including programs for developing speed and anaerobic endurance, refer to the work of Janssen (2001).

For a review of studies investigating the similarities and differences between endurance training and high-intensity interval training (HIT), see the article by Milanović, Sporiš, and Weston (2015). Their key points identify the influence of the comparative group's fitness status on the magnitude of change induced through the two styles of training. Regardless, HIT is reported as improving aerobic capacity more so than does traditional continuous endurance training.

As highlighted in a review regarding the potential of HIT programs, Kessler, Sisson, and Short (2012) differentiated between **sprint interval training (SIT)** and **aerobic interval training (AIT)**. SIT is typically based on iterative combinations of 30 sec maximal exertion sprints and extended recovery interludes (approximately 4 min) on a stationary cycle. AIT is based on iterations of near maximal (80%-95% $\dot{V}O_2$ max) 4 min bouts of treadmill or cycling exercise followed by 3 to 4 min recovery periods, and it appears to have broader application for nonathlete, sedentary, and clinical populations. However, the SIT and AIT protocols tend to vary widely in exercise session volume and number of exercise sessions. Both SIT and AIT protocols show similar if not larger increases in maximal aerobic capacity and insulin sensitivity compared with counterparts engaging in the standard continuous moderate-intensity exercise. This trend is pervasive even though the SIT and AIT groups exercise just a fraction of the time recommended by the ACSM and American Heart Association (150 min/wk). For example, Gillen and associates (2016) reported that 12 wk of stationary cycling increases $\dot{V}O_2$ peak by 19% regardless of group assignment. Of note, their moderate-intensity continuous (MIC) cycling group exercised five times longer each week than did their SIT cycling group. However, the MIC cycling group (3.75-5.0 hr/wk) in the 6 wk study conducted by Fisher and colleagues (2015) had greater improvements in their cardiorespiratory fitness than did the HIT cycling group (60 min/wk) even though both cycling programs improved cardiometabolic parameters in overweight, inactive men.

HDL-C and body fat percentage have been favorably altered by AIT, as has blood pressure in those not already undergoing treatment for hypertension. However, a dose-response relationship is evident as the duration of the HIT protocols on these cardiovascular risk factors varies. Kessler, Sisson, and Short (2012) also outlined the need for exercise session supervision early on in the HIT programs, which are rigorous and may not be appropriate for everyone. On the other hand, Gosselin and colleagues (2012) reported that HIT exercise is as physiologically taxing as moderate-intensity (70% $\dot{V}O_2$ max) steady-state exercise for physically active adults (20-30 yr).

Thirteen inactive yet healthy men (35-45 yr; BMI: 25-30 kg/m^2) underwent an AIT intervention that consisted of a 10 min warm-up (70% HRmax) and four 4 min bouts of treadmill running at incline and at 90% HRmax. Treadmill activity (3 min bouts at 70% HRmax) separated the near maximal periods of exertion. The study period covered 10 wk, with three sessions per week. Aerobic capacity increased by 13%, and systolic and diastolic blood pressures decreased, as did fasting blood glucose. However, only body fat, total cholesterol, and LDL-cholesterol values had decreased significantly after 10 wk (Tjønna et al. 2013).

Recreationally active men served as their own controls in an investigation comparing high-intensity (90% $\dot{V}O_2$ max) interval treadmill running (6 reps × 3 min·rep^{-1}) interspersed with moderate-intensity (50% $\dot{V}O_2$ max) active recovery (6 reps × 3 min·rep^{-1}) against a 50 min continuous treadmill running bout at moderate intensity (70% $\dot{V}O_2$ max). Along with the 7 min warm-up and cool-down periods, the high-intensity protocol involved approximately 50 min of exercise. Although the %HRmax, %$\dot{V}O_2$ max, and total energy expenditure were similar, RPE and perceived enjoyment were significantly higher for the high-intensity interval running protocol (Bartlett et al. 2011). An increased sense of enjoyment with exercise may lead to increased exercise adherence, although this needs to be investigated in less fit indi-

viduals. Consequently, research on longer duration interventions are needed to determine if adherence and long-term physiological gains are possible with AIT and SIT programs.

Treading and Spinning

Treading and **Spinning** are two examples of interval training that are popular offerings in fitness clubs because of the variety and enjoyment they offer. These group classes involve walking, jogging, and running at various speeds and grades on a treadmill (treading) or stationary cycling at various cadences and resistances (Spinning). A typical treading or Spinning workout consists of 1:1 or 1.5:1 work-recovery intervals, or stages, that are repeated for a specified duration. For example, a 30 min treading class may consist of six stages. Each stage lasts 5 min (i.e., 3 min work interval and 2 min recovery interval). Participants can advance the intensity of the work interval by increasing the treadmill speed or grade. During the recovery interval, both the speed and grade of the treadmill are decreased (e.g., 2.5 mph [4 km·hr^{-1}] and 0% grade). Instructors individualize and adapt the workouts for their clients by adjusting the duration of the work-recovery intervals and varying the speed and grade. Caution is urged for novice Spinning participants as the leg muscles may experience a trauma that releases cell contents into the bloodstream. This condition, exertional rhabdomyolysis, appears in medical literature and is being identified in some individuals following their first Spinning class (Brogan et al. 2017). Some researchers have suggested separate beginner-level familiarization classes to provide a controlled adaptation to the rigors of Spinning (de Melo dos Santos et al. 2015).

In one study, researchers designed 30 min treading workouts for walkers and runners (Nichols, Sherman, and Abbott 2000). They reported that the average intensity of the walking protocol was 40% to 49% $\dot{V}O_2$ max for male and female walkers, respectively. For the running protocol, the average intensity of the work intervals was 76% to 80% $\dot{V}O_2$ max for male and female runners, respectively. The researchers suggest that these average intensities, as well as the duration of the workout (30 min), are sufficient to meet ACSM recommendations for an aerobic exercise prescription. Although both treading and Spinning classes are offered in fitness

---

An Interval Training Prescription to Develop Aerobic Endurance

Sets: One

Repetitions: Three to seven

Distance: 1,100 yd (1,105 m)

Intensity: 70% to 85% $\dot{V}O_2$ max

Time: 3 to 5 min

Rest-relief interval: 1.5 to 2 min

centers coast to coast, there is very little research about their acute and long-term training effects on cardiorespiratory fitness.

Circuit Resistance Training

Use of circuit resistance training for the development of aerobic fitness, as well as muscular strength and tone, has received much attention. An example of a circuit resistance training program is presented in chapter 7 (see figure 7.1). Circuit resistance training usually consists of several circuits of resistance training with a minimal amount of rest between the exercise stations (15-20 sec). Alternatively, instead of rest, you can have your clients perform 1 to 3 min of aerobic exercise between each station. The aerobic stations may include activities such as stationary cycling, jogging in place, rope skipping, stair climbing, bench stepping, and rowing. This modification of the circuit is known as **super circuit resistance training**.

Gettman and Pollock (1981) reviewed the research on the physiological benefits of circuit resistance training. Because it produces only a 5% increase in aerobic capacity as compared with a 15% to 25% increase from other forms of aerobic training, the authors concluded that circuit resistance training is more suited for the maintenance stage of an aerobic exercise program than for developing aerobic fitness. Newer research indicates that 5 wk of high-intensity circuit resistance training (three sessions per week) using body weight exercises improves aerobic capacity (11%) for young sedentary women (Myers et al. 2015). The improvement in aerobic capacity (~8%) in recreationally active women completing 4 wk of circuit resistance training using body weight exercises was similar to the ~7% improvement reported for women performing 30 min of treadmill running at 85% HRmax (McRae et al. 2012). Both groups in the McRae study exercised four times per week. In addition to increasing the aerobic capacity of young women, high-intensity circuit resistance training using body weight exercises increases muscular endurance.

PERSONALIZED EXERCISE PROGRAMS

The aerobic exercise prescription should be individualized to meet each client's training goals and interests. To do this, you need to consider the client's age, gender, physical fitness level, and exercise preferences. This section presents a sample case study and examples of individualized exercise prescriptions to illustrate how the exercise prescription may be personalized for each client.

CASE STUDY

Like any preventive or therapeutic intervention, exercise should be prescribed carefully. You must be able to evaluate a client's medical history, medical condition, physical fitness status, lifestyle characteristics, and interests before designing the exercise program. In addition, to test your ability to extract, analyze, and evaluate all pertinent information needed to design a safe exercise program for the client, many professional certification examinations require that you be able to analyze a case study. For these reasons, this section includes a sample case study.

A case study is a written narrative that summarizes client information you will need in order to develop an accurate and safe individualized exercise prescription (Porter 1988). Important elements to focus on when reading and analyzing a case study are listed in Essential Elements of a Case Study. First, determine if medical clearance is needed for the client by assessing signs and symptoms of cardiovascular, metabolic, and renal disease (see Appendix A.3) and physical activity history in the past 3 mo. Then identify the client's coronary heart disease (CHD) risk factors by focusing on information provided about age, family history of CHD, blood lipid profile (total cholesterol, high- and low-density lipoprotein cholesterol [HDL-C and LDL-C]), blood glucose levels, resting BP, physical activity, body fat level, and smoking. Become familiar with ideal or typical values for various blood chemistry tests so you will be able to recognize normal or abnormal test results. Remember that each of the following factors places individuals at greater risk for CHD:

- Triglycerides ≥150 mg·dl^{-1}
- Total cholesterol ≥200 mg·dl^{-1}
- LDL-cholesterol ≥130 mg·dl^{-1}
- HDL-cholesterol <40 mg·dl^{-1}
- Total cholesterol/HDL ratio >5.0
- Blood glucose ≥110 mg·dl^{-1}
- Systolic BP ≥130 or diastolic BP ≥80 mmHg

SAMPLE CASE STUDY

A 28 yr old female police officer (5 ft 5 in. or 165.1 cm; 140 lb or 63.6 kg; 28% body fat) has enrolled in the adult fitness program. Her job demands a fairly high level of physical fitness—a level she was able to achieve 6 yr ago when she passed the physical fitness test battery used by the police department. Before becoming a police officer, she jogged 20 min, usually three times a week. Since starting her job, she has had little or no time for exercise and has gained 15 lb (6.8 kg). She is divorced, and she works 8 hr a day and takes care of two children, ages 7 and 9. At least three times a week, she and the children dine out, usually at fast food restaurants like Burger King and Taco Bell. She reports that her job, along with the sole responsibility for raising her two children, is quite stressful. Occasionally she experiences headaches and a tightness in the back of her neck. Usually in the evening she has one glass of wine to relax.

Her medical history reveals that she smoked one pack of cigarettes a day for 4 yr while she was in college. She quit smoking 3 yr ago. Over the past 2 yr, she has tried some quick weight loss diets, with little success. She was hospitalized on two occasions to give birth to her children. She reports that her father died of heart disease when he was 52 and that her older brother has high blood pressure. Recently she had her blood chemistry analyzed because she was feeling light-headed and dizzy after eating. In an attempt to lose weight, she eats only one large meal a day, at dinnertime. Results of the blood analysis were total cholesterol = 220 mg·dl^{-1}; triglycerides = 98 mg·dl^{-1}; glucose = 82 mg·dl^{-1}; high-density lipoprotein cholesterol = 37 mg·dl^{-1}; and total cholesterol/high-density lipoprotein cholesterol ratio = 5.9.

The exercise evaluation yielded the following data:

- Mode, protocol: Treadmill, modified Bruce
- Resting data: HR = 75 bpm; BP = 140/82 mmHg
- Endpoint: Stage 4 (2.5 mph [4 km·hr^{-1}], 12% grade). Test terminated because of fatigue.

Stage	METs	Duration (min)	HR (bpm)	BP (mmHg)	RPE
1	2.3	3	126	145/78	8
2	3.5	3	142	160/78	11
3	4.6	3	165	172/80	14
4	7.0	3	190	189/82	18

Analysis

1. Evaluate the client's need for medical clearance and the client's CHD risk profile. Be certain to address each of the positive and negative risk factors.

2. Describe any special problems or limitations that need to be considered in designing an exercise program for this client.

3. Were the HR, BP, and RPE responses to the GXT normal? Explain.

4. What is the client's functional aerobic capacity in METs? Categorize her cardiorespiratory fitness level (see table 4.1).

5. Plot the HR versus METs on graph paper.

6. From the graph, determine the client's target HR zone for the aerobic exercise program. What HRs and RPEs correspond to 60%, 70%, and 75% of the client's $\dot{V}O_2R$?

7. The client expressed an interest in walking outside on a level track to develop aerobic fitness. Calculate her walking speed for each of the following training intensities: 60%, 70%, and 75% $\dot{V}O_2R$. Use the ACSM equations presented in table 4.3.

8. In addition to starting an aerobic exercise program, what suggestions do you have for this client for modifying her lifestyle?

See appendix B.5 for answers to these questions.

SAMPLE CYCLING PROGRAM

Client Data

Age:	27 yr
Gender:	Female
Body weight:	70 kg (154 lb)
Resting heart rate:	67 bpm
Maximal heart rate:	195 bpm (measured)
$\dot{V}O_2$max:	26 ml·kg^{-1}·min^{-1} (measured); 7.4 METs
Graded exercise test:	Cycle ergometer
Initial cardiorespiratory fitness level:	Poor

Exercise Prescription

Mode:	Stationary cycling
Intensity:	60%-80% $\dot{V}O_2$R
	16.8-21.4 ml·kg^{-1}·min^{-1}
	4.8-6.1 METs
Exercise heart rates (from figure 5.3):	139 bpm minimum
	168 bpm maximum
RPE:	5-8 (OMNI scale)
Duration:	40-60 min
Frequency:	4 or 5 days/wk

Phase (wk)	Intensity %$\dot{V}O_2$R	METs	HR (bpm)	RPE	Power output (W)	Resistance (kg)	Pedal rate (rpm)	Net kcal·min^{-1}	Time (min)	Frequency	Weekly net expenditure (kcal)
INITIAL											
1	60	4.8	139	5	63	1.3	50	4.7	40	4	752
2	60	4.8	139	5	63	1.3	50	4.7	**45**	4	846
3	**65**	5.2	150	5-6	73	1.5	50	5.2	45	4	936
4	65	5.2	150	5-6	73	1.5	50	5.2	**50**	4	1,040
IMPROVEMENT											
5-8	65-**70**	5.2-5.5	150-155	5-6	73-80	1.5-1.6	50	5.2-5.5	50	4	1,040-1,103
9-12	65-70	5.2-5.5	150-155	5-6	73-80	1.5-1.6	50	5.2-5.5	**55**	4	1,144-1,210
13-16	70-**75**	5.5-5.8	152-162	6-7	80-86	1.6-1.7	50	5.5-5.9	55	4	1,210-1,298
17-20	75	5.8	162	7	86	1.7	50	5.9	60	4	1,416
21-24	75	5.8	162	7	86	1.7	50	5.9	**60**	5	1,770
25-28	**80**	6.1	168	8	93	1.9	50	6.2	60	5	1,874
MAINTENANCE											
24+											
Cycling	80	6.1	168	8	93	1.9	50	6.2	60	3	1,116
Low-impact aerobics	65% HRR	5.0	150	6-7	—	—	—	4.9	60	1	294
Tennis	—	7.0	—	7-8	—	—	—	7.4	60	1	440

Note: Values in boldface indicate training variables that are increased during each stage of the exercise progression.

Pay close attention to information about the client's medical history and physical examination results. These may reveal signs or symptoms of CHD, particularly if shortness of breath, chest discomfort, or leg cramps are reported or if high BP is detected. It is also important to note the types of medication the client is using. Drugs such as digitalis, beta-blockers, diuretics, vasodilators, bronchodilators, and insulin may alter the body's physiological responses during exercise and could affect the HR and BP responses reported for the GXT. Keep in mind that exercise programs need to be modified for individuals with musculoskeletal disorders such as arthritis, low back pain, osteoporosis, and chondromalacia. Next, be certain to key in on information regarding the client's lifestyle. Factors such as smoking, lack of physical activity, or diets high in saturated fats or cholesterol increase the risk of CHD, atherosclerosis, and hypertension. You can often target these factors for modification; they also help you assess the likelihood of the client's adherence to the exercise program (see table 3.3).

Examine the BP, HR, and RPE data for the GXT used to assess the client's functional aerobic capacity and cardiorespiratory fitness level. You need to be acutely aware of the normal and abnormal physiological responses to graded exercise. After assessing the client's CHD risk and cardiorespiratory fitness level, you can design an aerobic exercise program using a personalized exercise prescription of intensity, frequency, duration, mode, volume, and progression. To write the exercise prescription, use the results from the GXT (HR, RPE, functional MET capacity).

The sample case study is provided to test your ability to evaluate the need for medical clearance prior to exercise, risk factors, and GXT results and to prescribe an accurate and safe aerobic exercise program for this individual. See the results of the case study analysis in appendix B.5.

SAMPLE CYCLING PROGRAM

The sample cycling program later in this chapter shows a personalized program for a 27 yr old female who was given a maximal GXT on a stationary cycle ergometer. Her measured $\dot{V}O_2$ max is 7.4 METs. The exercise intensity is based on a percentage of her $\dot{V}O_2$ reserve (%$\dot{V}O_2$R), and the target exercise HRs

corresponding to 60% (4.8 METs) and 80% $\dot{V}O_2$R (6.1 METs) are 139 bpm and 168 bpm, respectively (see figure 5.3). Thus, the training exercise HR should fall within this HR range. During the initial stage of the exercise program, the woman will cycle at a work rate corresponding to 60% $\dot{V}O_2$R (4.8 METs) for 2 wk.

During weeks 1 and 2, the exercise duration is increased by 5 min/wk (from 40 to 45 min). During the third week, relative exercise intensity rather than duration is increased by 5% (from 60% $\dot{V}O_2$R to 65% $\dot{V}O_2$R). The work rate corresponding to an exercise intensity is calculated using the ACSM formulas for leg ergometry (see table 4.3). For example, the work rate corresponding to 60% $\dot{V}O_2$R (4.8 METs or 16.8 ml·kg^{-1}·min^{-1}) is calculated as follows:

$$\dot{V}O_2 \ (ml·kg^{-1}·min^{-1}) = W / M \times 1.8 + 3.5 + 3.5$$

where W = work rate in kgm·min^{-1}
and M = body mass in kg.

$$16.8 = W / 70 \ kg \times 1.8 + 7.0$$

$$16.8 - 7.0 = W / 70 \ kg \times 1.8$$

$$9.8 \times 70 \ kg / 1.8 = 381 \ kgm·min^{-1}$$

To calculate the resistance setting corresponding to 381 kgm·min^{-1} for a cycling cadence of 50 rpm, divide the work rate by the total distance the flywheel travels: 381 / 50 rpm × 6 = 1.27 kg, or 1.3 kg.

To calculate the net energy cost (kcal·min^{-1}) of cycling, subtract the resting $\dot{V}O_2$ (1 MET) from the gross $\dot{V}O_2$ for each intensity. Convert this net MET value to kcal·min^{-1} using the following formula:

$$kcal·min^{-1} = METs \times 3.5 \times body \ mass \ (kg) / 200$$

(e.g., 4.8 − 1.0 = 3.8 METs; 3.8 × 3.5 × 70 kg / 200

$$= 4.7 \ kcal·min^{-1})$$

In the initial stages of the program, the weekly net energy expenditure is between 752 and 1,040 kcal. In the improvement stage, the exercise intensity, duration, and frequency are progressively increased, and the weekly net caloric expenditure ranges between 1,040 and 1,874 kcal. Only one variable—intensity, duration, or frequency—should be increased at a time. The variable that is increased during each stage of the progression for this exercise program is indicated by boldface. During the improvement stage, this client's net caloric expenditure due to exercise

ESSENTIAL ELEMENTS OF A CASE STUDY

Demographic Factors

- Age
- Gender
- Ethnicity
- Occupation
- Height
- Body weight
- Family history of coronary heart disease

Medical History

Present Symptoms

- Dyspnea or shortness of breath
- Angina or chest pain
- Leg cramps or claudication
- Musculoskeletal problems or limitations
- Medications

Past History

- Diseases
- Injuries
- Surgeries
- Lab tests

Lifestyle Assessment

- Alcohol and caffeine intake
- Smoking
- Nutritional intake, eating patterns
- Physical activity patterns and interests
- Sleeping habits
- Occupational stress level
- Mental status, family lifestyle

Physical Examination

- Blood pressure
- Heart and lung sounds
- Orthopedic problems or limitations

Laboratory Tests (Ideal or Typical Values)

- Triglycerides (<150 mg·dl^{-1})
- Total cholesterol (<200 mg·dl^{-1})
- LDL-cholesterol (<100 mg·dl^{-1})
- HDL-cholesterol (>40 mg·dl^{-1})
- Total cholesterol/HDL-cholesterol (<3.5)
- Blood glucose (60-99 mg·dl^{-1})
- Hemoglobin:
    13.5-17.5 g·dl^{-1} (men)
    11.5-15.5 g·dl^{-1} (women)
- Hematocrit:
    40%-52% (men)
    36%-48% (women)
- Potassium (3.5-5.5 meq·dl^{-1})
- Blood urea nitrogen (4-24 mg·dl^{-1})
- Creatinine (0.3-1.4 mg·dl^{-1})
- Iron:
    40-190 mg·dl^{-1} (men)
    35-180 mg·dl^{-1} (women)
- Calcium (8.5-10.5 mg·dl^{-1})

Physical Fitness Evaluation

- Cardiorespiratory fitness (HR, BP, $\dot{V}O_2$max)
- Body composition (% body fat)
- Musculoskeletal fitness (muscle and bone strength)
- Flexibility
- Balance

meets the caloric threshold of between 1,000 and 2,000 kcal·wk⁻¹ from physical activity recommended by the ACSM (2018). In the maintenance phase, tennis and aerobic dancing are added to give variety and to supplement the cycling program. The ACSM (2018) guidelines were followed to calculate each component of this exercise prescription.

SAMPLE JOGGING PROGRAM

The sample jogging program later in this chapter is designed for a 29 yr old male who has an excellent cardiorespiratory fitness level. Since a GXT could not be administered, the $\dot{V}O_2$ max was predicted from performance on the 12 min distance run test. The maximal HR was predicted using the formula 220 − age. Because this client is accustomed to jogging and his cardiorespiratory fitness level is classified as excellent, he is exempted from the initial stage and enters the improvement stage of the program immediately. During this time (20 wk), the exercise intensity is increased from 70% to 85% of the estimated $\dot{V}O_2R$. The speed corresponding to each MET intensity is calculated using the ACSM formulas for running on a level course (see table 4.3).

The intensity, duration, and frequency of the exercise sessions provide a weekly net caloric expenditure between 1,010 and 2,170 kcal. During the first 4 wk of the program, this client's net rate of energy expenditure due to exercise is 10.2 kcal·min⁻¹ (8.3 METs × 3.5 × 70 kg / 200 = 10.2 kcal·min⁻¹); thus, he will expend approximately 1,010 kcal, jogging 33 min at a pace of 11:06 min·mi⁻¹ three times per week (33 min × 10.2 kcal·min⁻¹ × 3). To figure the distance covered, the exercise duration is divided by the running pace: 33 min / 11.1 min·mi⁻¹ = 3 mi (5 km). During the improvement stage, the frequency of exercise sessions gradually progresses from 3 to 5 days/wk. During the maintenance stage, the running is reduced to 3 days/wk, and handball and basketball are added to the aerobic exercise program. The ACSM (2018) guidelines were followed to calculate each component of this exercise prescription.

SAMPLE MULTIMODAL EXERCISE PROGRAM

Some clients prefer to engage in a variety of exercise modes (**cross-training**) to develop their cardiore-spiratory fitness (see the example in the Sample Multimodal Exercise Program later in the chapter). In these cases, it is difficult to systematically prescribe increments in exercise intensity using METs or target HRs. Although MET equivalents for various activities are available (see appendix E.3), typically a range of values is given, making it difficult for you to accurately prescribe work rates corresponding to specific intensity recommendations in an exercise prescription. Also, the HR response to a given MET level is highly dependent on the exercise mode.

The degree of muscle mass involved in the activity, as well as whether the body weight is supported during exercise, can affect the HR response to a prescribed exercise intensity. For example, whole-body exercise modes, such as Nordic skiing and aerobic dancing, involve both upper and lower body musculature. These produce higher submaximal HRs than lower body exercise modes (e.g., cycling and jogging). Also, at any given exercise intensity, the HR response during weight-bearing exercise such as jogging is greater than that for non-weight-bearing exercise (e.g., cycling).

Therefore, you should use RPEs to progressively increase exercise intensity throughout the improvement stage of a multimodal aerobic exercise program (see table 4.2). To use the RPE safely and effectively, you will need to teach your clients to focus on and learn to monitor important exertional cues such as breathing effort (rate and depth of breathing) and muscular sensations (e.g., pain, warmth, and fatigue). Guidelines for developing multimodal exercise prescriptions are presented in this section.

For **multimodal exercise programs**, you should set exercise frequency and weekly net caloric expenditure goals for each client (see the example in Sample Multimodal Exercise Program later in the chapter). Provide your clients with estimates of net energy expenditure (kcal·min⁻¹) for each of the aerobic activities they select for their exercise prescriptions. The exercise duration to achieve a specified weekly net caloric expenditure goal will vary depending on the activity mode chosen for each exercise session. Any combination of type A, B, or C activities can be used, provided the client is able to maintain the prescribed RPE intensity for at least 20 min.

Flexibility is the key to successful multimodal exercise prescriptions. Clients should be free not only to select exercise modes of interest but also to decide on various combinations of frequency and duration as long as they meet the caloric thresholds specified in their exercise prescriptions for each week.

The primary advantages of multimodal exercise programs over single-mode (e.g., jogging or cycling) programs for many of your clients are

- greater likelihood of engaging in a safe and effective exercise program,
- overall greater enjoyment of physical activity and exercise,
- better understanding of how their bodies respond to exercise,
- more direct involvement and sense of control in developing and monitoring their exercise programs, and
- increased likelihood of incorporating physical activity and exercise into their lifestyles.

Guidelines for Multimodal Exercise Prescriptions

- **Modes:** Select at least three per week from type A and B activities.
- **Frequency:** Three to seven sessions a week. Engage in either type A, B, or C activities at least three times per week.
- **Intensity:** Rating of perceived exertion between 5 and 9 on 10-point OMNI scale.
- **Duration:** At least 15 min, preferably 20 to 30 min. Duration depends on energy cost ($kcal \cdot min^{-1}$) of exercise mode.
- **Caloric expenditure:** 1,000 to 2,000 $kcal \cdot wk^{-1}$. Group C and D activities can be used to reach the weekly caloric expenditure goal, but they cannot be counted as one of the required aerobic activities.

SAMPLE HIT EXERCISE PROGRAM

The sample HIT program later in this chapter is designed for a 34 yr old, recreationally active male who has a fair cardiorespiratory fitness level and a limited amount of time per week to dedicate to aerobic training. Since he is satisfied with his body weight, his main goal is to improve his aerobic capacity. His $\dot{V}O_2max$ was predicted from a multistage treadmill test, and his maximal HR was predicted using the formula 220 – age. Because this client is undertaking his first HIT exercise program and his cardiorespiratory fitness level is classified as fair, he is starting his program 5% above the exercise intensity targeted by the end (60% $\dot{V}O_2R$) of the standard initial conditioning stage. During the first 2 wk of his treadmill routine, the work and active recovery (rest) intervals are performed at 65% and 35% of his estimated $\dot{V}O_2R$, respectively. With the work and rest intervals both being 1 min in duration, his work-to-rest ratio is 1:1; he is initially scheduled to complete 15 repetitions per session three times per week. While the frequency and total duration of his exercise sessions remain constant, the intensity and duration of the work interval are systematically manipulated throughout the remaining 11 wk of the program, as is the work-to-rest ratio (principle of progression). The average net $kcal \cdot min^{-1}$ expended in week 1 is calculated as follows: Work: [(7 METs × 3.5 ml $kg^{-1} \cdot min^{-1}$ × 97.7 kg) / 200] = 11.97 $kcal \cdot min^{-1}$; Rest: [(4.3 METs × 3.5 ml $kg^{-1} \cdot min^{-1}$ × 97.7 kg) / 200] = 7.35 $kcal \cdot min^{-1}$; average net $kcal \cdot min^{-1}$ = [(11.97 × 15 min) + (7.35 × 15 min)] / 30 min = 9.7. This represents the respective contributions of the work and rest intervals.

The 2 wk block arrangement of exercise sessions provides a weekly net caloric expenditure between 869 and 1,041 kcal and the opportunity to manipulate one programmatic variable at a time. As he advances through the improvement stage, adjustments are made to the intensity of the work interval, work-to-rest ratio, and number of repetitions. His ability to tolerate the progression must be closely monitored and his program adjusted accordingly. A reassessment of his estimated $\dot{V}O_2max$ is recommended after the sixth week. For additional information on the potential improvements in aerobic capacity or cardiometabolic disease risk following high-intensity interval training interventions, refer to the work of Bacon and colleagues (2013) and Kessler, Sisson, and Short (2012), respectively.

SAMPLE JOGGING PROGRAM

Client Data

Age:	29 yr
Gender:	Male
Body weight:	70 kg (154 lb)
Resting heart rate:	50 bpm
Maximal heart rate:	191 bpm (age predicted)
$\dot{V}O_2max$:	45 ml·kg^{-1}·min^{-1} (predicted); 12.9 METs
Graded exercise test:	None
Initial cardiorespiratory fitness level:	Excellent

Exercise Prescription

Mode:	Jogging and running
Intensity:	70%-85% $\dot{V}O_2R$
	32.5-38.8 ml·kg^{-1}·min^{-1}
	9.3-11.1 METs
Exercise heart rates:	149 bpm minimum (70% HRR)
	170 bpm maximum (85% HRR)
RPE:	6-9 (OMNI scale)
Duration:	33-35 min
Frequency:	3-5 days/wk

Phase (wk)	Intensity % $\dot{V}O_2R$	METs	HR (bpm)	RPE	Pace: mph (min·mi^{-1})	Distance (miles)	Net kcal·min^{-1}	Time (min)	Frequency	Weekly net expenditure (kcal)
IMPROVEMENT										
1-4	70	9.3	149	6	5.4 (11:06)	3.0	10.2	33	3	1,010
5-8	70-**80**	9.3-10.5	149-163	6-7	5.4-6.2 (9:40)	3.0-3.4	10.2-11.6	33	3	1,010-1,148
9-12	70-80	9.3-10.5	149-163	6-7	5.4-6.2 (9:40)	3.0-3.4	10.2-11.6	33	**4**	1,347-1,531
13-16	80-**85**	10.5-11.1	163-170	7-9	6.2-6.6 (9:05)	3.4-3.6	11.6-12.4	33	4	1,531-1,637
17-20	80-85	10.5-11.1	163-170	7-9	6.2-6.6 (9:05)	3.4-3.8	11.6-12.4	33-35	**5**	1,914-2,170
MAINTENANCE										
21+										
Jogging	85	11.2	170	7-9	6.6 (9:05)	3.8	12.4	35	3	1,302
Handball	60	8.0	—	6-7	—	—	9.2	60	1	552
Basketball	60	8.0	—	6-7	—	—	9.2	60	1	552

Note: Values in boldface indicate training variables that are increased during each stage of the exercise progression.

SAMPLE MULTIMODAL EXERCISE PROGRAM

Client Data

Age:	44 yr
Sex:	Female
Weight:	68 kg (150 lb)
Resting heart rate:	70 bpm
Maximal heart rate:	170 bpm
$\dot{V}O_2$max:	30 ml·kg^{-1}·min^{-1}
	8.6 METs
Graded exercise test:	Treadmill maximal GXT (Bruce protocol)
Initial cardiorespiratory fitness level:	Fair

Exercise Prescription

Modes and estimates of gross caloric expenditure (METs) and net caloric expenditure (*kcal·min^{-1}*)[a]:	Stationary cycling (100 W): 5.5 METs; 5.4 kcal·min^{-1}
	Rowing (100 W): 7.0 METs; 7.1 kcal·min^{-1}
	Swimming (moderate effort): 7.0 METs; 7.1 kcal·min^{-1}
	Stair climbing (machine): 9.0 METs; 9.5 kcal·min^{-1}
	In-line skating: 12.5 METs; 13.7 kcal·min^{-1}
	Hiking: 6.0 METs; 5.9 kcal·min^{-1}
	Resistance training (free weights, machines): 3.0 METs; 2.4 kcal·min^{-1}
Intensity:	RPE: 5-9 (OMNI scale)
Duration:	20-60 min
Frequency:	3-5 days/wk
Weekly caloric expenditure:	500-1,250 kcal·wk^{-1}

Phase (wk)	Intensity (RPE)	Minimal duration (min)	Minimal frequency	Average kcal per workout	Weekly caloric goal
INITIAL					
1-2	5	20	3	133	500
3-4	5	25	3	200	600
IMPROVEMENT					
5-8	6	25	3	200	700
9-12	6	30	3	233	800
13-16	6-7	30	4	225	900
17-20	7-8	30	4	250	1,000
21-24	8-9	30	5	250	1,250
MAINTENANCE					
24+	8-9	30	5	250	1,250

(continued)

Sample Multimodel Exercise Program *(continued)*

Week 1	Activity	Net kcal·min⁻¹ estimates	Time (min)	Frequency	Kcal per workout (net)	Activity type[b]
Monday	Stationary cycling	5.4	20	1	108	A
Wednesday	In-line skating	13.7	10	1	137	C
Friday	Stair climbing	9.5	30	1	285	B
		Totals[c]:	60	3	530	3
		Goals:	60	3	500	3
WEEK 21						
Monday	Swimming	7.1	35	1	248	C
Tuesday	Rowing	7.1	35	1	248	B
Wednesday	Stair climbing	9.5	30	1	285	B
Friday	Resistance training	2.4	40	1	96	D
Sunday	Hiking	5.9	60	1	354	D
		Totals[c]:	200	5	1,231	4
		Goals:	150	5	1,250	4

[a]Gross MET levels for activities from Ainsworth and colleagues (2000); net energy expenditure in kcal·min⁻¹ = net MET level × 3.5 × BM (kg) / 200.

[b]Check all type A and B activities.

[c]Compare weekly totals to weekly goals.

SAMPLE HIT PROGRAM

Client Data

Age:	34 yr
Gender:	Male
Body weight:	97.7 kg (215 lb)
Resting heart rate:	72 bpm
Maximal heart rate:	186 bpm (predicted)
$\dot{V}O_2$max:	36 ml·kg^{-1}·min^{-1} (predicted);10.3 METs
Graded exercise test:	Treadmill
Initial cardiorespiratory fitness level:	Fair

Exercise Prescription

Mode:	Treadmill
Intensity:	Work periods: 65% to 75% $\dot{V}O_2$R
	Rest periods: 35% $\dot{V}O_2$R
	Work periods: 15-20 min
	Rest periods: 10-15 min
Frequency:	3 days/wk
Weekly caloric expenditure:	869-1,041 kcal·wk^{-1}

Phase (wk)	Intensity %$\dot{V}O_2$R	METs	Rest %$\dot{V}O_2$R	Work duration (min)	Rest duration (min)	Work:rest ratio	Repetitions	Frequency	Time (min)	Net kcal·min^{-1}	Expenditure per session (kcal)	Weekly net expenditure (kcal)
1-2	65	7.0	35	1.0	1.0	1:1	15	3	30	9.7	289.8	869
3-4	65	7.0	35	**1.5**	1.0	1.5:1	12	3	30	10.1	303.7	911
5-6	**70**	7.2	35	1.0	1.0	1:1	15	3	30	10.1	302.6	908
7-8	70	7.2	35	**1.5**	1.0	1.5:1	12	3	30	10.6	319.0	957
9-10	**75**	7.7	35	1.5	1.0	1.5:1	12	3	30	11.1	334.4	1,003
11-12	75	7.7	35	**2.0**	1.0	2:1	10	3	30	11.6	347.1	1,041

Note: Values in boldface indicate training variables that are increased during each stage of the exercise progression.

Key Points

▶ Always personalize cardiorespiratory exercise programs to meet the needs, interests, and abilities of each participant.

▶ The exercise prescription includes mode, frequency, intensity, duration, volume, and progression (FITT-VP principle) of exercise.

▶ Aerobic endurance activities involving large muscle groups are well suited for developing cardiorespiratory fitness. Type A and B activities such as walking, jogging, and cycling allow the individual to maintain steady-state exercise intensities and are not highly dependent on skill.

▶ Exercise intensity can be prescribed using the HR, $\dot{V}O_2$R, or RPE methods, or a combination of these methods.

▶ For the average healthy person, the traditional cardiorespiratory exercise program should be at a moderate intensity of 40% to <60% $\dot{V}O_2$R, a duration of 30 to 60 min, and a frequency of 5 days/wk.

▶ More fit individuals can exercise at a vigorous intensity of ≥60% to 90% $\dot{V}O_2$R, 20 to 60 min/day, 3 day/wk.

▶ The cardiorespiratory exercise program includes three stages of progression: initial conditioning, improvement, and maintenance.

▶ Each exercise session includes a warm-up, aerobic conditioning exercise, and a cool-down.

▶ Continuous and discontinuous training methods are equally effective for improving cardiorespiratory fitness.

▶ AIT and SIT training programs may provide similar or better improvements in cardiometabolic factors in less time compared with continuous moderate-intensity programs. Additionally, they may improve adherence and increase enjoyment of exercise.

▶ Multimodal exercise prescriptions use a variety of type A, B, and C aerobic activities to improve cardiorespiratory endurance.

Key Terms

Learn the definition for each of the following key terms. Definitions of key terms can be found in the glossary.

aerobic interval training (AIT)

caloric threshold

continuous training

counting talk test (CTT)

cross-training

discontinuous training

FITT-VP principle

heart rate reserve (HRR)

high-intensity interval training

interval training

Karvonen method

lactate threshold

MET·min

multimodal exercise program

percent heart rate maximum (%HRmax)

percent heart rate reserve (%HRR) method

percent $\dot{V}O_2$max reserve (%$\dot{V}O_2$R)

pulmonary ventilation

Spinning

sprint interval training (SIT)

super circuit resistance training

talk test

treading

type A activities

type B activities

type C activities

type D activities

ventilatory threshold

volume of exercise

$\dot{V}O_2$reserve ($\dot{V}O_2$R)

Review Questions

In addition to being able to define each of the key terms, test your knowledge and understanding of the material by answering the following review questions.

1. Name the four components of any aerobic exercise prescription.

2. What are the guidelines for an exercise prescription for improved health?

3. What are the guidelines for an exercise prescription for cardiorespiratory fitness?

4. Identify the three parts of an aerobic exercise workout and state the purpose of each part.

5. To classify an aerobic exercise mode as either type A, B, C, or D activity, what criteria are used?

6. Give three examples each for type A, B, C, and D aerobic activities.

7. Describe three methods used to prescribe intensity for an aerobic exercise prescription.

8. Describe potential advantages of mixing non-load-bearing aerobic exercises into a load-bearing aerobic exercise program.

9. Using the $\dot{V}O_2$reserve method, calculate the target $\dot{V}O_2$ for a client whose $\dot{V}O_2$max is 12 METs and relative exercise intensity is 70% $\dot{V}O_2$R.

10. Which method of prescribing intensity (%HRR or %HRmax) corresponds 1:1 with the % $\dot{V}O_2R$ method?

11. What are the limitations of using HR methods to monitor intensity of aerobic exercise?

12. Describe how RPEs can be used to prescribe and monitor the intensity of aerobic exercise.

13. Describe how your clients can use the talk test to monitor exercise intensity during their aerobic exercise workouts.

14. How does the talk test differ from the counting talk test?

15. What target caloric thresholds are recommended by ACSM for aerobic exercise workouts and weekly caloric expenditure from physical activity and exercise?

16. What is the recommended frequency of activity and exercise for improved health benefits? For improved cardiorespiratory fitness?

17. Name the three stages of a cardiorespiratory exercise program. For the average individual, what is the typical length (in weeks) of each stage?

18. What is the difference between continuous and discontinuous aerobic exercise training? Give examples of continuous and discontinuous training methods.

19. Compare the health benefits of aerobic interval training, sprint interval training, and continuous moderate-intensity exercise training programs.

20. What are the essential elements of a client case study?

CHAPTER 6

Assessing Muscular Fitness

KEY QUESTIONS

▶ How are strength, muscular endurance, and power assessed?

▶ How does the type of muscle action (concentric, eccentric, static, or isokinetic) affect force production?

▶ What test protocols can be used to assess a client's muscular fitness?

▶ What are the advantages and limitations of using free weights and exercise machines to assess muscular strength?

▶ What are sources of measurement error for muscular fitness tests, and how are they controlled?

▶ What are the recommended procedures for administering 1-RM strength tests?

▶ Is it safe to give 1-RM strength tests to children and older adults?

▶ What tests can be used to assess the functional strength of older adults?

Muscular strength and endurance are two important components of muscular fitness. Minimal levels of muscular fitness are needed to perform activities of daily living, to maintain functional independence as one ages, and to partake in active leisure-time pursuits without undue stress or fatigue. Adequate levels of muscular fitness lessen the chance of developing low back problems, osteoporotic fractures, and musculoskeletal injuries. Traditionally, muscular power has not been routinely assessed in health and fitness programs. However, the American College of Sports Medicine (2018) now includes power along with muscular strength and endurance to collectively define muscular fitness. In addition to being critical for success in many athletic endeavors, muscular power might actually be more important than muscular strength for preventing slip-related falls (Han and Yang 2015).

This chapter describes a variety of laboratory and field tests for assessing all forms of muscular strength, endurance, and muscular power. In addition, the chapter compares types of exercise machines, addresses factors affecting muscular fitness tests, discusses sources of measurement error, and provides guidelines for testing muscular fitness of children and older adults.

DEFINITION OF TERMS

Muscular strength is defined as the ability of a muscle group to develop maximal contractile force against a resistance in a single contraction. The force generated by a muscle or muscle group, however, is highly dependent on the velocity of movement. Maximal force is produced when the limb is not rotating (i.e., zero velocity). As the speed of joint rotation increases, the muscular force decreases. Thus, *strength for dynamic movements* is defined as the maximal force generated in a single contraction at a specified velocity (Knuttgen and Kraemer 1987). **Muscular endurance** is the ability of a muscle group to exert submaximal force for extended periods. **Muscular power** is the muscle's ability to exert force per unit of time, or the rate of performing work.

Figure 6.1 summarizes the different types of muscle actions. Both strength and muscular endurance can be assessed for static and dynamic actions. If the resistance is immovable, the action is **static or isometric** (*iso*, same; *metric*, length), and there is no visible movement of the joint. **Dynamic actions**, in which there is visible joint movement, are classified as either auxotonic, isokinetic, or variable resistance.

Traditional resistance training with free weights is classified as **isotonic** (*iso*, same; *tonic*, tension) in many textbooks. However, the term *isotonic muscle action* is a misnomer because the tension produced by the muscle group fluctuates greatly even though the resistance is constant throughout the range of motion (ROM). This fluctuation in muscular force is due to the change in muscle length and angle of pull as the bony lever is moved, creating a strength curve that is unique for each muscle group. For example, the strength of the knee flexors is maximal at 160° to 170° (see figure 6.2). The correct term for describing the muscle action when lifting with free weights is *auxotonic*, defined as variable tensions caused by changing velocities and joint angles.

Auxotonic muscle action can be either concentric or eccentric (see figure 6.3*a*). If the resistance is less than the force produced by the muscle group, the muscle action is **concentric**, allowing the muscle to shorten as it exerts tension to move the bony lever. The muscle is also capable of exerting tension while lengthening. This is known as **eccentric muscle action**, and it typically occurs when the muscles produce a braking force to decelerate rapidly moving body segments or to resist gravity (e.g., slowly lowering a barbell).

In auxotonic (concentric and eccentric) dynamic exercise, because of the change in mechanical and physiological advantage as the limb is moved, the muscle group is not contracting maximally throughout the ROM. Thus, the greatest resistance that can be used during regular, dynamic exercise is equal to the maximum weight that can be moved at the weakest point in the ROM.

Video 6.1

Video 6.2

Video 6.3

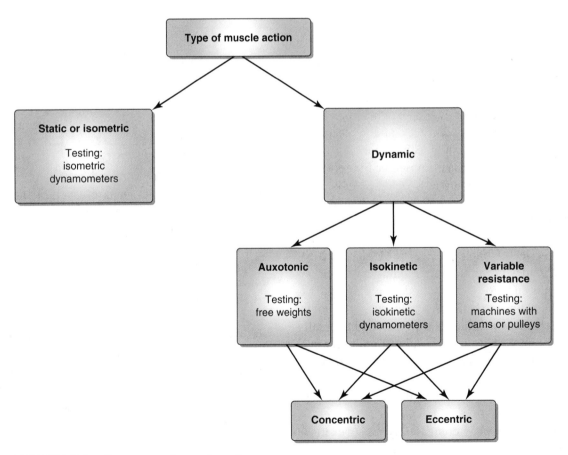

FIGURE 6.1 Summary of muscle actions.

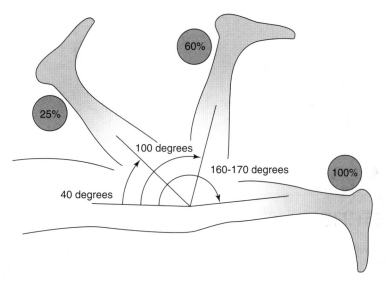

FIGURE 6.2 Strength variations in relation to knee joint angle.

In an attempt to overcome this deficiency, equipment manufacturers have designed variable-resistance machines that vary the resistance during the ROM. These machines have a moving connection (i.e., lever, cam, or pulley) between the resistance and the point of force application. As the weight is lifted, the mechanical advantage of the machine decreases. Therefore, more force must be applied to continue moving the resistance. The variable-resistance mode of exercise attempts to match the force capability of the musculoskeletal system throughout the ROM. However, many variable-resistance exercise machines fail to match the strength curves of different muscle groups.

Isokinetic muscle action (see figure 6.3b) is a maximal contraction of a muscle group at a constant velocity throughout the entire range of joint motion (*iso*, same; *kinetic*, motion). The velocity of contraction is controlled mechanically so that the limb rotates at a set velocity (e.g., 120°·sec^{-1}). Electromechanical devices vary the resistance to match the muscular force produced at each point in the ROM. Thus, isokinetic exercise machines allow the muscle group to encounter variable but maximal resistances during the movement.

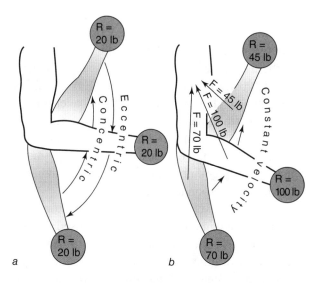

FIGURE 6.3 (a) Concentric and eccentric components of auxotonic muscle action and (b) isokinetic muscle action.

STRENGTH AND MUSCULAR ENDURANCE ASSESSMENT

Measures of static or dynamic strength and endurance are used to establish baseline values before training, monitor progress during training, and assess the overall effectiveness of resistance training and exercise rehabilitation programs. Static strength and muscular endurance are measured using dynamometers. Free weights (barbells and dumbbells), as well as constant-resistance, variable-resistance, and isokinetic exercise machines, are used to assess dynamic strength and endurance (see table 6.1). The testing procedures vary depending on the type of test (i.e., strength or endurance) and equipment.

ISOMETRIC MUSCLE TESTING USING DYNAMOMETERS

Isometric strength is measured as the maximum force exerted in a single contraction against an immovable resistance (i.e., maximum voluntary contraction, or MVC). For many years, spring-loaded dynamometers have been used to measure static strength and endurance of grip squeezing muscles and leg and back muscles (see figure 6.4). The handgrip dynamometer has an adjustable handle to fit the size of the hand and measures forces between 0 and 100 kg in 1 kg increments (0-220 lb in 2.2 lb increments). The back and leg dynamometer consists of a scale that measures forces ranging from 0 to 2,500 lb in 10 lb increments (0-1,134 kg in 4.5 kg increments). As force is applied to the dynamometer, the spring is compressed and moves the indicator needle a corresponding amount.

An alternative to spring-loaded dynamometers, hydraulic dynamometers can also be used to measure isometric grip strength. These instruments have a sealed hydraulic system that measures force (in lb or kg) on a gauge dial. The Jamar grip dynamometer is widely used and has excellent validity and reliability (Roberts et al. 2011). The American Society of Hand Therapists (ASHT; 1992) recommends the following standardized testing procedures:

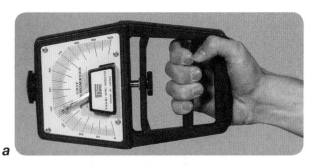

a

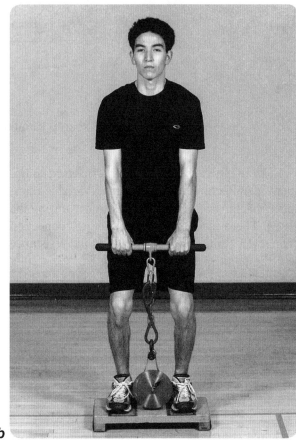

b

FIGURE 6.4 Spring-loaded dynamometers for measuring static strength and endurance: (*a*) handgrip dynamometer and (*b*) back and leg dynamometer.

Table 6.1 **Strength Training Modes**

Testing mode	Equipment	Measure*
Static	Isometric dynamometers	MVC (kg or N)

Dynamic
  Constant resistance
  Variable resistance
	Free weights (barbells and dumbbells) and exercise machines
	Exercise machines
		1-RM (lb or kg)
		NA

Isokinetic	Isokinetic machines	Peak torque (Nm or ft-lb)

*MVC = maximum voluntary contraction; N = newton; NA = not applicable; Nm = newton-meter; ft-lb = foot-pound.

1. Client is seated.

2. Shoulders are adducted and neutrally rotated. The elbow of the testing arm is flexed at 90° with the forearm in a neutral position.

3. Wrist is dorsiflexed between 0° and 30°.

4. Administer three trials for each hand and record the mean of three trials.

However, Roberts and colleagues (2011) reported that testing protocols for assessing grip strength vary widely. Therefore, they proposed a more detailed testing protocol based on the ASHT guidelines. This revised protocol standardizes leg and forearm position, encouragement and assessor training, and summary measures (i.e., use the best score from six trials). Norms for the Jamar grip dynamometer are available for women and men, ages 20 to 80+ yr (Bohannon et al. 2006; Peters et al. 2011).

The Jamar is widely regarded as the gold standard for handgrip dynamometers among clinicians. However, the resolution of the Jamar is too large to detect small changes in strength, and it may not be appropriate for individuals with a weak MVC. Hogrel (2015) recently reported on a dynamometer called the Myogrip with a 10 g resolution and an accuracy of 50 g. This dynamometer is recommended for very weak clients, and Hogrel provided norms for males and females aged 5 to 80 yr.

Grip Strength Testing Procedures

Video 6.4

Before using the handgrip dynamometer, adjust the handgrip size to a position that is comfortable for the individual. Alternatively, you can measure the hand width with a caliper and use this value to set the optimum grip size (Montoye and Faulkner 1964). The individual stands erect, with the arm and forearm positioned as follows (Fess 1992): shoulder adducted and neutrally rotated, elbow flexed at 90°, forearm in the neutral position, and wrist in slight extension (0° to 30°). For some test protocols, however, the client must keep the arm straight and slightly abducted for measurement of the grip strength of each hand (Canadian Society for Exercise Physiology 2003). The individual squeezes the dynamometer as hard as possible using one brief maximal contraction and no extraneous body movement. Administer three trials for each hand, allowing a 1 min rest between trials, and use the best score as the client's static strength.

Grip Endurance Testing Procedures

Video 6.5

Once the grip size is adjusted, instruct the client to squeeze the handle as hard as possible and to continue squeezing for 1 min. Record the initial force and the final force exerted at the end of 1 min. The greater the endurance, the lower the rate and degree of decline in force. The relative endurance score is the final force divided by the initial force times 100.

Alternatively, you can assess static grip endurance by having your client exert a submaximal force, which is a given percentage of the individual's **maximum voluntary contraction (MVC)** strength (e.g., 50% MVC). The relative endurance score is the time this force level is maintained. During the test, the client must watch the dial of the dynamometer and adjust the amount of force exerted as necessary in order to maintain the appropriate submaximal force level.

Leg Strength Testing Procedures

Using the back and leg dynamometer, the individual stands on the platform with trunk erect and the knees flexed to an angle of 130° to 140°. The client holds the hand bar using a pronated grip and positions it across the thighs by adjusting the length of the chain (see figure 6.4b). If a belt is available, attach it to each end of the hand bar after positioning the belt around the client's hips. The belt helps stabilize the bar and reduces the stress placed on the hands during the leg lift. Without using the back, the client slowly exerts as much force as possible while extending the knees. The maximum indicator needle remains at the peak force achieved. Administer two or three trials with a 1 min rest interval. Divide the maximum score (in pounds) by 2.2 to convert it to kilograms.

Back Strength Testing Procedures

Using the back and leg dynamometer, the individual stands on the platform with the knees fully extended and the head and trunk erect. The client grasps the hand bar using a pronated grip with the right hand and a supinated grip with the left. Position the hand bar across the client's thighs. Without leaning backward, the client pulls the hand bar straight upward using the back muscles. Instruct the client to roll the shoulders backward during the pull, to avoid flexing the trunk, and to keep the head and trunk erect during the test. Administer two trials with a 1 min rest between the trials. Divide the maximum score (in pounds) by 2.2 to convert it to kilograms.

Static Strength Norms for Spring-Loaded Dynamometers

Grip strength norms for each hand are presented in table 6.2. You can also use norms developed for men and women to assess your clients' static strength for each dynamometric test item (see table 6.2). Calculate the total strength score by adding the right grip, left grip, leg strength, and back strength scores. Before doing this, convert the leg and back strength scores (measured in pounds) to kilograms. To calculate the relative strength score, divide the total strength score by body mass (expressed in kilograms).

ISOMETRIC MUSCLE TESTING USING DIGITAL HANDHELD DYNAMOMETRY

Handheld dynamometry is a convenient method for measuring the isometric strength of the upper and lower body musculature. Compared against isokinetic testing (Kin-Com, Biodex, and Cybex), handheld dynamometry has moderate to good validity (Stark et al. 2011) and excellent reliability for most muscle groups (Lu et al. 2011). You can use handheld dynamometers that provide a digital display of force production to assess the isometric strength of 11 muscle groups (see figure 6.5, a and b). This handheld dynamometer digitally displays force measurements up to a maximum of 1334 newtons (300 lb in 0.1 lb increments). For this type of testing, place the dynamometer on the limb and hold it stationary while the client exerts maximum force against it. Administer two trials and use either the average or best score for each muscle group. Appendix C.1 describes standardized test protocols for the 11 muscle groups. Performance norms for adults (20-79 yr) and children (4-16 yr) are available (see Andrews, Thomas, and Bohannon 1996; Beenakker et al. 2001; Bohannon 1997; van den Beld et al. 2006).

Table 6.2 Static Strength Norms

Classification	Left grip (kg)	Right grip (kg)	Back strength (kg)	Leg strength (kg)	Total strength (kg)	Relative strength*
MEN						
Excellent	>68	>70	>209	>241	>587	>7.50
Good	56-67	62-69	177-208	214-240	508-586	7.10-7.49
Average	43-55	48-61	126-176	160-213	375-507	5.21-7.09
Below average	39-42	41-47	91-125	137-159	307-374	4.81-5.20
Poor	<39	<41	<91	<137	<307	<4.81
WOMEN						
Excellent	>37	>41	>111	>136	>324	>5.50
Good	34-36	38-40	98-110	114-135	282-323	4.80-5.49
Average	22-33	25-37	52-97	66-113	164-281	2.90-4.79
Below average	18-21	22-24	39-51	49-65	117-163	2.10-2.89
Poor	<18	<22	<39	<49	<117	<2.10

*Relative strength is determined by dividing total strength by body mass (kg).

For persons over age 50, reduce scores by 10% to adjust for muscle tissue loss due to aging.

Data from Corbin et al. 1978.

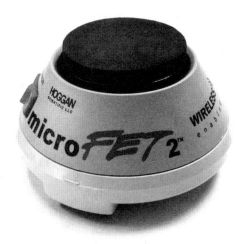

a

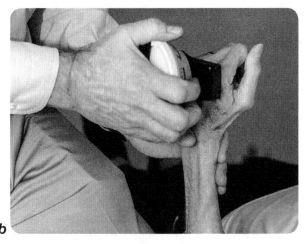

b

FIGURE 6.5 (a) Handheld dynamometer for measuring isometric strength and (b) the hand being tested.

Courtesy of Hoggan Scientific, LLC.

ISOMETRIC MUSCLE TESTING USING CLINICAL METHODS

Several clinical tests have been developed to measure the isometric endurance of core muscles used to stabilize the spine. Two of the most popular tests are the Kraus-Weber test for the trunk flexors and the Sorensen test for the trunk extensors (Biering-Sorensen 1984; Kraus 1970). For these tests, clients must maintain their trunk and lower extremities in a certain position for as long as possible. Over the years, the tests have been modified to reduce the risk of low back pain or injury resulting from hyperextension of the lumbar spine during testing

(Ito et al. 1996; McGill, Childs, and Liebenson 1999; Reiman et al. 2010).

To assess the isometric endurance of the trunk flexors, you can use the V-sit test. For this test, the trunk is reclined 60° above the horizontal plane, the knees and hips are flexed 90°, and the feet are stabilized. A wooden triangular supporting wedge is positioned behind the client to ensure that the torso is reclined to 60°. To start the test, the supporting wedge is moved away from the client. The client maintains the V-sit position for as long as possible. Endurance time (in seconds) is measured with a stopwatch (McGill, Childs, and Liebenson 1999). The test-retest reliability of the V-sit test is high ($r = .92$).

For the trunk extensor test, the client lies prone on the bench with the lower body strapped to the bench at the ankles, knees, and hips. The upper body is extended over the edge of the bench. The bench height is 25 cm. The arms are folded across the chest and the upper body is lifted until the trunk is horizontal to the floor. The client maintains this position for as long as possible. Endurance time (in seconds) is measured with a stopwatch. The test is terminated when the client's upper body touches the floor (McGill, Childs, and Liebenson 1999).

In addition to the trunk flexors and extensors, the lateral flexors of the spine are important for lumbar stabilization. The side bridge test can be used to assess the isometric endurance of the lateral flexors. For this test, the client elevates the torso from a side-lying position and supports this position on one elbow and forearm. The upper leg crosses in front of the lower leg for additional support. The non-weight-bearing arm is held across the chest, with the hand placed on the opposite shoulder. The client maintains a straight line position with the hips off the mat for as long as possible. Endurance time (in seconds) is measured with a stopwatch. The test is terminated when the hips return to the mat.

One disadvantage of the side bridge test is that some clients terminate the test because of upper extremity fatigue or pain. To avoid this shortcoming, Greene and colleagues (2012) developed a novel side-support test with the feet elevated on a 15 cm padded stool. To ensure that the torso is aligned properly, a horizontal reference rod of the alignment apparatus is placed on the greater trochanter of the top leg and fixed at this height. The client is instructed to maintain contact with the reference rod and hold this position for as long as possible

Video 6.6

during the test. The test is terminated when contact with the rod is lost for longer than 2 sec or when the client lowers the hips to the mat. Moderate to high correlations ($r = .59$-$.75$) were reported between this test and the traditional side bridge test, and the test-retest reliability was good. This modification may be a suitable alternative for clients with upper extremity pain or weakness.

For average endurance times for the trunk flexor, trunk extensor, and trunk lateral flexor tests for healthy men and women, see the work by McGill, Childs, and Liebenson (1999). Additionally, they provide average ratios of endurance times, normalized to the trunk extensor, that may be used to identify muscle endurance imbalances around the torso. Table 6.3 presents percentile norms for time to fatigue for the forearm plank for university students (Strand et al. 2014).

DYNAMIC MUSCLE TESTING USING CONSTANT-RESISTANCE AND VARIABLE-RESISTANCE MODES

Although either a **constant-resistance** (auxotonic muscle action) or a **variable-resistance exercise** mode can be used to assess dynamic (concentric and eccentric) muscle strength and endurance, you will be better served if you use either free weights or constant-resistance exercise machines.

A major disadvantage of free weights, dumbbells, and constant-resistance exercise machines, however, is that they measure dynamic strength only at the weakest point in the ROM. The reason is that the resistance cannot be varied to account for fluctuations in muscular force caused by the changing mechanical advantage (angle of pull of muscle) and physiological advantage (length of muscle) of the musculoskeletal system during the movement.

A major disadvantage of variable-resistance machines is that it is difficult to assess the client's maximal force or strength because the resistance is modified by the levers, pulleys, and cams, causing the movement velocity to vary. Variable-resistance exercise machines, therefore, have limited usefulness for maximal testing. Still, these types of machines are well suited for resistance training.

Although free weights and constant-resistance exercise machines are generally recommended for muscular fitness testing, there are advantages and limitations to each of these modalities. Compared with exercise machines, free weights require more neuromuscular coordination in order to stabilize body parts and maintain balance during lifting of the barbell or dumbbell. Although exercise machines may reduce the need for spotting during the test, these machines limit the individual's range of joint motion and plane of movement. Also, some exercise machines have relatively large weight plate increments, so you must attach smaller weights to the weight stack in order to accurately measure a client's strength.

Table 6.3 Percentile Scores for the Forearm Plank

Percentile	Male	Female
90th	201	142
80th	157	108
70th	137	95
60th	122	84
50th	110	72
40th	97	63
30th	89	58
20th	79	48
10th	62	35

Note: Score is measured in seconds.

Adapted by permission from S.L. Strand et al., "Norms for an Isometric Muscle Endurance Test," *Journal of Human Kinetics* 40 (2014): 93-102.

Last, some machines cannot accommodate individuals with short limbs; you may need to use child-sized machines to standardize their starting positions for testing. Clients with long limbs or large body and limb circumferences (e.g., some bodybuilders or obese clients) also may have difficulty using standard exercise machines. Body size and weight increments are less of a problem with free weights.

To overcome some of these limitations, **free-motion machines** that provide constant and variable resistance in multiple planes have been developed. These machines have adjustable seats, lever arms, and cable pulleys that can be set to exercise muscle groups in multiple planes. They are easy to get in and out of, they can accommodate smaller or larger individuals, and they have smaller weight increments (5 lb or 2.3 kg) than do older standard machines (typically 10 lb or 4.5 kg). When using free-motion exercise machines for muscular fitness testing, take care to adjust the plane of movement and the seat so that you simulate the starting and ending body positions that were used to develop test norms for older constant-resistance machines. If you use free-motion machines to monitor the progress of your clients, make certain that you use the same settings (i.e., seat and plane-of-movement adjustments) for each test session.

Dynamic Strength Tests

Force plates paired with linear transducers are used to obtain direct (i.e., gold standard) measures of muscular force and power. Cost of equipment, however, limits the usefulness of this method beyond the laboratory setting. With improved technology, new devices for assessing dynamic muscle force and power are being developed and validated against gold standard measures. Two such devices are the Tendo Weightlifting Analyzer System and the Myotest accelerometer.

The Tendo system is a linear transducer that can be attached to the end of a barbell. Measurements of peak velocity, average velocity, peak power, and average power were evaluated simultaneously by Tendo and an isoinertial dynamometer to assess the reliability and validity of Tendo during bench press and squat exercises. The intra-class correlation coefficients for reliability were .922 to .988 and for validity were .853 to .989 (Gar-

nacho-Castano, Lopez-Lastra, and Mate-Munoz 2015). The researchers also noted that the random errors and biases were low, and they concluded that the Tendo system was reliable and valid for measuring movement velocity and estimating power during resistance exercises. Similarly, the Myotest triaxial accelerometer has excellent validity ($r = .85$-$.99$) for calculating force, velocity, and power during dynamic exercise (Casartelli, Muller, and Maffiuletti 2010; Crewther et al. 2011; Thompson and Bemben 1999). This accelerometer also demonstrated high concurrent validity and reliability for measuring dynamic strength and power of men and women performing squat and bench press exercises (Comstock et al. 2011). In light of their small size, ease of use, and portability, the Tendo and Myotest are practical devices you can use in the field to evaluate lifting velocity, muscle force, and power.

However, more commonly in field settings, dynamic strength is measured as the **one-repetition maximum (1-RM)**, which is the maximum weight that can be lifted for one complete repetition of the movement. The 1-RM strength value is obtained through trial and error.

Although 1-RM strength tests can be safely administered to individuals of all ages, you should take precautions to decrease the risk of injury when clients attempt to lift maximal loads. Be certain that your clients warm up before attempting the lift, and start with a weight that is below their expected 1-RM. When you administer these tests, you should spot your clients and closely monitor their lifting technique and breathing. The National Strength and Conditioning Association (NSCA) outlines guidelines for spotting (see Tips for Spotting Free Weight Exercise).

The American College of Sports Medicine (2018) recommends the bench press and leg press (upper plate of constant-resistance exercise machine) for assessing strength of the upper and lower body, respectively. To determine **relative strength**, divide the 1-RM values by the client's body mass. Norms for men and women are provided in tables 6.4 and 6.5.

Another test of dynamic strength includes six test items: bench press, arm curl, latissimus pull, leg press, leg extension, and leg curl. For each exercise, express and evaluate the 1-RM as a percentage of

TIPS FOR SPOTTING FREE WEIGHT EXERCISE

1. The primary role of the spotter is to help protect the client from injury.

2. With the exception of power exercises, free weight exercises performed with the bar moving over the head, on the back, in front of the shoulders, or passing over the face require one or more spotters (e.g., bench press, lying triceps extensions, and front squat).

3. The spotter should be at least as strong and at least as tall as the client performing the exercise.

4. Overhead exercises and exercises where the bar is placed on the back or in front of the shoulders should be performed inside a power rack.

5. When spotting over-the-face exercises, use an alternated grip that is narrower than the client's when grasping the bar to lift or lower it. Use a supinated grip to spot the bar during the exercise.

6. When spotting heavy loads, establish a stable base of support and a flat-back position.

7. For dumbbell exercises, spot as close to the dumbbell as possible (e.g., for dumbbell flys, spot at the wrists, not at the elbows).

8. Spotters typically help the client move the barbell or dumbbells to the proper starting position (i.e., liftoff or moving the bar from the upright supports to client's hands and extended elbows).

9. Most clients need just enough help to successfully complete a repetition. During 1-RM attempts, however, the spotter should be prepared to take the bar immediately if the client cannot complete the repetition.

Video 6.7

Based on National Strength and Conditioning Association (2016).

Table 6.4 Age-Gender Norms for 1-RM Bench Press (1-RM/BM)

Percentile rankings* for men	AGE				
	20-29 yr	30-39 yr	40-49 yr	50-59 yr	60+ yr
90	1.48	1.24	1.10	0.97	0.89
80	1.32	1.12	1.00	0.90	0.82
70	1.22	1.04	0.93	0.84	0.77
60	1.14	0.98	0.88	0.79	0.72
50	1.06	0.93	0.84	0.75	0.68
40	0.99	0.88	0.80	0.71	0.66
30	0.93	0.83	0.76	0.68	0.63
20	0.88	0.78	0.72	0.63	0.57
10	0.80	0.71	0.65	0.57	0.53

Percentile rankings* for women	AGE					
	20-29 yr	30-39 yr	40-49 yr	50-59 yr	60-69 yr	70+ yr
90	0.54	0.49	0.46	0.40	0.41	0.44
80	0.49	0.45	0.40	0.37	0.38	0.39
70	0.42	0.42	0.38	0.35	0.36	0.33
60	0.41	0.41	0.37	0.33	0.32	0.31
50	0.40	0.38	0.34	0.31	0.30	0.27
40	0.37	0.37	0.32	0.28	0.29	0.25
30	0.35	0.34	0.30	0.26	0.28	0.24
20	0.33	0.32	0.27	0.23	0.26	0.21
10	0.30	0.27	0.23	0.19	0.25	0.20

*Descriptors for percentile rankings: 90 = well above average; 70 = above average; 50 = average; 30 = below average; 10 = well below average.

Data for women provided by the Women's Exercise Research Center, The George Washington University Medical Center, Washington, DC, 1998. Data for men provided by The Cooper Institute for Aerobics Research, *The Physical Fitness Specialist Manual*, The Cooper Institute, Dallas, TX, 2005.

Table 6.5   Age-Gender Norms for 1-RM Leg Press (1-RM/BM)

Percentile rankings* for men	AGE				
	20-29 yr	30-39 yr	40-49 yr	50-59 yr	60+ yr
90	2.27	2.07	1.92	1.80	1.73
80	2.13	1.93	1.82	1.71	1.62
70	2.05	1.85	1.74	1.64	1.56
60	1.97	1.77	1.68	1.58	1.49
50	1.91	1.71	1.62	1.52	1.43
40	1.83	1.65	1.57	1.46	1.38
30	1.74	1.59	1.51	1.39	1.30
20	1.63	1.52	1.44	1.32	1.25
10	1.51	1.43	1.35	1.22	1.16

Percentile rankings* for women	AGE					
	20-29 yr	30-39 yr	40-49 yr	50-59 yr	60-69 yr	70+ yr
90	2.05	1.73	1.63	1.51	1.40	1.27
80	1.66	1.50	1.46	1.30	1.25	1.12
70	1.42	1.47	1.35	1.24	1.18	1.10
60	1.36	1.32	1.26	1.18	1.15	0.95
50	1.32	1.26	1.19	1.09	1.08	0.89
40	1.25	1.21	1.12	1.03	1.04	0.83
30	1.23	1.16	1.03	0.95	0.98	0.82
20	1.13	1.09	0.94	0.86	0.94	0.79
10	1.02	0.94	0.76	0.75	0.84	0.75

*Descriptors for percentile rankings: 90 = well above average; 70 = above average; 50 = average; 30 = below average; 10 = well below average.

Data for women provided by the Women's Exercise Research Center, The George Washington University Medical Center, Washington, DC, 1998. Data for men provided by The Cooper Institute for Aerobics Research, *The Physical Fitness Specialist Manual,* The Cooper Institute, Dallas, TX, 2005.

body mass. For example, if a 120 lb (54.5 kg) woman bench presses 60 lb (27.2 kg), her ratio of strength to body mass is 0.50 (60 divided by 120), and she scores 3 points for that exercise. Follow this procedure for each exercise, and then add the total points to determine the individual's overall strength and fitness category. Strength-to-body-mass ratios with corresponding point values for college-age men and women are presented in table 6.6.

Dynamic Muscle Endurance Tests

You can assess your clients' dynamic muscle endurance by having them perform as many repetitions as possible using a weight that is a set percentage of their body weight or maximum strength (1-RM). Pollock, Wilmore, and Fox (1978) recommend using a weight that is 70% of the 1-RM value for each exercise. Although norms for this test have not been established, these authors suggest, on the basis of their testing and research findings, that the average individual should be able to complete 12 to 15 repetitions.

The YMCA (Golding 2000) recommends using a bench press test to assess dynamic muscular endurance of the upper body. For this absolute endurance test, use a flat bench and barbell. The client performs as many repetitions as possible at a set cadence of 30 repetitions per minute. Use a metronome to establish the exercise cadence. Male clients lift an 80 lb (36.4 kg) barbell, whereas female clients use a 35 lb (15.9 kg) barbell. Terminate the test when the client is unable to maintain the exercise cadence. Table 6.7 presents norms for this test.

Table 6.6 Strength-to-Body-Mass Ratios for Selected 1-RM Tests

Bench press	Arm curl	Lat pull-down	Leg press	Leg extension	Leg curl	Points
MEN						
1.50	0.70	1.20	3.00	0.80	0.70	10
1.40	0.65	1.15	2.80	0.75	0.65	9
1.30	0.60	1.10	2.60	0.70	0.60	8
1.20	0.55	1.05	2.40	0.65	0.55	7
1.10	0.50	1.00	2.20	0.60	0.50	6
1.00	0.45	0.95	2.00	0.55	0.45	5
0.90	0.40	0.90	1.80	0.50	0.40	4
0.80	0.35	0.85	1.60	0.45	0.35	3
0.70	0.30	0.80	1.40	0.40	0.30	2
0.60	0.25	0.75	1.20	0.35	0.25	1
WOMEN						
0.90	0.50	0.85	2.70	0.70	0.60	10
0.85	0.45	0.80	2.50	0.65	0.55	9
0.80	0.42	0.75	2.30	0.60	0.52	8
0.70	0.38	0.73	2.10	0.55	0.50	7
0.65	0.35	0.70	2.00	0.52	0.45	6
0.60	0.32	0.65	1.80	0.50	0.40	5
0.55	0.28	0.63	1.60	0.45	0.35	4
0.50	0.25	0.60	1.40	0.40	0.30	3
0.45	0.21	0.55	1.20	0.35	0.25	2
0.35	0.18	0.50	1.00	0.30	0.20	1

Total points			Strength fitness category[a]			
48-60			Excellent			
37-47			Good			
25-36			Average			
13-24			Fair			
0-12			Poor			

[a]Based on data compiled by V. Heyward from 250 college-age men and women.

Video
6.8

Steps for 1-RM Maximum Testing

The following basic steps are recommended for 1-RM testing.

- Have your client warm up by completing 5 to 10 repetitions of the exercise at 40% to 60% of the estimated 1-RM.

- Have the client rest for 1 min. This is followed by 3 to 5 repetitions of the exercise at 60% to 80% of the estimated 1-RM.

- Have the client rest for 2 min and attempt the 1-RM lift. If successful, increase the weight conservatively. Both the ACSM (2018) and the NSCA (2016) recommend increases of 5% to 10% for upper body exercise and 10% to 20% for lower body exercise. The client should rest 2 to 4 min before attempting the next weight increment. Follow this procedure until the client fails to complete the lift. The 1-RM typically is achieved within three to five trials.

- Record the 1-RM value as the maximum weight lifted for the last successful trial.

Alternatively, you can use a test battery consisting of seven items to assess dynamic muscular endurance. Select the weight to be lifted using a set percentage of the individual's body mass. The client lifts this weight up to a maximum of 15 repetitions. Table 6.8 provides percentages for each test item, as well as the scoring system and norms for college-age men and women.

Table 6.7 Muscular Endurance Norms for Bench Press

| Percentile | AGE GROUP (YR) | | | | | |
	18-25 yr	26-35 yr	36-45 yr	46-55 yr	56-65 yr	>65 yr
MEN						
95	49	48	41	33	28	22
75	34	30	26	21	17	12
50	26	22	20	13	10	8
25	17	16	12	8	4	3
5	5	4	2	1	0	0
WOMEN						
95	49	46	41	33	29	22
75	30	29	26	20	17	12
50	21	21	17	12	9	6
25	13	13	10	6	4	2
5	2	2	1	0	0	0

Note: Score is number of repetitions completed using 80 lb barbell for men and 35 lb barbell for women.

Data from YMCA of the USA 2000.

Table 6.8 Dynamic Muscular Endurance Test Battery

| % BODY MASS TO BE LIFTED | | | |
Exercise	Men	Women	Repetitions (max = 15)
Arm curl	0.33	0.25	_____
Bench press	0.66	0.50	_____
Lat pull-down	0.66	0.50	_____
Triceps extension	0.33	0.33	_____
Leg extension	0.50	0.50	_____
Leg curl	0.33	0.33	_____
Bent-knee sit-up			_____
			Total repetitions (max = 105) = _____

Total repetitions	Fitness category*
91-105	Excellent
77-90	Very good
63-76	Good
49-62	Fair
35-48	Poor
<35	Very poor

*Based on data compiled by V. Heyward from 250 college-age men and women.

DYNAMIC ISOKINETIC MUSCLE TESTING

Isokinetic dynamometers provide an accurate and reliable assessment of strength, endurance, and power of muscle groups (see figure 6.6). The speed of limb movement is kept at a constant preselected velocity. Any increase in muscular force produces an increased resistance rather than increased acceleration of the limb. Thus, fluctuations in muscular force throughout the ROM are matched by an equal counterforce, or **accommodating resistance**.

Video 6.9

Isokinetic dynamometers measure muscular torque production at speeds of $0°$ to $300°·sec^{-1}$. From the recorded output, you can evaluate peak torque, total work, and power. Some less expensive isokinetic dynamometers lack this recording capability, but these are suitable for training and rehabilitation exercise. Table 6.9 summarizes isokinetic test protocols for assessing strength, endurance, and power.

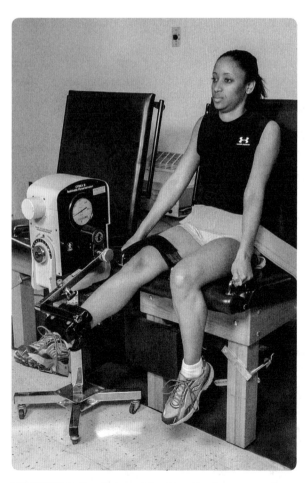

FIGURE 6.6 Cybex II isokinetic dynamometer.

CALISTHENIC-TYPE STRENGTH AND MUSCULAR ENDURANCE TESTS

In certain field situations, you may not have access to dynamometers, free weights, or exercise machines to assess muscular fitness. As an alternative, you may use calisthenic-type strength and endurance tests to assess your clients' strength and muscular endurance.

Calisthenic-Type Strength Tests

You can measure dynamic strength using calisthenic-type exercises by determining the maximum weight, in excess of body mass, that an individual can lift for one repetition of the movement. Because strength is related to the size and body mass of the individual, Johnson and Nelson (1986) recommend using relative strength scores. For each test, attach weight plates (2.5, 5, 10, and 25 lb or 1, 2.3, 4.5, and 11.4 kg) to the individual. The relative strength score is the amount of additional weight divided by the body mass. For example, if a 150 lb (68.2 kg) man successfully performs one pull-up with a 30 lb (13.6 kg) weight attached to the waist belt, his relative strength score is 0.20 (30 lb / 150 lb). Test protocols and performance norms for the pull-up, sit-up, and bench squat, as well as dip strength, are described elsewhere (Johnson and Nelson 1986).

Calisthenic-Type Endurance Tests

You can assess dynamic muscular endurance by measuring the maximum number of repetitions of various calisthenic exercises. Pull-up, push-up, and trunk curl (partial curl-up) tests are widely used for this purpose.

Pull-Up Tests

Pull-up tests may be used to measure the dynamic endurance of the arm and shoulder girdle muscles for individuals who are able to lift their body weight. For clients who are unable to perform even one pull-up, you can use modified pull-up and flexed-arm hang tests. Baumgartner (1978) developed a modified pull-up that uses an incline board (at a

Video 6.10

Table 6.9 Isokinetic Test Protocols

Isokinetic tests	Speed setting	Protocol	Measure
Strength	30° or 60°·sec⁻¹	Two submax practice trials followed by three maximal trials	Peak torque (ft-lb or Nm)
Endurance	120°-180°·sec⁻¹	One maximal trial	Number of repetitions until torque reaches 50% of initial torque value
Power	120°-300°·sec⁻¹	Two submax practice trials followed by three maximal trials	Peak torque (ft-lb or Nm)

ft-lb = foot-pound; Nm = newton-meter; 1 ft-lb = 0.138 Nm.

30° angle to the floor) with a pull-up bar at the top. A modified scooter board slides along garage door tracks attached to the incline board (Baumgartner et al. 1984). While lying prone on the scooter board, the client pulls up until the chin is over the pull-up bar. Detailed testing procedures, equipment designs, and performance norms for children, adolescents, and college-age women and men are available (see Baumgartner 1978; Baumgartner et al. 1984).

The flexed-arm hang test is scored as the amount of time the client maintains the flexed-arm hanging position (i.e., supporting the body weight with the chin over the pull-up bar). Traditionally, a pronated grip on the pull-up bar is used (i.e., overgrip); however, variations of the flexed-arm hang test include using a supinated grip (i.e., undergrip). Although the flexed-arm hang tests isometric endurance of the arm and shoulder girdle musculature, it has been used for more than three decades as a measure of upper body strength. One study of college women showed that flexed-arm hang time relates more to relative strength (1-RM / body mass) than to absolute strength (1-RM) or to dynamic muscle endurance (measured as repetitions to failure at 70% 1-RM) (Clemons et al. 2004).

Video 6.11

Push-Up Tests

The ACSM (2018) and Canadian Society for Exercise Physiology (CSEP; 2013) recommend using a push-up test to assess endurance of the upper body musculature. To start, clients lie prone on the mat with their legs together and hands pointing forward under the shoulders. Clients push up from the mat by fully extending the elbows and by using either the toes (for males) or the knees (for females) as the pivot point. The upper body should be kept in a straight line and the head should be kept up. The client returns to the down position, touching the chin to the mat. The stomach and thighs should not touch the mat. Clients perform as many consecutive repetitions (no rest between repetitions) as possible; there is no time limit. Repetitions not meeting the stated criteria should not be counted. Terminate the test when the client strains forcibly or is unable to maintain proper push-up technique over two consecutive repetitions; record the total number of correctly executed repetitions. Table 6.10 provides age-gender norms for the push-up test.

Trunk Curl Tests

Traditionally, abdominal muscle endurance tests (e.g., trunk curls, partial curl-ups, and sit-ups) were commonly included in health-related fitness test batteries to identify clients at risk for low back pain or injury because of weak abdominal muscles. However, the validity of these tests as measures of abdominal strength or endurance and as predictors of low back pain is questionable. Most trunk curl tests are poorly related to abdominal strength ($r_{x,y}$ = −.21-.36) and only moderately related to abdominal endurance ($r_{x,y}$ = .46-.50) (Knudson 2001; Knudson and Johnston 1995). Also, Jackson and colleagues (1998) found no relationship between sit-up test scores and incidence of low back pain. For these reasons, the current ACSM guidelines (2018) no longer include the curl-up test as a measure of muscular endurance.

Core Stability Tests

The Sahrmann Core Stability Test (Sahrmann 2002) is an excellent tool for assessing the core stability of your clients. Core stability is the ability of the trunk musculature to stabilize the spine and maintain optimal spinal alignment during movement. The transversus abdominis and multifidus are two deep-seated abdominal and spinal muscles.

Table 6.10 Age-Gender Norms for Push-Up Test

	AGE (YR)					
	15-19 yr	**20-29 yr**	**30-39 yr**	**40-49 yr**	**50-59 yr**	**60-69 yr**
MEN						
Excellent	≥39	≥36	≥30	≥25	≥21	≥18
Very good	29-38	29-35	22-29	17-24	13-20	11-17
Good	23-28	22-28	17-21	13-16	10-12	8-10
Fair	18-22	17-21	12-16	10-12	7-9	5-7
Needs improvement	≤17	≤16	≤11	≤9	≤6	≤4
WOMEN						
Excellent	≥33	≥30	≥27	≥24	≥21	≥17
Very good	25-32	21-29	20-26	15-23	11-20	12-16
Good	18-24	15-20	13-19	11-14	7-10	5-11
Fair	12-17	10-14	8-12	5-10	2-6	2-4
Needs improvement	≤11	≤9	≤7	≤4	≤1	≤1

Source: Canadian Physical Activity Training for Health (CSEP-PATH®). 2013. Used with permission of the Canadian Society for Exercise Physiology.

Weakness in these muscles may be linked to low back pain and injury.

The Sahrmann Core Stability Test (see table 6.11) may be used to assess and grade your clients' levels of core stability. The test consists of series of movements that are performed while maintaining lumbopelvic stability in a neutral position. You may use a blood pressure cuff under the client's back to determine if there is any movement of the spine by watching for pressure changes during the movement. Alternatively, you can have the client place the hands beneath the lower back to feel for any changes in pressure during the movement.

MUSCULAR POWER ASSESSMENT

A baseline measure of muscular power, followed by subsequent tests, can be used to monitor the progress of a client as well as the effectiveness of a training program for improving this muscular fitness variable. Power is the rate of work and is calculated as work divided by time. The vertical jump and standing long jump, or broad jump, are often used as field measures of muscular power, even though time is not typically measured during these assessments.

VERTICAL JUMP

Video 6.12

The vertical jump test can be performed without specialized equipment. A jumping client with colored chalk on the fingers touches a point as high as possible on a wall; use a measuring tape to determine jump height. Using a commercially available device, such as the Vertec, makes measurement easier. The Vertec resembles a volleyball standard with colored, movable horizontal plastic vanes spaced at 0.5 in. increments. For ease of rapid measurement, red vanes are spaced 6 in. apart, blue vanes are at 1 in. increments, and white vanes denote a 0.5 in. change. There are several variations of the vertical jump, such as the drop-step jump and the static jump, but the **countermovement jump (CMJ)** is the most commonly used version for assessing muscular power. The CMJ using the Vertec is explained here (see Steps for Vertical Jump Testing Using the Vertec), and norms for the CMJ are available in table 6.12.

Alternatively, a switch mat or contact mat can be used to assess vertical jump rather than the Vertec. The client simply stands on the mat and performs the CMJ as previously described, landing back on the mat. The contact mat automatically measures the flight time and the jump height based on the amount of time the client was in the air. Consequently, it is

Table 6.11 Sahrmann Core Stability Test

Level 1	Begin in supine, hook-lying position while hollowing abdomen. Slowly raise 1 leg to 100° of hip flexion with comfortable knee flexion. Bring opposite leg up to same position.
Level 2	From hip-flexed position, slowly lower 1 leg until heel contacts ground. Slide out leg to fully extend the knee. Return to starting flexed position.
Level 3	From hip-flexed position, slowly lower 1 leg until heel is 12 cm above ground. Slide out leg to fully extend the knee. Return to starting flexed position.
Level 4	From hip-flexed position, slowly lower both legs until heel contacts ground. Slide out legs to fully extend the knee. Return to starting flexed position.
Level 5	From hip-flexed position, slowly lower both legs until heels are 12 cm above ground. Slide out leg to fully extend the knee. Return to starting flexed position.

Table 6.12 Age-Gender Norms for Countermovement Vertical Jump

	15-19 yr	20-29 yr	30-39 yr	40-49 yr	50-59 yr	60-69 yr
MEN: JUMP HEIGHT (cm)						
Excellent	≥56	≥58	≥52	≥43	≥41	≥33
Very good	51-55	54-57	46-51	36-42	34-40	29-32
Good	46-50	48-53	40-45	32-35	28-33	25-28
Fair	42-45	42-47	31-39	26-31	18-27	18-24
Needs improvement	≤41	≤41	≤30	≤25	≤17	≤17
WOMEN: JUMP HEIGHT (cm)						
Excellent	≥40	≥38	≥36	≥31	≥25	≥19
Very good	36-39	34-37	32-35	27-30	21-24	15-18
Good	32-35	29-33	28-31	23-26	16-20	11-14
Fair	28-31	25-28	24-27	18-22	10-15	7-10
Needs improvement	≤27	≤24	≤23	≤17	≤9	≤6
MEN: POWER (W)						
Excellent	≥4,644	≥5,094	≥4,860	≥4,320	≥4,019	≥3,764
Very good	4,185-4,643	4,640-5,093	4,389-4,859	3,700-4,319	3,567-4,018	3,291-3,763
Good	3,858-4,184	4,297-4,639	3,967-4,388	3,242-3,699	2,937-3,566	2,843-3,290
Fair	3,323-3,857	3,775-4,296	3,485-3,966	2,708-3,241	2,512-2,936	2,383-2,842
Needs improvement	≤3,322	≤3,774	≤3,484	≤2,707	≤2,511	≤2,382
WOMEN: POWER (W)						
Excellent	≥3,167	≥3,250	≥3,193	≥2,675	≥2,559	≥2,475
Very good	2,795-3,166	2,804-3,249	2,550-3,192	2,288-2,674	2,161-2,558	1,718-2,474
Good	2,399-2,794	2,478-2,803	2,335-2,549	2,101-2,287	1,701-2,160	1,317-1,717
Fair	2,156-2,398	2,271-2,477	2,147-2,334	1,688-2,100	1,386-1,700	1,198-1,316
Needs improvement	≤2,155	≤2,270	≤2,146	≤1,687	≤1,385	≤1,197

cm = centimeters, W = watts

Data from Payne et al. 2000.

Steps for Vertical Jump Testing Using the Vertec

The following basic steps are recommended for CMJ testing.

1. The examiner adjusts the height of the movable vanes to be within the client's reach height, with the bottom vane at a known height.

2. The client stands flat-footed and reaches as high as possible with the dominant hand to push the vanes forward. This is recorded as the reach height.

3. The examiner readjusts the height of the vane stack to be within the estimated jump height of the client, again with the bottom vane at a known height.

4. Without a preparatory step or a step backward, the client performs a ballistic countermovement by quickly flexing the hips and knees and swinging the arms backward before exploding upward. During the jump, the dominant arm should reach as high as possible and swat or tap the vanes at the maximal height of reach.

5. The examiner records the height of the highest vane that was moved. This is the jump height. The client's vertical jump is the difference between the jump height and the reach height.

6. The best of three trials to the nearest 0.5 in. (each vane) is used.

---

important to instruct the jumper to avoid tucking the knees while airborne. Additionally, accelerometers, such as the Myotest previously described in the Dynamic Strength Tests section, can be used to measure vertical jump.

Researchers have compared the various technologies for measuring the CMJ. Nuzzo, Anning, and Scharfenberg (2011) compared the reliability of the Myotest, Vertec, and Just Jump, a contact mat. The best intrasession and intersession reliability occurred with the Myotest. Intrasession reliability was .91 (intraclass correlation) and .95 for females and males, respectively, and intersession reliability was .88 to .92. They noted that better jumpers tended to have greater fluctuations in jump scores across testing sessions, and this was more pronounced with the Vertec. Validity of the CMJ varies by the technology used. Leard and colleagues (2007) reported that both the Vertec ($r = .906$) and Just Jump contact mat ($r = .967$) were highly correlated with motion analysis, but the mean jump heights were significantly less for the Vertec (0.3937 m) compared with the contact mat (0.4420 m) and the motion analysis (0.4369 m). One research team reported that both the contact mat and Vertec recorded significantly lower jump heights than their criterion method of a laboratory force plate (Buckthorpe, Morris, and Folland 2012), while another research group found that the methods that rely on flight time (contact mat and accelerom-

eter) systematically record lower values than the Vertec (Magnusdottir, Porgilsson, and Karlsson 2014). In yet another comparison study, Whitmer and colleagues (2015) reported that a jump mat, but not a force plate, was in agreement with the Vertec. When taken together, these studies suggest that the CMJ is a reliable measure of muscular power, but the same testing device should be used when comparing subsequent tests against baseline measures.

Typically, the client's jump height is sufficient information for most examiners. However, prediction equations are available to convert jump height into peak power. Normative data for peak power from the CMJ are available in table 6.12. Sayers and colleagues (1999) derived the following equation to estimate peak power from a CMJ:

$$\text{peak power (W)} = 51.9 \times \text{CMJ (cm)} + 48.9 \times \text{body mass (kg)} - 2,007$$

Unfortunately, there is considerable variability in this equation ($R^2 = .78$; $SEE = 561.5$ W). Consequently, the researchers recommend using a static jump with a pause at the bottom of the bent-knee position before jumping, as this reduces the variability observed in CMJ. The static jump equation has less variability ($R^2 = .88$; $SEE = 372.9$ W) and is as follows:

$$\text{peak power (W)} = 60.7 \times \text{static jump (cm)} + 45.3 \times \text{body mass (kg)} - 2,055$$

STANDING LONG JUMP

An alternative power test to the vertical jump is the standing long jump. For this test, the client places both feet behind a taped line. Without any preparatory steps or drop-steps, the client swings the arms backward and then propels himself forward, jumping horizontally as far as possible. The client must stick the landing; the trial is discarded if the client falls forward. The jump distance is measured from the starting line to the back of the heel of the foot that landed closest to the starting line. The best of three trials is used. The standing long jump is moderately correlated with other power tests, such as the vertical jump and peak torque knee extension, as well as track and field performances in the sprint and jumping events (Almuzaini and Fleck 2008).

SOURCES OF MEASUREMENT ERROR IN MUSCULAR FITNESS TESTING

The validity and reliability of strength, muscular endurance, and power measures are affected by client factors, equipment, technician skill, and environmental factors. You must control each of these factors to ensure the accuracy and precision of muscular fitness scores.

CLIENT FACTORS

Before measuring a client's strength, muscular endurance, or power, familiarize the individual with the equipment and testing procedures. Clients with limited or no prior weightlifting experience need time to practice each lift to control for the effects of learning on performance. You should give even experienced weightlifters time to practice so you can correct any improper lifting techniques prior to testing.

Muscular fitness tests require clients to give a maximal effort. Therefore, clients should get adequate sleep before performing these tests, and you should restrict the use of drugs and medications that may adversely affect their performance. It is also important that you motivate your clients during testing by encouraging them to do their best

and giving them positive feedback after each trial. Adequate rest between trials is necessary in order for clients to obtain scores that truly represent their maximal effort.

EQUIPMENT

The design of testing equipment may also affect test scores. Most of the dynamic strength and muscular endurance protocols and norms presented in this chapter were developed using constant-resistance exercise machines. Therefore, you should not use free weights or variable-resistance machines when administering these tests. It is also important to calibrate the equipment and make sure it is in proper working condition prior to testing. Inspection and maintenance of equipment will increase accuracy and decrease risk of accidents. When selecting exercise machines, make sure the equipment can be properly adjusted to accommodate varying limb lengths and body sizes. Use equipment specifically designed for smaller individuals when testing children and smaller adults.

TECHNICIAN SKILL

All strength testing should be done by qualified, trained technicians who are knowledgeable about proper lifting and spotting techniques and familiar with standardized testing procedures. Explain and demonstrate the proper lifting technique and then correct any performance errors you see as the client practices. During the test, clients may inadvertently cheat by moving extraneous body parts to help lift the weight. Carefully observe the client during the test, focusing on the grip used and the starting position. The type of grip (pronated vs. supinated) has a substantial effect on performance. For example, using a narrow grip instead of a wide grip during a lat pull-down exercise increases the amount of weight that can be lifted. Likewise, the client will be able to produce more force during an arm curl using a supinated grip compared with a pronated grip.

The client's starting position may also affect strength scores. During the bench press, for example, eccentric movement (i.e., lowering the weight) prior to the concentric phase of the lift will increase maximal muscular force because of the stretch reflex and the tendency for the client to bounce the weight off the chest. To obtain accurate assessments of the client's strength, it is important to standardize starting positions and to follow all testing procedures carefully.

ENVIRONMENTAL FACTORS

Factors such as room temperature and humidity may affect test scores. The room temperature should be 70 to 74 °F (21 to 23 °C) to maximize subject comfort during testing. Ideally, you want a quiet, clean environment with limited distractions (not an overcrowded weight room, for example). When assessing improvements due to training, remember to pretest and posttest your clients at the same time of day to control for diurnal variations in strength.

ADDITIONAL CONSIDERATIONS FOR MUSCULAR FITNESS TESTING

This section addresses a number of additional factors and questions regarding the testing and evaluation of muscular fitness.

How can I estimate my clients' 1-RM?

Although 1-RM tests can be safely administered to clients of all ages, sometimes it is preferable to estimate the 1-RM. One-repetition maximum testing can be time consuming, especially for a large group of clients. Some clients may take 15 min to complete a 1-RM test (multiple attempts and rests). Also, the 1-RM may be underestimated for clients with little or no exercise experience because they are unaccustomed to or may be apprehensive about lifting heavy loads. In these cases, it may be more suitable and practical to estimate 1-RM.

You can estimate the 1-RM of your clients from submaximal muscle endurance tests. Research demonstrates a strong relationship between muscle endurance (measured as the number of repetitions to fatigue) and the percentage of 1-RM lifted (Brzycki 1993). Muscular strength (1-RM) therefore can be predicted from muscular endurance tests with a fair degree of accuracy (Ball and Rose 1991; Braith et al. 1993; Desgorces et al. 2010; Invergo, Ball, and

Looney 1991; Kuramoto and Payne 1995; Mayhew et al. 1992). The most frequently used prediction equations assume an inverse linear relationship between the %1-RM and number of repetitions performed, and they are typically based on the number of repetitions to fatigue in one set. For example, the Brzycki (1993) equation can be used to estimate 1-RM of men. This equation can be used for any combination of submaximal weights and repetitions to fatigue providing the repetitions to fatigue do not exceed 10.

$$1\text{-RM} = \text{weight lifted (lb)} / [1.0278 - (\text{reps to fatigue} \times 0.0278)]$$

For example, if your client completes seven repetitions to fatigue during a bench press exercise using a 100 lb (45 kg) barbell, the estimated 1-RM is calculated as follows:

$$1\text{-RM} = 100 \text{ lb} / [1.0278 - (7 \text{ reps} \times 0.0278)]$$
$$= 120 \text{ lb (54.5 kg)}$$

Brzycki (2000) also suggested using a prediction equation based on the number of repetitions to fatigue obtained in two submaximal sets to estimate 1-RM. Any two submaximal sets can be used as long as the number of reps to fatigue does not exceed 10. For example, you can determine the client's 5-RM value, or the maximum weight that can be lifted for 5 reps (e.g., 120 lb [55 kg] for 5 reps), and the 10-RM value (e.g., 80 lb [36 kg] for 10 reps) and use them in the following equation:

$$\text{predicted 1-RM} = [(SM_1 - SM_2) / (REP_2 - REP_1)] \times (REP_1 - 1) + SM_1$$
$$= [(120 - 80) / (10 - 5)] \times (5 - 1) + 120$$
$$= 152 \text{ lb}$$

In this equation, SM_1 and REP_1 represent the heavier submaximal weight (120 lb) and the respective number of repetitions (5) completed, and SM_2 and REP_2 correspond to the lighter submaximal weight (80 lb) and the respective number of repetitions (10) performed.

Alternatively, you can use the average number of repetitions corresponding to various percentages of 1-RM (see table 6.13). This technique and the Brzycki (1993) equation yield similar 1-RM estimates for lifts between 2-RM and 10-RM. To estimate

Table 6.13 Average Number of Repetitions and %1-RM Values

Repetitions	%1-RM*
1	100
2	95
3	93
4	90
5	87
6	85
7	83
8	80
9	77
10	75
12	70
14	65
15-20	60

*These values may vary slightly for different muscle groups and ages.

Adapted by permission from J.M. Sheppard and N.T. Triplett, Program Design for Resistance Training. In *Essentials of Strength Training and Conditioning,* 4th ed., edited by G.G. Haff and N.T. Triplett for the National Strength and Conditioning Association (Champaign, IL: Human Kinetics, 2016), 452.

the 1-RM from 2-RM to 10-RM values, divide the weight lifted by the respective %1-RM, expressed as a decimal (%1-RM / 100). For example, a client lifting 100 lb (45.4 kg) for 8 repetitions would have an estimated 1-RM of 125 lb (56.7 kg):

$$1\text{-RM} = 100 \text{ lb} / 0.80 \text{ or } 125 \text{ lb } (56.7 \text{ kg})$$

Also, gender-specific prediction equations can be used to estimate upper body strength (i.e., the 1-RM bench press) from the YMCA bench press test (see table 6.7) in younger clients (22-36 yr) (Kim, Mayhew, and Peterson 2002):

For Men

$$\text{predicted 1-RM (kg)} = (1.55 \times \text{YMCA test repetitions}) + 37.9$$

$$r = .87; SEE = 8.0 \text{ kg}$$

For Women

$$\text{predicted 1-RM (kg)} = (0.31 \times \text{YMCA test repetitions}) + 19.2$$

$$r = .87; SEE = 3.2 \text{ kg}$$

For example, if a 25 yr old female's YMCA bench press test score is 30 reps, her estimated 1-RM bench press strength is calculated as follows:

$$\text{predicted 1-RM (kg)} = (0.31 \times 30 \text{ reps}) + 19.2$$

$$= 28.5 \text{ kg } (62.8 \text{ lb})$$

Additionally, Desgorces and colleagues (2010) developed equations to predict %1-RM from the number of repetitions to failure for bench press exercise. They noted that predictive accuracy was improved using a model based on a nonlinear relationship (curve fitting two-function exponential decay) between %1-RM values and number of repetitions to failure, with a reduced number of repetitions (1-12 reps), performed at relatively high intensities (75%-85% 1-RM), yielding the best prediction. They developed two specific %1-RM prediction equations for male athletes—one for high-strength athletes (powerlifters and racquetball players) and another for high-endurance athletes (swimmers and rowers). A third equation based on the total population combined was also developed ($r^2 = .97$; $SEE = 3.4$).

$$\%1\text{-RM} = 79.3412^{\exp(-0.0302 \times \text{reps to failure})} + 20.7706$$

$$r = .98 \text{ and } SEE = 3.4 \text{ % 1-RM}$$

Mayhew and colleagues (2011) reported that the Desgorces prediction equation accurately (<5% error) predicted strength changes (%1-RM bench press) of untrained men and women following a 12 wk periodization resistance training program.

How is muscle balance assessed?

Muscle strength is important for joint stability; however, a strength imbalance between opposing muscle groups (e.g., quadriceps femoris and hamstrings) may compromise joint stability and increase the risk of musculoskeletal injury. For this reason, experts recommend maintaining a balance in strength between agonist and antagonist muscle groups.

Muscle balance ratios differ among muscle groups and are affected by the force-velocity of muscle groups at specific joints. To control limb velocity during muscle balance testing, you will do best to use isokinetic dynamometers. In field settings, however, you may obtain a crude index of muscle balance by comparing 1-RM values of muscle groups. Based on isokinetic tests of peak torque production at slow speeds ($30°$-$60°$·sec^{-1}), the muscle balance ratios shown in table 6.14 are recommended for agonist and antagonist muscle groups.

Muscle balance between other pairs of muscle groups is also important. The difference in strength between contralateral (right vs. left sides) muscle groups should be no more than 15%, and the strength-to-body-mass (BM) ratio of the upper body (bench press 1-RM / BM) should be at least 40% of lower body relative strength (leg press 1-RM / BM). If you detect imbalances, prescribe additional exercises for the weaker muscle groups.

Can strength or muscular endurance be assessed by a single test?

Strength and endurance are specific to the muscle group, the type of muscular contraction (static or dynamic), the speed of muscular contraction (slow or fast), and the joint angle being tested (static contraction). There is no single test to evaluate total body muscle strength or endurance. Minimally, the strength test battery should include a measure of abdominal, lower extremity, and upper extremity strength. In addition, if the individual trains dynamically, select a dynamic, not static, test to assess strength or endurance levels before and after training.

You should also use caution in selecting test items to measure muscle strength. The maximum number of sit-ups, pull-ups, or push-ups that an individual can perform measures muscular endurance, yet maximum-repetition tests have been included in some strength test batteries. This may lead to misinterpretation of the test results.

Should absolute or relative measures be used to classify a client's muscle strength?

A direct relationship exists between body size and muscle strength. Generally, larger individuals have more muscle mass, and therefore greater strength, than smaller individuals with less muscle mass.

Because strength directly relates to the body mass and lean body mass of the individual, you should express the test results in relative terms (e.g., 1-RM / BM). This is especially true in comparing a client's score to group norms and in comparing groups or individuals differing in body size and composition (e.g., men vs. women or older vs. younger adults).

Use relative strength scores for assessing individual improvement from training. As a result of resistance training, some individuals may gain body

Table 6.14 Muscle Balance Ratios

Muscle groups	Muscle balance ratio
Hip extensors and flexors	1:1
Elbow extensors and flexors	1:1
Trunk extensors and flexors	1:1
Ankle inverters and evertors	1:1
Shoulder flexors and extensors	2:3
Knee extensors and flexors	3:2
Shoulder internal and external rotators	3:2
Ankle plantar flexors and dorsiflexors	3:1

weight while others may lose weight, especially if they are using resistance training as part of a program for weight gain or loss. If you compare the client's relative strength scores (from pre- and posttest training), you will be able to evaluate the change in strength that is independent of a change in body weight.

How can the influence of strength on muscular endurance be controlled?

Performance on some endurance tests (e.g., pull-ups and push-ups) is highly dependent on the strength of the individual. It is recommended that you use relative endurance tests that are proportional to the individual's body mass or maximum strength to assess muscle endurance. You cannot use a pull-up test to assess muscular endurance if the individual is not strong enough to lift the body weight for one repetition of that exercise. Therefore, select a modified or submaximal (percentage of body weight) endurance test.

Are there comprehensive norms that can be used to classify muscular fitness levels of diverse population subgroups?

Strength norms for women (20-82 yr) were developed for the bench press (1-RM), leg press (1-RM), static grip strength, and push-up tests (Brown and Miller 1998). These norms are based on data obtained from 304 independent-living women attending wellness classes at a university medical center. However, there is a lack of up-to-date endurance norms for men and strength and endurance norms for older men. New norms need to be established for this population in particular.

MUSCULAR FITNESS TESTING OF OLDER ADULTS

It is important to accurately assess the muscular fitness of older individuals. Adequate strength in the upper and lower body lessens risk of falls and of injuries associated with falling, reduces age-related loss of bone mineral, maintains lean body tissue, improves glucose utilization, and prevents obesity. Moderate to high levels of muscular strength enable older adults to maintain their functional independence and to perform activities of daily living as well as fitness and recreational activities. This section addresses tests you can use to assess the muscular strength and physical performance of older clients.

STRENGTH TESTING OF OLDER ADULTS

Experts agree that it is safe to administer 1-RM tests to older adults if proper procedures (see Steps for 1-RM Maximum Testing earlier in the chapter) are followed (Shaw, McCully, and Posner 1995). The risk of injury is low, with only 2.4% of older adults (55-80 yr) experiencing an injury during 1-RM assessment (Salem, Wang, and Sigward 2002; Shaw, McCully, and Posner 1995). Salem and colleagues (2002) suggested that at least one pretesting session (i.e., a practice 1-RM test session) is necessary to establish stable baseline 1-RM values for older adults.

Alternatively, you can estimate the 1-RM of older clients from submaximal muscular endurance tests. Kuramoto and Payne (1995) developed prediction equations to estimate 1-RM from a submaximal endurance test in middle-aged and older women. For this endurance protocol, the client completes as many repetitions as possible using a weight equivalent to 45% of her body mass. To estimate 1-RM, use the following equations:

Middle-Aged Women (40-50 yr)

$$1\text{-RM} = (1.06 \times \text{weight lifted in kg}) + (0.58 \times \text{reps}) - (0.20 \times \text{age}) - 3.41$$

$$r = .94; SEE = 1.85 \text{ kg}$$

Older Women (60-70 yr)

$$1\text{-RM} = (0.92 \times \text{weight lifted in kg}) + (0.79 \times \text{reps}) - 3.73$$

$$r = .90; SEE = 2.04 \text{ kg}$$

Knutzen, Brilla, and Caine (1999) tested the validity of selected 1-RM prediction equations for older women (mean age = 69 yr) and men (mean age = 73 yr). On average, these prediction equations underestimated the actual 1-RM for 11 different constant-resistance machine exercises. For exercises such as the biceps curl, the lateral row, the bench press, and ankle plantar and dorsiflexion, the predicted values were on average 0.5 to 3.0 kg less than the actual 1-RM values. However, larger differences (as much as a 10 kg underestimation) were noted for the triceps press-down, the supine leg press, and the hip flexion, extension, abduction, and adduction exercises. The Brzycki (1993) equation gave a closer estimate of actual 1-RMs for hip exercises (extension, flexion, adduction, and abduction) than the other equations evaluated; the Wathen (1994) equation, $1\text{-RM} = 100 \times \text{weight lifted} / [48.8 + 53.8^{-0.075 \text{ (reps)}}]$, most closely estimates 1-RM for all upper body exercises, the leg press, and dorsiflexion exercises. The authors concluded that the actual and predicted 1-RM are close enough to warrant using these prediction equations to determine resistance training intensities (i.e., %1-RMs) for older adults. In addition, given that the predicted 1-RM values were consistently less than the actual 1-RM values, the resistance training intensity will not likely exceed the prescribed value.

FUNCTIONAL FITNESS TESTING OF OLDER ADULTS

Functional fitness is the ability to perform everyday activities safely and independently without undue fatigue (Rikli and Jones 2013). Functional fitness is multidimensional, requiring aerobic endurance, flexibility, balance, agility, and muscular strength. Older individuals with moderate to high functional fitness have the ability to perform normal **activities of daily living (ADLs)** such as getting out of a chair or car, climbing stairs, shopping, dressing, and bathing; these individuals are able to stay strong, active, and independent as they age.

The Senior Fitness Test (Rikli and Jones 2013) assesses the physical capacity and functional fitness of older adults (60-94 yr). This test battery includes two measures of muscular strength: (1) an arm (biceps) curl for upper body strength (figure 6.7) and (2) a 30 sec chair stand for lower body strength (figure 6.8). The ACSM (2018) recommends using these two test items to safely assess the muscular fitness of most older adults.

ARM CURL TEST

Purpose: Assess upper body strength.

Application: Measure ability to perform ADLs such as lifting and carrying groceries, grandchildren, and pets.

Equipment: You will need a folding or straight-back chair, a stopwatch, and a 5 lb (2.27 kg) dumbbell for women or an 8 lb (3.63 kg) dumbbell for men.

Test procedures: The client sits in the chair with the back straight and the feet flat on the floor. The client holds the dumbbell in the dominant hand using a neutral (handshake) grip and lets this arm hang down at the side (see figure 6.7). For each repetition, the client curls the weight by fully flexing the elbow while supinating the forearm and returns the weight to the starting position by fully extending the elbow and pronating the forearm. Instruct your client to keep the upper arm in contact with the trunk during the test. Have your client perform as many repetitions as possible in 30 sec. Administer one trial.

Scoring: Count the number of repetitions executed in 30 sec. If the forearm is more than halfway up when the time expires, count the move as a complete repetition. Use table 6.15 to determine your client's percentile ranking.

Safety tips: Before testing, demonstrate the exercise for your client. Have your client perform one or two repetitions of the exercise without a dumbbell to check body position and lifting technique. Stop the test if the client complains of pain.

Validity and reliability: Arm curl test scores were moderately related ($r_{x,y}$ = .84 for men and .79 for women) to combined 1-RM values for the chest, upper back, and biceps (criterion-related validity). Average arm curl test scores of physically active older adults were significantly greater than those of sedentary older adults (construct validity). Test-retest reliability was .81.

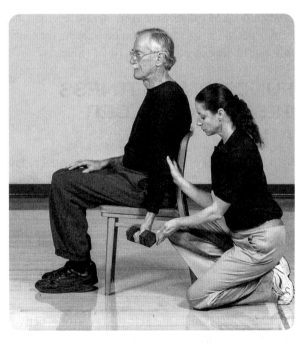 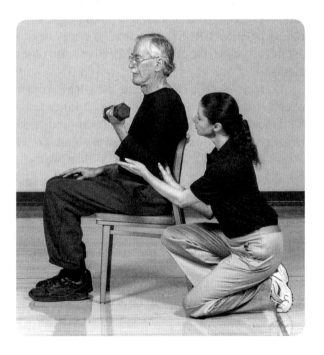

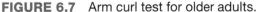

FIGURE 6.7 Arm curl test for older adults.

Table 6.15   Arm Curl Test Norms for Older Adults

Percentile rank	60-64 YR F	60-64 YR M	65-69 YR F	65-69 YR M	70-74 YR F	70-74 YR M	75-79 YR F	75-79 YR M	80-84 YR F	80-84 YR M	85-89 YR F	85-89 YR M	90-94 YR F	90-94 YR M
95	24	27	22	27	22	26	21	24	20	23	18	21	17	18
90	22	25	21	25	20	24	20	22	18	22	17	19	16	16
85	21	24	20	24	19	23	19	21	17	20	16	18	15	16
80	20	23	19	23	18	22	18	20	16	20	15	17	14	15
75	19	22	18	21	17	21	17	19	16	19	15	17	13	14
70	18	21	17	21	17	20	16	19	15	18	14	16	13	14
65	18	21	17	20	16	19	16	18	15	18	14	15	12	13
60	17	20	16	20	16	19	15	17	14	17	13	15	12	13
55	17	20	16	19	15	18	15	17	14	17	13	14	11	12
50	16	19	15	18	14	17	14	16	13	16	12	14	11	12
45	16	18	15	18	14	17	13	16	12	15	12	13	10	12
40	15	18	14	17	13	16	13	15	12	15	11	13	10	11
35	14	17	14	16	13	15	12	14	11	14	11	12	9	11
30	14	17	13	16	12	15	12	14	11	14	10	11	9	10
25	13	16	12	15	12	14	11	13	10	13	10	11	8	10
20	12	15	12	14	11	13	10	12	10	12	9	10	8	9
15	11	14	11	13	10	12	9	11	9	12	8	9	7	8
10	10	13	10	12	9	11	8	10	8	10	7	8	6	8
5	9	11	8	10	8	9	7	9	6	9	6	7	5	6

F = females; M = males.

Note: Values represent number of repetitions in 30 sec.

Adapted by permission from R. Rikli and C. Jones, *Senior Fitness Test Manual,* 2nd ed. (Champaign, IL: Human Kinetics, 2013), 155.

30 SEC CHAIR STAND TEST

Purpose: Assess lower body strength.

Application: Measure ability to perform ADLs such as climbing stairs, walking, and getting out of a chair, bathtub, or car.

Equipment: You will need a folding or straight-back chair (seat height = 17 in. or 43 cm) and a stopwatch.

Test procedures: Place the chair against a wall to prevent slipping. Instruct your client to sit erect in the chair with the feet flat on the floor and the arms crossed at the wrists and held against the chest (see figure 6.8). For each repetition, the client rises to a full stand and then returns to the fully seated starting position. Have your

client perform as many repetitions as possible in 30 sec. Administer one trial.

Scoring: Count the number of repetitions executed in 30 sec. If the client is more than half-way up when the time expires, count the move as a full stand. Use table 6.16 to determine the client's percentile ranking.

Safety tips: Brace the chair against a wall, watch for balance problems, and stop the test if the client complains of pain. Before testing, demonstrate the movement slowly to show proper form. Have your client perform one or two repetitions to check body position (fully standing and fully seated) for the test.

Validity and reliability: Scores for the chair stand test were moderately related to the 1-RM leg press (criterion-related validity) in older men ($r_{x,y}$ = .78) and women ($r_{x,y}$ = .71). Average

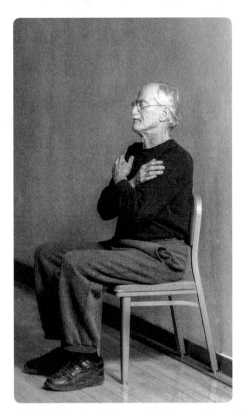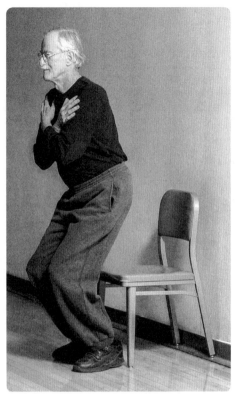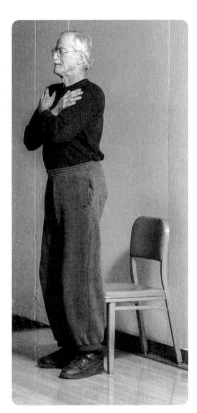

FIGURE 6.8 30 sec chair stand test for older adults

Table 6.16 30 Sec Chair Stand Test Norms for Older Adults

Percentile rank	60-64 YR		65-69 YR		70-74 YR		75-79 YR		80-84 YR		85-89 YR		90-94 YR	
	F	M	F	M	F	M	F	M	F	M	F	M	F	M
95	21	23	19	23	19	21	19	21	18	19	17	19	16	16
90	20	22	18	21	18	20	17	20	17	17	15	17	15	15
85	19	21	17	20	17	19	16	18	16	16	14	16	13	14
80	18	20	16	19	16	18	16	18	15	16	14	15	12	13
75	17	19	16	18	15	17	15	17	14	15	13	14	11	12
70	17	19	15	18	15	17	14	16	13	14	12	13	11	12
65	16	18	15	17	14	16	14	16	13	14	12	13	10	11
60	16	17	14	16	14	16	13	15	12	13	11	12	9	11
55	15	17	14	16	13	15	13	15	12	13	11	12	9	10
50	15	16	14	15	13	14	12	14	11	12	10	11	8	10
45	14	16	13	15	12	14	12	13	11	12	10	11	7	9
40	14	15	13	14	12	13	12	13	10	11	9	10	7	9
35	13	15	12	13	11	13	11	12	10	11	9	9	6	8
30	12	14	12	13	11	12	11	12	9	10	8	9	5	8
25	12	14	11	12	10	11	10	11	9	10	8	8	4	7
20	11	13	11	11	10	11	9	10	8	9	7	7	4	7
15	10	12	10	11	9	10	9	10	7	8	6	6	3	6
10	9	11	9	9	8	9	8	8	6	7	5	5	1	5
5	8	9	8	8	7	8	6	7	4	6	4	4	0	3

F = females; M = males.

Note: Values represent number of repetitions.

Adapted by permission from R. Rikli and C. Jones, *Senior Fitness Test Manual*, 2nd ed. (Champaign, IL: Human Kinetics, 2013), 155.

scores were lower for older adults (80+ yr) than for relatively younger adults (60-69 yr) and higher for physically active older adults compared with sedentary older adults (construct validity). Test-retest reliability was .86 and .92 for older men and women, respectively.

LOWER BODY POWER TEST

Purpose: Assess lower body power.

Application: Muscular power declines at a faster rate than muscular strength and endurance, and power is a stronger predictor of impaired mobility and functional limitations than these other muscle fitness variables (Reid and Fielding 2012). Having more power may help prevent slip-related falls (Han and Yang 2015).

Equipment: You will need a Tendo (described in Dynamic Strength Tests section earlier in the chapter), a belt, a folding or straight-back chair, and a scale to measure body mass.

Test procedures: Measure the client's body mass. Attach the Tendo to the client's waist with the belt. Place the chair against the wall to prevent slipping, and have the client sit in the chair with arms crossed over the chest. Similar to the 30 sec chair stand test, have the client rise to a full standing position, but this time do only one repetition as quickly as possible. The client completes at least three repetitions, with complete recovery (60 sec) between each effort.

Scoring: Power is assessed from the Tendo unit from the vertical velocity (m·sec^{-1}) and the mass moved (kg). Record the best trial.

Safety tips: Brace the chair against a wall, watch for balance problems, and stop the test if the client complains of pain. Before testing, demonstrate the movement slowly to show proper form. Have your client perform one or two repetitions to check body position (fully standing and fully seated) for the test.

Validity and reliability: Norms have not yet been established. However, Gray and Paulson (2014) administered this test to 20 older adults (>65 yr). Relative power measured by Tendo (5.34 ± 1.67 W·kg^{-1}) was similar to power obtained by measuring changes in center of mass from motion analysis (5.39 ± 1.73 W·kg^{-1}), and the two measures were strongly correlated ($r = .76$). Cronbach's alpha for 10 repeated trials was .98, suggesting excellent reliability.

MUSCULAR FITNESS TESTING OF CHILDREN

In the past, experts questioned whether or not it was safe to use 1-RM tests to evaluate children. A major concern was the risk of growth plate fractures when the children attempted to lift heavy weights. Experts now agree it is safe to administer 1-RM tests to children (6-12 yr) if appropriate procedures are followed (Faigenbaum, Milliken, and Westcott 2003).

Results from 1-RM tests may be used to establish baselines for evaluating the progress of children in resistance training programs. You can also use these values to plan a personalized resistance training program for each child, to identify muscle imbalances, and to provide motivation. One shortcoming of 1-RM testing is that it must be closely supervised (one on one) to ensure safety, which limits its usefulness in physical education classes and youth sport programs. Also, child-sized exercise machines must be used; the safety of 1-RM testing using other modes (e.g., dumbbells or barbells) has not been adequately established.

Generally speaking, the same tests described in this chapter for assessing the muscular strength, endurance, and power of adults can be applied to youth, albeit with some modifications and norms that are age appropriate. In a study that assessed the power, speed, and agility of athletic preadolescent youth, Jones and Lorenzo (2013) suggested a test battery that included vertical jump, standing long jump, proagility shuttle run, and 20 yd sprint. In another study that compared a variety of field-based muscular fitness tests against the criterion measure of isokinetic strength in 126 adolescents (14.4 ± 1.7 yr), Artero, España-Romero, et al. (2012) determined that handgrip strength and standing long jump had the highest associations to the criterion measure. For standing long jump norms for youth (10-18 yr), see Saint-Maurice and colleagues (2015) and Catley and Tomkinson (2013).

1-RM TESTING GUIDELINES FOR CHILDREN

The following steps are recommended for 1-RM testing of children (Faigenbaum, Milliken, and Westcott 2003):

1. Have a certified, experienced exercise professional administer and closely supervise (one on one) all tests.

2. Before testing, familiarize the child with proper lifting techniques (i.e., proper breathing and controlled movements), allow him to practice these techniques, and answer any questions he may have.

3. Have the child warm up by performing 10 min of low- to moderate-intensity aerobic exercise and stretching.

4. Use dynamic, constant-resistance exercise machines designed specifically for children or individuals with small body frames.

5. Before the 1-RM lift, instruct the child to perform six repetitions with a relatively light load followed by three repetitions with a heavier load. Then gradually increase the weight and have the child attempt the 1-RM lift. Allow at least 2 min of rest between the series of single repetitions with increasing loads. Follow this procedure until the child fails to complete the full ROM of the exercise for at least two attempts. The 1-RM is typically achieved within 7 to 11 trials.

6. Record the 1-RM as the maximum weight lifted for the last successful trial.

7. After testing, have the child stretch the exercised muscle groups for 5 min.

Key Points

▶ Strength is the ability of a muscle group to exert maximal contractile force against a resistance in a single contraction.

▶ Muscular endurance is the ability of a muscle group to exert submaximal force for an extended duration.

▶ Muscular power is the ability of a muscle group to exert force rapidly.

▶ Both strength and muscular endurance are specific to the muscle group and to the type of muscle action—static, concentric, eccentric, or isokinetic.

▶ The greatest resistance that can be used during dynamic, concentric muscle action with a constant-resistance exercise mode is equal to the maximum weight that can be moved at the weakest point in the ROM.

▶ Dynamometers are used to measure static strength and endurance.

▶ Constant-resistance modes of exercise (free weights and exercise machines) are used to assess dynamic (i.e., concentric and eccentric) strength and endurance.

▶ The accommodating-resistance mode of exercise is used to assess isokinetic strength, endurance, and power.

▶ Free-motion machines allow muscle groups to be exercised in multiple planes.

▶ Calisthenic-type exercise tests provide a crude index of strength and endurance but can be used when other equipment is not available.

▶ Strength should be expressed relative to the body mass or lean body mass of the individual.

▶ Muscular endurance tests should take into account the body mass or maximal strength of the individual.

▶ The countermovement vertical jump test is a commonly used field method to assess muscular power.

▶ Test batteries should include a minimum of three items that measure upper body, lower body, and abdominal strength or endurance.

▶ It is important to follow standardized testing procedures and to control extraneous variables (e.g., motivation level, time of testing, isolation of body parts, and joint angles) when assessing strength, muscular endurance, and power.

▶ It is safe to give 1-RM strength tests to children and older adults if appropriate testing procedures are followed.

▶ Although strength can be predicted from submaximal endurance tests, 1-RM assessments are preferable.

▶ Use the arm curl test and the 30 sec chair stand test to assess the functional strength of older clients.

Key Terms

Learn the definition of each of the following key terms. Definitions of terms can be found in the glossary.

accommodating-resistance exercise

activities of daily living (ADLs)

auxotonic muscle action

concentric muscle action

constant-resistance exercise

countermovement jump (CMJ)

dynamic muscle action

eccentric muscle action

free-motion machines

functional fitness

isokinetic muscle action

isometric muscle action

isotonic muscle action

maximum voluntary contraction (MVC)

muscular endurance

muscular power

muscular strength

one-repetition maximum (1-RM)

relative strength

static muscle action

variable-resistance exercise

Review Questions

In addition to being able to define each of the key terms, test your knowledge and understanding of the material by answering the following review questions.

1. During dynamic movement, why does muscle force production fluctuate throughout the ROM?

2. Name two methods for assessing static strength and muscular endurance.

3. How do constant-resistance, variable-resistance, accommodating-resistance, and free-motion exercise machines differ?

4. Why are strength test scores typically expressed relative to the client's body mass?

5. Describe the recommended procedures for administering 1-RM strength tests.

6. Describe the recommended procedures for administering the vertical jump test.

7. Identify three sources of measurement error for muscular fitness testing. What can you do to control these potential errors?

8. Is it safe to give 1-RM tests to children and older adults?

9. Describe two tests that can be used to assess the functional strength of older adults.

10. Why is it important to assess muscle balance?

11. In terms of the specificity principle, explain why a single test cannot be used to adequately assess your clients' overall strength. Minimally, what muscle groups should be tested to evaluate overall strength?

12. Identify the test items recommended by ACSM for assessing your clients' upper and lower body strength.

13. For certain clients, you may choose not to administer 1-RM strength tests. Describe how you could obtain an estimate of their strength instead.

CHAPTER 7

Designing Resistance Training Programs

KEY QUESTIONS

▶ How do training principles specifically apply to the design of resistance training programs?

▶ How are resistance training programs modified to optimize the development of strength, muscular endurance, muscle power, or muscle size?

▶ What factors do I need to consider when designing individualized exercise prescriptions?

▶ Is resistance training recommended for children, adolescents, and older adults?

▶ What methods can be used to design advanced resistance training programs?

▶ What are the outcomes and health benefits derived from resistance training?

▶ What is the cause of delayed-onset muscle soreness, and can it be prevented?

Muscular strength and endurance are important for the overall health and physical fitness of your clients, enabling them to engage in physically active leisure-time pursuits, to perform activities of daily living more easily, and to maintain functional independence later in life. Resistance training is a systematic program of exercise for development of the muscular system. Although the primary outcome of resistance training is improved strength and muscular endurance, a number of health benefits are also derived from this form of exercise. Resistance exercise builds bone mass, thereby counteracting the loss of bone mineral (osteoporosis) and risk of falls as one ages. This form of training also lowers blood pressure in hypertensive individuals, reduces body fat levels, and may prevent the development of low back syndrome.

Moderate-intensity aerobic exercise receives most of the attention for lowering the risk of all-cause mortality (see chapter 1), but some public health professionals are promoting a paradigm shift to higher-intensity activity with a greater emphasis on resistance training (Steele et al. 2017).

Although resistance training has long been widely used by bodybuilders, powerlifters, and competitive athletes to develop strength and muscle size, participation in weightlifting by individuals of all ages and levels of athletic interest has increased dramatically over the past 30 yr. The popularity and widespread appeal of weightlifting exercise for general muscle conditioning gives exercise specialists and personal trainers the challenge of developing resistance training programs that can meet the diverse needs of their clients.

This chapter shows you how to apply basic training principles (see chapter 3) to the design of resistance training programs for novice, intermediate, and advanced weightlifters. The chapter also presents guidelines for developing muscle strength, muscle endurance, muscle size, and muscle power. The chapter addresses various models of periodization, functional training exercise progressions, and guidelines for youth resistance training.

TYPES OF RESISTANCE TRAINING

Muscular fitness can be improved using various types of resistance training—isometric (static), dynamic (concentric and eccentric), and isokinetic. Although there are general guidelines for designing isometric, dynamic, and isokinetic resistance training programs, each exercise prescription should be individualized to meet the specific needs and goals of your clients.

ISOMETRIC TRAINING

In 1953, Hettinger and Muller reported that people produce significant gains in isometric strength (5% per week) by holding one 6 sec contraction at two-thirds of maximum intensity, 5 days/wk. This type of training became popular in the late 1950s and early 1960s because the exercises could be performed anywhere and at any time with little or no equipment. A major disadvantage is that strength gains are specific to the joint angle used during training. Thus, to increase strength throughout the range of motion, the exercise needs to be performed at a number of different joint angles (e.g., 30°, 60°, 90°, 120°, and 180° of knee flexion).

Isometric exercise is widely used in rehabilitation programs to counteract strength loss and muscle atrophy, especially in cases in which the limb is temporarily immobilized. This type of training, however, is contraindicated for coronary-prone and hypertensive individuals because the static contraction may produce large increases in intrathoracic pressure. This reduces the venous return to the heart, increases the work of the heart, and causes a substantial rise in blood pressure.

After further research, Hettinger and Muller modified their original exercise prescription. Table 7.1 presents the general guidelines for designing training programs for isometric strength and endurance development. For descriptions and illustrations of isometric exercises for various muscle groups, see appendix C.3.

DYNAMIC RESISTANCE TRAINING

Dynamic resistance training is suitable for developing muscular fitness of men and women of all ages, as well as children. This type of resistance training involves concentric and eccentric actions of the muscle group performed against a constant or variable resistance. Typically, free weights (barbells and dumbbells) and constant- or variable-resistance machines are used for resistance training.

Several important concepts used to prescribe dynamic resistance training programs are intensity, repetitions, sets, training volume, and order of exercises (Fleck and Kraemer 2014). Intensity is expressed either as a percentage of the individual's one-repetition maximum (%1-RM) or as the **repetition maximum (RM)**, which is the maximum weight the person can lift for a given number of repetitions of an exercise (e.g., 8-RM equals the maximum weight the person can lift for 8 repetitions). For the number of repetitions (1-15) corresponding to various percentages of 1-RM (60%-100%), see table 6.15.

Intensity is inversely related to repetitions. In other words, individuals are able to perform more **repetitions** using lighter resistance or weights and fewer repetitions using heavier resistance. A **set** consists of a given number of consecutive repetitions of the exercise. **Training volume** is the total amount of weight lifted during the workout and is calculated by summing the products of the weight lifted, repetitions, and sets for each exercise.

The optimal training stimulus for developing muscular strength or endurance is controversial. Some research supports the conventional prescription of **high-intensity–low-repetition** resistance exercise for strength development and **low-intensity–high-repetition** exercise for muscular endur-

Table 7.1 Guidelines for Designing Isometric Training Programs

Type	Intensity	Duration	Repetitions	Frequency (days/wk)	Length of program
Isometric strength	100% MVC	5 sec per contraction	5-10	5	4 wk or more
Isometric endurance	60% MVC or less	Until fatigued	1 per session	5	4 wk or more

MVC = maximum voluntary contraction.

ance (Kraemer and Ratamess 2004; Ratamess et al. 2009). To develop muscle strength and muscle mass, the American College of Sports Medicine (ACSM; 2018) recommends selecting a resistance that allows the individual to complete 8 to 12 repetitions per set; to improve muscular endurance, a lower resistance (≤50% 1-RM) and higher number of repetitions (15-25) are recommended. Table 7.2 summarizes the ACSM (2018) guidelines for the resistance training of healthy populations.

Although this training stimulus may be sufficient for beginner and novice lifters, experts recommend that resistance training programs be tailored to the specific goals of intermediate and advanced lifters (Kraemer and Ratamess 2004; Ratamess et al. 2009). You can design programs to optimize the development of muscle strength, size (hypertrophy), endurance, or power by varying the intensity, repetitions, sets, and frequency of training. Tables 7.3 through 7.5 present guidelines for designing programs for novice, intermediate, and advanced weightlifters. For descriptions of dynamic resistance training exercises, see appendix C.4. Also, see the online video for additional information on grip and body position variations and common weightlifting errors and corrections.

Video 7.1-7.8

Intensity

As previously mentioned, the %1-RM and RM are widely used to estimate intensity for resistance training programs. The %1-RM, however, may not accurately estimate intensity because the number of repetitions performed at a given %1-RM varies among single-joint and multijoint exercises and among upper body and lower body exercises (Marocolo et al. 2016). Still, many experts endorse the %1-RM to prescribe intensity (Ratamess et al. 2009). Alternatively, Naclerio and colleagues (2011) demonstrated that the intensity of bench press exercise can be controlled and monitored using the OMNI-resistance exercise RPE scale (see appendix B.4)

The mean optimal intensity for developing strength ranges between 60% and 100% 1-RM. At these intensities, most individuals are able to perform 1 to 12 repetitions (1-RM to 12-RM). The client's experience with resistance training dictates the optimal intensity for developing strength. Generally, you should prescribe intensities of 60% to 70% 1-RM for novice lifters, 70% to 80% 1-RM for intermediate lifters, and 80% to 100% 1-RM for advanced lifters (Kraemer and Ratamess 2004; Ratamess et al. 2009). Meta-analyses support these recommendations. Rhea and colleagues (2003a) reported that the optimal intensity for strength gains in untrained (<1 yr of resistance training) and trained (>1 yr) lifters differs (60% 1-RM and 80% 1-RM, respectively). For competitive athletes (college and professional), the optimal training intensity is 85% 1-RM (Peterson, Rhea, and Alvar 2004). Keep in mind that these intensities are averages. Throughout the strength training program, intensity needs to be varied for continued improvement.

To develop muscular endurance, prescribe an intensity of ≤50% 1-RM (American College of Sports Medicine 2018). Although low to moderate intensity best suits muscle endurance and toning, it also brings some strength gains. The degree and rate of strength gain, however, will be less than that experienced with a program that optimizes strength development (specificity principle).

Table 7.2 ACSM Guidelines for Resistance Training of Healthy Populations

Goal	Intensity[a]	Repetitions	Sets[b]	Frequency	Number of exercises[c]
Muscle strength and muscle mass	60%-80% 1-RM	8-12	2-4	2-3 nonconsecutive days/wk	8-10
Muscle endurance	≤50% 1-RM	15-25	≤2	2-3 nonconsecutive days/wk	8-10

[a]To point of momentary muscular fatigue or failure.

[b]Allow 2-3 min rest between sets.

[c]Perform a different exercise for a specific muscle group every two or three sessions.

Based on ACSM 2018.

Table 7.3 Guidelines for Resistance Training Programs for Novice Lifters

Goal	Intensity	Volume	Velocity	Frequency	Rest interval
Strength	60%-70% 1-RM	2-4 sets of 8-12 reps	Slow to moderate	2 or 3 days/wk	2-3 min MJ; 1-2 min SJ
Hypertrophy	70%-85% 1-RM	1-3 sets of 8-12 reps	Slow to moderate	2 or 3 days/wk	1-2 min
Endurance	≤50% 1-RM	≤2 sets of 15-20 reps	Slow	2 or 3 days/wk	<1 min
Power	85%-100% 1-RM for force, 30%-60% 1-RM for upper body, and 0%-60% 1-RM for lower body exercises for velocity	2-4 sets of 8-12 reps	Moderate	2 or 3 days/wk	2-3 min for core exercises (MJ); 1-2 min for SJ

MJ = multijoint exercise; SJ = single-joint exercise.

Data from Ratamess et al. 2009.

Table 7.4 Guidelines for Resistance Training Programs for Intermediate Lifters

Goal	Intensity	Volume	Velocity	Frequency	Rest interval
Strength	70%-80% 1-RM	1-3 sets of 6-12 reps	Moderate	3 days/wk for whole-body workouts; 4 days/wk for split workouts	2-3 min MJ; 1-2 min SJ
Hypertrophy	70%-85% 1-RM	1-3 sets of 8-12 reps	Slow to moderate	3 or 4 days/wk	1-2 min
Endurance	50%-70% 1-RM	1-3 sets of 10-15 reps	Slow to moderate	3 or 4 days/wk	<1 min
Power	85%-100% 1-RM for force, 30%-60% 1-RM for upper body, and 0%-60% 1-RM for lower body exercises for velocity	1-3 sets of 3-6 reps	Moderate	2-4 days/wk	2-3 min for core exercises (MJ); 1-2 min for SJ

MJ = multijoint exercise; SJ = single-joint exercise.

Data from Ratamess et al. 2009.

Table 7.5 Guidelines for Resistance Training Programs for Advanced Lifters

Goal	Intensity	Volume	Velocity	Frequency	Rest interval
Strength	80%-100% 1-RM, periodized	Multiple sets of 1-12 reps, periodized	Slow to fast	4-6 days/wk	2-3 min MJ; 1-2 min SJ
Hypertrophy	70%-100% 1-RM	3-6 sets of 1-12 reps,* periodized	Slow to moderate	4-6 days/wk	2-3 min MJ; 1-2 min SJ
Endurance	30%-80% 1-RM	Multiple sets of 10-25 reps, periodized	Slow for 10-15 reps; moderate to fast for 15-25 reps	4-6 days/wk	<1 min for 10-15 reps; 1-2 min for 15-25 reps
Power	85%-100% 1-RM for force; 30%-60% 1-RM for velocity	3-6 sets of 1-6 reps, periodized	Fast	4-6 days/wk	2-3 min MJ; 1-2 min SJ

MJ = multijoint exercise; SJ = single-joint exercise.

*Greater emphasis on 6-RM to 12-RM.

Note: For power, emphasize MJ exercises. For strength, hypertrophy, and endurance, use both MJ and SJ exercises; perform MJ before SJ exercises. Exercise larger muscle groups before smaller muscle groups.

Data from Ratamess et al. 2009.

Sets

The optimal number of sets for improving muscular strength is controversial and depends on the client's goal; one to three sets for children, older adults, and novice lifters are recommended (Ratamess et al. 2009). A major advantage of single-set programs is that they require much less time for a training session than do multiple-set programs (20 vs. 50 min), potentially increasing your clients' compliance. Some studies suggest that single sets (one set per exercise) are just as effective as multiple sets (two or three sets per exercise) for increasing the strength of untrained and recreational lifters during the first 3 to 4 mo of resistance training (Feigenbaum and Pollock 1999; Frohlich, Emrich, and Schmidtbleicher 2010; Hass et al. 2000).

However, the results from analyses of resistance training studies do not support prescribing single-set programs to develop strength (Rhea et al. 2003a) or hypertrophy (Krieger 2010) in untrained and trained recreational lifters. Traditionally, a set refers to the number of consecutive repetitions performed for a specific exercise; however, Rhea and colleagues (2003a) noted that the total number of sets performed for a specific muscle group is a better indicator of training stress than sets per exercise. Using this definition of sets, they reported that an average of four sets during each training session optimizes strength development in untrained and trained lifters. For single-set programs, the authors suggest prescribing multiple exercises for a specific muscle group in order to reach the goal of four sets. The ACSM (2018) stated that each set should be performed to the point of volitional fatigue for each exercise (see table 7.2).

Multiple sets using periodization are recommended for serious athletes, powerlifters, and bodybuilders engaging in advanced strength training and hypertrophy programs (Frohlich, Emrich, and Schmidtbleicher 2010; Ratamess et al. 2009). To optimize the strength gains of collegiate and professional athletes, an average of eight sets per muscle group is recommended (Peterson, Rhea, and Alvar 2004).

Frequency

Muscular fitness may improve from exercising just 1 day/wk, especially in clients with below-average muscular fitness. Recent research, however, suggests that the optimal frequency of strength training for untrained individuals is 3 days/wk. For healthy populations, the ACSM (2018) recommends 2 or 3 nonconsecutive days per week. For advanced lifters, four to six training sessions per week and split routines are recommended (Ratamess et al. 2009). To optimize the strength gains of trained recreational lifters and competitive athletes, each muscle group should be exercised twice a week (Rhea et al. 2003a; Peterson, Rhea, and Alvar 2004; Ratamess et al. 2009). Advanced lifters and competitive athletes who train 4 to 6 days/wk can accomplish this goal by using split routines (see Variations for Frequency). You should prescribe 48 hr of rest between workouts of the same muscle groups to allow the muscles to recuperate and to prevent injury from overtraining.

Volume

Training volume is the sum of the repetitions performed during each training session multiplied by the resistance used (Ratamess et al. 2009). Throughout a resistance training program, volume and intensity must be systematically increased (progression principle) to avoid plateaus and to ensure continued strength improvements. You can alter training volume by changing the number of exercises performed for each session, the number of repetitions performed for each set, or the number of sets performed for each exercise. Several models of periodized training can be used to systematically vary volume and intensity (see Periodization).

Order of Exercises

A well-rounded resistance training program should include at least one exercise for each of the major muscle groups in the body. In this way, **muscle balance**—that is, the ratio of strength between opposing muscle groups (agonists vs. antagonists), contralateral muscle groups (right vs. left side), and upper and lower body muscle groups—can be maintained. Order the exercises so that the client first executes multijoint exercises—such as the seated leg press, bench press, and lat pull-down—that involve larger muscles (e.g., gluteus maximus, pectoralis major, and latissimus dorsi) and more muscle groups. Then have the client progress to single-joint exercises for smaller muscle groups (see table 7.6). To avoid muscle fatigue in novice weightlifters, arrange the order so that successive exercises do not involve the same muscle group. This allows time for the muscle to recover.

Rest

The amount of rest taken between sets and exercises is another variable to consider when designing resistance training programs. The recommended rest between sets and exercises depends on exercise intensity: A lower intensity requires shorter rests and a higher intensity longer rests (see table 7.7). Short rest intervals may compromise the number of repetitions that can be completed (Ratamess et al. 2009), and the ACSM recommends a rest interval of 2 to 3 min between sets (American College of Sports Medicine 2018). In strength or power training, rests should last 3 to 5 min to allow resynthesis of adenosine triphosphate (ATP) and creatine phosphate (CrP) and to prevent metabolic acidosis (Kraemer 2003).

Dynamic Resistance Training Methods

You can use a variety of methods to design dynamic resistance training programs. The majority of these methods are best suited for advanced programs. Each uses a different approach for prescribing sets, order of exercises, or frequency of workouts.

Variations for Sets

You can use either a single set or multiple sets of exercise. For multiple sets, you may choose to have your clients consecutively perform a designated number of sets (usually three or more) at a constant intensity (e.g., 10-RM) for each exercise. Alternatively, you may have your clients perform one set of three different exercises for the same muscle group. For example, instead of three consecutive sets of barbell curls for the elbow flexors, you may prescribe one set of incline dumbbell curls, one set of hammer curls, and one set of barbell curls. This adds variety to the program and changes the training stimulus because different muscles or parts of a muscle are used to perform each of these exercises.

A client performing multiple sets of a given exercise may choose to lift the same weight for each set

Table 7.6 Example of Exercise Order for a Basic Resistance Training Program

Body segment	Type of exercise*	Joint actions	Exercise
1. Hips and thighs	Multijoint	Hip extension and knee extension	Seated leg press
2. Chest	Multijoint	Shoulder horizontal flexion and elbow extension	Flat bench press
3. Upper back and mid back	Multijoint	Shoulder extension/adduction and elbow flexion	Lat pull-down
4. Legs	Single joint	Knee extension	Leg extension
5. Shoulders and upper arms	Multijoint	Shoulder abduction and elbow flexion	Upright row
6. Lower back	Multijoint	Trunk extension and hip extension	Back extension
7. Upper arms	Single joint	Elbow extension	Triceps push-down
8. Legs	Single joint	Knee flexion	Leg curl
9. Upper arms	Single joint	Elbow flexion	Arm curl
10. Calves	Single joint	Ankle plantar flexion	Toe raise
11. Forearms	Single joint	Wrist flexion and extension	Wrist curl
12. Abdomen	Single joint	Trunk flexion	Curl-up

*Multijoint exercises involving larger muscle groups are followed by single-joint exercises for smaller muscle groups.

Table 7.7 Exercise Intensity and Recommended Rest Periods

Intensity	%1-RM	Length of rest
>13-RM	<65%	<1 min
11-RM to 13-RM	65%-74%	1-2 min
8-RM to 10-RM	75%-80%	2-3 min
5-RM to 7-RM	81%-87%	3-5 min
<5-RM	>87%	>5 min

Data from Kraemer 2003.

or to vary the intensity of each set by lifting progressively heavier weights (light to heavy sets) or lighter weights (heavy to light sets). **Pyramiding** is a light to heavy system in which the client performs as many as six sets of each exercise. In the first set, the client lifts a relatively lighter weight for 10 to 12 repetitions (10-RM to 12-RM). In subsequent sets the individual lifts progressively heavier weights (i.e., 8-RM, 6-RM, and 4-RM). Because this involves such a large volume of work, you should prescribe the pyramid system for experienced weightlifters only. Bodybuilders commonly use this system to develop muscle size. Although pyramiding adds variety to a resistance training program, it might not be any more effective than performing multiple sets with the same weight. When training volume is equal, there is no difference between multiple sets and pyramiding for muscular strength, muscle damage, or hormonal responses in either healthy young men (Charro et al. 2010) or older women (Ribeiro, Schoenfeld, et al. 2017).

Variations for Order and Number of Exercises

Exercise scientists generally recommend ordering the exercises so that large muscle groups are exercised at the beginning of the workout, with progression to smaller muscle groups later in the workout. To maximize the overload of muscle groups, however, some clients may choose to preexhaust muscle groups by reversing this order. To do this, the individual fatigues smaller muscles by using single-joint exercises prior to performing multijoint exercises.

When you prescribe two or more exercises for a specific muscle group, instruct the average individual to alternate muscle groups so that the muscle can rest and recover between exercises. For example, your client should not perform leg press and leg extension exercises consecutively because the quadriceps femoris is used in both of these exercises. Instead, intersperse one or more exercises using different muscle groups between these two exercises.

In contrast, many advanced weightlifters prefer to do **compound sets** or **tri-sets** in order to completely fatigue a targeted muscle group. To use this training system, the client performs two exercises (compound sets) or three exercises (tri-sets) consecutively for the same muscle group, with little or no rest between the exercises.

Many bodybuilders also use a training system called **supersetting**. For supersets, the client exercises agonist and antagonist muscle groups consecutively without resting. For example, to superset the hamstrings and quadriceps femoris, follow a leg curl set immediately with a leg extension set. Balsamo and colleagues (2012) compared the effects of different superset exercise sequences for the quadriceps femoris (leg extensions) and hamstrings (leg curls) on total training volume and perceived exertion. They reported that total training volume is increased and the RPE is decreased when leg curls preceded leg extensions. Further research is warranted to identify optimal exercise sequences for other agonist-antagonist muscle groups. Weakley and colleagues (2017) suggested that supersets and tri-sets can enhance training efficiency and reduce training time, but these routines are more fatiguing than normal multiset routines and may require additional posttraining recovery.

Variations for Frequency

Traditionally for advanced resistance training programs, exercise scientists have recommended resistance training 3 days/wk on alternate days (e.g., M-W-F) to give the muscles time to recover. For individuals who want to resistance train 4 to 6 days/wk, prescribe a split routine. With a **split routine**, you are targeting different muscle groups on consecutive days, thereby allowing at least 1 day of recovery for each muscle group. For example, a bodybuilder may exercise the chest and shoulders on Monday and Thursday, the hips and legs on Tuesday and Friday, and the back and arms on Wednesday and Saturday. Ribeiro, Schoenfeld, Silva, and colleagues (2015) demonstrated that the muscular strength and fat-free mass gains of elite bodybuilders were similar for four sessions per week compared with six sessions per week.

Periodization

Periodization systematically varies the intensity and volume of resistance training. The goal of periodization is twofold: (1) to maximize the response of the neuromuscular system (i.e., gains in strength, endurance, power, and hypertrophy) by systematically changing the training or exercise stimulus and (2) to minimize overtraining and injury by planning rest and recovery. A recent meta-analysis showed that periodized resistance training programs are indeed more effective than nonperiodized training plans for increasing 1-RM (Williams et al. 2017). The training stimulus may be varied by manipulations in one or more of the following program elements:

- Training volume (number of sets, repetitions, or exercises)
- Training intensity (amount of resistance)
- Type of muscle action (concentric, eccentric, or isometric)
- Training frequency

Given the number of variables, there are numerous possibilities for designing periodized programs. Researchers have identified combinations that optimize the training stimulus for developing strength and muscular endurance (Rhea et al. 2002, 2003b).

Three common periodization models are linear periodization (LP), reverse linear periodization (RLP), and undulating periodization (UP). All periodized training programs are divided into periods, or cycles; however, the duration and the training stimulus differ depending on the model used.

Classic Linear Periodization Model

The classic **linear periodization (LP)** model is divided into three types of cycles. The **macrocycle** (usually 9-12 mo) is divided into mesocycles that last 3 to 4 mo. **Mesocycles** are subdivided into **microcycles** lasting 1 to 4 wk. Within and between cycles, training intensity increases as training volume decreases. For example, a 3 mo (12 wk) mesocycle can be divided into three 4 wk microcycles as follows: During weeks 1 through 4, three sets are performed at 12-RM, or 70% 1-RM; during weeks 5 through 8, three sets are performed at 10-RM, or 75% 1-RM; and during weeks 9 through 12, three sets are performed at 8-RM, or 80% 1-RM (see Sample Linear Periodized Resistance Training Program for Intermediate Lifter later in the chapter). The training intensity increases from 70% 1-RM (12-RM) to 80% 1-RM (8-RM) while the training volume systematically decreases because of the progressive reduction in the number of repetitions (from 12 to 8) performed during each microcycle.

Reverse Linear Periodization Model

The **reverse linear periodization (RLP)** model reverses the progression of the LP training stimulus. Between and within cycles, training intensity decreases as training volume increases. The RLP configuration of the mesocycles and microcycles is as follows: weeks 1 through 4, three sets at 80% 1-RM (8-RM); weeks 5 through 8, three sets at 75% 1-RM (10-RM); and weeks 9 through 12, three sets at 70% 1-RM (12-RM). As you can see, the training intensity decreases from 80% to 70% 1-RM (8-RM to 12-RM) as the training volume increases (from 8-12 reps) during the three progressive microcycles.

Undulating Periodization Model

Compared with those in LP and RLP, the microcycles for **undulating periodization (UP)** are considerably shorter (biweekly, weekly, or even daily) so that the training stimulus (intensity and volume) changes frequently. The client may progress from high volume, low intensity to low volume, high intensity in the same week. For example, in a 3 days/wk UP program, the individual may perform three sets of 8-RM (high volume, low intensity) on day 1, three sets of 6-RM on day 2, and three sets of 4-RM on day 3 (low volume, high intensity). In subsequent microcycles (each week), this training stimulus could be repeated or could be varied to change the order of the training stimulus (e.g., day 1 = 4-RM, day 2 = 6-RM, and day 3 = 8-RM). Frequently changing the volume and intensity subjects the exercising muscles to a different training stimulus on a daily or weekly basis. As such, UP may prevent plateaus in training and maintain the client's interest and motivation for long-term resistance training.

Circuit Resistance Training

Circuit resistance training is a method of dynamic resistance training that increases strength, muscular endurance, and cardiorespiratory endurance (Gettman and Pollock 1981). Circuit resistance training compares favorably with traditional resistance training programs for increasing muscle strength of untrained adults, especially if low-repetition, high-resistance exercises are used (Gettman et al. 1978; Wilmore et al. 1978). Recent reviews concluded that circuit training can be effective for increasing muscular strength of adults 18-65 yr (Muñoz-Martinez et al. 2017) as well as middle-aged and older adults (Buch et al. 2017). Additionally, Alcaraz and colleagues (2011) reported that high-resistance training (3-RM to 6-RM; six sets; 35 sec interset rest) was as effective as traditional resistance training for improving upper and lower body 1-RM strength and power in resistance-trained men.

A circuit resistance training program usually has 10 to 15 stations per circuit (see figure 7.1). The circuit is repeated two or three times so that the total time of continuous exercise is 20 to 30 min. At each exercise

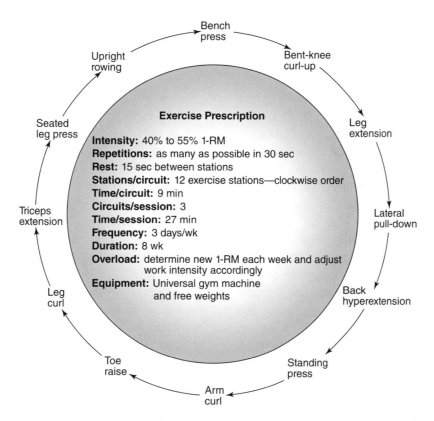

FIGURE 7.1 Sample circuit resistance training program. 1-RM = 1-repetition maximum.

station, select a resistance that fatigues the muscle group in approximately 30 sec (as many repetitions as possible at approximately 40% to 55% of 1-RM). Include a 15 to 20 sec rest period between exercise stations. Circuit resistance training is usually performed 3 days/wk for at least 6 wk. This method of training is ideal for clients with a limited amount of time for exercise. As mentioned in chapter 5, you can add aerobic exercise stations to the circuit between each weightlifting station (i.e., super circuit resistance training) to obtain additional cardiorespiratory benefits.

Eccentric Training

Traditional dynamic resistance training includes both concentric and eccentric muscle actions. However, one can train with higher forces and velocities when the load is limited to eccentric muscle action only (Cowell, Cronin, and Brughelli 2012). **Eccentric training** has the potential to improve strength, hypertrophy, and performance as well as aid in tendon and muscle injury rehabilitation (Cowell, Cronin, and Brughelli 2012). Thus, it is not sur-

prising that several manufacturers have designed eccentric training devices. One such device is the Eccentron, which looks like a recumbent stair stepper. However, instead of pushing down on the pedals, the exerciser must resist the movement of the pedals toward him. This action simulates downhill walking or running. Numerous other eccentric training machines have been developed. These range from isokinetic devices that apply an eccentric force, to weight machines that reduce the load during the concentric phase and increase it during the eccentric phase, to eccentric cycle ergometers. See the review by Tinwala and colleagues (2017) for an explanation of the technology as well as the advantages and disadvantages of various negative-resistance training devices. Unfortunately, there is still a lack of peer-reviewed literature comparing these devices against traditional resistance training.

Several researchers have proposed training plans using eccentric training devices. Eccentric training is appealing because of the potential for high force production at a very low energy cost (e.g., the energy

Video
7.9

cost of walking downhill is only about a quarter of the cost of walking uphill) (Hoppeler 2016; LaStayo et al. 2014). This mode of training is distinctively different from other forms of eccentric exercise, such as plyometrics or eccentric overload with free weights. Hoppeler (2016) coined the term *moderate-load eccentric exercise* to describe progressive exercise performed on motorized ergometers that allow for controlled application of eccentric loads. Hoppeler recommended initial negative loads of 50 to 75 W for 5 to 10 min, eventually progressing to negative loads of 400 to 500 W for 20 to 30 min, three times per week, in rehabilitation settings. In comparison, plyometric exercises can produce negative loads of several thousand watts and are inherently more dangerous, placing the exerciser at increased risk for muscle damage. According to Hoppeler (2016), delayed-onset muscle soreness (DOMS) can largely be prevented with the progressive protocols of moderate-load eccentric training. LaStayo and colleagues (2014) described the potential rehabilitative applications of this type of eccentric training in older adults, cancer survivors, and those with cardiopulmonary, metabolic, neurologic, and orthopedic disorders.

CORE STABILITY AND FUNCTIONAL TRAINING

Core stability training is widely promoted in fitness settings to improve functional capacity (activities of daily living and occupational tasks) and sport skills performance of healthy individuals. **Core stability** is the ability to maintain the ideal alignment of the neck, spine, scapulae, and pelvis while performing an exercise or a sport skill. Abdominal bracing is more effective than abdominal hollowing in optimizing spinal stability. Traditional core stability training includes resistance exercises performed on unstable surfaces (e.g., wobble board, balance disc, and Swiss ball).

Compared with exercise on stable surfaces (e.g., ground-based free weights), exercising on unstable surfaces is thought to enhance the activation of the core and limb muscles but may decrease force, power, velocity, and range of motion during the resistance exercise. In contrast, some researchers believe that multijoint free weight exercises actually engage the core more than core-specific exercises (Martus-

cello et al. 2013). Regardless, core stability training performed on unstable surfaces may be better suited for developing muscular endurance than muscle strength and power (Willardson 2008). Instability resistance training, however, can play an important role in periodized training programs and rehabilitation programs. Also, nonathletes who prefer not to use ground-based free weights to achieve muscular fitness may receive health-related benefits from resistance training on instability devices (Behm et al. 2010b). For more on this topic, see Core Stability Testing and Training for Low Back Pain in chapter 11. The muscles and their functional contribution to core stability are presented in Core Stability Muscles and Function.

For years, functional training has been widely used in physical rehabilitation programs to improve joint stability, neuromuscular control, flexibility, and muscular fitness (strength and endurance) of injured clients. Functional training programs typically include four types of exercise:

1. Spinal stabilization exercises to improve stability of the spine during movement
2. Proprioception and balance exercises to enhance neuromuscular coordination
3. Resistance exercises to develop muscular fitness
4. Flexibility exercises to regain range of movement

Functional training has gained popularity and recognition, especially in health and fitness clubs. Usually the goal of functional training is to train and develop muscles so that performing everyday activities is easier, safer, and more efficient (Yoke and Kennedy 2004). However, some studies have examined the efficacy of functional training for improving sport performance (Thompson, Cobb, and Blackwell 2007).

Functional training is a system of exercise progressions for specific muscle groups that uses a six-step approach developed by Yoke and Kennedy (2004). The difficulty level (strength) and skill level (balance and coordination) of specific exercises are rated, with 1 representing the least difficult exercises (requiring less strength and skill) and 6 the most difficult exercises (requiring more strength and skill). As the difficulty of the exercises pro-

CORE STABILITY MUSCLES AND FUNCTION

Muscles	Location	Function
Multifidus, rotators, intertransversales, interspinalis	Between adjacent vertebrae	Maintain core stability by contracting in response to sudden changes in posture
Transversus abdominis, internal abdominal obliques, quadratus lumborum	Transverse processes of lumbar vertebrae	Stabilize the spine by drawing in umbilicus and increasing compressive forces between bodies of lumbar vertebrae
Rectus abdominis, external abdominal obliques, erector spinae, latissimus dorsi	Pelvic girdle and rib cage	Maintain core stability during performance of heavy ground-based movements with free weights (e.g., squats)
Hip flexors, extensors, adductors, and abductors	Pelvis and lumbar vertebrae to femur	Produce pelvic tilt that results in movement of lumbar spine, affecting core stability

gresses, greater strength, balance, core stability, and coordination are required. The hardest exercises (6 rating) require the most core stability. To maintain proper postural alignment, the strength of the core muscle groups (erector spinae and abdominal prime movers and stabilizers) needs to be developed (**core strengthening**). Because core stability is dynamic, changing with body position during exercise, isolated core strengthening does not automatically increase core stability unless it is accompanied by motor skill training (Yessis 2003). Functional exercise progressions develop the strength and function of all muscle groups, not just core muscles. For an outline and example of functional exercise progressions, see Functional Exercise Progressions: Six-Step Approach and Example.

It is not necessary for every client to progress to the most difficult levels (5 and 6) on the exercise continuum. Safety is of utmost importance. Be certain that your clients are able to perform exercises with proper form and postural alignment for the duration of the set before progressing to the next level. Your clients' ability to perform each level of exercise depends on their fitness and skill levels. Level 6 exercises should challenge competitive athletes or very fit individuals with excellent balance, strength, motor skill, and core stability. Although functional training potentially adds variety and challenge to workouts, research is needed to compare its effectiveness against conventional strength and muscular endurance training. Improvements in strength, endurance, balance, flexibility, and coordination as well as in functional performance of everyday tasks

need to be evaluated. For more information, detailed descriptions, and illustrations of functional exercise progressions for all muscle groups, see Yoke and Kennedy (2004).

EXTREME CONDITIONING PROGRAMS

High-intensity functional training, or extreme conditioning programs, typically consists of high-intensity and high-volume activities with short recovery periods between exercises (Knapik 2015). Additionally, these programs place an emphasis on multijoint exercises, functional movements, body resistance, and variety to target multiple joint angles. Examples of extreme conditioning programs include CrossFit, Insanity, and P90X. Insanity and P90X are home-based exercise programs; exercisers follow a series of DVDs for the workouts. CrossFit-affiliated gyms are available worldwide, but daily workouts are posted online for those who want to train on their own. Given that high-intensity interval training, body weight training, strength training, and functional fitness were ranked numbers 1, 4, 5, and 10, respectively, on the list of worldwide fitness trends for 2018 (Thompson 2017), it is not surprising that extreme conditioning programs that incorporate aspects of all these trends are popular.

Despite the popularity of these programs and anecdotal reports of their effectiveness, peer-reviewed research comparing extreme functional training against traditional resistance training is limited. Heinrich and colleagues (2014) compared

FUNCTIONAL EXERCISE PROGRESSIONS: SIX-STEP APPROACH AND EXAMPLE

Step	Aim	Body position, resistance	Example for knee extensors
1. Isolate and educate	Teach client to focus on individual muscle action and to selectively contract or isolate the specific muscle group	Lying supine or prone on bench or floor	Lying supine with knees bent, hips flexed to 45°, and arms at sides, client extends the knee one leg at a time.
2. Add resistance	Increase resistance by using exercise machines, longer lever length, or elastic tubing	Sitting on bench or floor	Sitting upright on a bench with elastic tubing attached to the ankle, client extends the knee one leg at a time.
3. Add functional training positions	Decrease supporting base to require greater use of stabilizing muscles	Sitting or standing	Supported at low back level by a stability ball pressed against the wall, with pelvis and spine in neutral position, feet shoulder-width apart and far enough away from wall so that knees flex no more than 90° during exercise, client squats, not allowing hips to drop below the knees.
4. Combine increased function with resistance	Overload core stabilizers in functional positions	Using exercise machines, free weights, or elastic exercise bands to increase resistance	With exercise band attached to ankles, client stands in upright, neutral spine position, balancing on support leg with exercise leg flexed at hip and knee slightly flexed. Client flexes the hip while extending the knee of the exercise leg.
5. Exercise multiple muscle groups with increased resistance and core challenge	Increase demand on strength, balance, coordination, and core stability	Using multijoint exercise machines to increase resistance	Using seated, lying, or standing leg press machine, client extends hips and knees simultaneously.
6. Add balance, increased function, speed, or rotation	Increase demand on balance, speed, and joint rotation	Using smaller or moving base of support such as stability balls and balance boards or discs; using free weights (barbells or dumbbells) to increase resistance	Standing in upright position with one hand on wall or support bar and holding dumbbell in other hand, client extends hip and places one leg on stability ball. Client rolls the back leg backward on the ball, flexing the knee (no more than 90°) of the opposite leg while keeping the pelvis and spine in a neutral position and the shoulders and hips squared. Client returns to starting position by extending the knee of exercising leg and rolling opposite leg forward on top of the ball.

previously inactive CrossFit participants with a group engaged in moderate-intensity aerobic and resistance training. Each group exercised three times a week. At the conclusion of the 8 wk study, CrossFit participants reported higher enjoyment and planned to continue the same exercise more so than those engaged in the moderate-intensity workouts. Additionally, in a randomized controlled trial conducted in a secondary school in Australia, researchers concluded that a CrossFit program was feasible, enjoyable, and effective for improving health-related fitness in adolescents (Eather, Morgan, and Lubans 2016).

Some fitness experts, including a consortium for health and military performance and the ACSM (Bergeron et al. 2011), have questioned the safety of extreme conditioning programs. Epidemiological injury surveys of CrossFit exercisers in the United States (Weisenthal et al. 2014) and Brazil (Sprey et al. 2016) reported injury rates of 19% and 31%, respectively. Although these injury statistics sound alarming, recent research indicates that the injury rates for participants of extreme conditioning programs are comparable to other resistance training programs (Aune and Powers 2017; Grier et al. 2013; Montalvo et al. 2017); the injury incidence reported for CrossFit ranges from 2.1 to 2.3 per 1,000 athlete training hours (Montalvo et al. 2017; Moran et al. 2017). Weisenthal et al. (2014) noted that the injury rate was significantly reduced when a trainer was involved in the workout.

As with all training programs, a well-planned stepwise approach to increasing frequency, intensity, and duration is a prudent strategy when prescribing an extreme conditioning program. With careful planning, extreme conditioning programs can be safe alternatives or supplements to traditional resistance training.

ISOKINETIC TRAINING

Isokinetic exercise combines the advantages of dynamic (full range of motion) and static (maximum force exerted) exercise. Since the resistance is accommodating, isokinetic training overcomes the problems associated with using either a constant- or variable-resistance exercise mode. You can use isokinetic training to increase strength, power, and muscular endurance. Isokinetic training involves dynamic shortening contractions of the muscle group against an accommodating resistance that matches the force produced by the muscle group throughout the entire range of motion. The speed of the movement is controlled mechanically by the isokinetic exercise device. Isokinetic dynamometers are used for isokinetic training. If this equipment is not available, exercises can be done with a partner who offers accommodating resistance to the movement. The speed of the movement, however, is not precisely controlled.

Isokinetic training is done at speeds that vary between 24° and 300°·sec^{-1}, depending on the needs of the individual. The carryover effect appears to be greater when a person trains at faster speeds (180°-300°·sec^{-1}) as compared with slower speeds (30°-60°·sec^{-1}). In some studies, strength gains have been limited to velocities at or below the training velocity (Lesmes et al. 1978; Moffroid and Whipple 1970). Other researchers have reported significant strength gains at all testing velocities (30°-300°·sec^{-1}) for high-velocity training groups (240°-300°·sec^{-1}) (Coyle et al. 1981; Jenkins, Thackaberry, and Killian 1984). Recent isokinetic research with older adults resulted in velocity-specific training improvements in both low-velocity (75°·sec^{-1}) and high-velocity (240°·sec^{-1}) groups, but the carryover of improvements into other velocities was greater for the high-velocity group (Englund et al. 2017). Table 7.8 presents general guidelines for designing isokinetic training programs for the development of strength and endurance.

A major advantage of isokinetic training over traditional forms of training is that little or no muscle soreness results because the muscles do not contract eccentrically when performing traditional isokinetic training, and eccentric muscle action is thought to produce more muscle soreness than other muscle actions (see Muscular Soreness later in this chapter). For example, when performing knee extension and flexion on an isokinetic device, the client performs a concentric muscle action of the quadriceps (kicking the leg out) followed by a concentric muscle action of the hamstrings (forcibly pulling the leg back to the starting position) for extension and flexion, respectively. This differs from auxotonic dynamic training with free weights in which an eccentric action of the quadriceps is needed to act as a braking force as the lower leg returns to the starting position. However, when the goal of training is an increase in muscle size, traditional isokinetic exercise that

Table 7.8 Guidelines for Designing Isokinetic Training Programs

Type	Intensity	Repetitions	Sets	Speed	Frequency	Length of program
Isokinetic strength	Maximum contraction	2-15	3	24°-180°·sec^{-1}	3-5 days/wk	6 wk or more
Isokinetic endurance	Maximum contraction	Until fatigued	1	≥180°·sec^{-1}	3-5 days/wk	6 wk or more

involves only concentric muscle actions is not the best choice. Although muscle hypertrophy can be achieved with concentric exercise only (Cadore et al. 2014; Moore, Young, and Phillips 2012), research by Farthing and Chilibeck (2003) demonstrated that eccentric muscle action performed at a fast velocity is the most effective method for muscle hypertrophy. A combination of eccentric and concentric actions is recommended when the goal is to increase muscle hypertrophy (Schoenfeld et al. 2017).

DEVELOPING RESISTANCE TRAINING PROGRAMS

Before designing a resistance training program for a client, review training principles and determine how each of these principles can be incorporated into your client's program. The training program needs to be individualized. By varying the combination of intensity, duration, and frequency of exercise, you can develop programs that meet the unique goals and needs of each client. Be sure to follow guidelines and recommendations for resistance training programs (see tables 7.2 through 7.5), as well as specific recommendations and precautions, when developing resistance training programs for children and older adults. See Steps for Developing a Resistance Training Program.

APPLICATION OF TRAINING PRINCIPLES TO RESISTANCE EXERCISE

To develop effective resistance training programs, you must apply each of the training principles presented in chapter 3 (see Basic Principles for Exercise Program Design). This section reviews some of the more pertinent training principles and outlines how they are applied to the design of resistance training programs.

Specificity Principle

The development of muscular fitness is specific to the muscle group that is exercised, the type of muscle action, and training intensity. To increase the dynamic strength of the elbow flexors, for example, you must select exercises that involve the concentric and eccentric actions of that particular muscle group. For strength, the person performs exercises at a high intensity with low repetitions; exercising at a low intensity with high repetitions stimulates the development of muscular endurance.

Strength and endurance gains are also specific to the speed and range of motion used during the training. With isometric training, strength gains at angles other than the training angle are typically 50% less than those at the exercised angle. Similarly, as previously noted, strength gains in isokinetic

Steps for Developing a Resistance Training Program

The following steps, used to design the sample dynamic resistance training programs, provide an outline of how you should proceed.

1. In consultation with your client, identify the primary goal of the program (i.e., strength, muscular endurance, muscle size, or muscle toning), and ask the client how much time she is willing to commit to this program.

2. Based on your client's goal, time commitment, and access to equipment, determine the type of resistance training program (i.e., dynamic, static, or isokinetic).

3. Using results from your client's muscular fitness assessment, identify specific muscle groups that need to be targeted in the exercise prescription.

4. In addition to core exercises for the major muscle groups, select exercises for those muscle groups targeted in step 3.

5. For novice weightlifters, order the exercises so the same muscle group is not exercised consecutively.

6. Based on your client's goal, determine appropriate starting loads, repetitions, and sets for each exercise.

7. Set guidelines for progressively overloading each muscle group.

training may be limited to velocities at or below the training velocity (Lesmes et al. 1978; Moffroid and Whipple 1970).

Overload Principle

To promote strength and endurance gains, it is necessary to exercise the muscle group at workloads that are greater than normal for the client. The exercise intensity should be at least 60% of maximum to stimulate the development of strength. Clients may achieve more rapid strength gains, however, by exercising the muscle at or near maximum (80%-100%) resistance. To stimulate endurance gains, intensities as low as 30% of maximum may be used; however, at low intensities the muscle group should be exercised to the point of fatigue.

Progression Principle

Generally, throughout a resistance training program, you must periodically increase the training volume, or total amount of work performed, to continue overloading the muscle so that the person can make further improvements in strength and muscular endurance. The progression needs to be gradual because doing too much too soon may cause musculoskeletal injuries and excessive muscle soreness. Typically you progressively overload muscle groups by increasing the resistance or amount of weight lifted. As clients adapt to the training stimulus, they will be able to perform more repetitions at the prescribed resistance. Thus, the number of repetitions a client is able to perform will indicate when it is necessary to increase the resistance throughout the training program. In addition to increasing resistance, you may progressively overload muscle groups by increasing the total number of repetitions performed at a selected intensity, altering the speed of movement (slow, moderate, fast pace), and varying the duration of rest periods between sets of exercises (Ratamess et al. 2009).

Additional Principles

Individuals with lower initial strength will show greater relative gains and a faster rate of improvement in response to resistance training than those starting out with higher strength levels (principles of initial values and interindividual variability). However, the rate of improvement slows, and eventually plateaus, as clients progress through the program and move closer to their genetic ceiling (principle of diminishing returns). Also, when an individual stops resistance training, the physiological adaptations and improvements in muscle structure and function are reversed (principle of reversibility). Using periodization techniques (see Periodization), you can lessen the effects of detraining on athletes and maintain strength gains during the competitive period by manipulating the intensity and volume of the resistance training exercise (see Haff 2016).

GENERAL PROCEDURES AND SAMPLE RESISTANCE TRAINING PROGRAMS

After assessing a client's muscular fitness, you can individualize the resistance training exercise prescription to meet the client's individual needs and interests by using the steps outlined in this section.

The first example (see Sample Resistance Training Program for Older Adult) describes a beginning resistance training program developed for a 70 yr old man with no previous weightlifting experience. The primary goal for this program is to develop adequate muscular fitness so the client can retain functional independence. During the first 4 wk of training, low-intensity (30%-40% 1-RM), high-repetition (15-20 reps) exercises familiarize the client with weightlifting exercise and reduce the chance of injury and excessive muscle soreness. The client gradually increases the resistance so that by the end of this phase, the exercise intensity is 50% 1-RM. After 8 wk, the intensity starts at 50% 1-RM and gradually increases to 75% 1-RM. The client does one or two sets of 10 to 15 repetitions for each exercise. To overload the muscles during this phase, he increases the resistance gradually, but only after he is able to complete 15 or more repetitions at the prescribed relative intensity. This program includes multijoint exercises, weight-bearing calisthenics, and stair climbing. The client exercises two times a week, allowing at least 2 days of rest between each workout. Additionally, muscle power training can be incorporated using light to moderate loads (30%-60% 1-RM) for one to three sets of 6 to 10 repetitions (American College of Sports Medicine 2018).

The second program (see Sample Linear Periodized Resistance Training Program for Intermediate

Client Data

Age: 70 yr

Gender: Male

Body weight: 160 lb (72.7 kg)

Program goal: Muscle fitness and functional independence

Time commitment: 20-30 min per workout

Equipment: Exercise machines

Intensity: 30%-50% 1-RM for first 8 wk; 50%-75% 1-RM thereafter

Frequency: 2 days/wk; at least 48 hr between workouts

Duration: 16 wk or longer

Overload: Increase reps first; increase resistance only when able to complete >15 reps

Rest: 2-3 min between exercises

Exercise[a]	1-RM (lb)[b]	Weeks[c]	Intensity[d] (%1-RM)	Weight (lb)	Repetitions	Sets	Muscle groups
Leg press (seated)	180	1-4	30-40	55-70	15-20	1	Hip extensors
		5-8	40-50	70-90	15-20	1	Knee extensors
		9-12	50-60	90-110	10-15	1	
		13-16	60-75	110-135	10-15	1	
Chest flys (seated)	90	1-4	30-40	30-36	15-20	1	Shoulder horizontal flexors
		5-8	40-50	36-45	15-20	1	Elbow extensors
		9-12	50-60	45-54	10-15	1	
		13-16	60-75	54-68	10-15	1	
Leg curl (seated)	45	1-4	30-40	13-18	15-20	1	Knee flexors
		5-8	40-50	18-22	15-20	1	
		9-12	50-60	22-27	10-15	1	
		13-16	60-75	27-34	10-15	1	
Lat pull-down	100	1-4	30-40	30-40	15-20	1	Shoulder extensors
		5-8	40-50	40-50	15-20	1	Elbow flexors
		9-12	50-60	50-60	10-15	1	
		13-16	60-75	60-75	10-15	1	
Shoulder press (seated)	50	1-4	30-40	15-20	15-20	1	Shoulder flexors and adductors
		5-8	40-50	20-25	15-20	1	
		9-12	50-60	25-30	10-15	1	
		13-16	60-75	30-38	10-15	1	
Heel (calf) raises (seated)	90	1-4	30-40	27-36	15-20	1	Ankle plantar flexors
		5-8	40-50	36-45	15-20	1	
		9-12	50-60	45-54	10-15	1	
		13-16	60-75	54-68	10-15	1	
Abdominal curl	—	1-4	—	Body weight	5-10	1 or 2	Trunk flexors
		5-8			10-15	1 or 2	
		9-12			15-20	1 or 2	
		13-16			20-25	1 or 2	

[a]Multijoint exercise machines are used for most exercises. Seated and lying (instead of standing) positions are recommended to stabilize the body while lifting. Do exercises in the order listed.

[b]1 lb = 0.45 kg.

[c]During first 2 wk, closely monitor and supervise workouts. Initial training phase lasts 8 wk.

[d]Intensity is gradually increased every 2 wk, only after client is able to do more than the prescribed number of repetitions at each target intensity.

SAMPLE LINEAR PERIODIZED RESISTANCE TRAINING PROGRAM FOR INTERMEDIATE LIFTER

Client Data

Age: 25 yr

Gender: Female

Body weight: 155 lb (70.4 kg)

Program goal: Muscle strength

Time commitment: 50-60 min per workout

Equipment: Variable resistance machines and free weights

Cycles: 3; each microcycle = 4 wk

Intensity: 70%-80% 1-RM

Repetitions: 8-12

Sets: 3

Rest: 1-2 min for 70% 1-RM; 2-3 min for 75%-80% 1-RM

Frequency: 3 days/wk, alternate days

Duration: 12 wk or longer

Exercise[a]	1-RM (lb)[b]	Cycle 1 wk 1-4			Cycle 2 wk 5-8			Cycle 3 wk 9-12			Sets	Muscle groups
		Int	Wt[b]	Rep	Int	Wt[b]	Rep	Int	Wt[b]	Rep		
Leg press	200	70	140	12	75	150	10	80	160	8	3	Hip extensors, knee extensors
Bench press[c]	100	70	70	12	75	75	10	80	80	8	3	Shoulder flexors and adductors, elbow extensors
Leg curl (lying)	80	70	55	12	75	60	10	80	65	8	3	Knee flexors
Lat pull-down	140	70	100	12	75	105	10	80	110	8	3	Shoulder extensors and adductors, elbow flexors
Dumbbell fly[c] (flat bench)	40	70	25	12	75	30	10	80	35	8	3	Shoulder flexors and adductors
Heel (calf) raise (standing)	160	70	110	12	75	120	10	80	130	8	3	Ankle plantar flexors
Abdominal curl	—									25	3	Trunk flexors
Arm curl[c] (incline bench)	40	70	25	12	75	30	10	80	35	8	3	Elbow flexors
Lateral raise (dumbbell)	25	70	15	12	75	15-20	10	80	20	8	3	Shoulder abductors
Triceps press-down	60	70	40	12	75	45	10	80	50	8	3	Elbow extensors
Hammer curl[c] (dumbbells)	40	70	25	12	75	30	10	80	35	8	3	Elbow flexors

Int = %1-RM; Wt = weight lifted; Rep = number of repetitions.

[a]Do exercises in order listed, using larger muscle groups first. Perform multijoint exercises before single-joint exercises. Other exercises that work the same muscle groups may be substituted to add variety to the program (see appendix C.4, Dynamic Resistance Training Exercises).

[b]1 lb = 0.45 kg; weight is to nearest 5 lb increment for most exercises.

[c]Two exercises are prescribed for each of the weaker muscle groups (shoulder flexors and elbow flexors) identified from client's strength assessment.

Lifter) is for a 25 yr old woman whose primary goal is to improve muscle strength. This client is an experienced weightlifter. Results from her 1-RM tests indicated that her upper body strength (particularly the shoulder flexor and forearm flexor muscle groups) is below average. Therefore, two exercises are prescribed for each of the weaker muscle groups. The strength of all other muscle groups is average or above average; therefore, only one exercise is prescribed for each of these muscle groups. Given her initial strength levels and weightlifting experience, the prescription is for three sets of each exercise; and the exercise intensity is set at 70% to 80% 1-RM to maximize the development of strength. The client completes about 8 to 12 repetitions at the prescribed intensity for each microcycle. She devotes 50 to 60 min, 3 days/wk, to her workouts.

The third example (see Sample Undulating Periodized Resistance Training Program for Body-builder) illustrates an advanced resistance training program developed for an experienced weightlifter (28 yr old male with superior strength) whose long-term goal is competitive bodybuilding. He engages in a high-volume UP training program. The intensity (70%-85% 1-RM) and moderate repetitions (6-12) vary systematically throughout each macro- and microcycle to maximize the development of muscle size. To achieve a high training volume, he performs three exercises for each muscle group and three or four sets of each exercise. To effectively overload the muscles, he performs the exercises for each muscle group consecutively (tri-sets) with little or no rest between the sets. He lifts weights 6 days/wk, splitting the routine so he is not exercising the same muscle groups on consecutive days. With this routine, each muscle group is exercised two times a week.

SAMPLE UNDULATING PERIODIZED RESISTANCE TRAINING PROGRAM FOR BODYBUILDER

Client Data

Age: 28 yr	*Microcycles:* 4; each microcycle = 1 wk
Gender: Male	*Intensity:* 70%-85% 1-RM
Body weight: 190 lb (86.2 kg)	*Repetitions:* 6-12
Program goal: Hypertrophy	*Sets:* 3 or 4
Time commitment: 90 min per workout	*Rest:* 1 min rest between tri-sets
Equipment: Free weights and exercise machines	*Frequency:* 6 days/wk, split routine
Mesocycles: 4; each mesocycle = 1 mo	*Duration:* 24 wk or longer

UP Mesocycles and Microcycles

	Intensity	Volume
MONTH 1		
Week 1	70% 1-RM	3 or 4 sets; 12 reps
Week 2	75% 1-RM	3 or 4 sets; 10 reps
Week 3	80% 1-RM	3 or 4 sets; 8 reps
Week 4	85% 1-RM	3 or 4 sets; 6 reps

	Intensity	Volume
MONTH 2		
Week 1	75% 1-RM	3 or 4 sets; 10 reps
Week 2	80% 1-RM	3 or 4 sets; 8 reps
Week 3	85% 1-RM	3 or 4 sets; 6 reps
Week 4	70% 1-RM	3 or 4 sets; 12 reps
MONTH 3		
Week 1	80% 1-RM	3 or 4 sets; 8 reps
Week 2	85% 1-RM	3 or 4 sets; 6 reps
Week 3	70% 1-RM	3 or 4 sets; 12 reps
Week 4	75% 1-RM	3 or 4 sets; 10 reps
MONTH 4		
Week 1	85% 1-RM	3 or 4 sets; 6 reps
Week 2	80% 1-RM	3 or 4 sets; 8 reps
Week 3	75% 1-RM	3 or 4 sets; 10 reps
Week 4	70% 1-RM	3 or 4 sets; 12 reps

Split Routine Using Tri-Sets

Exercises	1-RM (lb)[c]	Muscles
MONDAY AND THURSDAY[a]		
Chest[b]		
Flat bench press (barbell)	250	Pectoralis major (midsternal portion); triceps brachii
Incline dumbbell fly	80	Pectoralis major (clavicular portion); anterior deltoid
Decline bench press (barbell)	180	Pectoralis major (lower sternal portion)
Shoulders[b]		
Upright row (barbell)	140	Middle deltoid
Front dumbbell raises	80	Anterior deltoid
Posterior cable pull (horizontal plane)	100	Posterior deltoid
TUESDAY AND FRIDAY[a]		
Hips and thighs[a]		
First tri-set		
Squats (Smith machine)	300	Gluteus maximus; quadriceps femoris; upper hamstrings
Leg extension (machine)	150	Quadriceps femoris
Leg curl (standing, unilateral, machine)	90	Hamstrings (mid to lower portions)
Second tri-set		
Leg press (seated)	400	Gluteus maximus; quadriceps femoris; upper hamstrings
Leg curl (lying)	130	Hamstrings (mid to lower portions)
Glute-ham raise	—	Gluteus maximus; hamstrings
Legs and calves[b]		
Standing calf (heel) raise	250	Gastrocnemius; soleus
Ankle flexion exercise (seated)	90	Tibialis anterior

(continued)

Sample Undulating Periodized Resistance Training Program for Bodybuilder *(continued)*

Exercises	1-RM (lb)[c]	Muscles
Seated calf raise	180	Soleus; gastrocnemius
WEDNESDAY AND SATURDAY[a]		
Back[b]		
Lat pull-down (wide grip)	225	Latissimus dorsi (lateral portion); biceps brachii; brachialis
Seated row (narrow grip)	240	Latissimus dorsi (mid portion); biceps brachii; brachialis
Dumbbell row	90	Latissimus dorsi (mid portion); biceps brachii; brachialis
Elbow flexors[b]		
Standing barbell curl	130	Biceps brachii; brachialis; brachioradialis
Preacher curl (dumbbells)	100	Biceps brachii (mid portion); brachialis
Hammer curl (dumbbells)	80	Brachioradialis; brachialis
Elbow extensors[b]		
Lying triceps extension (barbell)	120	Triceps brachii (long head)
Triceps push-down (cables)	150	Triceps brachii (short and lateral heads)
Triceps pull-down with lateral flair (cables)	130	Triceps brachii (lateral head)

[a]Other exercises that work the same muscles may be substituted on the second day to add variety to the program (see appendix C.4, Dynamic Resistance Training Exercises).

[b]For tri-sets, the three exercises listed are performed consecutively without rest, then the tri-set is repeated for the prescribed number of sets for that muscle group (1 min rest between sets).

[c]1 lb = 0.45 kg.

Several excellent references deal with the design of advanced resistance training programs (Fleck and Kraemer 2014; Kraemer and Fleck 2007; National Strength and Conditioning Association 2016, 2017).

DESIGNING RESISTANCE TRAINING PROGRAMS FOR CHILDREN

Children and adolescents can safely participate in resistance training if special precautions and recommended guidelines are carefully followed. Because children are anatomically and physiologically immature, high-resistance training programs are not typically recommended for them. Most experts agree that to lessen the risk of injury (e.g., epiphyseal growth plate fractures) to developing bones and joints, exercise intensity should not exceed 80% 1-RM, which equates to 8 to 15 repetitions per set. Faigenbaum and colleagues (1999) reported that high-repetition–moderate-intensity training (one set, 13-RM to 15-RM) was more effective than low-repetition–high-intensity training (one set, 6-RM to 8-RM) for improving the strength and muscle endurance of children (5-12 yr) during the initial training phase (8 wk).

Strength gains in resistance-trained children result from neural adaptations (e.g., increased activation of motor units and coordination) rather than from hypertrophy (Guy and Micheli 2001). In addition, resistance training positively affects the bone mineral density of the femoral neck in adolescent girls ages 14 to 17 yr (Nichols, Sanborn, and Love 2001), and there appears to be a dose-response relationship between weight-bearing activity and bone health in this population (Ishikawa et al. 2013). Furthermore, experts recommend strength training for youth to develop an adequate strength foundation prior to power training (e.g., plyometrics) (Behm et al. 2017). There is no evidence that children lose flexibility when they resistance train (Guy and Micheli 2001). Resistance training is safe and beneficial for youth, especially when the established training guidelines are followed (see Youth Resistance Training Guidelines). These guidelines are based primarily on recommendations outlined in the Canadian Society for Exercise Physiology position paper on resistance training for children and adolescents (Behm et al. 2008) and the National Strength and Conditioning Association position paper on youth resistance training (Faigenbaum et al. 2009).

Youth Resistance Training Guidelines

- Provide qualified instruction and supervision.
- Provide an exercise environment that is safe and free of hazards.
- Teach clients about the benefits and risks of strength training.
- Design a comprehensive program that focuses on developing muscular fitness and motor skills.
- Begin each workout with a 5 to 10 min warm-up.
- Select 8 to 12 multijoint exercises for major muscle groups; include exercises for the abdominal muscles and lower back.
- Use equipment that is appropriate for the size, strength, and maturity of the child.
- Start with one or two sets of 8 to 15 repetitions with light to moderate load (~60% 1-RM) for each exercise.
- Slowly progress to three or four sets at 60% to 80% 1-RM, or 8-RM to 15-RM, depending on the child's needs and goals; as strength improves, increase the number of repetitions before increasing resistance.
- Increase resistance gradually and only when the child can perform the specified number of repetitions with good form.
- Reduce the resistance for prepubescent children who cannot perform a minimum of eight repetitions with good form.
- Prescribe low-repetition exercises (fewer than eight reps) for mature adolescents only.
- Focus on correct exercise technique (slow and smooth movements and breathing) instead of amount of weight lifted.
- Train two or three times per week on nonconsecutive days.
- Closely supervise the child in the event of a failed repetition.
- Monitor progress (e.g., use workout logs), listen to the child's concerns, and answer questions.
- Systematically vary the training program to keep it fresh and challenging by adding new exercises, changing the number of sets and repetitions, and incorporating calisthenics as well as exercises using elastic tubing and fitness balls.
- Focus on participation and provide positive reinforcement.

Adapted from Behm et al. 2008.

DESIGNING RESISTANCE TRAINING PROGRAMS FOR OLDER ADULTS

Resistance training provides many health benefits, especially for older adults. The primary goal of the resistance training program is to develop sufficient muscular fitness so that older adults may carry out activities of daily living (ADLs) without undue stress or fatigue and may retain their functional independence. To achieve these goals, age-related losses in muscle mass (**sarcopenia**) and muscle strength (**dynapenia**) must be counteracted. Experts agree that resistance training is the most effective mode of exercise to maintain and to improve strength and muscle mass in older adults (Garber et al. 2011; Peterson et al. 2010; Peterson and Gordon 2011; Romo-Perez, Schwingel, and Chodzko-Zajko 2011;

Tremblay et al. 2011). Candow and associates (2011) reported that 22 wk of whole-body resistance training (3 days/wk) was sufficient not only in attenuating age-related deficits in lean body tissue and upper and lower body strength of older (60-71 yr) men but also in realizing strength levels comparable to those of untrained, younger men.

Over the years, researchers have discovered that muscular strength in older adults can be improved by lifting 1, 2, or 3 days/wk (Taaffe et al. 1999), at low or high intensities (Vincent et al. 2002), and with either nonperiodized or UP programs (Hunter et al. 2001). Using results from meta-analyses of studies investigating resistance training and strength gains, Peterson and colleagues (2010, 2011) concluded that the higher the training volume, the greater the absolute and relative improvement in strength and lean body mass of older adults. In a more recent meta-analysis, Borde, Hortobagyi, and Granacher (2015) concurred that a dose-response relationship exists, with the largest effects for the longest training periods (50-53 wk). The most effective resistance training program for older adults appears to consist of two or three sessions a week of seven to nine repetitions of each exercise (two or three sets), at an intensity of 51% to 69% of 1-RM, with 60 to 120 sec rest between sets.

Muscle power (strength × speed of contraction) is a significant predictor of ability to perform ADLs. With aging, both strength and power decline because of atrophy of slow and fast muscle fibers. Muscle power declines at a relatively faster rate (3%-4% per yr after age 60) than strength (1%-2% per yr). Some experts suggest that resistance training of older persons should emphasize the development of power by using fast-velocity resistance exercise (Forbes, Little, and Candow 2012; Porter 2006). In fact, a recent meta-analysis indicates that fast-velocity resistance training is superior to traditional resistance training for increasing lower body muscle power in middle-aged and older adults (Straight et al. 2016). For fast-velocity exercise, the concentric phase of the exercise is performed as quickly as possible, and the eccentric phase should take about 2 sec.

In addition to increasing strength, power, and muscular endurance, resistance training may improve the performance of functional tasks such as lifting and reaching, rising from the floor or a chair to a standing position, stair climbing, and walking (Henwood and Taaffe 2003; Messier et al. 2000; Schot et al. 2003; Vincent et al. 2002). Also, the postural sway and balance of older, osteoarthritic adults were improved by participation in either long-term resistance training or aerobic walking (Messier et al. 2000). Muscle strength and power likely contribute to balance performance; however, a cause-and-effect relationship between muscle function and balance performance cannot yet be made (Orr 2010). Improved strength and balance may help prevent falls and injuries in older adults.

For older adults, the ACSM (Garber et al. 2011) recommends resistance training 2 days/wk at moderate intensity (40%-50% 1-RM; 10-15 reps) to improve strength and at a lower intensity (20%-50% 1-RM) to improve power. Although resistance training guidelines for older adults vary among organizations, the consensus is that older adults should exercise the major muscle groups of the body at least 2 days/wk on nonconsecutive days. Most suggest prescribing two or three sets of 8 to 10 different exercises at intensities ranging between 8-RM and 15-RM (Peterson and Gordon 2011; Romo-Perez, Schwingel, and Chodzko-Zajko 2011; Tremblay et al. 2011). As with your younger clients, the training volume needs to be varied and gradually increased over time (progression principle). For a detailed example of a 6 mo progressive resistance training program for healthy, older adults, see Peterson (2010) or Peterson and Gordon (2011).

The ACSM (2018) recommends moderate-intensity (rating of perceived exertion [RPE] = 5 or 6) to vigorous-intensity (RPE = 7 or 8) exercise at least 2 days/wk to improve the muscular fitness of older adults; prescribe one to three sets of 8 to 12 repetitions for 8 to 10 different exercises each workout.

In addition to the general guidelines for designing resistance training programs for healthy adults (see table 7.2), the following guidelines and precautions are recommended for older adults:

- During the first few weeks of training, use minimal resistance for all exercises.
- Instruct older adults about proper weightlifting and breathing techniques.
- Trained exercise leaders who have experience working with older adults should closely supervise and monitor each client's weightlifting techniques and resistance training program during the first few exercise sessions.
- Prescribe multijoint, rather than single-joint, exercises.
- Use exercise machines to stabilize body position and control the range of joint motion. Avoid using free weights with older adults.
- Each exercise session should last approximately 20 to 30 min and should not exceed 60 min.
- Older adults should rate their perceived exertion during exercise. Ratings of perceived exertion should be 5 or 6 (moderate) or 7 or 8 (vigorous).
- Prescribe at least two sets of 8 to 15 repetitions for 8 to 10 different exercises for the major muscle groups.
- Train at least 2 days/wk, allowing at least 48 hr of rest between the exercise workouts.

- Discourage clients with arthritis from lifting weights when they are actively experiencing joint pain or inflammation.
- When clients are returning to resistance training following a layoff of more than 3 wk, they should start with a low resistance that is less than 50% of the weight they were lifting prior to the layoff.

COMMON QUESTIONS ABOUT RESISTANCE TRAINING

Because of the popularity of resistance training, there is an overwhelming amount of information about the subject in professional journals as well as in popular magazines and newspapers. This section presents common questions that exercise professionals may have about designing resistance training programs and addresses questions and concerns your clients may pose.

PROGRAM DESIGN

There are numerous ways to make small alterations to resistance training programs. Considerable deliberation exists, even among fitness professionals, whether or not these variations offer any meaningful benefit over traditional weightlifting. This section addresses the efficacy of some of the most commonly applied variations to traditional resistance training programs.

Which resistance training method, nonperiodized or periodized, is better?

The answer depends on the client's initial training status and goals. During the first stage (4 wk) of resistance training, both nonperiodized and periodized multiple-set programs increase the muscular fitness of untrained and novice lifters (Baker, Wilson, and Carlyon 1994); however, a varied training stimulus is needed for continued improvements in muscle strength and endurance during long-term (>4 wk) training (Fleck 1999; Marx et al. 2001). Kell (2011) reported that periodized training (12 wk; 3 or 4 days/wk) significantly improved the strength of men and women who had nonperiodized training experience. In contrast, nonperiodized, LP, and UP resistance training programs were equally effective at improving the physical function and health (systolic blood pressure, body composition, maximal strength, functional capacity, balance confidence, and blood biomarkers) of untrained older adults (Conlon et al. 2016). Periodized training is highly recommended for intermediate and advanced lifters; nonperiodized training may be more appropriate for clients just starting a weightlifting program or who are primarily interested in maintaining strength and muscle tone. Varying workouts daily (UP training) helps prevent boredom and maintain exercise compliance.

Which periodization model is best?

The answer depends on the client's training goal. One research team conducted two studies to assess the effectiveness of different types of periodized programs (LP, RLP, and daily UP) for increasing the strength and local muscular endurance of young, resistance-trained women and men (Rhea et al. 2002, 2003b). The researchers reported that daily UP was superior to LP for developing the strength of young men who trained 3 days/wk for 12 wk. For endurance gains, there were no statistically significant differences across the three plans. Analysis of effect sizes, however, indicated that RLP was more effective than either LP or daily UP for increasing the muscular endurance of women and men who trained 2 days/wk for 15 wk. Other researchers also noted that daily UP programs are more effective than LP programs for increasing strength, muscle endurance, and muscle thickness in untrained males (Miranda et al. 2011; Simao et al. 2012). However, a more recent meta-analysis revealed no significant differences in the effectiveness of LP versus UP on upper or lower body strength (Harries, Lubans, and Callister 2015).

Is single-set training as effective as multiple-set training?

Some research suggests that single-set training is as effective as multiple-set training for increasing the strength of untrained individuals during the initial stage of resistance training. However, the majority of recent research on this topic indicates a dose-response relationship for training volume and strength gains. Ribeiro, Schoenfeld, Pina, et al. (2015) reported greater strength gains in the chest press (26.6% vs. 20.3%) and knee extension (23.9%

vs. 16.2%) when three sets were executed compared with a single-set resistance training program (12 wk) for older women. Likewise, Radaelli and colleagues (2015) reported a dose-response relationship for one, three, and five sets for strength gains, muscular endurance, and hypertrophy in previously untrained men who lifted three times a week for 6 mo. Finally, a recent meta-analysis by Ralston and associates (2017) concluded that moderate and high weekly sets were superior to low weekly sets for producing strength increases in novice, intermediate, and advanced lifters.

Is it better to train using fixed-form or free-form exercise machines?

Both fixed-form and free-form resistance exercise machines may be used to improve muscular fitness. Fixed-form devices limit the range of motion and plane of motion during the resistance exercise (e.g., a leg extension machine that allows flexion and extension in sagittal plane only). In contrast, free-form exercise machines allow movement in multiple planes (e.g., chest fly machine that allows press or fly movements in horizontal and oblique planes). One study compared the effects of 16 wk of fixed-form training and free-form training on strength and balance of sedentary men and women (Spennewyn 2008). The improvement in overall strength of the free-form training group (116%) was significantly greater than that of the fixed-form training group (58%). Also, overall balance performance improved 245% and 49%, respectively, for the free-form and fixed-form training groups. In contrast, Balachandran and colleagues (2016) recently reported that although both standing cable training and seated machine training improved physical performance in adults ≥ 65 yr, there were no significant differences between training interventions.

Are abdominal training devices more effective than traditional calisthenic exercises for strengthening abdominal muscles?

There is little scientific evidence justifying manufacturers' claims that abdominal training devices improve strength more effectively than simply performing calisthenic exercises without these devices (e.g., curl-ups). These devices purportedly overload the abdominal muscles by adding resistance (e.g., abdominal belts) and isolate the abdominal musculature by supporting the head, neck, or back. However, studies using electromyography (EMG) show that exercising with these devices does not increase the muscle activity of the abdominal prime movers (rectus abdominis and external abdominal oblique muscles) more than exercising without the devices (American Council on Exercise 1997; Demont et al. 1999; Francis et al. 2001). Although research does not support the use of abdominal trainers, they can add variety to conventional abdominal exercises and may even improve some clients' adherence to the abdominal exercise regimen.

To progressively overload (increase the training stimulus of) the abdominal muscles, you can have your clients modify body position (e.g., perform abdominal curls on a decline bench rather than on a flat bench), hold a weight across the chest, or change arm positions. Abdominal exercises become more difficult as the arms move from along the sides to behind the head to overhead.

How can stability balls, medicine balls, resistance bands, and suspension systems be used to improve a client's fitness?

Stability balls, medicine balls, resistance bands, and suspension training can be used in a variety of ways to improve muscular strength, power, core stability, flexibility, and static and dynamic balance. For example, performing a plank from a suspended position using the TRX suspension system resulted in greater abdominal muscle activation than a plank done on the floor (Byrne et al. 2014), and performing a pike on instability devices elicited higher percentages of MVC than when done on stable ground (Snarr et al. 2016). Calisthenic exercises such as abdominal crunches and back extensions can be performed while clients are lying on the ball; dumbbell exercises can be performed while they are lying supine or prone or sitting on the ball. Stability and medicine ball exercises are used to train the body as a linked system, starting with the core muscle groups. Use of resistance bands and tubing allows the individual to train the muscles with exercises that simulate the movement patterns of a specific sport. For more information about stability ball, resistance band, and suspension training, see Goldenberg and Twist (2016), Page and Ellenbecker (2011), and Dawes (2017), respectively.

Does performing the curl-up on an unstable surface increase the challenge for the abdominal muscles?

Another way to increase the training stimulus for developing abdominal muscular fitness is to perform curl-up exercises on an unstable surface. Vera-Garcia, Grenier, and McGill (2000) studied the EMG activity of the abdominal muscles (upper and lower rectus abdominis and internal and external abdominal obliques) during four types of curl-ups: curl-ups on a stable bench, curl-ups on a gym ball with feet flat on the floor, curl-ups on a gym ball with feet on a bench, and curl-ups on a wobble board. Curl-ups performed with instability devices (gym ball and wobble board) doubled the EMG activity of the rectus abdominis and quadrupled the activity of the external oblique muscles. In terms of maintaining whole-body stability, the curl-up on the gym ball with the feet flat on the floor was the most demanding, as evidenced by increased EMG activity in all the abdominal muscles. Curl-ups with the upper body supported on the wobble board produced the most EMG activity in the upper rectus abdominis. Although exercising on an unstable surface increases abdominal muscle activity and coactivation, it also increases loads on the spine. In rehabilitation programs, curl-ups on movable surfaces should be used only with clients who can tolerate higher spinal loads (Vera-Garcia, Grenier, and McGill 2000).

What is whole-body vibration training and how does it work?

Over 50 yr ago, scientists explored the idea of using vibration loading to prevent bone mineral loss and muscle atrophy in astronauts during space travel. Today **whole-body vibration (WBV)** exercise devices can be found in fitness and rehabilitation centers throughout the world. WBV exercise involves positioning the body on a motorized platform that produces vibratory signals at a set frequency and amplitude. Frequency is measured in hertz (Hz) and usually ranges from 20 to 60 Hz. At 35 Hz, for example, the targeted muscles will contract and relax 35 times per second. Amplitude, or the vertical displacement of the platform during vibrations, is measured in millimeters. Intensity is a direct function of the frequency and amplitude. These oscillating vibrations are transmitted to the weight-bearing muscles and bones. The body parts in direct contact with the surface of the platform will receive the greatest amount of vibration. Typically, the client stands on the platform holding the handles and performs lower body exercises such as squats, lunges, calf raises, or light jumping. Alternatively, the arms or feet may be placed on the platform for upper body and abdominal exercises such as push-ups, triceps dips, side support, abdominal planks, and static stretches.

Vibration devices vary in how the oscillating signals are delivered to the body. For synchronous WBV devices, the vibration is applied to the right and left foot simultaneously, whereas side-alternating models apply the vibration sequentially to the right and left foot. In the fitness setting, low-magnitude vibratory platforms are usually used. For these devices, the magnitude of acceleration due to gravity ($1 g = 9.81 m·sec^{-2}$) is less than 1 g. High-magnitude devices provide an acceleration greater than 1 g and may cause musculoskeletal and neural damage, posing a health risk (Abercromby et al. 2007; Judex and Rubin 2010). These high-intensity WBV devices are not regulated by the Food and Drug Administration and are more commonly used in clinical rehabilitation settings. WBV exercise, even at low intensities, is contraindicated for pregnant women or individuals with thrombosis, seizures, pacemakers, or other electronic implants (Albasini, Krause, and Rembitzki 2010).

The frequency, intensity, and duration of WBV sessions used in training studies vary greatly. Frequency of training sessions varies between one and seven per wk and their duration can last from 6 wk to 18 mo. The peak acceleration of the vibration platform is usually less than 1 g, with intensity of the oscillating signals varying from 10 to 60 Hz (frequency) and 0.05 to 8 mm (amplitude). The vibration signal is delivered in bouts lasting anywhere from 30 sec to 10 min (Lau et al. 2011). The disparity in training protocols and lack of standardization of methods complicate the synthesis, application, and ability to generalize research findings. To address this issue, the International Society of Musculoskeletal and Neuronal Interactions developed a set of recommendations for describing methods used in WBV training intervention studies (Rauch et al. 2010).

Vibration loading produces small changes in muscle length that stimulate a **tonic vibration reflex**. This reflex activates muscle spindles and alpha motor neurons, causing the muscles to contract (Torvinen et al. 2002). Torvinen and colleagues examined the long-term (4 mo) effects of vibration training combined with unloaded static and dynamic exercises on strength, power, and balance. They noted that the greatest relative gains in isometric leg extension strength and in leg power (measured by the vertical jump) occurred after the first 2 mo of training. Gains in strength and power during the last 2 mo of training were minimal. Thus, it appears that vibration training elicits a neural response and adaptation (recruitment of motor units through the activation of muscle spindles) similar to that observed during the early stages of conventional resistance training. When compared against a standard fitness program (combined aerobic and resistance training) and conventional resistance training (exercise machines) in women, vibration training during unloaded static and dynamic exercises produced similar gains in isometric, isokinetic, and dynamic strength over 3 to 4 mo (Delecluse, Roelants, and Verschueren 2003; Roelants et al. 2004). However, Abercromby and colleagues (2007) reported that more than 10 min a day of whole-body vibration training may have adverse health effects. Vibration training warrants further study, especially to determine its applicability in improving strength, flexibility, and possibly even balance in elderly individuals in order to prevent falls, as well as to identify any long-term potential health hazards for this form of training.

Is whole-body vibration training as effective as traditional resistance training for improving musculoskeletal fitness of my clients?

Over the past two decades, research has examined the potential of using whole-body vibration as a method for improving muscular strength, explosive power, bone density, body composition, balance, mobility, and postural control (McBride et al. 2010). Additionally, the usefulness of WBV for attenuating muscle soreness due to eccentric exercise and for reducing low back pain has been addressed. Only studies dealing with effects of WBV on musculoskeletal parameters are summarized in this section. Findings relative to body composition, balance, mobility, postural control, and low back pain are addressed in later chapters. Much of the research focuses on older adults, in light of age-related declines in muscle strength (dynapenia), muscle mass (sarcopenia), and bone mineral (osteoporosis). For specific guidelines for using WBV in the treatment of low back pain, osteoporosis and osteopenia, balance disorders, sarcopenia, and dynapenia, see Albasini, Krause, and Rembitzki (2010).

For older clients, the addition of WBV to resistance training augments the positive effects of resistance training on muscle strength (Bemben et al. 2010; Bogaerts et al. 2009) and muscle hypertrophy (Machado et al. 2010). Vibration training is suggested as a "skilling up" activity in older people with low function until they are able to perform conventional exercises (Rogan et al. 2015). In some cases, WBV training is even more effective than resistance training alone for increasing muscle strength and power of older women (Lau et al. 2011; von Stengel et al. 2012). Medium frequency and medium duration (40 Hz × 360 sec) was more effective than low frequency and long duration (20 Hz × 720 sec) or high frequency and short duration (60 Hz × 240 sec) for improving the isokinetic knee extension of older adults (Wei et al. 2016).

For younger, well-trained adults, supplementing resistance training with WBV does not augment strength gains or corticospinal excitability induced by resistance training alone (Artero, Espada-Fuentes, et al. 2012; Weier and Kidgell 2012). WBV, however, does have an additive effect on muscular power in well-trained athletes (Fort et al. 2012; Ronnestad et al. 2012).

The effects of WBV training on bone mineral density (BMD) vary. In a study of older postmenopausal women, von Stengel, Kemmler, Bebenek, and colleagues (2011) reported that the BMD of the lumbar spine increases significantly following 12 mo of WBV training. In contrast, others have shown little or no change in BMD of the femur, spine, and hip with WBV training. In fact, a number of review articles and meta-analyses of published literature concluded that WBV training does not lead to a clinically important increase in BMD of postmenopausal women (Cheung and Giangregorio 2012; Lau et al. 2011; von Stengel, Kemmler, Engelke, et al. 2011; Wysocki et al. 2011; Xu, Lombardi et al. 2016). At this time, WBV should not replace usual treatments for osteoporosis; however, further research should examine the efficacy of using WBV as an adjunct therapy for osteoporosis, sarcopenia, and dynapenia.

Is kettlebell training a safe and effective method to enhance my clients' muscular fitness?

In the United States, kettlebell exercise has emerged as a popular mode of exercise training with purported claims of improved muscular strength and endurance as well as cardiorespiratory fitness and body composition. Otto and colleagues (2012) reported that 6 wk of **kettlebell training** significantly improves the muscular strength (1-RM back squat) and power (1-RM power clean) of healthy young men; however, traditional resistance training (weightlifting) produces greater improvements in strength compared with kettlebell training. Likewise, Lake and Lauder (2012) noted that 6 wk of kettlebell training (12 min bouts; 30 sec exercise, 30 sec rest using 12 kg [BW <70 kg] and 16 kg [BW >70 kg] kettlebells) produces a 9.8% increase in maximum strength (1-RM half-squat) and a 19.8% increase in explosive strength (height of vertical jump) in young men.

Because of the unique shape of kettlebells, the client needs to learn how to control and stabilize the weight of the kettlebell during exercise. Thus, some kettlebell exercises are well suited for functional training of strength and stability for carrying a suitcase or grocery bag (Liebenson 2011). For an overview of the effects of kettlebell training on strength, power, and aerobic fitness, as well as the biomechanics of this unique mode of muscular fitness training, see the review by Beardsley and Contreras (2014).

Given that kettlebell exercises involve a lot of swinging and bending movements, is kettlebell exercise contraindicated for clients with neck and low back pain?

Jay and colleagues (2011) investigated the efficacy of using kettlebell training to improve trunk extensor strength and to lessen low back and neck pain of adults engaging in occupations with a high prevalence of musculoskeletal pain symptoms. The training group performed full-body ballistic kettlebell exercises, 3 days/wk for 8 wk. Compared with a control group, kettlebell training reduced pain in the neck and shoulders (−2.1 points) and low back (−1.4 points). The training group also showed a significant increase in trunk extensor strength. Although an isolated lumbar extension generates a greater level of lumbar fatigue, kettlebell swings are still an effective method for strengthening the lumbar extensors (Edinborough, Fisher, and Steele 2016).

McGill and Marshall (2012) measured spinal compression and shear loads during kettlebell swings. This exercise creates a hip-hinge squat pattern with cycles of rapid muscle activation and relaxation for the low back extensors (50% MVC [maximum voluntary contraction]) and gluteal muscles (80% MVC) when using a 16 kg kettlebell. Unlike the anterior shear produced during traditional lower body weightlifting exercises, kettlebell swings create a posterior shear of the L4 vertebrae on the L5 vertebrae. This observation lends support to anecdotal reports that kettlebell exercise may be useful in restoring and improving low back health and function (McGill and Marshall 2012).

CLIENT CONCERNS

This section poses typical questions that clients have for their fitness professionals regarding strength training and muscle hypertrophy.

Is it OK to lift weights every day?

During weightlifting, you are exercising your muscles at greater than normal workloads, producing microscopic tears in the muscle cells and connective tissues. Your body responds by producing new muscle proteins, which causes muscle growth and increased strength. For these changes to occur, you need to rest the exercised muscles between workouts. Most people show substantial improvements in strength when they lift weights every other day, just two or three times a week. If you lift weights every day, you run the risk of overtraining your muscles. Overtraining may cause muscle strains, tendinitis, bursitis, and other muscle and joint injuries. Experienced weightlifters who work out every day split their exercise routine so they do not exercise the same muscle groups on consecutive days. A split routine reduces the risk of excessive muscle soreness and overuse injuries if you lift weights every day.

Can I use calisthenic exercises like push-ups and pull-ups to improve my strength?

You can use calisthenic exercises to increase your strength. Exercise professionals often prescribe push-ups and pull-ups in addition to free weight and machine exercises to strengthen the chest, arm, and back muscles. When you do calisthenics, your body weight provides the resistance. If you are unable to lift your body weight, you will need to modify the calisthenic exercise. For example, doing push-ups with your body weight supported by your knees and hands is easier than doing standard push-ups with your body fully extended and your weight supported by your hands and feet. As your strength improves, you may increase the difficulty of the push-up by placing your hands wider than shoulder-width apart.

If you are unable to lift your body weight, you can modify pull-ups by using a spotter or resistance band. As you pull up, assist your movement by extending your knees as the spotter supports your lower legs or ankles. Alternatively, stretching a resistance band from the bar to your knees or feet can help propel you upward during a pull-up. To increase the difficulty of a pull-up, place your hands wider than shoulder-width apart and use an overhand (pronated) grip instead of an underhand (supinated) grip.

I have followed my exercise prescription closely, but over the last several weeks I haven't seen any change in my strength. What should I do?

At the beginning of your program, your strength gains were dramatic and rapid because your initial strength level was less than it is now. As your muscles adapt to the training stimulus, you may reach a plateau, or a point where you can't seem to improve further. It may be helpful if you periodically alter the training stimulus more frequently (weekly or even daily) by changing your combination of intensity, repetitions, and sets (ask your personal trainer about a periodized program). For example, if you are presently doing high-intensity–low-repetition exercises during each workout, you may want to decrease your intensity (from 80% to 70% 1-RM) and increase your repetitions (from 6-8 to 10-12) for several days. Selecting different exercises for the muscle groups may also help.

Will I become muscle bound and lose flexibility if I lift weights?

It is a common misconception that resistance training decreases joint flexibility. Studies of elite bodybuilders and powerlifters indicate that these athletes have excellent flexibility. Resistance training has been shown to improve or at least preserve flexibility in young men and women (Ribeiro, Campos-Filho et al. 2017). One study showed that resistance training

actually increased the flexibility of elderly women, and training three times a week resulted in greater hip flexion than twice a week (Carneiro et al. 2015). The key to remaining flexible during resistance training is to perform each exercise throughout the entire range of motion. Also, statically stretching the muscle groups after each workout may help you maintain flexibility.

Will resistance training help me lose weight and fat?

Resistance training positively alters your body composition and preserves your lean body tissues. Although your body weight may not change, your lean body mass (muscle and bone) increases and your body fat decreases. Given that muscle tissue is more metabolically active (burns more calories) than fat tissue, the increase in muscle size and lean body mass helps maintain your resting metabolic rate when you are on a weight loss diet. Exercise science and nutrition professionals recommend using resistance training combined with aerobic exercise to maximize the loss of body fat and to maintain lean body tissues.

Will my strength improve if I train aerobically at the same time that I am resistance training?

If you concurrently participate in aerobic and resistance training, your muscle growth and strength improvement may be lessened because of the increased energy demands and protein requirements of endurance training. In a meta-analysis of studies addressing this question, Wilson and associates (2012) reported that doing resistance training concurrently with running significantly lessens strength gains and hypertrophy. The frequency and duration of endurance training were negatively related to hypertrophy, strength, and power. However, recent research suggests that concurrent training does not necessarily interfere with muscular strength and hypertrophy (Murach and Bagley 2016). The type and sequence of training might moderate any interference effect. For example, combining HIT with resistance training did not diminish knee extensor or elbow flexor strength gains in premenopausal women training for 8 wk compared with those who participated only in resistance training (Gentil et al. 2017). Additionally, there is some evidence that performing resistance training before aerobic training during concurrent sessions aids in retaining muscle strength (Alves et al. 2016; Murlasits, Kneffel, and Thalib 2017). Although the potential interference is an important consideration for competitive bodybuilders and power athletes, your decision to participate in both forms of training depends on your overall exercise program goal. If your goal is improved health or weight loss, experts recommend including both aerobic and resistance training in your program.

Are protein and amino acid supplements necessary to maximize muscle growth and strength during resistance training?

Although the protein needs of resistance-trained individuals (1.6-1.8 g·kg⁻¹ each day) are higher than the recommended dietary allowance for inactive individuals (0.8 g·kg⁻¹ each day), for most individuals, a well-balanced diet containing 12% to 25% protein will meet increased protein needs during resistance training. However, if your goal is to augment muscle hypertrophy and strength gains beyond those produced from resistance training alone, whole protein or amino acid supplementation, consumed close to the time you engage in resistance exercise, may dramatically enhance the acute anabolic response to the exercise (Hayes and Cribb 2008). There is a synergistic relationship between resistance training and protein intake that triggers muscle protein synthesis and muscle hypertrophy (Guimaraes-Ferreira et al. 2014). According to a review by Stark and colleagues (2012), pre- and postworkout protein supplementation increases lean mass, muscle hypertrophy, strength, physical performance, and recovery.

The timing of protein intake is critical for optimizing muscle growth in response to resistance training. In a frequently cited study of elderly men who resistance trained over 12 wk, those who took a protein-carbohydrate supplement immediately after exercise (within 5 min) had greater gains in muscle hypertrophy, lean body mass, and muscular strength than those who ingested the supplement 2 hr after the training session (Esmarck et al. 2001).

What types of protein and amino supplements are most effective for augmenting muscle and strength development in response to resistance training?

The type of protein consumed may influence the anabolic response to resistance training. Whey protein supplements (i.e., >80% protein concentrates or >90% protein isolates) are widely used among athletes to increase muscle mass. Whey protein supplements are the richest source of branched-chain amino acids, particularly leucine, which is a regulator of muscle protein synthesis (Hayes and Cribb 2008). In a study comparing the effects of whey protein and casein supplements in athletic individuals engaging in a 10 wk resistance training program, the group taking whey protein isolates (1.5 g·kg⁻¹·day⁻¹) had a fivefold better gain in fat-free mass and better gains in strength compared with the group taking an equivalent daily dose of casein supplements (Cribb et al. 2006). The optimal postworkout supplement for protein synthesis provides at least 3 g of leucine per serving, combined with a fast-acting carbohydrate such as maltodextrin or glucose; the preworkout supplement should combine dextrose with essential amino acids (Stark et al. 2012).

Will creatine supplements enhance strength and muscle size during resistance training?

According to the International Society for Sports Nutrition, creatine monohydrate is an effective ergogenic supplement for increasing lean body mass and high-intensity exercise capacity in athletes (Kreider et al. 2010). Over 300 studies have tested the effects of creatine supplementation on performance. Overall, the data suggest that creatine supplementation can improve the performance of high-intensity exercise lasting less than 30 sec (Branch 2003; Rawson and Clarkson 2003). Studies demonstrate that creatine supplementation combined with resistance training increases muscular strength, body mass, fat-free mass, muscle fiber size, and training volume in healthy young adults as well as in older women and men (Brose, Parise, and Tarnopolsky 2003; Cribb et al. 2007; Nissen and Sharp 2003). However, differences in skeletal muscle morphology may affect hypertrophy responses (i.e., changes in lean body mass, fiber-specific hypertrophy, and contractile protein content) to resistance training (Cribb et al. 2007). Creatine supplements increase muscle creatine, but there is much interindividual variability in the response (Rawson and Clarkson 2003). Theoretically, an increase in muscle creatine enhances training volume and decreases the amount of recovery time needed between sets and exercises. The increased training stimulus improves the physiological adaptation to resistance training for some individuals (i.e., they experience a greater gain in muscle mass and strength).

In addition, researchers have compared the separate and combined effects of creatine monohydrate and whey protein supplementation on strength and muscle hypertrophy improvements with resistance training. After 10 or 11 wk of resistance training, both creatine and whey protein supplements resulted in significant improvements in strength compared with values in a control group. However, the addition of creatine monohydrate (0.1-0.3 g·kg^{-1}·day^{-1}) to the whey protein supplement (1.5 g·kg^{-1}·day^{-1}) produced much greater gains in body weight, lean body mass, and muscle hypertrophy than whey protein alone (Cribb, Williams, and Hayes 2007; Cribb et al. 2007). Thus, if the goal of the resistance training program is to maximize gains in muscle mass and body weight along with strength improvement, the addition of creatine monohydrate to a whey protein supplement is recommended (Hayes and Cribb 2008). In addition to creatine monohydrate, other creatine forms are now being promoted as potential ergogenic aids. For a summary of these other creatine forms, see the review by Andres and colleagues (2017).

Is it safe to take creatine supplements?

Creatine is a widely studied supplement. Although anecdotal reports associate creatine supplementation with muscle cramping, gastrointestinal distress, soft tissue injuries, and impaired renal function, the available evidence from controlled studies indicates that creatine is safe when taken in recommended doses (Andres et al. 2017; Cooper et al. 2012). In a recent review that cites policy statements from several food safety agencies, Andres and colleagues (2017) concluded that a 3 g·day^{-1} intake of creatine is unlikely to pose any health risk, and even much higher doses associated with creatine loading (5-10 g·day^{-1}) have been used with no adverse effects. However, they recommend that people with impaired kidney function, pregnant or breastfeeding women, and children obtain medical advice before supplementing with creatine. Similarly, Cooper and associates (2012) concluded that creatine supplementation appears to be safe, but they cautioned that the effects of prolonged use are still largely unknown.

Do β-hydroxy-β-methylbutyrate (HMB)

supplements increase lean body mass and muscle strength?

β-hydroxy-β-methylbutyrate (HMB) is a metabolite of the amino acid leucine. HMB has a potent anticatabolic effect on skeletal muscle by inhibiting muscle protein breakdown and enhancing protein synthesis (Zanchi et al. 2011). HMB also reduces muscle damage associated with resistance training. In a meta-analysis of dietary supplements, Nissen and Sharp (2003) reported that HMB is one of only two supplements (the other being creatine) that significantly increases the lean body mass and muscular strength of individuals engaging in resistance training. Several double-blind, placebo-controlled studies were all in agreement that HMB was effective at increasing lean mass and strength in trained individuals during a 12 wk supplementation and strength training period (Ferreira et al. 2013, 2015; Lowery et al. 2016; Wilson et al. 2014). Furthermore, these different investigators all discovered that HMB appears to attenuate markers of muscle damage (e.g., creatine kinase) during periods of overreaching or intense training (Ferreira et al. 2013, 2015; Lowery et al. 2016; Wilson et al. 2014).

Studies have examined the effect of combining HMB with creatine (Jowko, Ostaszewski, and Jank 2001; O'Connor and Crowe 2007) or whey protein (Kraemer et al. 2015; Shirato et al. 2016), with varying results. Over a 3 wk strength training program, Jowko, Ostaszewski, and Jank (2001) found that a group taking the HMB-creatine combination had greater gains in strength and lean body mass than participants taking only creatine or only HMB. In contrast, O'Connor and Crowe (2007) reported that neither HMB alone or in combination with creatine was effective at increasing strength, power, or lean mass of trained athletes over a 6 wk training period. The combination of HMB with whey protein offered no benefit over HMB alone or whey protein alone at inhibiting muscle strength loss and soreness or decreasing muscle damage markers following a bout of eccentric exercise (Shirato et al. 2016). However, Kraemer and colleagues (2015) reported that the recovery benefits of whey protein are enhanced with the addition of HMB. Compared with whey protein only, the HMB-whey combination resulted in reductions in markers of muscle damage (creatine kinase and interleukin-6) induced by 3 consecutive days of intense resistance exercise.

EFFECTS OF RESISTANCE TRAINING PROGRAMS

Resistance training improves muscular fitness by increasing strength, muscular endurance, and power. This section addresses the morphological, biochemical, and neurological effects of resistance training.

MORPHOLOGICAL EFFECTS OF RESISTANCE TRAINING ON THE MUSCULOSKELETAL SYSTEM

Resistance training leads to morphological adaptations in skeletal muscles and bone. Structural changes in muscle fibers account for a large portion of the strength gains resulting from resistance training. Increases in bone mineral content and bone density improve bone health. The following questions deal with these adaptations.

What is exercise-induced muscle hypertrophy?

One effect of strength training is an increase in the size of the muscle tissue. This adaptation, known as **exercise-induced hypertrophy**, results from an increase in the total amount of contractile protein, the number and size of myofibrils per fiber, and the amount of connective tissue surrounding the muscle fibers (Goldberg et al. 1975). With heavy resistance training, fast (type II) muscle fibers show a twofold greater increase in size than slow (type I) fibers (Kosek et al. 2006). An increase in protein synthesis and myogenic satellite cell proliferation are two major processes leading to hypertrophy. Although these two processes are initiated immediately following a client's first bout of resistance training exercise, it typically takes 4 to 6 wk of intensive training to observe a measurable amount of hypertrophy in untrained adults (Seynnes, de Boer, and Narici 2007). For more information on how resistance training influences gene and protein synthesis leading to muscle hypertrophy, see the review by McGlory, Devries, and Phillips (2017).

Is it possible to increase the number of muscle fibers by resistance training?

Heavy resistance training has been reported to produce an increase in the number of muscle fibers (i.e., hyperplasia) in animals due to longitudinal splitting and satellite cell proliferation (Antonio and Gonyea 1993; Edgerton 1970; Gonyea, Ericson, and Bonde-Petersen 1977). Such processes, however, have not been clearly demonstrated in human skeletal muscle tissue (Taylor and Wilkinson 1986; Tesch 1988). Although some data suggest that human skeletal muscle has the potential to increase muscle fiber number (Alway et al. 1989; Sjostrom et al. 1992), hyperplasia probably contributes less than 5% to overall muscle growth in response to heavy resistance training (Kraemer, Fleck, and Evans 1996). The major factor contributing to exercise-induced hypertrophy for humans, apparently, is an increase in the size of existing muscle fibers.

Does resistance training alter muscle fiber type from slow-twitch to fast-twitch?

One way to classify muscle fibers is by identifying the myosin heavy chain isoforms present in individual fibers. Three different isoforms of myosin heavy chain (MHC) proteins are MHC I, MHC IIA, and MHC IIX (formerly called type IIB). Pure muscle fibers contain only one type of isoform. Hybrid muscle fibers contain a mix of MHC I and MHC IIA or MHC IIA and MHC IIX. MHC I fibers are the slowest contracting fibers, and MHC IIX are the fastest contracting fibers; the contractile speed of hybrid fibers is somewhere between these two (Andersen and Aagaard 2010; Harridge 2007). Heavy resistance training decreases the expression of MHC IIX and simultaneously increases the expression of MHC IIA fibers, but MHC I fibers are relatively unaffected (Fry 2004; Andersen and Aagaard 2000). Thus, strength training appears to affect only the relative amount and size of MHC IIA and IIX fast fibers, with no change in the contractile characteristics of MHC I slow fibers (Andersen and Aagaard 2010).

Is the relationship between muscle size and strength the same for men and women?

Muscle strength is directly related to the cross-sectional area of the muscle tissue. Ikai and Fukunaga

(1968) noted that the static strength per unit of cross-sectional area of the elbow flexors was similar for young men and women. These values ranged between 4.5 and 8.9 kg·cm²; average values were 6.2 and 6.7 kg·cm² for women and men, respectively. Cureton and colleagues (1988) also reported that the dynamic strength per unit of cross-sectional area (CSA) was similar for men and women. Posttraining ratios of elbow flexor or extensor strength to upper arm CSA were 1.65 kg·cm² and 1.85 kg·cm², respectively, for men and women. Likewise, the posttraining ratios for leg strength to thigh CSA were 1.10 kg·cm² for men and 0.90 kg·cm² for women.

Is there a limit to the degree of hypertrophy in response to resistance training?

A ceiling, or plateau, effect appears to exist in the degree of hypertrophy attainable. As mentioned previously, the two major processes responsible for muscle hypertrophy are protein synthesis and satellite cell proliferation. This ceiling effect may be related to the client's ability to activate the pool of satellite cells and to add new nuclei to the muscle cells. The amount of cellular hypertrophy for moderate and extreme responders following a 16 wk resistance training program typically ranges between 25% to 75% of the cross-sectional area of the muscle tissue (Petrella et al. 2008). In light of the amount of interindividual variation in the degree of hypertrophy in response to resistance training, it is important to closely examine the client's training background and to modify the resistance training exercise prescription accordingly (Andersen and Aagaard 2010).

How much do women's muscles hypertrophy in response to resistance training?

In the past, it was believed that resistance training produced less muscle hypertrophy in women than in men even though their relative strength gains were similar, but muscle hypertrophy was assessed indirectly using anthropometric and body composition measures. However, Cureton and colleagues (1988), using computerized tomography to directly assess muscle hypertrophy in a heavy resistance training program (70%-90% 1-RM, 3 days/wk for 16 wk), found significant increases in CSA of the upper arms of women (5 cm² or 23%) as well as men (7 cm² or 15%). Although absolute change in muscle volume was greater in men, the relative degree of hypertrophy (% change) was similar for men and women (Cureton et al. 1988). Research confirms this observation. Walts and colleagues (2008) reported that 10 wk of strength training resulted in similar relative gains in muscle volume of the knee extensors of Caucasian and African-American men (9%) and women (7.5%). Today experts agree that the relative increases in fiber size are similar for women and men when the training stimulus is the same (Deschenes and Kraemer 2002).

Is it possible for older adults to increase the size of their muscles by resistance training?

For many years it was thought that strength gains from resistance training in older individuals were due primarily to neural adaptation rather than muscle hypertrophy (Moritani and deVries 1979). However, it is now well accepted that exercise-induced hypertrophy appears to be an important mechanism underlying strength gains in older women and men. This implies that older adults can effectively counter age-related loss in muscle mass by participating in a vigorous resistance training program. However, these size gains take time to become apparent. Recently, Lixandrao and colleagues (2016), using ultrasound, took weekly cross-sectional measurements of the vastus lateralis muscle of older adults who were doing four sets of 10 repetitions of the leg press at 70% to 80% 1-RM twice a week. Muscle mass accrual was not observable until after 18 sessions (9 wk).

Raue and colleagues (2012) identified and compared gene sets responsible for eliciting a growth response to resistance training in young (24 yr) and old (84 yr) adults. Approximately 660 genes are affected by resistance training during the 1st and 36th training sessions. These genes are termed the **transcriptome signature of resistance exercise** (Raue et al. 2012) and are correlated with gains in muscle size and strength. The number of genes responding to acute resistance exercise in untrained and trained muscles decreased in young adults but stayed fairly constant in old adults, thereby suggesting a lack of training response in older adults. The skeletal muscle of young adults was more responsive to resistance exercise at the gene level compared with that of older adults. After 12 wk of resistance training, however, a greater number of genes changed expression in old vs. young adults. This finding indicated that some cell types in old muscle are capable of adapting to resistance training. The resistance exercise gene response was more pronounced in MHC IIA fibers than in MHC I fibers. This study provides insight into understanding the molecular basis for increases in muscle size in response to resistance exercise (hypertrophy), as well as decreases in muscle size (atrophy) due to aging and lack of physical exercise.

Does resistance training improve bone health and joint integrity?

Resistance training has beneficial effects on bone health that may decrease the risk of osteoporosis and bone fractures, particularly in women. This form of training may help achieve the highest possible peak bone mass in premenopausal women and may aid in maintaining and increasing bone in postmenopausal women and older adults (Layne and Nelson 1999). In a recent systematic review and meta-analysis, Xu, Lombardi, and colleagues (2016) concluded that combining impact exercise with resistance training was the best exercise strategy to preserve and improve bone mineral density in pre- and postmenopausal women. In a long-term study of postmenopausal women (45-65 yr), muscle strength and bone mineral density improved significantly (25%-75%) after 1 yr of resistance training (two sets; 6-RM to 8-RM; 70%-80% 1-RM; 2 days/wk). Women who lifted weights consistently for over 4 yr had significant changes in bone mineral density at the femur and lumbar spine sites. The researchers concluded that women who maintained bone density lifted weights two or more times per week (Metcalfe 2010). Evidence suggests that resistance training and higher-intensity weight-bearing activities (not walking) may slow the decline in bone loss even if there

SUMMARY OF EFFECTS OF RESISTANCE TRAINING

Morphological Factors

- Muscle hypertrophy due to increase in contractile proteins, number and size of myofibrils, connective tissues, and size of MHC II muscle fibers
- No change in relative amounts of MHC I and MHC II muscle fibers
- Conversion of MHC IIX to MHC IIA fast fibers
- Little or no change in the number of muscle fibers (<5%)
- Increase in size and strength of ligaments and tendons
- Increase in bone density and bone strength
- Increase in muscle capillary density

Neural Factors

- Increase in motor unit activation and recruitment
- Increase in discharge frequency of motor neurons
- Decrease in neural inhibition
- Increase in corticospinal excitability

Biochemical Factors

- Minor increase in ATP and CrP stores
- Minor increase in creatine phosphokinase (CPK), myosin adenosine triphosphatase (ATPase), and myokinase activity
- Decrease in mitochondrial volume density
- Increase in testosterone, growth hormone, insulin-like growth factor (IGF-I), and catecholamines during resistance training exercises
- Enhanced fat oxidation and fat availability during submaximal cycle ergometer exercise following resistance exercise

Additional Factors

- Little or no change in body mass
- Increase in fat-free mass
- Decrease in fat mass and relative body fat
- Improved bone health increases with exercise intensity
- Changes in the transcriptome signature of genes

is no significant increase in bone mineral density. Improvements in bone mineral density appear to be site specific; the greater changes occur in bones to which the exercising muscles attach. Experts agree that resistance training has a more potent effect on bone health than do weight-bearing aerobic exercises such as walking and jogging (Layne and Nelson 1999); this is true for men as well as women (Bolam, Van Uffelen, and Taaffe 2013).

Resistance training also improves the size and strength of ligaments and tendons (Edgerton 1973; Fleck and Falkel 1986; Tipton et al. 1975). These changes may increase joint stability, thereby reducing the risk of sprains and dislocations.

BIOCHEMICAL EFFECTS OF RESISTANCE TRAINING

The morphological changes in skeletal muscles due to resistance training are caused by hormones. This section addresses questions regarding hormonal responses to resistance exercise, as well as changes in the metabolic profile of skeletal muscles.

What causes the increase in muscle size with resistance training?

Exercise-induced hypertrophy occurs through hormonal mechanisms. Anabolic (protein building) hormones such as testosterone, growth hormone, and insulin-like growth hormone increase in response to heavy resistance exercise and interact to promote protein synthesis. The magnitude of testosterone and growth hormone release, however, appears to be related to the size of the muscle groups used, the exercise intensity (%1-RM), and the length of rest between sets, with larger increases observed for high-intensity (5-RM to 10-RM) exercise and short (1 min) rest periods involving large muscle groups (Kraemer et al. 1991). In men, high-intensity resistance training produces significant increases in testosterone and growth hormone, but testosterone appears to be the principal muscle-building hormone (Deschenes and Kraemer 2002). Levels of catecholamines (norepinephrine, epinephrine, and dopamine), which augment the release of testosterone and insulin-like growth factor, also increase in men in response to heavy resistance exercise (Kraemer et al. 1987). In women, growth hormone is likely the most potent muscle-building hormone

(Deschenes and Kraemer 2002). For more information on insulin-like growth factor, growth hormone, and testosterone and their role in skeletal muscle hypertrophy, see the review by Schoenfeld (2013).

Does resistance training alter the metabolic profile of skeletal muscles?

Although high-intensity resistance training results in substantial increases in muscle proteins, it appears to have little or no effect on muscle substrate stores and enzymes involved with the generation of adenosine triphosphate (ATP). Although stores of ATP and CrP may increase significantly in response to strength training (MacDougall et al. 1979), the changes are not large enough to have practical significance. Strength training produces only minor alterations in myosin adenosine triphosphatase (ATPase) activity (Tesch 1992) and other ATP turnover enzymes, such as creatine phosphokinase (CPK), in response to strength training (Costill et al. 1979; Komi et al. 1978; Thorstensson et al. 1976). Strength training using heavy resistance and explosive exercises results in decreased activities for hexokinase, myofibrillar ATPase, and citrate synthase (Tesch 1988).

Does resistance training decrease aerobic capacity and endurance performance?

This is somewhat controversial. The mitochondrial volume density following heavy resistance training has been reported to decrease as a consequence of a disproportionate increase of contractile protein in comparison with mitochondria. In theory, this could be detrimental to aerobic capacity and endurance performance. In similar studies of untrained men, one research team found that $\dot{V}O_2$peak increased equally in groups who trained only aerobically or with a combination of strength and endurance training (McCarthy et al. 1995), while another research team reported that $\dot{V}O_2$peak increased only in the endurance training group (Glowacki et al. 2004). For young elite cyclists, $\dot{V}O_2$max remained unchanged after 16 wk of concurrent strength and endurance training, but 45 min time trial performance improved 8% only with concurrent training, not endurance training (Aagaard et al. 2011). They attributed the improved endurance capacity to an increased proportion of type IIA muscle fibers, while capillarization remained unchanged. Similarly, adding lower body resistance exercise to well-trained female duathletes improved their running and cycling performance compared with an endurance-only training group (Vikmoen et al. 2017). However, Psilander and colleagues (2015) found that concurrent training did not enhance aerobic capacity or endurance in moderately trained cyclists. Their combined endurance-strength training group increased leg strength (19%), sprint power (5%), and short-term endurance (9%), but only the endurance group increased muscle citrate synthase activity (11%), lactate threshold (3%), and long-term endurance (4%).

NEUROLOGICAL EFFECTS OF RESISTANCE TRAINING

In addition to muscle hypertrophy, neural adaptations significantly contribute to strength gains, especially during the initial stages of resistance training. This section addresses questions regarding neural adaptations to short- and long-term resistance training.

What changes in neural function occur in response to resistance training?

The nervous system responds to resistance training by increasing the activation and recruitment of motor units (the alpha motor neuron and all the muscle fibers it innervates) and by decreasing the coaction of antagonistic muscle groups (Sale 1988). Recruiting additional motor units as well as increasing the frequency of firing results in greater muscular force production. Some evidence suggests that the central drive from higher neural centers (e.g., motor cortex of the brain) changes and that the number of neurotransmitters and postsynaptic receptors at the neuromuscular junction increases (Deschenes and Kraemer 2002). These changes facilitate the activation and recruitment of additional motor units, thereby increasing force production.

Transcranial magnetic stimulation (TMS) has been used to assess the strength of neural signals between the motor cortex and skeletal muscles (Kidgell and Pearce 2011). With this technique, adaptations in the central nervous system in response to strength training can be studied. In one study using TMS, strength improved after 4 wk of isometric strength training because of decreased cortical inhibition, thereby improving the corticospinal drive

to the motor unit pool (Carroll et al. 2009). This increase in MVC with a decrease in cortical inhibition that coincides with resistance training has been observed in both young and older adults (Christie and Kamen 2014). Kidgell and colleagues (2010) reported that strength gains (28% in trained arm and 19% in untrained contralateral arm) in response to resistance training (four sets; six to eight repetitions at 80% 1-RM) are related to increased corticospinal excitability (53% and 33% increase, respectively, in trained and untrained arms). Findings from TMS studies suggest that neural adaptations in response to strength training occur at the cortical, spinal, and motor unit levels. Manipulation of the load, timing of repetitions, and precision of movement (ballistic vs. controlled) modulate central nervous system adaptations (Kidgell and Pearce 2011).

At what stage during resistance training does neural adaptation occur?

In the past, it was believed that neural adaptations are primarily responsible for strength gains only during the initial stage (first 2-8 wk) of resistance training. At about 8 to 10 wk of resistance training, muscle hypertrophy contributes more than neural adaptation to strength gains, but hypertrophy eventually levels off (Sale 1988). Evidence suggests that muscle hypertrophy is finite and may be limited to no more than 12 mo (Deschenes and Kraemer 2002). Given that long-term resistance training (>6 mo) continues to increase strength without hypertrophy, experts now believe a secondary phase of neural adaptation is most likely responsible for strength gains occurring between 6 and 12 mo of training (Deschenes and Kraemer 2002).

What role do neural factors play in age-related loss of muscle strength?

The term *sarcopenia*, or age-related loss in muscle mass, has also been used to define age-related loss in muscle strength. This implies that changes in muscle mass are fully responsible for changes in strength. According to Clark and Manini (2008), longitudinal studies indicate that age-related changes in muscle mass account for less than 5% of the change in strength with aging. Changes in muscle mass and strength do not follow the same time course, suggesting that neural factors, along with changes in muscle factors (e.g., muscle architecture, fiber type transformations, and electro-contractile coupling), may modulate age-related loss of strength. They recommend using the term *dynapenia* to refer to age-related loss in strength, and they proposed a screening algorithm to help define and identify dynapenia (Manini and Clark 2012). Although it is difficult to identify specific neural mechanisms associated with dynapenia, changes in supraspinal drive, coactivation of antagonist muscles, muscle synergism, and maximal spinal cord output may mediate strength loss with aging (Clark and Manini 2008).

MUSCULAR SORENESS

Muscular soreness may develop as a result of resistance training because isolated muscle groups are being overloaded beyond normal use. **Acute-onset muscle soreness** occurs during or immediately following the exercise and is usually caused by ischemia and the accumulation of metabolic waste products in the muscle tissue. The pain and discomfort may persist up to 1 hr after the cessation of the exercise.

In **delayed-onset muscle soreness (DOMS)**, the pain occurs 24 to 48 hr after exercise. Although the causes of DOMS are not known (Armstrong 1984; Smith 1991), it appears to be related to the type of muscle action. Eccentric exercise produces a greater degree of delayed muscular soreness than either concentric or isometric exercise (Byrnes, Clarkson, and Katch 1985; Schwane et al. 1983; Talag 1973). Little or no muscular soreness occurs with isokinetic exercise (Byrnes, Clarkson, and Katch 1985). This most likely reflects the fact that isokinetic exercise devices offer no resistance to the recovery phase of the movement and therefore the muscle does not contract eccentrically. For a better understanding of eccentric muscle action and its role in DOMS, see the review by Hyldahl and Hubal (2014).

THEORIES OF DELAYED-ONSET MUSCLE SORENESS

Although the precise causes of DOMS remain unclear, several theories have been proposed. The more widely recognized theories suggest that exer-

cise, particularly eccentric exercise, causes damage to skeletal muscle cells and connective tissues, producing an acute inflammation.

Connective Tissue Damage

Abraham (1977) extensively studied the factors related to DOMS produced by resistance training. He suggested that DOMS most likely results from disruption in the connective tissue of the muscle and its tendinous attachments. Abraham noted that urinary excretion of hydroxyproline, a specific by-product of connective tissue breakdown, was higher in subjects who experienced muscular soreness than in those who did not. Because a significant rise in urinary hydroxyproline levels indicates an increase in both collagen degradation and synthesis, he concluded that more strenuous exercise damages the connective tissue, which increases the degradation of collagen and creates an imbalance in collagen metabolism. To compensate for this imbalance, the rate of collagen synthesis increases.

Skeletal Muscle Damage

Researchers have assessed skeletal muscle damage induced through exercise. **Exercise-induced muscle damage (EIMD)** may occur when individuals engage in eccentric exercise or exercise to which they are unaccustomed. The muscle damage results in decreased force production and increased passive tension, as well as increased muscle soreness, swelling, and intramuscular proteins in the blood (Howatson and van Someren 2008). Much of the research on EIMD has focused on the effects of eccentric exercise on muscle damage and soreness. Regardless of the speed or intensity of muscle action, eccentric exercise injures both the contractile and cytoskeletal components of myofibrils as well as the excitation coupling system; this is especially true for novel exercise (Howatson and van Someren 2008).

Friden, Sjostrom, and Ekblom (1983) observed structural damage to myofibrillar Z bands resulting from eccentric exercise. Proske and Morgan (2001) pointed out that disruption of the sarcomere organization within the skeletal muscle is most likely the cause of the decreased active tension and force production that follows a series of intense eccentric muscle actions. Mackey and colleagues (2008) reported that electrically stimulated isometric muscle actions may also produce muscle damage at the sarcomere level. Z-line disruption and microphage infiltration provided direct evidence of damage to myofibers and sarcomeres. More research is needed to assess the effects of various types of muscle action, as well as high- and low-impact eccentric exercise (e.g., downhill running and eccentric cycle exercise), on muscle damage (Friden 2002).

Researchers have also examined markers of muscle damage such as serum CPK, lactate dehydrogenase, and myoglobin. Schwane and colleagues (1983) noted a significant increase in plasma CPK levels produced by downhill running. They suggested that the mechanical stress from eccentric exercise causes cellular damage, resulting in an enzyme efflux. Clarkson and colleagues (1986) reported similar increases in serum CPK levels following concentric (37.6%), eccentric (35.8%), and isometric (34%) arm curl exercises. They concluded that muscle damage occurred with all three types of muscle actions; however, the subjects perceived greater muscle soreness with eccentric and isometric exercises. Likewise, Byrnes, Clarkson, and Katch (1985) observed that both concentric and eccentric resistance training elevated serum CPK levels, but that individuals who trained concentrically did not develop DOMS. In contrast to all of this evidence implicating muscle damage, recent research suggests that muscle fiber damage is not essential for DOMS; rather neurotrophic factors produced by satellite cells play a key role (Mizumura and Taguchi 2016).

Armstrong's Model of Delayed-Onset Muscle Soreness

On the basis of an extensive literature review, Armstrong (1984) proposed the following model of the development of DOMS:

1. The structural proteins in muscle cells and connective tissue are disrupted by high mechanical forces produced during exercise, especially eccentric exercise.

2. Structural damage to the sarcolemma alters the permeability of the cell membrane, allowing a net influx of calcium from the interstitial space. Abnormally high levels of calcium inhibit cellular respiration, thereby lessening the cell's ability to produce ATP for active removal of calcium from the cell.

3. High calcium levels within the cell activate a calcium-dependent proteolytic enzyme that degrades Z discs, troponin, and tropomyosin.

4. This progressive destruction of the sarcolemma (postexercise) allows intracellular components to diffuse into the interstitial space and plasma. These substances attract monocytes and activate mast cells and histocytes in the injured area.

5. Histamine, kinins, and potassium accumulate in the interstitial space because of the active phagocytosis and cellular necrosis. These substances, as well as increased tissue edema and temperature, may stimulate pain receptors, resulting in the sensation of DOMS.

Acute Inflammation Theory

Smith (1991) suggested that acute inflammation, in response to muscle cell and connective damage caused by eccentric exercise, is the primary mechanism underlying DOMS. Many of the signs and symptoms of acute inflammation, such as pain, swelling, and loss of function, are also present with DOMS. On the basis of research about acute inflammation and DOMS, Smith proposed the following sequence of events:

1. Connective tissue and muscle tissue disruption occurs during eccentric exercise, especially when the individual is not accustomed to eccentric exercise.

2. Within a few hours, neutrophils in the blood are elevated and migrate to the site of injury for several hours postinjury.

3. Monocytes also migrate to the injured tissues for 6 to 12 hr postinjury.

4. Macrophages synthesize prostaglandins (series E).

5. The prostaglandins sensitize type III and IV pain afferents, resulting in the sensation of pain in response to intramuscular pressure caused by movement or palpation.

6. The combination of increased pressure and hypersensitization produces the sensation of DOMS.

In summary, it appears that there is no single mechanism or theory to explain DOMS. In a review article, Lewis, Ruby, and Bush-Joseph (2012) concluded that the culmination of six different mechanisms underlie muscle soreness. DOMS starts with microtrauma to the muscles and connective tissues. This trauma is followed by inflammation and shifts of fluids and electrolytes, causing the pain and discomfort associated with DOMS. Furthermore, interindividual genetic variation exists in response to EIMD such that individuals with certain genotypes experience greater muscle damage following exercise (Baumert et al. 2016).

PREVENTION OF EXERCISE-INDUCED MUSCLE DAMAGE AND MUSCULAR SORENESS

Given that eccentric muscle action is an integral part of human locomotion, physical activities, and sport, researchers have explored myriad intervention strategies to lessen the negative effects of eccentric muscle actions and to treat EIMD. These approaches include nutrition (e.g., antioxidants, carbohydrate-protein supplements, and β-hydroxy-β-methylbutyrate) and pharmacological strategies (e.g., aspirin, ibuprofen, and naproxen); manual (e.g., massage and cryotherapy), neuromuscular (e.g., transcutaneous electrical nerve stimulation [TENS] and ultrasound), and whole-body vibration therapies; and exercise (e.g., prior bouts of isometric or eccentric exercise and stretching). Some evidence suggests that cold water immersion (cryotherapy) may reduce DOMS after exercise (Bleakley et al. 2012; Lynch and Barry 2012). Likewise, whole-body vibration therapy prior to eccentric exercise reduces muscle inflammation, strength loss, and DOMS symptoms (Aminian-Far et al. 2011; Broadbent et al. 2010; Imtiyaz, Veqar, and Shareef 2014). Performing isometric MVCs in the weeks preceding a bout of maximal eccentric contractions reduced soreness and creatine kinase concentration (Tseng et al. 2016). Additionally, a single bout of low-volume, high-intensity eccentric exercise has been consistently shown to have a

positive effect on reducing EIMD. Howatson and van Someren (2008) provide an excellent review of research dealing with the prevention and treatment of EIMD.

For many years, slow static stretching exercises were recommended to warm up major muscle groups at the start of a resistance training workout. It was believed that this form of stretching prevented muscle injury and soreness (deVries 1961). However, evidence suggests that stretching prior to physical activity does not prevent injury (Pope et al. 2000). Also, stretching before, after, or before and after exercise does not produce clinically significant reductions in delayed-onset muscle soreness (Henschke and Lin 2011; Herbert, de Noronha, and Kamper 2011). In fact, stretching before resistance exercise may actually decrease strength and force production (Rubini, Costa, and Gomes 2007). Therefore, stretching immediately prior to resistance exercise is not recommended. Instead of performing static stretching, your clients should warm up by completing 5 to 10 repetitions of the exercise at a low intensity (e.g., 40% 1-RM).

Law and Herbert (2007) reported that low-intensity exercise (i.e., warm-up) prior to unaccustomed eccentric exercise (e.g., walking backward downhill on an inclined treadmill for 30 min) reduced muscle soreness up to 48 hr after exercise. In contrast, neither low-intensity cool-down exercise nor stretching after exercise reduces muscle soreness (Herbert and de Noronha 2007; Herbert, de Noronha, and Kamper 2011; Law and Herbert 2007).

Using a gradual progression of exercise intensity at the beginning of a resistance training program may also help prevent muscular soreness. Some experts suggest using 12-RM to 15-RM during the beginning phases of strength training. Make sure your clients gradually increase exercise intensity throughout the resistance training program. Avoiding eccentric actions during dynamic resistance training may also lessen the chance of muscular soreness. An assistant or exercise partner should return the weight to the starting position.

Key Points

▸ The specificity principle states that muscular fitness development is specific to the muscle group, type of muscle action, training intensity, speed, and range of movement.

▸ The overload principle states that the muscle group must be exercised at greater than normal workloads to promote development of muscular strength and endurance.

▸ For nonperiodized resistance training programs, the training volume must be progressively increased to overload the muscle groups for continued gains in strength and muscular endurance.

▸ In most programs, resistance training exercises should be ordered so that successive exercises do not involve the same muscle group. For advanced programs, however, exercises for the same muscle group should be done consecutively.

▸ Dynamic resistance training can be used to develop muscular strength, power, size, or endurance by modifying the intensity, repetitions, sets, and frequency of the exercise.

▸ Periodization programs can result in greater changes in strength than nonperiodized resistance training programs.

▸ Strength and endurance gains resulting from resistance training are due to morphological, neurological, and biochemical changes in the muscle tissue.

▸ Eccentric exercise produces a greater degree of DOMS than either concentric, isometric, or isokinetic exercise.

▸ Little or no muscular soreness is produced by isokinetic training.

▸ The precise cause of DOMS is unknown; however, connective tissue and muscle damage, as well as acute inflammation, have been proposed as possible causes.

Key Terms

Learn the definition of each of the following key terms. Definitions of terms can be found in the glossary.

acute-onset muscle soreness

β-hydroxy-β-methylbutyrate (HMB)

compound sets

core stability

core strengthening

delayed-onset muscle soreness (DOMS)

dynapenia

eccentric training

exercise-induced hypertrophy

exercise-induced muscle damage (EIMD)

functional training

high intensity–low repetition

kettlebell training

linear periodization (LP)

low intensity–high repetition

macrocycle

mesocycle

microcycle

muscle balance

periodization

pyramiding

repetition maximum (RM)

repetitions

reverse linear periodization (RLP)

sarcopenia

set

split routine

supersetting

tonic vibration reflex

training volume

transcranial magnetic stimulation (TMS)

transcriptome signature of resistance exercise

tri-sets

undulating periodization (UP)

whole-body vibration (WBV)

Review Questions

In addition to being able to define each of the key terms, test your knowledge and understanding of the material by answering the following review questions.

1. What are the health benefits of resistance training?

2. Name three general types of resistance training. Which one is best suited for physical therapy rehabilitation programs?

3. Describe the ACSM guidelines for designing resistance training programs for healthy adults. What modifications are necessary when you are planning resistance training programs for children and older adults?

4. Describe how the basic exercise prescriptions for strength training and muscular endurance training programs differ.

5. Describe how you can increase training volume for advanced strength training and hypertrophy programs.

6. Describe two methods of varying sets for advanced strength training programs.

7. Explain two methods an advanced weightlifter can use to completely fatigue a targeted muscle group.

8. Describe three periodization models. How do they differ?

9. How does moderate-load eccentric training differ from plyometric training?

10. What is the major advantage of isokinetic training compared with traditional forms of resistance training?

11. Explain how the specificity, overload, and progression principles are applied in the design of resistance training programs.

12. What will you tell your clients if they ask about supplementing their resistance training with creatine?

13. Explain what causes the exercise-induced hypertrophy resulting from resistance training. In the time course of a resistance training program, when is this morphological adaptation most likely to occur?

14. Describe the potential effects of resistance training on bone health.

15. What neural adaptations account for initial strength gains during resistance training? When are these changes most likely to be observed during the time course of resistance training?

16. Define sarcopenia and dynapenia. Identify muscle morphological and neurological mechanisms responsible for dynapenia.

17. Describe one theory of DOMS. What can you instruct your clients to do to help prevent and relieve muscle soreness caused by resistance training?

CHAPTER 8

Assessing Body Composition

KEY QUESTIONS

▶ Why is it important to measure body composition, and how are body composition measures used by health and fitness professionals?

▶ What are the standards for classifying body fat levels?

▶ What is the difference between two-component and multicomponent body composition models?

▶ What are the guidelines and limitations of the hydrostatic weighing method?

▶ Is air displacement plethysmography as accurate as hydrostatic weighing?

▶ Is dual-energy X-ray absorptiometry considered a gold standard method for measuring body composition?

▶ What are the guidelines, limitations, and sources of measurement error for the skinfold method?

▶ Is ultrasound a suitable alternative to the skinfold method for assessing body composition in field settings?

▶ What is bioelectrical impedance analysis? What factors affect the accuracy of this method?

▶ Can circumferences and skeletal diameters be used to accurately assess body composition?

▶ What anthropometric indices can be used to identify at-risk individuals?

Body composition is a key component of an individual's health and physical fitness profile. Obesity is a serious health problem that contributes to reduced life expectancy by increasing one's risk of developing coronary artery disease, hypertension, type 2 diabetes, obstructive pulmonary disease, osteoarthritis, and certain types of cancer. Too little body fat also poses a health risk because the body needs a certain amount of fat for normal physiological functions. Essential lipids, such as phospholipids, are needed for cell membrane formation; nonessential lipids, like triglycerides found in adipose tissue, provide thermal insulation and store metabolic fuel (free fatty acids). In addition, lipids are involved in the transport and storage of fat-soluble vitamins (A, D, E, and K) and in the functioning of the nervous system, the menstrual cycle, and the reproductive system, as well as in growth and maturation during pubescence. Thus, too little body fatness, as found in individuals with eating disorders (e.g., anorexia nervosa), exercise addiction, and certain diseases such as cystic fibrosis, can lead to serious physiological dysfunction.

This chapter describes standardized testing procedures for reference methods (hydrostatic weighing, air displacement plethysmography, and dual-energy X-ray absorptiometry) and field methods (skinfold, ultrasound, bioimpedance, and anthropometry) for assessing body composition. For each method, you will learn to identify potential sources of measurement error as well as ways to minimize these errors.

CLASSIFICATION AND USES OF BODY COMPOSITION MEASURES

To classify level of body fatness, the **relative body fat (%BF)** is used. Table 8.1 presents %BF ranges, by decade of life, for men and women. It is important to recall that these data are based on skinfolds, and the skinfold measures are reported to be within ± 3.5% BF of a hydrostatic weighing reference. The minimal, average, and obesity fat values vary with age, gender, and activity status. For example, the average or median %BF values for adult men and women (20-29 yr) are approximately 15.0% for men and 20% for women. The corresponding minimal recommended fat values are 3% and 10%, respectively. Body fat percentages above 22% for men and 28% for women exceed what is believed to be healthy.

In addition to classifying your client's %BF and disease risk, body composition measures are useful for

- estimating a healthy body weight and formulating nutritional considerations and exercise prescriptions (see chapter 9);
- estimating competitive body weight for athletes participating in sports that use body weight classifications for competition (e.g., wrestling and bodybuilding);
- monitoring the growth of children and adolescents and identifying those at risk because of under- or overfatness; and
- assessing changes in body composition associated with aging, malnutrition, and certain diseases, as well as the effectiveness of nutrition and exercise interventions in counteracting these changes.

BODY COMPOSITION MODELS

To make the most valid assessment of body composition for your clients, it is necessary to understand the underlying theoretical models. You may recall that

Table 8.1 Body Fat Percentage Categories for Adults[1] and Children[2] by Decade of Life

Age	Very lean	Lean	Average	Over fat	Obese
MALES					
6-18	6-9	10-17	18-28	29-35	>35
20-29	4-7	8-12	13-17	18-23	>23
30-39	7-11	12-16	17-20	21-25	>25
40-49	9-13	14-18	19-22	23-26	>26
50-59	11-15	16-20	21-23	24-28	>28
60-69	12-17	18-21	22-24	25-29	>29
70-79	14-16	17-21	22-24	25-29	>29
FEMALES					
6-18	9-16	17-22	23-29	30-34	>34
20-29	11-15	16-18	19-22	23-28	>28
30-39	11-16	17-19	20-23	24-30	>30
40-49	12-17	18-21	22-25	26-32	>32
50-59	13-19	20-24	25-28	29-34	>34
60-69	14-20	21-25	26-29	30-35	>35
70-79	11-18	19-24	25-28	29-35	>35

Adapted by permission from [1] The Cooper Institute, *Physical Fitness Assessments and Norms for Adults and Law Enforcement* (Dallas: Cooper Institute, 2013) and from [2] Laurson, Eisenmann, and Welk 2011.

the body is composed of water, protein, minerals, and fat. The two-component model of body composition (Brozek et al. 1963; Siri 1961) divides the body into a fat component and a **fat-free body (FFB)** component. The FFB consists of all residual chemicals and tissues including water, muscle (protein), and bone (mineral). The **two-component model** of body composition makes the following five assumptions:

1. The density of fat is 0.901 g·cc^{-1}.
2. The density of the FFB is 1.100 g·cc^{-1}.
3. The densities of fat and the FFB components (water, protein, mineral) are the same for all individuals.
4. The densities of the various tissues composing the FFB are constant within an individual, and their proportional contribution to the lean component remains constant.
5. The individual being measured differs from the reference body only in the amount of fat; the FFB of the reference body is assumed to be 73.8% water, 19.4% protein, and 6.8% mineral.

This two-component model is the foundation for the **hydrodensitometry** (underwater weighing) method. With use of the assumed proportions of water, mineral, and protein and their respective densities, equations were derived to convert an individual's total body density (Db) from hydrostatic weighing into relative body fat proportions (%BF). Two commonly used equations are the Siri (1961) equation, %BF = (4.95 / Db − 4.50) × 100, and the equation of Brozek and colleagues (1963), %BF = (4.57 / Db − 4.142) × 100. These two equations yield similar %BF estimates for body densities ranging from 1.0300 to 1.0900 g·cc^{-1}. For example, if a client's measured Db is 1.0500 g·cc^{-1}, the %BF estimates obtained by plugging this value into the Siri and Brozek equations are 21.4% and 21.0%, respectively.

Generally, two-component (2C) model equations provide accurate estimates of %BF as long as the basic assumptions of the model are met. However, there is no guarantee that the FFB composition of an individual within a certain population subgroup will exactly match the values assumed for the reference body. Researchers have reported that FFB density varies with age, gender, ethnicity, level of body fatness, and physical activity level, depending mainly on the relative proportion of water and mineral composing the FFB (Baumgartner et al. 1991; Wil-

liams, Going, et al. 1993). For example, the average FFB density of black women and black men (~1.106 g·cc^{-1}) is greater than 1.10 g·cc^{-1} because of their higher mineral content (~7.3% FFB) or relative body protein (or both) (Cote and Adams 1993; Ortiz et al. 1992; Wagner and Heyward 2001). Because of this difference in FFB density, the body fat of blacks will be systematically underestimated when 2C model equations are used to estimate %BF. In fact, negative %BF values were reported for professional football players whose measured Db exceeded 1.10 g·cc^{-1} (Adams et al. 1982). Likewise, the FFB density of white children is estimated to be only 1.086 g·cc^{-1} because of their relative lower mineral values (5.2% FFB) and higher body water values (76.6% FFB) compared with the reference body (Lohman, Boileau, and Slaughter 1984). Also, the average density of the FFB of elderly white men and women is 1.098 g·cc^{-1} because of the relatively low body mineral value (6.2% FFB) in this population (Heymsfield et al. 1989). Thus, the relative body fat of children and persons who are elderly will be systematically overestimated using 2C model equations.

For certain population subgroups, therefore, scientists have applied **multicomponent models** of body composition based on measured total body water and bone mineral values. With the multicomponent approach, you can avoid systematic errors in estimating body fat by replacing the reference body with population-specific reference bodies that take into account the age (e.g., for children, for persons who are elderly), gender, and ethnicity of the individual. Table 8.2 provides population-specific formulas for converting Db to %BF. You will note that population-specific conversion formulas do not yet exist for all age groups within each ethnic group. You may have to use the age-specific conversion formula developed for white males and females in these cases. Also, you can use the population-specific conversion formulas for anorexic and obese females only when it is obvious that your client is either anorexic or obese.

REFERENCE METHODS FOR ASSESSING BODY COMPOSITION

In many laboratory and clinical settings, **densitometry** and dual-energy X-ray absorptiometry are used

Table 8.2 Population-Specific Two-Component Model Formulas for Converting Body Density to Percent Body Fat

Population	Age (yr)	Gender	%BF[a]	FFB[d] (g·cc⁻¹)[b]
RACE OR ETHNICITY				
African-American	9-17	Female	(5.24 / Db) − 4.82	1.088
	19-45	Male	(4.86 / Db) − 4.39	1.106
	24-79	Female	(4.85 / Db) − 4.39	1.106
American Indian	18-62	Male	(4.97 / Db) − 4.52	1.099
	18-60	Female	(4.81 / Db) − 4.34	1.108
Japanese Native	18-48	Male	(4.97 / Db) − 4.52	1.099
		Female	(4.76 / Db) − 4.28	1.111
	61-78	Male	(4.87 / Db) − 4.41	1.105
		Female	(4.95 / Db) − 4.50	1.100
Singaporean (Chinese, Indian, Malay)		Male	(4.94 / Db) − 4.48	1.102
		Female	(4.84 / Db) − 4.37	1.107
White	8-12	Male	(5.27 / Db) − 4.85	1.086
		Female	(5.27 / Db) − 4.85	1.086
	13-17	Male	(5.12 / Db) − 4.69	1.092
		Female	(5.19 / Db) − 4.76	1.090
	18-59	Male	(4.95 / Db) − 4.50	1.100
		Female	(4.96 / Db) − 4.51	1.101
	60-90	Male	(4.97 / Db) − 4.52	1.099
		Female	(5.02 / Db) − 4.57	1.098
Hispanic	20-40	Male	NA	NA
		Female	(4.87 / Db) − 4.41	1.105
ATHLETES				
Resistance trained	24 ± 4	Male	(5.21 / Db) − 4.78	1.089
	35 ± 6	Female	(4.97 / Db) − 4.52	1.099
Endurance trained	21 ± 2	Male	(5.03 / Db) − 4.59	1.097
	21 ± 4	Female	(4.95 / Db) − 4.50	1.100
All sports	18-22	Male	(5.12 / Db) − 4.68	1.093
	18-22	Female	(4.97 / Db) − 4.52	1.099
CLINICAL POPULATIONS				
Anorexia nervosa	15-44	Female	(4.96 / Db) − 4.51	1.101
Obesity	17-62	Female	(4.95 / Db) − 4.50	1.100
Spinal cord injury (paraplegic or quadriplegic)	18-73	Male	(4.67 / Db) − 4.18	1.116
		Female	(4.70 / Db) − 4.22	1.114

FFB_d = fat-free body density; Db = body density; %BF = percent body fat; NA = no data available for this population subgroup.

[a]Multiply value by 100 to calculate %BF.

[b]FFB_d based on average values reported in selected research articles.

to obtain reference measures of body composition. For densitometric methods, total **body density (Db)** is estimated from the ratio of body mass to body volume (Db = BM / BV). Body volume is usually measured using either hydrostatic weighing or air displacement plethysmography.

HYDROSTATIC WEIGHING

Hydrostatic weighing (HW) is a valid, reliable, and widely used laboratory method for assessing total Db. Hydrostatic weighing provides an estimate of total **body volume (BV)** from the water displaced by the body's volume. According to **Archimedes' principle**, weight of a body under water is directly proportional to the volume of water displaced by the body's volume. For calculating Db, body mass is divided by body volume. The total Db is a function of the amounts of muscle, bone, water, and fat in the body.

Using Hydrostatic Weighing

Determine BV by totally submerging the body in an underwater weighing tank or pool and measuring the **underwater weight (UWW)** of the body. To measure UWW, you can use either a chair attached to an HW scale (see figure 8.1) or a platform attached to load cells (see figure 8.2). Given that the weight loss under water is directly proportional to the volume of water displaced by the body's volume, the BV is equal to the **body mass (BM)** minus the UWW (see figure 8.3). The net UWW is the difference between the UWW and the weight of the chair or platform and its supporting equipment (i.e., tare weight). The BV must be corrected for the volume of air remaining in the lungs after a maximal expiration (i.e., **residual volume** or **RV**), as well as the volume of air in the gastrointestinal tract (GV). The GV is assumed to be 100 ml.

The RV is commonly measured using helium dilution, nitrogen washout, or oxygen dilution techniques. The RV is measured in liters and must be converted to kilograms (kg) in order to correct UWW. This is easy to do because 1 L of water weighs approximately 1 kg; therefore, the water weight per liter of RV is 1 kg. To correct the BV, you subtract the equivalent weight of the RV and the GV (100 ml or 0.1 kg). Since water density varies with water temperature, the BV is corrected for water density

(see figure 8.3). Under normal circumstances, the water temperature of the underwater weighing tank or swimming pool will be between 34 and 36 °C.

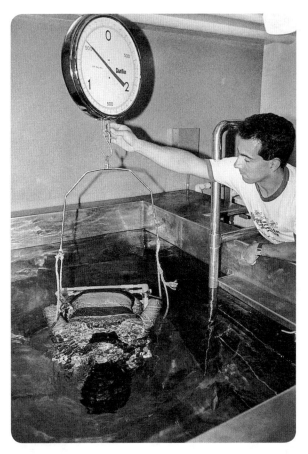

FIGURE 8.1 Hydrostatic weighing using scale and chair.

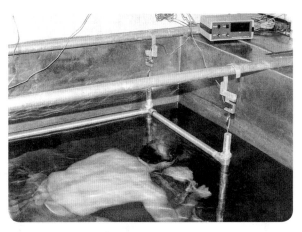

FIGURE 8.2 Hydrostatic weighing using load cells and platform.

HYDROSTATIC WEIGHING DATA

Name _____   Date _____

Gender _____

Ethnicity _____

Body mass (BM) _____ lb _____ kg   Age _____

I.   Measured RV: Estimated RV (select one equation from appendix D.1):
     (average 2 trials within 100 ml)
     Trial 1 _____ Trial 2 _____ Trial 3 _____
     Average measured RV = _____ L   Estimated RV = _____ L

II. Water temperature _____ ° C
     Water density _____ g·cc⁻¹

Temperature (C)	Density (g·cc⁻¹)
33°	0.9947
34°	0.9944
35°	0.9941
36°	0.9937
37°	0.9934

III. Gross underwater weight (in kg)

     Trial 1 _____   Trial 6 _____
     Trial 2 _____   Trial 7 _____
     Trial 3 _____   Trial 8 _____
     Trial 4 _____   Trial 9 _____
     Trial 5 _____   Trial 10 _____
     Average (3 trials within 0.1 kg)   _____ kg

IV. Tare weight (chair, platform, and supporting
     equipment)   _____ kg

V.   Net underwater weight
     gross UWW _____ – tare weight _____ =   _____ kg

VI. Body volume (BV)
     [(BM in kg – net UWW in kg) / water density] – (RV + GV)   BV = _____ L
     Note: GV assumed value = 100 ml or 0.1 L

VII. Body density = BM (kg) / BV (L)
     (carry out to 5 or 6 decimal places)   Db = _____ g·cc⁻¹

VIII. Percent body fat (select conversion formula from table 8.2)   BF = _____ %

IX. Fat weight = BM × %BF (decimal)
     _____ × _____   FW = _____ kg

X.   Fat-free mass = BM – FW
     _____ – _____   FFM = _____ kg

Comments and observations:

FIGURE 8.3 Hydrostatic weighing data collection form.

From A.L. Gibson, D.R. Wagner, and V.H. Heyward, 2019, *Advanced Fitness Assessment and Exercise Prescription,* 8th ed. (Champaign, IL: Human Kinetics).

The resulting equation for BV is

$$BV = [(BM - net\ UWW) / density\ of\ water] - (RV + GV)$$

Calculate body density (Db in $g \cdot cc^{-1}$) by dividing BM by BV: Db = BM / BV. After you calculate Db, you can convert it into **percent body fat (%BF)** by using the appropriate population-specific conversion formula (see table 8.2).

You should adhere to established guidelines when using the HW technique (see Guidelines for Hydrostatic Weighing).

In addition to the HW testing guidelines, following the suggestions in Tips for Minimizing Error in Hydrostatic Weighing may improve the accuracy of your underwater weighing measurements.

GUIDELINES FOR HYDROSTATIC WEIGHING

Video 8.1

Pretest Guidelines for Clients

- Do not eat or engage in strenuous exercise for at least 4 hr before your scheduled appointment.
- Avoid ingesting any gas-producing foods or beverages (e.g., baked beans, diet soda) for at least 12 hr before your test.
- Bring a towel and a tight-fitting, lightweight swimsuit.

Testing Procedure Guidelines

- Carefully calibrate the body weight scale and underwater weighing scale. To determine the accuracy of the underwater weighing scale, hang calibrated weights from the scale and check the corresponding scale values. To calibrate a load cell system, place weights on the platform and check the recorded values.
- Have your client use the restroom to void and change into a swimsuit.
- Measure the underwater weight of the chair or platform and of the supporting equipment and weight belt; the total is the **tare weight**.
- Measure your client's dry weight (weight in air) to the nearest 50 g.
- Check and record the water temperature of the tank just before the test; it should range between 34 and 36 °C. Use the constant values in figure 8.3 to determine the density of the water at that temperature.
- Instruct your client to shower and then enter the tank slowly, so that the water stays calm. Have the client gently submerge without touching the chair or weighing platform and rub hands over the body to eliminate air bubbles from the swimsuit, skin, and hair.
- Have the client kneel on the underwater weighing platform or sit in the chair. Your client may need to wear a scuba diving weight belt to facilitate the kneeling or sitting position. If RV is being measured simultaneously, insert the mouthpiece at this time. If RV is measured outside of the tank, administer the RV test prior to the HW test and before the client changes clothes and showers.
- Have the client take a few normal breaths and then exhale maximally while slowly bending forward at the waist to submerge the head. Check to make certain that the client's head, back, and hair are completely underwater and that the arms and feet are not touching the sides or bottom of the tank. Instruct the client to continue exhaling until RV is reached. The client needs to remain as still as possible during this procedure. A relaxed and motionless state under water will aid in an accurate reading of UWW.
- Record the highest stable weight with the client fully submerged at RV, then signal to the client that the trial is completed.
- Administer as many trials as needed to obtain three readings within ±100 g. Most clients achieve a consistent and maximal UWW in four or five trials (Bonge and Donnelly 1989). Average the three highest trials and record this value as the gross UWW.
- Determine the net UWW by subtracting the tare weight from the gross UWW. The net UWW is used to calculate body volume (see figure 8.3).

TIPS FOR MINIMIZING ERROR IN HYDROSTATIC WEIGHING

- Make sure clients adhere to all pretesting guidelines.
- Before each test session, check the calibration of the BW and UWW scales or load cells, and carefully calibrate the gas analyzers used to measure RV.
- Precisely measure BW to ±50 g, UWW to ±100 g, and RV to ±100 ml.
- Coach the client to maximally exhale and remain motionless under the water.
- Steady the underwater weighing apparatus as the client submerges, but remove your hand from the scale before actually reading the UWW.
- If possible, use a load cell system and measure RV and UWW simultaneously.
- Carry the calculated Db value out to five decimal places. Rounding off a Db of 1.07499 g·cc^{-1} to 1.07 g·cc^{-1} corresponds to a difference of 2.2% BF when converted with the Siri (1961) 2C model formula.
- If you are estimating %BF from Db with a 2C model, use the appropriate population-specific conversion formula (see table 8.2).

Special Considerations

Some clients may have difficulty performing the HW test using these standardized procedures. Accurate test results are highly dependent on the client's skill, cooperation, and motivation. This section addresses the use of modified HW procedures as well as other questions and concerns about this method.

What should I do when my client is unable to blow out all the air from the lungs or remain still while under water?

You will likely come across clients who are uncomfortable expelling all the air from their lungs during HW. In such cases, you can weigh these individuals at functional residual capacity (FRC) or total lung capacity (TLC) instead of RV. Thomas and Etheridge (1980) underwater-weighed 43 males, comparing the body densities measured at FRC (taken at the end of normal expiration while the person was submerged) and at RV (at the end of maximal expiration). The two methods yielded similar results. Similarly, Timson and Coffman (1984) reported that Db measured by HW at TLC (vital capacity + RV) was similar (less than 0.3% BF difference) to that measured at RV if TLC was measured in the water. However, when the TLC was measured out of the water, the method significantly overestimated Db. When using these modifications of the HW method, you must still measure RV in order to calculate the FRC or TLC of your client. Also, be certain to substitute the appropriate lung volume (FRC or TLC) for RV in the calculation of BV.

People uncomfortable under water tend to have difficulty being still while fully submerged. Your client's movement under water causes the arm of the scale to move. In addition to prolonging the time your client is under water, it may preclude your ability to confidently determine your client's underwater weight. The **damping technique** as described by Moon and colleagues (2011) reduces the magnitude of the swings in the scale arm until the client and chair become stable under water. Damping is performed by temporarily holding the moving part of the scale (where the chair attaches) to apply an upward force that counters the motion associated with submersion or movement in the chair. Gently releasing the hold prior to the end of the maximal exhalation maneuver allows the scale arm to stabilize for a more accurate measurement. The damping technique produced similar underwater weights compared with hydrodensitometric assessments made via load cell and without damping (Moon et al. 2011).

Because of their lower Db, clients with greater amounts of body fat are more buoyant than leaner individuals; therefore, they have more difficulty remaining motionless while under the water. To correct this problem, place a weighted scuba belt around the client's waist. Be certain to include the weight of the scuba belt when measuring and subtracting the tare weight of the HW system.

What should I do when my clients are afraid to put their face in the water or are not flexible enough to get their backs and heads completely submerged?

Occasionally, you will encounter clients who are extremely fearful of being submerged, who dislike facial contact with water, or who are unable to bend forward to assume the proper body position for HW. In such cases, a satisfactory alternative would be to weigh your clients at TLC while their heads remain above water level. Donnelly and colleagues (1988) compared this measure (i.e., TLCNS, or total lung capacity with head not submerged) to the criterion Db obtained from HW at RV for 75 men and 67 women. Vital capacity was measured with the subject submerged in the water to shoulder level. Regression analysis yielded the following equations for predicting Db at RV, using the Db determined at TLCNS as the predictor:

Males

$$Db \text{ at } RV = 0.5829(Db \text{ at } TLCNS) + 0.4059$$

$$r = .88; SEE = 0.0067 \text{ g·cc}^{-1}$$

Females

$$Db \text{ at } RV = 0.4745(Db \text{ at } TLCNS) + 0.5173$$

$$r = .85; SEE = 0.0061 \text{ g·cc}^{-1}$$

The correlations (r) between the actual Db at RV and the predicted Db at RV were high, and the standard errors of estimate (SEE) were within acceptable limits. These equations were cross-validated for an independent sample of 20 men and 20 women. The differences between the Db from HW at RV and the predicted Db from weighing at TLCNS were quite small (less than 0.0014 g·cc^{-1} or 0.7% BF). This method may be especially useful for HW of older adults, obese individuals with limited flexibility, and people with physical disabilities.

Will the accuracy of the HW test be affected if I estimate RV instead of measuring it?

Several prediction equations have been developed to estimate RV based on an individual's age, height, gender, and smoking status (see appendix D.1, Prediction Equations for Residual Volume). However, these RV prediction equations have large prediction errors $(SEE = 400\text{-}500 \text{ ml})$. When RV is measured, the precision of the HW method is excellent ($\leq$1% BF). However, this precision error increases substantially ($\pm$2.8%-3.7% BF) when RV is estimated (Morrow et al. 1986). Therefore, always measure RV when you are using the HW method.

When is the best time during the menstrual cycle to hydrostatically weigh my female clients?

Some women, particularly those whose body weight fluctuates widely during their menstrual cycles, may have significantly different estimates of Db and %BF when weighed hydrostatically at different times in their cycles. Bunt, Lohman, and Boileau (1989) reported that changes in total body water values due to water retention partly explain the differences in body weight and Db during a menstrual cycle. On the average, the relative body fat of the women was 24.8% at their lowest body weights, compared with an average of 27.6% BF at their peak body weights during their menstrual cycles. Because their low and peak body weights occurred at different times during the menstrual cycle (varied from 0 to 14 days prior to the onset of the next menses), the effect of total body water fluctuations cannot be routinely controlled by using the same day of the menstrual cycle for all women. However, when you are monitoring changes in body composition over time or establishing healthy body weight for a female client, it is recommended that you hydrostatically weigh her at the same time within her menstrual cycle and outside of the period of her perceived peak body weight.

AIR DISPLACEMENT PLETHYSMOGRAPHY

Air displacement plethysmography (ADP) is a method to assess body volume and density. This method uses air displacement instead of water displacement to estimate volume. Because ADP is quick (usually 5-10 min) and requires minimal client compliance and minimal technician skill, it is considered a viable alternative to hydrostatic weighing. The ADP method requires a whole-body plethysmograph such as the Bod Pod. The Bod Pod is a large, egg-shaped fiberglass chamber that uses air displacement and pressure-volume relationships to estimate body volume (see figure 8.4).

The Bod Pod system consists of two chambers: a front chamber in which the client sits during the measurement and a rear reference chamber. A molded fiberglass seat forms the wall between the two chambers, and a moving diaphragm mounted in this wall oscillates during testing (figure 8.5). The oscillating diaphragm creates small volume changes

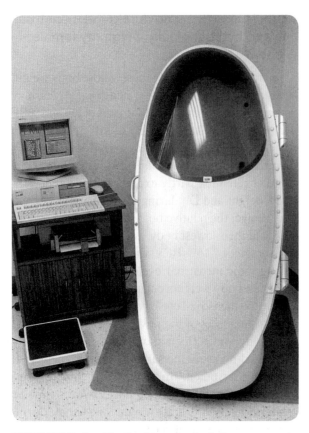

FIGURE 8.4 Air displacement plethysmograph.

between the two chambers. These changes are equal in magnitude but opposite in sign, and they produce small pressure fluctuations. The pressure-volume relationship is used to calculate the volume of the front chamber when it is empty and when the client is sitting in it. Body volume is calculated as the difference in the volume of the chamber with and without the client inside.

The principle underlying ADP centers on the relationship between pressure and volume. At a constant temperature (isothermal condition), volume (V) and pressure (P) are inversely related. According to **Boyle's law,**

$$P_1 / P_2 = V_2 / V_1,$$

where P_1 and V_1 represent one paired condition of pressure and volume and P_2 and V_2 represent another paired condition. P_1 and V_1 correspond to the pressure and volume of the Bod Pod when it is empty; P_2 and V_2 represent the pressure and volume of the Bod Pod when the client is in the chamber.

One assumption of the ADP method is that the Bod Pod controls the isothermal effects of clothing, hair, thoracic gas volume, and body surface area in the enclosed chamber. Bod Pod clients are tested

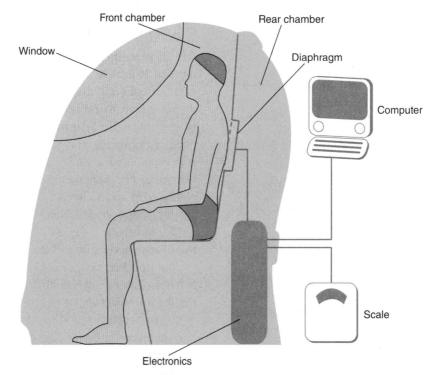

FIGURE 8.5 Two-chamber Bod Pod system.

while wearing minimal clothing (e.g., a swimsuit) and a swim cap to compress the hair. An estimate of the **body surface area**, calculated from the height and weight of the client, is used to correct for the isothermal effects at the body's surface. **Thoracic gas volume (TGV)** is the volume of air in the lungs (functional residual capacity) at midexhalation. The TGV is either directly measured or estimated by the Bod Pod to account for the isothermal conditions in the lungs. The Bod Pod software calculates the functional residual capacity at end exhalation by subtracting one-half of the exhaled tidal volume from the FRC measured at midexhalation.

Numerous studies have assessed the accuracy of the Bod Pod for measuring Db. Several researchers reported only small differences in average Db ($\leq$0.002 g·cc^{-1}) measured by the Bod Pod and HW (Fields et al. 2001; Vescovi et al. 2001; Yee et al. 2001). Some studies have reported slightly higher and statistically significant differences (0.003-0.007 g·cc^{-1}) in adults (Collins et al. 1999; Demerath et al. 2002; Dewit et al. 2000; Millard-Stafford et al. 2001; Wagner, Heyward, and Gibson 2000). In high school male athletes and collegiate track and field female athletes, the Bod Pod significantly underestimated average body density (Bentzur, Kravitz, and Lockner 2008; Moon et al. 2008).

Several studies, however, showed good group prediction errors (*SEE* $\leq$ 0.008 g·cc^{-1}) for adults (Fields, Hunter, and Goran 2000; Nunez et al. 1999; Wagner, Heyward, and Gibson 2000). Compared with multicomponent body composition models, the Bod Pod and HW methods have similar predictive accuracy (Fields et al. 2001). However, against a multicomponent reference model, ADP significantly overestimates fat-free mass of elite male rowers (Kendall et al. 2017). Regardless, since the Bod Pod is more accommodating than HW, there is much interest in further exploring the validity of the ADP method for estimating %BF in clinical populations and special populations such as children and older adults (Heyward and Wagner 2004).

Compared with dual-energy X-ray absorptiometry (DXA), ADP was strongly correlated (*r* = .88) and similar, on average, for body fat estimation; however, there may be large individual differences between the two methods, suggesting they are not interchangeable for young healthy women (Edwards, Simpson, and Buchholz 2011). Hurst and associates (2016) found no differences between %BF from DXA (Hologic QDR Discovery A) and Bod Pod for their large sample of adults (19-71 yr). However, the individual differences reflected by the limits of agreement were large (−6.1%-6.9% BF). Sex-specific differences were also noted. The Bod Pod underestimated the DXA %BF values for the lean men and overestimated the DXA %BF values for women with high levels of body fat. When looking at the entire sample, the opposite is true. ADP overestimated %BF for the lean participants while underestimating the DXA results for those having higher body fat levels (Hurst et al. 2016). Having recruited adults from the underweight, normal weight, and overweight/obese BMI categories, Lowry and Tomiyama (2015) compared %BF values between DXA (Lunar Prodigy) and ADP. Their results align somewhat with those of Hurst and colleagues by indicating that ADP overestimates %BF from DXA for those in the lower BMI ranges but, conversely, underestimates the DXA %BF of those in the higher BMI ranges. The magnitude of the significant mean differences was 7.6% and 2.1% for the underweight and overweight/obese participants, respectively.

More recently, Gibby and colleagues (2017) compared %BF values from ADP and HW against those from whole-body computed tomography (CT) for a sample that was predominantly male. Correlations between CT and the densitometry methods were strong (>.95), and the only reported mean differences involved comparisons with HW. On average, %BF from HW compared with ADP was lower by approximately 3.1%. The confidence interval (limits of agreement) for the densitometry method comparison was 1.28% to 4.28% BF, with ADP resulting in the higher %BF values. The two %BF conversion algorithms used with the CT significantly overestimated %BF from HW by 2.32% and 1.94%, respectively (Gibby et al. 2017).

Using the ADP Method

The Bod Pod is user friendly, providing computer prompts for each step of the procedure. Air displacement plethysmography is faster and easier than HW; researchers reported better compliance with ADP and a preference for ADP over HW among participants, including among children (Demerath et al. 2002; Dewit et al. 2000; Lockner et al. 2000). To increase the likelihood of accurate body composition assessments with ADP, give your client pretesting instructions before the scheduled appointment. These instructions are similar to those for HW (see Guidelines for Hydrostatic Weighing). For step-by-step instructions for Bod Pod testing, see Testing Procedures for the Bod Pod.

Special Considerations for the ADP Method

Accurate test results from the Bod Pod depend on a number of factors. The following questions address these factors.

How will the test results be affected if my client has excess body hair?

As mentioned earlier, isothermal air trapped in body hair may affect test results. For clients with beards, %BF may be underestimated by 1%; when scalp hair is exposed (no swim cap), relative body fat is underestimated by about 2.3% BF (Higgins et al. 2001). Wearing a tight-fitting swim cap and shaving excess facial and body hair ensure the most accurate estimate of body volume and Db.

Can I use the Bod Pod to measure the body composition of children?

During the 20 sec test, the client must remain very still, as the body volume estimate from the ADP method can vary if the client moves during testing. Fields and Goran (2000) commented that it took twice as long to measure children compared with adults, primarily because children move during the test. This was substantiated by Crook and colleagues (2012). They reported that the BV measurement took 50 sec for their sample of children aged 3 to 5 yr. As a result of children's tendency to move during the assessment, the test-retest reliability of the Bod Pod is lower in children ($r = .90$) than in adults ($r = .96$) (Demerath et al. 2002).

Also, several researchers commented that body size may affect Bod Pod estimates, with the largest effects seen in the smallest clients (Demerath et al. 2002; Lockner et al. 2000; Nunez et al. 1999; Rosendale and Bartok 2012). The Pea Pod was developed to assess the body composition of infants younger than 6 mo and weighing less than 8 kg. A pediatric option for the Bod Pod is now commercially

Video
8.2

TESTING PROCEDURES FOR THE BOD POD

- Instruct the client to change into dry, form-fitting swimwear and to completely void the bladder and bowels.
- Measure the client's height to the nearest centimeter and body weight to the nearest 5 g using the Bod Pod scale. These measures are used to calculate body surface area.
- Perform the two-point calibration: (a) baseline calibration with the chamber empty and (b) phantom calibration with a 50 L calibration cylinder. Be careful when handling the calibration cylinder; a dent in the cylinder alters its volume. If measuring TGV, attach the microbial filter and breathing tube according to the manufacturer's guidelines.
- Instruct your client to sit still and upright in the chamber, with the back against the wall and feet on the floor. Remind your client to breathe normally during the upcoming 20 sec test. Then close the door tightly.

- Follow the prompts and then open the door and close it again tightly; repeat the 20 sec test. If the two tests disagree by more than 150 ml, perform additional tests until two results agree within 150 ml; average these and use them to calculate raw BV.
- Open the door and instruct the client about the steps they need to follow during the TGV measurement. Be sure you give your client a nose clip or instructions on pinching the nostrils shut during the TGV measurement. All air exchange during the TGV measurement needs to take place via the single-use microbial filter and breathing tube.
- Instruct your client to follow the breathing cycle prompts and close the door. After a few tidal volume (normal) breathing cycles, the airway is occluded by the Bod Pod software. Guide your client through the puffing maneuver. If the computer-calculated figure of merit (indicating similar pressure signals in the airway and chamber) is not met, repeat this step.

available to address the smaller body size of young children. The pediatric option utilizes a smaller calibration cylinder (19.993 L), a booster seat, and special software modifications. Research, however, is not unanimous in terms of the accuracy of the pediatric modifications. Crook and associates (2012) reported that the pediatric option %BF estimates for children (3-5 yr) were weakly correlated ($r < .18$) to the reference measure calculated following isotope dilution. They also reported that the limits of agreement were large. Conversely, Fields and Allison (2012) reported that compared with a four-component (4C) reference measure, the pediatric option is reliable, precise, and accurate for estimating body fat levels of children aged 2 to 6 yr. It is important to note, however, that the BV parameter included in the 4C model was derived from the Bod Pod assessment (Fields and Allison 2012). This area requires further investigation.

Is it absolutely necessary that my client wear a swimsuit and swim cap during the Bod Pod test?

The original investigators of the Bod Pod recognized that the isothermal effect of clothing leads to an underestimation of body volume; they recommended that clients wear only a swimsuit and swim cap during testing to minimize this effect (Dempster and Aitkens 1995; McCrory et al. 1995). Silicone swim caps more thoroughly compress scalp hair compared with Lycra swim caps; for a sample of Caucasian women, the body fat percentage was an average of 1.2% higher when wearing the silicone swim cap (Peeters and Claessens 2011). More or loose-fitting clothing leads to a larger layer of isothermal air and a greater underestimation of body volume. For example, wearing a hospital gown instead of a swimsuit lowers %BF by about 5% (Fields et al. 2000). Thus, the clothing recommendation needs to be followed.

As long as they sit still, do I need to closely monitor how my clients are positioned inside the Bod Pod?

Deviations from the upright seated position may affect the volume of isothermal air in the pulmonary tree. This may cause an incorrect calculation of raw body volume. To test the influence of body position, Peeters (2012) assessed the body volume (at measured TGV) of young men in the standard seated position and in a forward leaning position (slight hip flexion, shoulders hanging, and back curved). Although the measured TGV did not differ by position, body volume was significantly smaller in the forward leaning position; the 86 ± 122 ml difference in body volume resulted in a small ($0.5\% \pm 0.7\%$) yet significant difference in body fat estimations. Consequently, to increase the test-retest reliability of your assessments, standardize your instructions to the client regarding body position (Peeters 2012). Adhering to this recommendation may prove critical in research studies.

Do I need to measure my client's TGV or can I use a predicted TGV?

Although McCrory and colleagues (1998) reported an insignificant difference (54 ml) between measured and predicted TGV, the *SEE* was large (442 ml). Some researchers have reported larger mean differences (344-400 ml) and *SEE*s (650 ml) (Collins et al. 1999; Lockner et al. 2000). Given that only 40% of the TGV value is used to calculate body volume, using a predicted TGV has a relatively smaller effect on Db and %BF compared with using a predicted RV for the HW method. Nevertheless, a measured TGV maximizes accuracy.

For top-level collegiate athletes at the extremes of the height distributions, Wagner (2015) recommends measuring TGV instead of predicting it. Although no significant difference between measured and predicted TGVs was reported for the athletes, there was a significant negative bias. This means the predicted TGV was larger than the measured TGV at small volumes, with the opposite being true for high volumes.

If I measure TGV, should I take one or more measurements?

To date, few researchers mention averaging multiple measurements of thoracic gas volume. Some that do, however, are suggesting that at least two TGV measurements be taken and averaged (Gibson, Roper, and Mermier 2016; Noreen and Lemon 2006; Tucker, Lechiminant, and Bailey 2014) even though doing so may increase the amount of time required. Notable individual between-trial differences in Db, BV, and %BF have been reported. If using Db from ADP in a multicomponent model, it is recommended that the average of multiple TGV measurements be used for Db calculations.

Do I need to closely monitor how my client breathes during the body volume and TGV measurement procedures?

Software revisions now guide the client through the tidal volume breathing cycles during TGV assessment. The client breathes in synchronization with the *in* and *out* prompts displayed on the computer screen, even if this is not her normal breathing pattern. However, if your Bod Pod does not have this software upgrade, then deviations in normal tidal breathing can affect body volume and %BF estimations.

For example, Tegenkamp and colleagues (2011) instructed their subjects to alter their tidal volume breathing patterns and found significant ($p < .001$) differences in %BF estimations as a result. During the body volume measurement procedure, deeper-than-normal breathing resulted in an average body fat percentage that was 2.1% lower. On the other hand, breathing more shallowly resulted in a %BF that was 2.2% higher. Differences in the opposite direction were recorded when breathing patterns were altered only during the TGV measurement. Shallower breathing underestimated body fat by an average of 3.4%, while deeper breathing increased body fat estimations by 3.7% (Tegenkamp et al. 2011). Standardizing instructions to your client regarding the need to inhale and exhale as normally as possible throughout the body volume and TGV measurements is important to obtain the best estimates of their body fat percentage.

Does the Bod Pod yield a valid and reliable measure of functional residual capacity?

Davis and colleagues (2007) compared FRC measures obtained from the Bod Pod and traditional gas dilution techniques in healthy males and females (18-50 yr). The FRC at midexpiration as measured by the Bod Pod was corrected to an end-exhalation volume by subtracting approximately one-half of the measured tidal volume. The mean difference between FRC from the Bod Pod and gas dilution FRC measures was −32 ml for males ($r = .925$; *SEE* = 0.246 L) and −23 ml for females ($r = .917$; *SEE* = 0.216 L). The test-retest reliability of the Bod Pod FRC was excellent ($r = .95$-.97). These results suggest that the Bod Pod provides a valid and reliable measure of FRC in healthy adults.

If I use both hydrostatic weighing and the Bod Pod to measure my client's body composition, which test should I give first?

The Bod Pod manufacturer recommends testing clients under resting conditions and when the body is dry. Although there are no known studies indicating the amount of error that may occur if these guidelines are violated, experts suggest adhering to these recommendations (Fields, Goran, and McCrory 2002). Thus, if a test battery includes both HW and ADP, administer the Bod Pod test first. If doing so is not possible, make certain your client is completely dry and fully recovered from the HW test before you administer the Bod Pod test.

Does exercise before Bod Pod testing affect the results?

The effect of an acute bout of exercise prior to body composition assessment via ADP was investigated by Harrop and Woodruff (2015). Compared with preexercise, 30 min of cycling at 75% HRmax (age predicted) resulted in numerous significant and sex-specific differences postexercise and during the repeat testing 2 hr postexercise. Similarly, Grossman and Deitrick (2015) compared ADP results at baseline against those acquired 2 hr after a resistance training workout lasting approximately 1 hr. Their finding of significant differences in %BF, body mass, BV, and FM supports the findings of Harrop and Woodruff (2015). The Bod Pod manufacturer's recommendation is that clients refrain from exercise for 2 hr before their ADP test. However, significant changes in body composition variables 2 hr postexercise indicate that refraining from exercise for only 2 hr is insufficient. Consequently, the accuracy of the ADP results may be affected.

Which model and equation should I use to convert Db to %BF?

Using a multicomponent model and a population-specific conversion formula increases the group and individual accuracy of %BF estimates. The default equation in the Bod Pod software is the Siri (1961) two-component model formula for non-black adults. A formula for black adults is also available. In field settings, these 2C conversion formulas may be appropriate for some clients with certain demographic characteristics. For other clients, you may need to select an appropriate population-specific 2C model formula (see table 8.2).

DUAL-ENERGY X-RAY ABSORPTIOMETRY

Dual-energy X-ray absorptiometry (DXA) is increasingly used as a reference method for body composition research (see figure 8.6), especially in clinical settings. This method yields estimates of bone mineral, fat, lean soft tissue, and visceral adipose tissue (VAT) mass. It is also possible to obtain estimates of these variables at the whole-body level and the regional (trunk and appendicular) level. Dual-energy X-ray absorptiometry is an attractive alternative to HW because it is safe and rapid, it requires minimal client cooperation, and, most important, it accounts for individual variability in bone mineral content. The time required per whole-body scan ranges from approximately 3 to 20 min, depending on the model, type of scan beam, and age of the DXA machine as well as the stature of the client (Bazzocchi et al. 2016).

The basic principle underlying DXA technology is that the attenuation of X-rays with high and low photon energies is measurable and dependent on the thickness, density, and chemical composition of the underlying tissue. The **attenuation**, or weakening, of X-rays through fat, lean tissue, and bone varies because of differences in the densities and chemical compositions of these tissues. The attenuation ratios for the high and low X-ray energies are thought to be constant for all individuals (Pietrobelli et al. 1996).

It is difficult to assess the validity of the DXA method because each of the three manufacturers of DXA instruments (General Electric, Hologic, and Norland) has developed its own models and software over the years. As researchers and clinicians have discovered, body composition results vary with manufacturer, model, and software version. Thus, some of the variability reported in DXA validation studies may be due to the different DXA scanners and software versions. Thus experts who have reviewed DXA studies have called for more standardization among manufacturers (Genton et al. 2002; Lohman 1996).

Some researchers have reported that the predictive accuracy of DXA is better than that of HW (Fields and Goran 2000; Friedl et al. 1992; Prior et al. 1997; Wagner and Heyward 2001; Withers et al. 1998). However, the opposite finding (that HW is more accurate than DXA) has also been reported (Bergsma-Kadijk, Baumeister, and Deurenberg 1996; Goran, Toth, and Poehlman 1998; Millard-Stafford et al. 2001). In a review of DXA

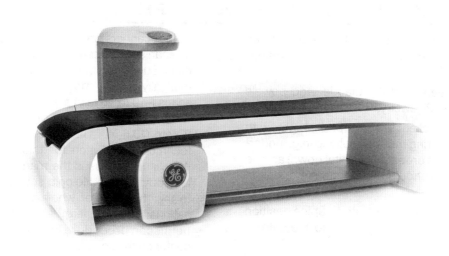

FIGURE 8.6 Dual-energy X-ray absorptiometer.
© 2006 General Electric Company

studies, Lohman and colleagues (2000) concluded that DXA estimates of %BF are within 1% to 3% of multicomponent model estimates.

Although some body composition prediction equations have been developed and validated with DXA as the reference method, further research is needed before DXA can be firmly established as the best reference method. Toombs and colleagues (2012), in their review of the metamorphosis of DXA technology, support the call for additional research using 4C and human cadaver criterion measures before labeling DXA as a gold standard for body composition assessment. Still, the DXA method is widely used in light of its availability, ease of use, and low radiation exposure (Yee and Gallagher 2008). Regardless, caution is urged when interpreting the results of DXA comparison studies given equivocal findings such as large intra-individual and significant group mean differences in body fat percentage compared with 4C measures (Toombs et al. 2012).

Using the DXA Method

The DXA method requires minimal client cooperation during the scan and minimal technical skill. However, to use the scanner to get precise and accurate DXA scans, proper training and client preparation are essential. Many states require that a licensed X-ray technician perform the scan under direct supervision of a medical doctor. For general procedures for DXA testing, see Basic Testing Procedures for DXA.

In terms of client preparation for DXA scanning, give the client a reminder call or send an email or text 24 hr before the appointment. In this reminder, instruct your client to arrive in a rested, fasted state with no fluid intake prior to the scan and to refrain from exercise until after the scan (Nana et al. 2015).

Special Considerations

The accuracy of DXA results depends on a number of factors. The following questions address some of these factors.

Will my client's body size and hydration state affect the test results?

In the past, the DXA method was not recommended for assessing the body composition of clients whose body dimensions exceed the length or width of the scanning bed. Techniques and software options are now available to accommodate people whose height or width is outside the scanning field. These options require repositioning the body on the scan bed and performing a half-body (hemiscan procedure)

BASIC TESTING PROCEDURES FOR DXA

- Before testing, calibrate the DXA scanner with a calibration marker provided by the manufacturer.
- Have the client void the bladder and bowels and remove all jewelry.
- Measure the client's height and weight, with the client wearing minimal clothing (e.g., underwear, wireless crop top, hospital gown) and no shoes. There should be no chlorine or salt in the clothing.
- Carefully guide the client into a supine position on the scanner bed for a head-to-toe anteroposterior scan.
- Use a skeletal anthropometer to accurately determine body thickness (see the Sagittal Abdominal Diameter section later in this chapter).

- Some scanners have different acquisition modes so scan speeds can be adjusted for body thickness. Such adjustments are usually made automatically by new model scanners. Slow speed scans (~10 to 15 min) are appropriate for clients with sagittal abdominal diameters exceeding 27 cm (10.6 in.). GE Lunar scanners alert the technician to switch to "thick" scan mode if the client surpasses the manufacturer's cutoff for body weight. Hologic scanners can switch to the "high power whole-body" mode (International Atomic Energy Association 2010). The **hemiscan procedure** (positioning the client off center on the scan table so one side of the body is completely within the scan field) can be used for clients too wide for the scan table. Resulting values are doubled to derive total body values (International Atomic Energy Association 2010).

Adapted from Nana et al. 2015; International Atomic Energy Association 2010.

analysis (Bazzocchi et al. 2016) or multiple partial body scans (Nana et al. 2015). The results of these partial scans need to be summed in order to estimate body composition.

In terms of hydration, DXA algorithms assume the adult FFB is consistently 73% water (Toomey, McCormack, and Jakeman 2017). Research has shown that small fluctuations in hydration have little effect on DXA estimates of fat mass or bone (Toomey, McCormack, and Jakeman 2017). Conversely, Nana and colleagues (2012) reported that many dietary factors affect regional body composition estimates more than they affect total and lean mass estimates. Consequently, DXA scan precision may be maximized if the client arrives in a fasted (Nana et al. 2015) and euhydrated (Rodriguez-Sanchez and Galloway 2015) state. For athletes, lean tissue mass assessment will be more accurate if they strictly adhere to pretest instructions regarding exercise, euhydration, and postexercise nutritional compensation (Toomey, McCormack, and Jakeman 2017).

Does it matter if my client has fasted and is rested when having a DXA scan?

As just mentioned, fasting prior to a DXA scan increases the accuracy of the body composition assessment and provides a level of standardization that is important for repeat measurements. An investigation of young adults revealed that performing activities of daily living (meal consumption and typical physical activity) before a DXA scan does not significantly influence body fat estimates (Nana et al. 2012). However, other regional and total body composition results are affected. Substantial increases in the mean estimate and typical error were noted in the regional and total lean mass as well as total body mass. For the women, eating prior to the DXA scan substantially increased the mean bone mineral content (BMC) values of the total body, trunk, and arms. To learn more about the influence of usual daily activities, meal consumption, and within- and between-day variability on DXA measurements, see the work of Nana and colleagues (2012). Nana and associates (2015) offer a best practice protocol for whole-body scanning of athletes and active people. This positioning protocol differs somewhat from the protocol used by NHANES (Centers for Disease Control and Prevention 2013). Kerr and associates (2016) reported that the two protocols are not interchangeable and that the measurement precision of the arms and trunk are increased with the positioning protocol of Nana and colleagues.

For client comfort and compliance, is DXA better than other reference methods?

According to anecdotal feedback on positioning protocols, participants in the study by Kerr's research team (2016) preferred the protocol of Nana and associates (2015) over the NHANES protocol. Compared with a 4C model reference, the new iDXA scanner (GE Healthcare Lunar) differed significantly in the calculations of fat mass (FM) for a sample of adults (Watson, Venables, and Murgatroyd 2017). The iDXA overestimates the reference FM of the participants whose FM values are below 32 kg and underestimates the reference when FM values exceed 32 kg.

Compared with other reference methods, DXA requires little client participation. The client does not need to perform the breathing maneuvers required for measuring RV for hydrostatic weighing and TGV for air displacement plethysmography. The BV component of a 4C model traditionally comes from a densitometric method (HW or ADP). Recently, a 4C model deriving its BV component from ADP was compared against a 4C model with the BV being derived from DXA (Smith-Ryan et al. 2017). There were no differences between 4C models for %BF, FM, and lean mass, although the limits of agreement for %BF were large (−5.33 to 7.01 %BF). In addition to eliminating client errors in UWW or ADP's thoracic gas volume measurements, the DXA body volume method may eventually provide all but the water component for a 4C reference measure of body fat. Additional research and cross-validation using each style of DXA machine is required before eliminating the densitometric assessment of body volume for multicomponent models.

How do the various DXA machines and software versions affect test results?

As mentioned earlier, variability among DXA technologies is a major source of error. Although all DXA equipment uses the same underlying physical principles, the instruments differ in their generation of high- and low-energy beams (filter or switching

BODY COMPOSITION ASSESSMENT USING 3D BODY SURFACE SCANNING

Historically used in the clothing industry, whole-body scanning with three-dimensional (3D) body surface scanners is gaining recognition as a quick, noninvasive, and precise automated method for quantifying anthropometric measures of length, circumference, and volume (Löffler-Wirth et al. 2016; Ng et al. 2016; Soileau et al. 2016). Device reliability is high regardless of operator skill level (Zancanaro et al. 2015). More expensive high-resolution laser-based systems are useful in clinical settings but may soon be rivaled by systems derived from inexpensive Microsoft Corporation Kinect devices. Soileau and colleagues (2016) compared 3D whole-body scanning results from a Kinect-based system against a laser-based system reference, ADP, and stadiometry for a sample of healthy adults and children. Differences in estimated height, waist circumference, body volume, and body surface area were small compared with reference measures. Conversely, smaller and more distal features had much larger differences. Although there are some anatomical feature acquisition issues yet to be resolved, whole-body 3D scanning holds promise as a valid and reliable method to quickly assess anthropometric measurements without the need to identify bony landmarks. In the future, using a Kinect-based system may prove suitable for field-based epidemiological use.

voltage), imaging geometry (pencil beam, fan beam, or narrow fan beam), X-ray detectors, calibration methodology, and algorithms (Genton et al. 2002). Comparisons of older (Lunar Prodigy) and newer (iDXA) scanners made by GE Healthcare indicate the correlation between the devices is strong, and there is no significant difference between means for whole-body values in samples of adults spanning the BMI range (Morrison et al. 2016; Reinhardt et al. 2017). However, in the Bland and Altman plots of individual variation, the %BF from iDXA is higher than from the Lunar Prodigy in lean adults; the opposite is true for heavier adults (Reinhardt et al. 2017). Reports of significant interdevice differences in regional (arms, legs, and torso) values also appear in the recent literature (Morrison et al. 2016; Oldroyd, Treadgold, and Hind 2017).

Because of technological differences, you should use the same DXA device and software version for longitudinal assessments or cross-sectional comparisons of body composition. If upgrading DXA machines or software, perform same-day scans of a representative sample using both versions. By doing so, you will have the information necessary to create a prediction equation useful in converting the older data, bringing it into alignment with results from the upgrade (Camhi et al. 2011). Equations to convert %BF values between the Lunar Prodigy and iDXA have been created and validated by multiple research teams (Oldroyd, Treadgold, and Hind 2017; Reinhardt et al. 2017). Likewise, Xu, Chafi, and colleagues (2016) developed equations to convert

%BF, BMD, BMC, and total mass values between the Hologic Discovery and iDXA scanners.

Is the DXA method safe for my clients, given that it uses X-rays to estimate body composition?

Even though two X-ray energies are passed through the body during a scan, the radiation exposure is very low. For example, a standard chest X-ray has a radiation dose of 50 microSeiverts (µSv), and a whole-body DXA scan is in the range of 0.2 to 0.5 µSv (Nana et al. 2015). Even so, the International Society for Clinical Densitometry does not recommend DXA scans for pregnant women. The radiation exposure depends on the scanner's manufacturer, model, and mode of scan. The scan mode is based on the anteroposterior thickness (sagittal abdominal diameter) of the client. Mode options are thin, standard, and thick. Mode selection is typically done automatically based on BMI, but it can be changed by the technician. The thicker the client, the slower the scan; this may slightly increase radiation exposure (Nana et al. 2015).

Is the DXA method recommended for estimating visceral adipose tissue (VAT)?

Computed tomography and magnetic resonance imaging (MRI) are considered the gold standards for VAT assessment, but both increase radiation exposure as compared with DXA. The Lunar Prodigy and iDXA fan-beam technology provides the ability to automatically and separately identify VAT from subcutaneous adipose tissue (SAT). In the VAT estimation study by Cheung's research team (2016), the Lunar Prodigy significantly underestimated VAT as compared with MRI for their sample of older men (61.6 ± 6.5 yr). The DXA-MRI and DXA-CT correlations were strong ($r > .80$); no comparison of mean differences between DXA and the CT was reported (Cheung et al. 2016). After comparing the two methods in a sample of 40 adults, Reinhardt and associates (2017) concluded the iDXA is a suitable alternative to MRI for assessing VAT in research studies. Consequently, both the Lunar Prodigy and iDXA offer a less expensive and safer option for VAT assessment.

FIELD METHODS FOR ASSESSING BODY COMPOSITION

In field settings, you can use more practical methods to estimate your clients' body composition. Your choices include skinfolds, ultrasound, bioelectrical impedance, and other types of anthropometric prediction equations. To use these methods and equations appropriately, you need to understand the basic assumptions and principles as well as the potential sources of measurement error for each method. You must closely follow standardized testing procedures, and you must practice in order to perfect your measurement techniques. For more detailed information about these field methods and how they are applied to various population subgroups, see Heyward and Wagner (2004) and Wagner (2013).

SKINFOLD METHOD

A **skinfold (SKF)** indirectly measures the thickness of subcutaneous adipose tissue. When you use the SKF method to estimate total Db in order to calculate relative body fat (%BF), certain basic relationships are assumed:

• *A SKF is a good measure of subcutaneous fat.* Research has demonstrated that the subcutaneous fat value obtained by SKF measurements at 12 sites is similar to the value obtained from magnetic resonance imaging (Hayes et al. 1988).

• *The distribution of fat subcutaneously and internally is similar for all individuals within each gender.* The validity of this assumption is question-

able. There are large interindividual differences in the patterning of subcutaneous adipose tissue within and between genders (Martin et al. 1985). Older subjects of the same gender and Db have proportionately less subcutaneous fat than their younger counterparts. Also, lean individuals have a higher proportion of internal fat, and the proportion of fat located internally decreases as overall body fatness increases (Lohman 1981).

• *Because there is a relationship between subcutaneous fat and total body fat, the sum of several SKFs can be used to estimate total body fat.* Research has established that SKF thicknesses at multiple sites measure a common body fat factor (Jackson and Pollock 1976; Quatrochi et al. 1992). It is assumed that approximately one-third of the total fat is located subcutaneously in men and women (Lohman 1981). However, there is considerable biological variation in subcutaneous, intramuscular, intermuscular, and internal organ fat deposits (Clarys et al. 1987), as well as in essential lipids in bone marrow and the central nervous system. Age, gender, and degree of fatness all affect variation in fat distribution (Lohman 1981).

• *There is a relationship between the sum of SKFs (ΣSKF) and Db.* This relationship is linear for homogeneous samples (population-specific SKF equations) but nonlinear over a wide range of Db (generalized SKF equations) for both men and women. A linear regression line depicting the relationship between the ΣSKF and Db will fit the data well only within a narrow range of body fatness values. Thus, you will get an inaccurate estimate if you use a population-specific equation to estimate the Db of a client who is not representative of the sample used to develop that equation (Jackson 1984).

• *Age is an independent predictor of Db for both men and women.* Using age and the quadratic expression of the sum of skinfolds (ΣSKF^2) accounts for more variance in Db of a heterogeneous population than using the ΣSKF^2 alone (Jackson 1984).

Using the Skinfold Method

Skinfold prediction equations are developed using either linear (population specific) or quadratic (generalized) regression models. There are well over 100 population-specific equations for predicting Db from various combinations of SKFs, circumferences, and bony diameters (Jackson and Pollock

1985). These equations were developed for relatively homogeneous populations, and they are assumed to be valid only for individuals having similar characteristics, such as age, gender, ethnicity, or level of physical activity. For example, an equation derived specifically for 18 to 21 yr old sedentary men would not be valid for predicting the Db of 35 to 45 yr old sedentary men. Population-specific equations are based on a linear relationship between SKF fat and Db (linear model); however, research shows a curvilinear relationship (quadratic model) between SKFs and Db across a large range of body fatness (see figure 8.7). Population-specific equations will tend to underestimate %BF in fatter subjects and overestimate it in leaner subjects.

Using the quadratic model, Jackson and colleagues (Jackson and Pollock 1978; Jackson, Pollock, and Ward 1980) developed generalized equations applicable to individuals varying greatly in age (18-60 yr) and body fatness (up to 45% BF). These equations also take into account the effect of age on the distribution of subcutaneous and internal fat. An advantage of the generalized equations is that you can use one equation, instead of several, to accurately estimate your clients' %BF.

Given that these generalized SKF equations were developed on predominately white adults, Jackson and colleagues (2009) cross-validated the equations with samples of young white, Hispanic, and African-American men and women (17-35 yr). The DXA method was used to obtain reference measures of %BF for 706 women and 423 men. Although the generalized SKF equations were highly correlated ($r = .91$) with $\%BF_{DXA}$, these equations lacked accuracy when applied to racially and ethnically diverse samples. New race-specific equations have been developed and reported. Practitioners who use the new DXA-based equations are urged to use ones that have undergone independent cross-validation.

Most equations use two or three SKFs to predict Db. Experts recommend using equations that have SKF measures from a variety of sites, including both upper and lower body sites (Martin et al. 1985). The Db is then converted to %BF using the

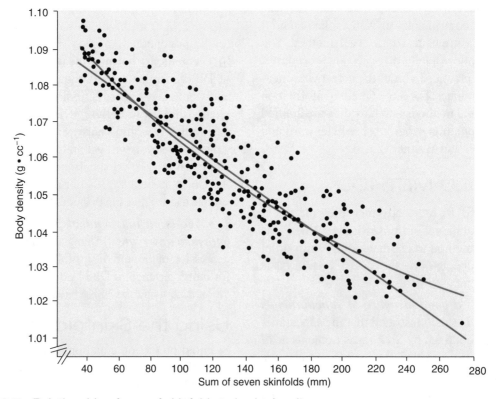

FIGURE 8.7 Relationship of sum of skinfolds to body density.

Reprinted from A.S. Jackson and M.L. Pollock, "Generalized Equations for Predicting Body Density of Men," *British Journal of Nutrition* 40 no. 3 (1978): 497-504. © 1978 The Nutrition Society. Reprinted with the permission of Cambridge University Press.

appropriate population-specific conversion formula (see table 8.2). Table 8.3 presents commonly used population-specific and generalized SKF prediction equations. Select the appropriate SKF equation and population-specific conversion formula in table 8.2 to estimate %BF based on physical demographics (e.g., age, gender, ethnicity, and physical activity level) of your clients. Using these equations, you can accurately estimate the %BF of your clients within the recommended value, ±3.5% BF (Lohman 1992).

Alternatively, nomograms exist for some SKF prediction equations. The nomogram in figure 8.8 was specifically developed for the Jackson sum-of-three-SKFs equations. To use this nomogram, plot the sum of three skinfolds (Σ3SKF) and age in the appropriate columns, and use a ruler to connect these two points. The corresponding %BF is read at the point where the connecting line intersects the %BF column on the nomogram.

Although nomograms are potential time-savers, you should be aware that this nomogram is based on a two-component body composition model, using the Siri equation to convert Db to %BF. In general, use this nomogram only to calculate %BF of clients with an estimated fat-free body density of 1.100 $g \cdot cc^{-1}$ (see table 8.2).

Skinfold Technique

It takes a great deal of time and practice to develop your skill as a skinfold technician. Following standardized procedures (see Standardized Procedures for Skinfold Measurements) will increase the accuracy and reliability of your measurements.

You will also be able to increase your skill by following the recommendations (see Recommendations for Skinfold Technicians) made by experts in the field (Jackson and Pollock 1985; Lohman et al. 1984; Pollock and Jackson 1984).

Table 8.3 Skinfold Prediction Equations

SKF sites	Population subgroups	Equation	Reference
Σ7SKF (chest + abdomen + thigh + triceps + subscapular + suprailiac + midaxilla)	Black or Hispanic women, 18-55 yr	Db $(g \cdot cc^{-1})^a$ = 1.0970 − 0.00046971(Σ7SKF) + 0.00000056$(Σ7SKF)^2$ − 0.00012828(age)	Jackson et al. (1980)
	Black men or male athletes, 18-61 yr	Db $(g \cdot cc^{-1})^a$ = 1.1120 − 0.00043499(Σ7SKF) + 0.00000055$(Σ7SKF)^2$ − 0.00028826(age)	Jackson and Pollock (1978)
Σ4SKF (triceps + anterior suprailiac + abdomen + thigh)	Female athletes, 18-29 yr	Db $(g \cdot cc^{-1})^a$ = 1.096095 − 0.0006952(Σ4SKF) + 0.0000011$(Σ4SKF)^2$ − 0.0000714(age)	Jackson et al. (1980)
Σ3SKF (triceps + suprailiac + thigh)	White or anorexic women, 18-55 yr	Db $(g \cdot cc^{-1})^a$ = 1.0994921 − 0.0009929(Σ3SKF) + 0.0000023$(Σ3SKF)^2$ − 0.0001392(age)	Jackson et al. (1980)
Σ3SKF (chest + abdomen + thigh)	White men, 18-61 yr	Db $(g \cdot cc^{-1})^a$ = 1.109380 − 0.0008267(Σ3SKF) + 0.0000016$(Σ3SKF)^2$ − 0.0002574(age)	Jackson and Pollock (1978)
Σ3SKF (abdomen + thigh + triceps)	Black or white collegiate male and female athletes, 18-34 yr	%BF = 8.997 + 0.2468(Σ3SKF) − 6.343(gender[b]) − 1.998(race[c])	Evans et al. (2005)
Σ2SKF (triceps + calf)	Black or white boys, 6-17 yr Black or white girls, 6-17 yr	%BF = 0.735(Σ2SKF) + 1.0 %BF = 0.610(Σ2SKF) + 5.1	Slaughter et al. (1988)

ΣSKF = sum of skinfolds (mm).

[a]Use population-specific conversion formulas to calculate %BF (percent body fat) from Db (body density).

[b]Male athletes = 1; female athletes = 0.

[c]Black athletes = 1; white athletes = 0.

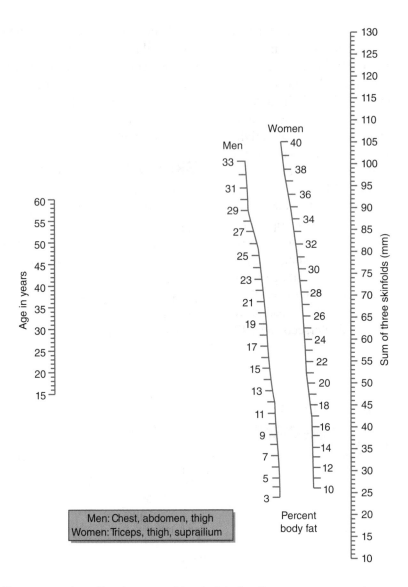

FIGURE 8.8 Nomogram to estimate percent body fat of college-age men and women using the Jackson sum-of-three-skinfolds equations.

From *A nomogram for the estimate of percent body fat from generalized equations,* by W.B. Baun, M.R. Baun, and P.B. Raven, 1981, Research Quarterly for Exercise and Sport, 52(3), pg. 382. Copyright 1981 by American Alliance for Health, Physical Education, and Dance, 1900 Association Drive, Reston, VA 20191.

In addition to perfecting your technical skills, you should develop your interpersonal skills when administering SKF and other anthropometric tests. For suggestions about developing interpersonal skills, see Tips for Developing Interpersonal Skills.

Sources of Measurement Error

The accuracy and precision of SKF measurements and the SKF method are affected by the technician's skill, the type of SKF caliper, and client factors. The following questions and responses address these sources of measurement error.

Is there high agreement among SKF values when the measurements are taken by two different technicians?

A major source of measurement error is differences between SKF technicians. Objectivity, or between-technician reliability, is improved when SKF technicians follow standardized testing procedures, practice taking SKFs together, and mark the SKF site (Pollock and Jackson 1984). A major cause of low intertester reliability is improper location and measurement of the SKF sites (Lohman et al. 1984). The amount of between-technician error depends on the SKF site, with larger errors reported for the abdomen (8.8%) and thigh (7.1%) sites than for the triceps (~3.0%), subscapular (~3.0%-5.0%), and suprailiac (~4%) sites (Lohman et al. 1984).

Are the anatomical descriptions for specific SKF sites the same for all SKF equations?

In the past, for some SKF sites, the anatomical location and direction of the fold have varied. For example, Behnke and Wilmore (1974) recommend measuring the abdominal SKF using a horizontal fold adjacent to the umbilicus; Jackson and Pollock (1978), however, recommend measuring a vertical fold taken 2 cm (0.8 in.) lateral to the umbilicus.

Inconsistencies such as this have led to confusion and lack of agreement among SKF technicians. As a result, groups of experts in the field of anthropometry have developed standardized testing procedures and detailed descriptions for identification and measurement of SKF sites (Harrison et al. 1988; Ross and Marfell-Jones 1991). Appendix D.2, Standardized Sites for Skinfold Measurements, summarizes some of the most commonly used sites as described in the *Anthropometric Standardization*

Reference Manual.

Although the objective is to have all SKF technicians follow standardized procedures and recommendations for site location and SKF measurements, you may not be able to do so under all circumstances. For example, if you are using the generalized equations of Jackson and Pollock (1978) and Jackson and colleagues (1980), the chest, midaxillary, subscapular, abdominal, and suprailiac SKFs will be located at sites that differ from those described in the *Anthropometric Standardization Reference Manual.* The descriptions for the sites used in these equations are presented in appendix D.3, Skinfold Sites for Jackson's Generalized Skinfold Equations.

How many measurements do I need to take at each SKF site?

A lack of intratechnician reliability or consistency of measurements by the SKF technician is another source of error for the SKF method. You need to practice your SKF technique on 50 to 100 clients to develop a high degree of skill and proficiency (Jackson and Pollock 1985). Take a minimum of two measurements at each site using a rotational order. If values vary from each other by more than 10%, take additional measurements and average the two trials that meet this criterion. Use this average value

Standardized Procedures for Skinfold Measurements

1. Take all SKF measurements on the right side of the body.
2. Carefully identify, measure, and mark the SKF site, especially if you are a novice SKF technician (see appendix D.2, Standardized Sites for Skinfold Measurements).
3. Grasp the SKF firmly between the thumb and index finger of your left hand. Lift the fold 1 cm (0.4 in.) above the site to be measured.
4. Lift the fold by placing the thumb and index finger 8 cm (~3 in.) apart on a line that is perpendicular to the long axis of the SKF. The long axis is parallel to the natural cleavage lines of the skin. For individuals with extremely large SKFs, you will need to separate your thumb and finger more than 8 cm in order to lift the fold.
5. Keep the fold elevated while you take the measurement.
6. Place the jaws of the caliper perpendicular to the fold, approximately 1 cm below the thumb and index finger and halfway between the crest and the base of the fold. Release the jaw pressure slowly.
7. Take the SKF measurement 3 sec after the pressure is released. The American College of Sports Medicine (ACSM 2018) recommends that you wait only 1 to 2 sec before reading the caliper.
8. Open the jaws of the caliper to remove it from the site. Close the jaws slowly to prevent damage or loss of calibration.

Recommendations for Skinfold Technicians

- Be meticulous when locating the anatomical landmarks used to identify the SKF site, when measuring the distance, and when marking the site with a surgical marking pen.
- Read the dial of the caliper to the nearest 0.1 mm (Harpenden or Holtain), 0.5 mm (Lange), or 1 mm (plastic calipers).
- Take a minimum of two measurements at each site. If values vary from each other by more than 2 mm, take additional measurements and use the average of two measurements within that range.
- Take SKF measurements in a rotational order (circuits) rather than taking consecutive readings at each site.
- Take the SKF measurements when the client's skin is dry and lotion free.

- Do not measure SKFs immediately after exercise because the shift in body fluid to the skin tends to increase the size of the SKF.
- Practice taking SKFs on 50 to 100 clients.
- Avoid using plastic calipers if you are an inexperienced SKF technician. Instead use metal calipers.
- Train with skilled SKF technicians and compare your results.
- Use a training videotape that demonstrates proper SKF techniques (Lohman 1987; Human Kinetics 1995).
- Seek additional training through workshops held at state, regional, and national conferences or through distance education courses.

TIPS FOR DEVELOPING INTERPERSONAL SKILLS

- Before the scheduled test session, instruct your clients to wear loose clothing that allows easy access to the measurement sites, such as shorts and a T-shirt or two-piece exercise gear.
- Often clients are apprehensive about having their SKFs measured, particularly when they are meeting you for the first time. During the testing, put your clients at ease by establishing good rapport (e.g., talk about some unrelated topic), projecting a sense of relaxed confidence, and creating a test environment that is friendly, private, safe, and comfortable.
- Perform the test in an uncluttered private room that holds a small table for calipers, pens, and clipboards and a chair for clients who are unstable standing or need to rest during the testing.

- Some clients feel more comfortable having their SKFs measured by a technician of the same gender. If this is not feasible, you could ask your clients if they would like another person of the same gender to observe the test.
- Educate your clients about the SKF test by talking about the purpose and use of the measurements, pointing to the SKF sites on your body, and demonstrating on yourself how the SKF is measured.
- Limit your verbal and facial reactions while collecting SKF data.

Based on Habash 2002.

in the SKF prediction equation. The ±10% value for duplicate measurements at each site is recommended as the standardized procedure in the *Anthropometric Standardized Reference Manual*.

However, if you are preparing to take an ACSM certification examination, you will need to modify this standardized procedure slightly by using the ACSM-recommended criterion for duplicate SKF measurements. The ACSM (2018) also suggests taking at least two measurements at each site in rotational order; however, these two measurements at a given site need to be within 2 mm of each other.

If you take more than two measurements to meet this criterion, average the two trials that are within ± 2 mm of each other, and use this value in the prediction equation to estimate Db and %BF. On the other hand, some researchers suggest taking three SKF measurements at each site and using the median (middle score) instead of the mean (average) (Ward and Anderson 1998).

What types of SKF calipers are available, and how do they differ?

A variety of high-quality metal and plastic calipers are offered for measuring SKF thickness (see figure 8.9). When choosing a caliper, you need to consider factors such as cost, durability, accuracy, and precision as well as which type of caliper was used for developing a specific SKF equation. Table 8.4 and figure 8.10 compare some of the basic characteristics of selected SKF calipers.

High-quality metal calipers are accurate and precise throughout the range of measurement. The Harpenden, Lange, Holtain, and Lafayette calipers

exert constant pressure (~7-8 g·mm^{-2}) over their range (0-60 mm). Calipers should not have tension that varies by more than 2.0 g·mm^{-2} throughout the range of measurement or exceeds 15 g·mm^{-2} (Edwards et al. 1955). Excessive tension and pressure cause client discomfort (pinching sensation) and significantly reduce the SKF measurement (Gruber et al. 1990). High-quality calipers also have excellent scale precision (e.g., 0.2 and 1.0 mm, respectively, for Harpenden and Lange).

Although the Harpenden and Lange SKF calipers have similar pressure characteristics, a number of researchers reported that SKFs measured with Harpenden calipers are significantly smaller than those measured with Lange calipers (Gruber et al. 1990; Lohman et al. 1984; Schmidt and Carter 1990). This difference translates into a systematic underestimation (~1.5% BF) of average %BF by the Harpenden calipers (Gruber et al. 1990). Even though the pressure is similar for the Lange (8.37 g·mm^{-2}) and Harpenden (8.25 g·mm^{-2}) calipers (Schmidt and Carter 1990), researchers noted that

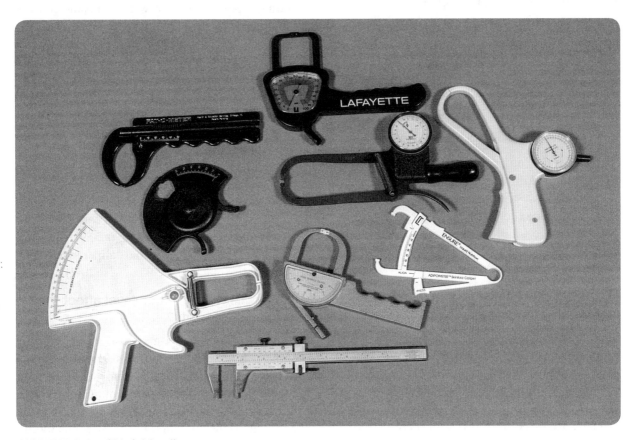

FIGURE 8.9 Skinfold calipers.

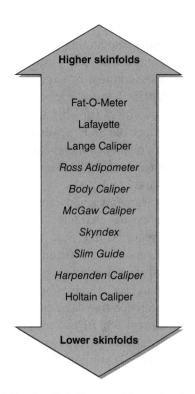

FIGURE 8.10 Relative ranking of values measured by various types of skinfold calipers. Calipers in italics give similar skinfold readings.

opening the jaws of the Harpenden caliper requires three times more force. Therefore, it is likely that the Harpenden compresses adipose tissue to a greater extent, resulting in SKF measurements smaller than those that the Lange caliper yields. The Cescorf skinfold caliper has a configuration and pressure characteristics similar to those of the Harpenden. As expected, skinfold thickness measurements at the nine sites assessed were significantly lower with a Cescorf caliper compared with a Lange caliper. This difference translates into an underestimation (5.2%-6.9% BF) of average %BF by the Cescorf calipers (Cyrino et al. 2003).

Are plastic SKF calipers as accurate as high-quality metal calipers?

Compared with high-quality calipers, some plastic calipers do not exert constant tension throughout the range of measurement and have less scale precision (~2 mm) and a smaller range of measurement (0-40 mm). Despite these differences, some plastic calipers compare well (see table 8.4) with more expensive high-quality metal calipers (Cataldo and Heyward

2000). Given that the type of caliper is a potential source of measurement error, follow these suggestions to minimize error:

- Use the same caliper when monitoring changes in a client's SKF thicknesses.
- Use the same type of caliper as was used in the development of the specific SKF prediction equation you have selected. If the same type of caliper is not available, use one that gives similar readings (see figure 8.10).
- Periodically check the accuracy of your caliper and calibrate if needed.

How accurate are the digital SKF calipers?

In an attempt to reduce, if not eliminate, the human errors introduced by an inexperienced or inattentive skinfold technician (e.g., failing to read the gauge after the proper time interval, misreading the gauge, miscalculating body density and %BF), efforts are under way to automate the skinfold thickness reading and calculation processes. A digital modification utilizing miniaturized sensor technology and transmission of a wireless signal to a computer running Liposoft 2008 software (Adipsmeter V1.0) is commercially available for Harpenden calipers (LipoTool). The standard skinfold thickness assessment protocol is programmed into the software application, thereby eliminating the technician's need to read the gauge or perform mathematical calculations. Amaral and colleagues (2011) investigated the validity and reliability of the LipoTool by comparing skinfold thickness results with those obtained using a standard Harpenden caliper. The mean difference between the two calipers was 0.3 mm, the associated limits of agreement ranged from −3.1 to 3.4 mm, and the correlation coefficients for the skinfold sites were all strong ($r > .91$). To learn more about this digital skinfold caliper system, see the work of Amaral and colleagues (2011).

Will my clients' hydration level affect the SKF measurements?

Skinfold measurements may also be affected by compressibility of the adipose tissue and hydration levels of your clients (Ward, Rempel, and Anderson 1999). Martin, Drinkwater, and Clarys (1992) reported that variation in SKF compressibility may be an important limitation of the SKF method. In addition, an accumulation of extracellular water

Table 8.4 Comparison of High-Quality Metal Calipers and Plastic SKF Calipers

Caliper type	Average pressure (g·mm⁻²)	Range (mm)	Scale precision (mm)	Accuracy	Durability	Relative cost[c]	Unique features	Supplier
METAL								
Harpenden (HA)	8.2	0-55	0.2	HA < LNG[a]	Excellent	$$$	—	Creative Health Products
Lange (LNG)	8.4	0-60	0.5	LNG > HA[a]	Excellent	$$	—	Creative Health Products
Lafayette (LF)	7.5	0-100	0.5	LF > LNG[a]	Excellent	$$$	Measurement range 0-100 mm	Creative Health Products
Skyndex (SKN)	7.3		0.5	SKN < LNG[a]; SKN ≈ HA[a]	Excellent	$$$	Skyndex I: built-in computer, Durnin and Womersley and Jackson and Pollock equations; Syndex II: digital readout but no computer	Creative Health Products
Holtain (HO)			0.2	HO < HA, LNG[b]	Excellent	$$$	—	Hotain, Ltd.
PLASTIC								
Accu-Measure (AM)	NR	0-60	1.0	NR	Fair	$	Can be used for self-assessment of body fat	Accu-Measure
Body Caliper (BC)	NR	0-60	1.0	BC ≈ HA[b]	Good	$$	Measurement scale on both sides of caliper; suitable for right- or left-handed technician	The Caliper Company
Fat-O-Meter (F)	5.6	0-40	2.0	F ≈ LNG[b]	Poor	$	—	Creative Health Products
Fat Track (FT)	NR	0-60	0.1	NR	Good	$$	Can be used for self-assessment of body fat, digital read-out, and Jackson and Pollock equations	Accu-Measure
McGaw (MG)	12.0	0-40	2.0	MG ≈ HA[b]; MG < LNG[b]	Fair	$	—	None available
Ross Adipometer (RA)	12.0	0-60	2.0	RA ≈ HA[b]; RA < LNG[b]	Fair	$	—	Ross Products Division
Slim Guide (SG)	7.5	0-80	1.0	SG ≈ HA ≈ SKN[a]; SG < LNG[a]	Good	$	—	Creative Health Products

NR = not reported; ≈ approximately equal.

[a]Determined by comparing dynamic compression of foam rubber models of human skinfolds.

[b]Determined by comparing skinfold thicknesses of individuals measured by a technician; thus, any differences include not only instrument error but also error associated with technician skill and client factors.

[c]Cost: $ = <$25 U.S.; $$ = $50-$200 U.S.; $$$ = >$200 U.S.

(edema) in the subcutaneous tissue—caused by factors such as peripheral vasodilation or certain diseases—may increase SKF thicknesses (Keys and Brozek 1953). This suggests that you should not measure SKFs immediately after exercise, especially in hot environments. Grossman and Deitrick (2015) measured SKF thicknesses at four sites immediately before and 2 hr following a resistance training workout about 60 min in duration. Although the postexercise SKF measurements were approximately 3 mm higher compared with baseline, no significant differences in ΣSKF or FFM were found. Also, most of the weight gain experienced by some women during their menstrual cycles is caused by water retention (Bunt et al. 1989). This theoretically could increase SKF thicknesses, particularly on the trunk and abdomen, but there continues to be no empirical data to support or refute this hypothesis.

Should SKFs be measured on the right or left side of the body?

Only small differences (up to 2 mm) between SKF thicknesses on the right and left sides of the body occur for the typical individual. The standard practice in the United States, as well as in European and developing countries, however, is to take SKF measurements on the right side of the body, as recommended in the *Anthropometric Standardization Reference Manual* (Lohman, Roche, and Martorell 1988) and by the International Society for the Advancement of Kinanthropometry (Norton et al. 2000) and ACSM (2018).

Should I use SKFs to measure the body fat of obese clients?

It is difficult, even for highly skilled SKF technicians, to accurately measure the SKF thickness of extremely obese individuals. Sometimes a client's SKF thickness exceeds the maximum aperture of the caliper, and the jaws of the caliper may slip off the fold during the measurement, resulting in a potentially embarrassing and awkward situation for you and your client. Therefore, avoid using the SKF method to measure body fat of extremely obese clients.

ULTRASOUND

Ultrasound technology is gaining ground in the body composition literature as a portable, noninvasive alternative to the skinfold thickness assessment technique. It may also be used for clinical purposes given its ability to assess adipose tissue thicknesses deep within the body (Bazzocchi et al. 2016). Wagner (2013) has published an informative review of ultrasound technology and its use in body composition assessment.

Ultrasound technology uses a handheld wand, or probe (see figure 8.11), with bidirectional (sending and receiving) sound transducers integrated with a computerized application. The pulsatile frequency of the ultrasound signals transmitted through the skin is generated by piezoelectric crystals within the transducer itself. The signal frequencies generated exceed what can be heard by the human ear and tend to range between 1 and 18 MHz. The signals are reflected back to the transducer when they encounter a tissue interface. Depending on the mode of ultrasound being used, the reflected signals are presented as a line drawing of peaks with different amplitudes or as a series of dots forming horizontal bands of differing brightness.

A-Mode Ultrasound

A-mode (amplitude mode) ultrasound devices use a single transducer to emit a narrow signal beam and

Video 8.3

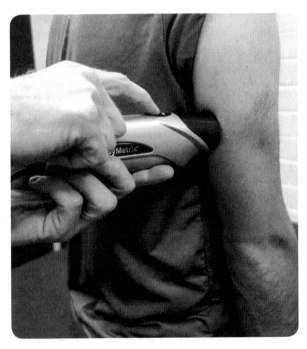

FIGURE 8.11   Handheld ultrasound probe.
Dale R. Wagner.

produce an image of amplitude-related spikes. The amplitude of the peaks reflects the tissue depths (see figure 8.12). The subcutaneous adipose tissue interface with skeletal muscle is defined as the midpoint of the highest peak (Smith-Ryan et al. 2014).

As an alternative to SKF measurements, the A-mode ultrasound uses the same sites as the SKF method. Reviewing the Using the Skinfold Method section of this chapter will refresh your familiarity with the skinfold sites and help you understand the direction of wand movement at each site. The conversions of site-specific subcutaneous fat thicknesses into %BF use proprietary conversions and prediction equations that mimic the traditional SKF prediction equations (Baranauskas et al. 2017).

B-Mode Ultrasound

B-mode (brightness modulation) ultrasound uses a linear array of transducers to create a two-dimensional image. The transducer interprets the reflected signals and presents those processed signals as dots on the graphical display on the computer screen. The brighter the dots, the stronger the signal reflections. The dots are depicted in an *x*- and *y*-axis format, with the point of axes

intersection (lower left of the graphic) being the highest value (mm). The uppermost portion of the screen (smallest mm value) represents the contact between the transducer and skin. A bright line or band of dots appears a bit below that and depicts the first tissue interface (subcutaneous fat with skeletal muscle). The distance (depth in mm) between the head of the probe and the tissue interface gives an indication of the time it takes the signal to leave and return to the transducer. The average thickness (mm) is calculated by the proprietary application and approximates one-half of the skinfold thickness at that site (Wagner 2013).

According to Müller and associates (2016), the skinfold sites defined by the International Society for the Advancement of Kinanthropometry are inappropriate for quantifying subcutaneous fat with B-mode ultrasound. As a result, they standardized a B-mode ultrasound technique that uses 8 sites and specific positioning of the client during the identification of measurement sites (see B-Mode Ultrasound Technique). All measurements are made with the client in a supine or side-lying position.

As explained by Wagner (2013), interpreting the results of an ultrasound scan is more difficult than

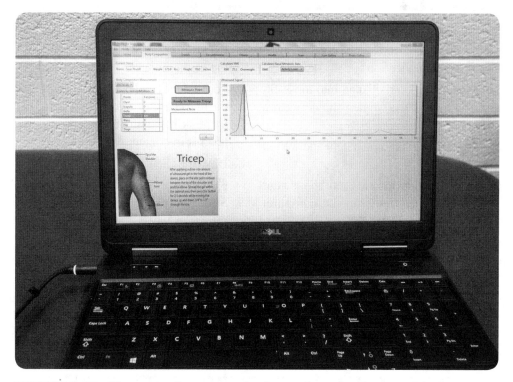

FIGURE 8.12 Tissue depth measured using an A-mode ultrasound device.

Dale R. Wagner.

performing the scan in the first place. Accurate identification of the interfaces is crucial. As the probe slides back and forth along the skin, a line of dots will be displayed on the computer screen. The various tissue interfaces will be identifiable as continuous brightly colored bands. With practice the technician should become proficient in identifying the borders of the various interfaces. Another skill required for interpreting ultrasound images is the accurate measurement of the tissue thicknesses, which depends on identification of the interface borders and the proper placement of the software's electronic calipers.

Sources of Measurement Error

The accuracy and precision of ultrasound measurements and the ultrasound method are directly related to the technician's skill, mode of ultrasound, signal frequency, and sound speed. The following questions and responses address these sources of measurement error.

What is the standardized technique to use with A-mode ultrasound?

Unlike for B-mode, there is not yet a standardized technique. The sites of measurement are the same as for skinfold thickness assessment. The computer software will alert the technician when repeat measurements are needed.

How much pressure should be applied to the skin with the probe?

Toomey and colleagues (2011) compared A-mode ultrasound measurements at several sites (triceps, abdomen, anterior thigh) using three different amounts of skin and subcutaneous adipose tissue compression. When the skin and underlying fat were compressed as much as possible, the subcutaneous adipose tissue result was lower (36%, 37%, and 25%, respectively) at each site tested as compared to when minimal compressive pressure was applied. Reducing the maximal amount of pressure by one-half resulted in thickness differences from minimal compression that were similar to those attained when

Standardized Procedures for B-Mode Ultrasound Technique

Standardized procedures for the B-mode ultrasound (Müller et al. 2016) are as follows.

1. Connect the ultrasound wand to the computer and open the software application.

2. Have your client void and change into loose-fitting shorts and a T-shirt; women should wear a sports bra.

3. Measure your client's standing height and weight while barefoot.

4. Enter the demographic information about your client into the proper fields on the computer screen.

5. Position your client as recommended, and then meticulously identify, measure, and mark the sites of interest on the right side of the body.

6. Center a dime-sized amount of conductive gel on the head of the probe. Störchle and associates (2017) suggest using a thick layer of conductive gel to help prevent overapplication of pressure;

the layer of gel will appear as a dark band at the top of the images.

7. Position the head of the probe lightly on the skin at the marked site, and hold the wand perpendicular to the skin. Be sure the entire surface of the probe head is in contact with the skin.

8. Have the client interrupt (stop) his breathing cycle at midpoint for all measurements on the torso.

9. Slide the probe linearly about 5 mm in each direction while following the long axis of the underlying muscle at that site.

10. Novice technicians are advised to save the image for subsequent analysis.

11. Repeat measurements at each site are recommended so that the average of two within ±1 mm is attained and recorded.

the tissues were maximally compressed (Toomey et al. 2011). Toomey and associates (2011) suggest applying just enough pressure so that the image begins to appear on the computer monitor.

How do signal frequency and sound speed affect measurement accuracy?

The frequency emitted by the transducer may be more important than the mode in that there is an inverse relationship between signal frequency and depth of penetration (Wagner 2013). However, with A-mode ultrasound, higher frequencies increase the resolution of the images (Smith-Ryan et al. 2014).

With B-mode ultrasound, image resolution nears 0.1 mm at 18 MHz; whereas at 6MHz resolution is approximately 0.3 mm (Störchle et al. 2017). Sound speed is also of utmost importance; the wrong speed introduces an error of approximately 6% BF (Müller et al. 2016). For thick layers of subcutaneous adipose tissue, use a slow sound speed (1,450 m·s^{-1}). Otherwise, a sound speed of 1,540 m·s^{-1} is appropriate.

How accurate is the ultrasound method in comparison to other reference methods?

Research comparing the results of ultrasound assessments against reference methods is limited but growing. Technician training, technology, and algorithms may need a bit more development.

When using A-mode ultrasound to assess subcutaneous thicknesses for subsequent conversion via equation into %BF, researchers report that the proprietary equations within the devices underestimate %BF from DXA in 12 to 17 yr olds (Ripka et al. 2016) and in comparison to a 4C model reference (Kendall et al. 2017). The study by the Smith-Ryan team (2014) recruited overweight and obese adults and compared A-mode ultrasound device derivations of %BF and FM to multicomponent model references. Siri's (1961) 3C model values were significantly underestimated by the seven-site assessment using a frequency of 2.5 MHz (Smith-Ryan et al. 2014).

O'Neill and colleagues (2016) used B-mode ultrasound to compare %BF results against those from an iDXA for a sample of elite male rowers. The B-mode underestimated the iDXA reference values for %BF while overestimating iDXA FFM. O'Neill's group improved the predictive accuracy of the B-mode ultrasound device by identifying significant measurement sites via multiple linear regression analyses and creating a new prediction equation. When this new equation [%BF = 0.476 × (Σ triceps, biceps, supraspinale, and anterior thigh)] was applied to the athletes in that study, ultrasound %BF (16.9%) was identical to the reference value, correlation was strong (r = .94), *SEE* acceptable (1.9%), and limits of agreement were good (3.7%). O'Neill indicated that the ultrasound method worked better for the athletes with less than 15% BF.

Smith-Ryan and colleagues (2016) again recruited overweight and obese adults to compare B-mode ultrasound %BF and FM values against a 4C reference model. Sex-specific comparisons indicated that the ultrasound method worked better for the men than the women in this study. No mean difference was found for the men, but ultrasound (frequency: 5-13 MHz) overestimated the reference %BF by 9.2% on average for the women. As noted by the authors, the men were leaner than the women.

Both A- and B-mode ultrasound devices demonstrate excellent reliability and moderately strong to strong correlations with multicomponent reference models while resulting in large limits of agreement (O'Neill et al. 2016; Ripka et al. 2016; Smith-Ryan et al. 2014, 2016). Comments by the Smith-Ryan teams indicate that ultrasound technology is worth considering for tracking body composition changes over time. The methodological differences between ultrasound and a 4C reference are smaller than those of other laboratory methods that take only a single measurement (e.g., ADP) (Smith-Ryan et al. 2014, 2016).

How does the ultrasound method compare to the results of SKFs and other 2C models?

The A-mode ultrasound results from the study by Wagner, Cain, and Clark (2016) showed strong correlations (r > .68) and small minimal differences (<2.0% BF) at each of the three sites (Jackson and Pollock 1978; Jackson, Pollock, and Ward 1980) measured. In what is apparently the first published intertester reliability study using ultrasound (Wagner, Cain, and Clark 2016), the two technicians attained better test-retest results with the A-mode ultrasound (*ICC* = .99; 95% confidence interval 0.98-0.99 mm) than with SKF (*ICC* = .97; 95% confidence interval 0.33-0.99 mm). The intertester differences varied by the athletes' sex and assessment method. Ultrasound differences were approximately 0.2% BF for both sexes, whereas SKF differences were close to 1.9% BF for the men and 3.3% BF for the women (Wagner, Cain, and Clark 2016).

Wagner's research group (2016) recruited NCAA Division I athletes for their study, in which they reported a strong correlation ($r > .92$), good *SEE* (2.6% BF), and fair *TE* (4.4% BF) but large limits of agreement when comparing A-mode ultrasound with ADP. A-mode ultrasound overestimated %BF from ADP in only 5 of the 45 participating athletes (22 men and 23 women). When comparing sex-specific results, no differences were found for the men. Their body fat percentages differed minimally (± 1.5% BF), and *TE* improved to 2.4%. Conversely, for the women, ultrasound overestimated %BF from ADP by approximately 5.0%, and *TE* increased to 5.5% BF (Wagner, Cain, and Clark 2016). Kendall and associates (2017) reported no differences in FFM estimations when comparing A-mode ultrasound (76.8 ± 9.1 kg) results to ADP (76.7 ± 9.5 kg) and to SKF (76.7 ± 9.0 kg) using the Jackson and Pollock (1978) three-site equation. Comparisons of A-mode ultrasound measurements and skinfold thicknesses acquired at the sex-specific sites for men (chest, abdomen, thigh) and women (triceps, suprailiac, thigh) (Jackson and Pollock 1978; Jackson, Pollock, and Ward 1980) resulted in similar group means (ultrasound: 18.2 ± 8.3% BF; SKF: 13.3 ± 7.1% BF; *SEE*: 7.5%; *TE*: >4.0%) for a small, predominantly Caucasian male sample of young adults (Loenneke et al. 2014).

Smith-Ryan and colleagues (2016) used the sex-specific seven-site assessments (Jackson and Pollock 1978; Jackson, Pollock, and Ward 1980) for a sample of overweight and obese adults (31.6 ± 5.2 kg·m^{-2}). There were nonsignificant differences for both the men (26.8 ± 4.1% vs. 29.8 ± 6.0% BF) and women (47.4 ± 6.9% vs. 39.8 ± 4.4% BF) with B-mode ultrasonography and SKF, respectively.

BIOELECTRICAL IMPEDANCE METHOD

Bioelectrical impedance analysis (BIA) is a rapid, noninvasive, and relatively inexpensive method for evaluating body composition in field settings. With this method, a low-level electrical current is passed through the client's body, and the **impedance (Z)**, or opposition to the flow of current, is measured with a BIA analyzer. You can estimate the individual's total body water (TBW) from the impedance measurement because the electrolytes in the body's water are excellent conductors of electrical current. When the volume of TBW is large, the current flows more easily through the body, with less **resistance (R)**. The resistance to current flow is greater in individuals with large amounts of body fat, since adipose tissue, with its relatively low water content, is a poor conductor of electrical current. Because the water content of the FFB component is relatively large (~73% water), **fat-free mass (FFM)** can be predicted from TBW estimates. Individuals with large FFM and TBW have less resistance to current flowing through their bodies than those with a smaller FFM.

Bioelectrical impedance indirectly estimates FFM and TBW. Therefore, the following assumptions are made about the geometric shape of the body and the relationship of impedance to the length and volume of the conductor.

• *The human body is shaped like a perfect cylinder with a uniform length and cross-sectional area.* Of course, this assumption is not entirely true. Because the body segments are not uniform in length or cross-sectional area, resistance to the flow of current through these body segments will differ.

• *Assuming the body is a perfect cylinder, at a fixed signal frequency (e.g., 50 kHz) the impedance (Z) to current flow through the body is directly related to the length (L) of the conductor (height) and inversely related to its cross-sectional area (A) [$Z = \rho(L/A)$, where ρ is the specific resistivity of the body's tissues and is assumed to be constant].* To express this relationship in terms of Z and the body's volume, instead of its cross-sectional area, the equation is multiplied by L/L: $Z = \rho(L/A)(L/L)$. $A \times L$ is equal to volume (V), so rearranging this equation yields $V = \rho L^2/Z$. Thus, the volume of the FFM or TBW of the body is directly related to L^2, or height squared (ht^2), and indirectly related to Z.

• *Biological tissues act as conductors or insulators, and the flow of current through the body will follow the path of least resistance.* Because the FFM contains large amounts of water (~73%) and electrolytes, it is a better conductor of electrical current than is fat. Fat is anhydrous and a poor conductor of electrical current. The total body impedance, measured at the constant frequency of 50 kHz, primarily reflects the volumes of the water and muscle compartments composing the FFM and the extracellular water volume (Kushner 1992).

• *Impedance is a function of resistance and reactance, where* $Z = \sqrt{(R2 + X_c^2)}$. Resistance (R) is a measure of pure opposition to current flow through the body; **reactance (X_c)** is the opposition to current flow caused by capacitance produced by the cell membrane (Kushner 1992). R is much larger than X_c (at a 50 kHz frequency) when whole-body impedance is measured; therefore, R is a better predictor of FFM and TBW than Z (Lohman 1989). For these reasons, the **resistance index (ht^2 / R)**, instead of ht^2 / Z, is often used in BIA models to predict FFM or TBW.

Using the Bioelectrical Impedance Analysis Method

The traditional BIA method measures whole-body resistance using a tetrapolar wrist-to-ankle electrode configuration at a single frequency for estimating TBW or FFM (figure 8.13). However, technological advances and changes in theoretical modeling have led to a number of variations in the traditional BIA method. These variations use sophisticated models to assess segmental body composition and fluid subcompartments, thereby improving the clinical usefulness of BIA. Also, user-friendly BIA analyzers designed for home use and individual monitoring of health and fitness use upper or lower body

impedance measures to estimate body composition (figure 8.14).

Whole-body bioimpedance measures (Z, R, and X_c) are used in BIA prediction equations to estimate TBW and FFM. These prediction equations are based on either population-specific or generalized models. A population-specific equation is valid for only those individuals whose physical characteristics match the sample from which the equation was derived. Researchers have developed equations specific to age (Deurenberg et al. 1990; Lohman 1992), ethnicity (Hastuti et al. 2016; Stolarczyk et al. 1994), body fatness (Gray et al. 1989; Segal et al. 1988), and level of physical activity (Houtkooper et al. 1989). Alternatively, generalized BIA equations have been developed for heterogeneous populations varying in age, gender, and body fatness (Deurenberg et al. 1990; Gray et al. 1989; Kyle et al. 2001; Kushner and Schoeller 1986; Lukaski and Bolonchuk 1988; Van Loan and Mayclin 1987).

Inexpensive lower body (foot-to-foot) and upper body (hand-to-hand) BIA devices are available and have been marketed for home use. Two manufacturers of these devices are Omron Healthcare and Tanita Corporation. The Tanita analyzers measure lower body impedance between the right and left legs as the individual stands on the analyzer's electrode plates (see figure 8.14a). The Omron Body Logic analyzer, which is handheld, measures upper body impedance between the right and left arms (see figure 8.14b). The Tanita and Omron analyzers estimate %BF and FFM using proprietary equations developed by the manufacturers. Typically, it is

Video 8.4

Video 8.5-8.6

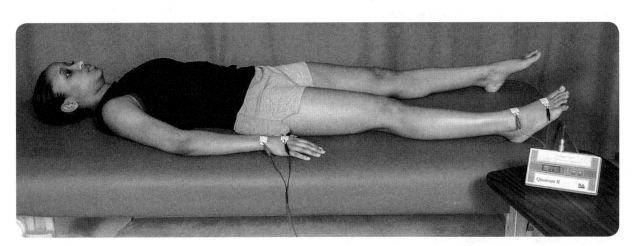

FIGURE 8.13 Bioelectrical impedance analysis electrode placement and client positioning.

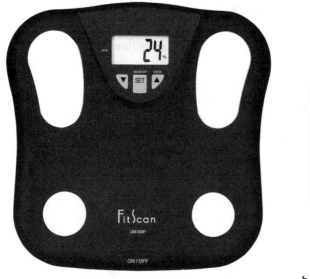

Courtesy of Tanita Corporation.

a

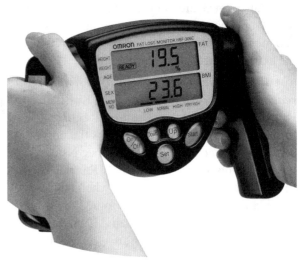

Courtesy of Omron Healthcare, Inc.

b

FIGURE 8.14 *(a)* Tanita and *(b)* Omron bioelectrical impedance analyzers.

not possible to obtain impedance (resistance and reactance) data from these analyzers. However, they do provide the general public with an inexpensive, simple, and reasonably accurate means of self-assessing body fat.

Table 8.5 presents commonly used population-specific and generalized BIA equations. With these equations, you can accurately estimate the

BIA PRETESTING CLIENT GUIDELINES

- No eating or drinking within 4 hr of the test.
- No moderate or vigorous exercise within 12 hr of the test.
- Void completely within 30 min of the test.
- Abstain from alcohol consumption within 48 hr of the test.
- Do not ingest diuretics, including caffeine, before the assessment unless they are prescribed by a physician.
- If you are in a stage of your menstrual cycle during which you perceive you are retaining water, postpone testing (female clients).

FFM of your clients within the recommended values, ±2.8 kg for women and ±3.5 kg for men (Lohman 1992). To use these equations, obtain R and X_c directly from your BIA analyzer. Estimate the %BF of your client by determining the **fat mass (FM)** (FM = BM − FFM) and dividing FM by the client's body mass [%BF = (FM / BM) × 100].

Experts recommend not using the FFM and %BF estimates obtained directly from your BIA analyzer (e.g., BMR, Holtain, RJL, or Valhalla) unless you know for sure which equations are programmed in the analyzer's computer software, obtain information from the manufacturer regarding the validity and accuracy of these equations, and determine that these equations are applicable to your clients.

Although the relative predictive accuracy of the BIA method is similar to that of the SKF method, BIA may be preferable in some settings for the following reasons:

- It does not require a high degree of technician skill.
- It is generally more comfortable and does not intrude as much on the client's privacy.
- It can be used to estimate body composition of obese individuals.

Table 8.5 Bioelectrical Impedance Analysis Prediction Equations

Population subgroup	%BF level[a]	Equation	Reference
American Indian, black, Hispanic, or white men, 17-62 yr	<20% BF	FFM (kg) = 0.00066360(ht^2) − 0.02117(R) + 0.62854(BM) − 0.12380(age) + 9.33285	Segal et al. (1988)
	≥20%	FFM (kg) = 0.00088580(ht^2) − 0.02999(R) + 0.42688(BM) − 0.07002(age) + 14.52435	Segal et al. (1988)
American Indian, black, Hispanic, or white women, 17-62 yr	<30%	FFM (kg) = 0.000646(ht^2) − 0.014(R) + 0.421(BM) + 10.4	Segal et al. (1988)
	≥30%	FFM (kg) = 0.00091186(ht^2) − 0.01466(R) + 0.29990(BM) − 0.07012(age) + 9.37938	Segal et al. (1988)
White boys and girls, 8-15 yr	NA	FFM (kg) = 0.62(ht^2/ R) + 0.21(BM) + 0.10(X_c) + 4.2	Lohman (1992)
White boys and girls, 10-19 yr	NA	FFM (kg) = 0.61(ht^2/ R) + 0.25(BM) + 1.31	Houtkooper et al. (1992)
Female athletes, 18-27 yr	NA	FFM (kg) = 0.282(ht) + 0.415(BM) − 0.037(R) + 0.096(X_c) − 9.734	Fornetti et al. (1999)
Male athletes, 19-40 yr	NA	FFM (kg) = 0.186(ht^2/ R) + 0.701(BM) + 1.949	Oppliger et al. (1991)

%BF = percent body fat; NA = not applicable; FFM = fat-free mass (kg); BM = body mass (kg); R = resistance (Ω); X_c = reactance (Ω); ht = height (cm).

[a]For clients who are obviously lean, use the <20% BF (men) and <30% BF (women) equations. For clients who are obviously obese, use the ≥20% BF (men) and ≥30% BF (women) equations. For clients who are not obviously lean or obese, calculate their FFM using both the lean and obese equations and then average the two FFM estimates.

Bioelectrical Impedance Analysis Technique

Bioelectrical impedance analysis accuracy highly depends on controlling the factors that may increase measurement error. Regardless of the BIA method being used (whole, upper, or lower body), your client must adhere to guidelines that control fluctuations in hydration status (see BIA Pretesting Client Guidelines).

Use standardized testing procedures to minimize error in the BIA method (see Standardized Procedures for the Whole-Body BIA Method).

Sources of Measurement Error

The accuracy and precision of the BIA method are affected by instrumentation, client factors, technician skill, environmental factors, and the prediction equation used to estimate FFM. The following questions address sources of BIA measurement error.

Can different types of whole-body BIA analyzers be used interchangeably?

Research demonstrates significant differences in whole-body resistance when different brands of single-frequency analyzers are used (Graves et al. 1989; Smye, Sutcliffe, and Pitt 1993). For example, Smye, Sutcliffe, and Pitt (1993) reported lower resistances (6% or 32-36 Ω) for the Holtain device compared with the Bodystat, RJL, and EZcomp analyzers. Graves and colleagues (1989) noted that the correlation between resistance values measured with the Valhalla and Bioelectrical Sciences (BES) analyzers was only $r = .59$; the average %BF estimated for men from one BIA equation differed by 6.3% using the resistances from these two instruments. Although there is a high correlation ($r = .99$) between resistances measured with the Valhalla and RJL analyzers, the Valhalla analyzer produces significantly higher resistances for men (~16 Ω) and women (~19 Ω), corresponding to a systematic underestimation of FFM in men (~1.3 kg) and women (~1.0 kg) (Graves et al. 1989). Also, differences may exist within a given model of analyzer. The Z values from three RJL (model 101) analyzers differed by 7 to 16 Ω, causing a difference in FFM of 2.1 kg for some individuals (Deurenberg, van der Kooy, and Leenan 1989).

Do upper and lower body BIA analyzers accurately estimate body composition?

The Tanita Corporation now markets more than 30 different adult models of body composition analyzers that vary in weight capacity, software, memory, and data output. The majority of these are lower body analyzers, but some offer whole-body and regional (segmental) analysis. Compared with two-component model estimates of FFM obtained from underwater weighing, Tanita analyzer estimates of the average FFM of heterogeneous adult samples are reasonably good (SEE = 3.5-3.7 kg) (Cable et al. 2001; Utter et al. 1999). Estimates by Tanita analyzers also agree well with SKF estimates of %BF in collegiate wrestlers (Utter et al. 2001) and with DXA estimates of FFM in children (Sung et al. 2001; Tyrrel et al. 2001). On the other hand, compared with DXA, Tanita underestimated %BF and FFM (kg) for a sample of college-age women (del Consuelo Velazquez-Alva et al. 2014). Compared with UWW estimates of the FFM of high school wrestlers, the prediction error for the Tanita analyzer (TBF-300WA) was larger than that of the SKF method (3.64 kg vs. 1.97 kg). Utter and colleagues (2005), therefore, recommend using the leg-to-leg Tanita analyzer only when trained SKF technicians are not available.

The Tanita BC 532 lower body analyzer utilizes two frequencies (50 kHz and 200 µA) to estimate %BF, FFM, and visceral fat. In a sample of 200 Chinese men and women ranging in age from 18 to 80 yr, Wang and colleagues (2013) investigated the predictive accuracy of the BC 532 as compared with reference measures from DXA (%BF and %FFM) and MRI (visceral fat). Even though the correlations were strong, the underestimation of $\%BF_{DXA}$ was significant for both the men (10.7%, r = .84) and women (6.1%, r = .86), as was the underestimation of %FFM (men: 1.4%, r = .84; women: 2.5%, r = .86). The reference visceral fat percentage from MRI was significantly overestimated (20.4%) in the men and underestimated (18.0%) in the women. The gender-specific visceral fat correlations were .81 and .86 for the men and women, respectively. The strength of correlations and magnitude of mean differences reported by Wang and associates (2013) may differ for other population subgroups using the BC 532.

In the late 1990s, Omron Healthcare developed a low-cost, hand-to-hand BIA analyzer for home use. Omron's proprietary equation was developed and cross-validated on a large heterogeneous sample from three laboratories using HW to obtain two-component model reference measures of %BF

and FFM (Loy et al. 1998). The group predictive accuracy *(SEE)* for estimating FFM was 3.9 kg for men and 2.9 kg for women. In an independent cross-validation of the Omron analyzer, Gibson and colleagues (2000) reported slightly smaller prediction errors (SEE = 2.9 kg for men and 2.2 kg for women). Loy and colleagues (1998) noted that the average FFM estimates from the Omron device are similar to values obtained with whole-body (RJL and Valhalla) analyzers. Last, in a study of Japanese men, the accuracy of upper body (Omron, HBF-300), lower body (Tanita, TBF-102), and whole-body (Selco, SIF-891) analyzers was compared against two-component model reference measures of %BF obtained from HW. The average difference between reference and predicted %BF values was slightly smaller for the Omron (2.2% BF) than for the whole-body (3.3% BF) and lower body (3.2% BF) analyzers (Demura et al. 2002). However, estimation errors from the Omron and Tanita devices tended to be greater at the lower and upper extremes of the %BF distribution.

Omron also developed BIA prediction equations to estimate the body composition of physically active adults. These equations are programmed in the HBF-306 Omron analyzer along with prediction equations for nonactive adults and children. The predictor variables in the manufacturer's equation for this unit are upper body impedance, age, gender, height, weight, and level of physical activity (i.e., athlete or nonathlete). The prediction errors for athletes (SEE = 3.8% and 3.6% BF for male and female athletes, respectively) were somewhat less than those for nonathletes (SEE = 4.5% BF) (K. Yamanoto, personal communication). Compared with a DXA reference method, the Omron HBF 300 model had good correlation for %BF (r = .74; SEE = 3.6% BF) and FFM (r = .84; SEE = 2.45 kg) for a sample of collegiate female athletes from three sports (Esco et al. 2011).

The Omron (HBF-306) model has been tested on ethnically diverse samples of European and Asian populations. Generally the group predictive accuracy is good for these subgroups, but individual prediction errors can be high (Deurenberg-Yap et al. 2001; Deurenberg and Deurenberg-Yap 2002). Deurenberg-Yap and colleagues (2001) noted that Omron data misclassified (gave false negatives) for 24% of the obese females and 44% of the obese

STANDARDIZED PROCEDURES FOR THE WHOLE-BODY BIA METHOD

1. Take bioimpedance measures on the right side of the body with the client lying supine on a nonconductive surface in a room with normal ambient temperature (~25 °C).

2. Clean the skin at the electrode sites with an alcohol pad.

3. Place the sensor (proximal) electrodes on (a) the dorsal surface of the wrist so that the upper border of the electrode bisects the head of the ulna and (b) the dorsal surface of the ankle so that the upper border of the electrode bisects the medial and lateral malleoli (see figure 8.13). You can use a measuring tape and surgical marking pen to mark these points for electrode placement.

4. Place the source (distal) electrodes at the bases of the second or third metacarpophalangeal joints of the hand and foot (see figure 8.13). Make certain there is at least 5 cm (~2 in.) between the proximal and distal electrodes.

5. Attach the lead wires to the appropriate electrodes. Red leads are attached to the wrist and ankle, and black leads are attached to the hand and foot.

6. Make certain the client's legs and arms are comfortably abducted, at about a 30° to 45° angle from the trunk. Ensure there is no contact between the arms and trunk and between the thighs, as contact will short-circuit the electrical path, dramatically affecting the impedance value.

---

males in their study. When the Omron estimates of %BF were compared with those of a multicomponent model, the *SEE* was 4.5% BF; the error in estimating %BF using the Omron analyzer was related to the age, body fatness, and ratio of arm span to height of the subjects (Deurenberg and Deurenberg-Yap 2002).

Esco and colleagues (2011) urged caution when using the Omron HBF 300 to estimate the body composition of athletic young women, given the magnitude of differences in estimating %BF (5% BF underestimation) and FFM (3.4 kg overestimation) compared with DXA. In comparing the Omron HBF 300 and Tanita TF 400 FS with each other as well as DXA for a sample of Caucasian women representing the entire spectrum of BMI values, Větrovska and coauthors (2014) reported that both BIA devices follow the same pattern of underestimating the DXA %BF values for the lower BMI ranges while overestimating the reference for those with BMI values >30 kg·m^{-2}. The Omron had the narrowest limits of agreement with DXA as long as the BMI values were <40 kg·m^{-2}. The Tanita, conversely, performed better in relation to the DXA when BMI exceeded 30 kg·m^{-2}, at which point DXA significantly overestimated the Omron and Tanita results. Below 30 kg·m^{-2} there were no significant differences compared with the reference method.

Compared with handheld and leg-to-leg BIA analyzers, does octapolar bioimpedance spectroscopy (BIS) provide a better estimate of body composition?

Bioimpedance spectroscopy (BIS) analyzers combine upper body, lower body, and whole-body bioimpedance to estimate FFM and %BF. The tactile eight-point system (four pairs of electrodes) from the line of InBody (manufactured by Biospace Co. Ltd.) and other vertical analyzer manufacturers has electrodes embedded into the analyzers' handles (thumb and arm) and floor scale (ball of foot and heel). Comparing estimates from the InBody720 and InBody320 BIS analyzers to multicomponent model estimates of %BF, Gibson and colleagues (2008) reported large prediction errors for samples of Hispanic, black, and white men (*SEE* = 5.2% BF) and women (*SEE* = 4.8% BF). The average %BF of the women was significantly overestimated by 2.5% to 3.0% BF for both BIS analyzers. Compared with a Lunar Prodigy Primo DXA, the InBody720 overestimated FFM ($p < .05$) and underestimated FM ($p < .05$) for a sample of healthy postmenopausal women. The methodological difference in FM estimation is more apparent at the upper ends of the Bland and Altman distribution (Gába et al. 2015).

Esco's research team (2015) compared whole-body and segmental results from an InBody720 and Lunar

Prodigy DXA for a sample of 45 female collegiate athletes. They reported significantly lower (3.3%) %BF and higher (~2.1 kg) FFM results from the InBody compared with the DXA, and the limits of agreement were large. Interestingly, the between-device comparisons of segmental lean soft tissue (FFM minus bone) were not significant for arms, legs, or torso. Thus, the authors commented that the InBody720 is a viable alternative to DXA for quantifying segmental lean soft tissue in athletic women.

Using DXA for the reference method, Anderson, Erceg, and Schroeder (2012) also investigated the ability of two eight-electrode InBody BIS analyzers (models 520 and 720) to assess total and regional body composition for 25 men and 25 women. Fat mass (FM) correlations were significant for both sexes ($r =$ .90-.98), as were lean body mass (LBM) correlations ($r =$ .83-.97). Overall, the prediction errors (SEEs) ranged from 2.5 to 2.8 kg for FM and 2.4 to 2.8 kg for FFM. The limits of agreement for FM were larger for the men. Anderson, Erceg, and Schroeder (2012) concluded that both of the InBody analyzers provide reliable and valid estimations of LBM and FM and can, therefore, be used interchangeably with DXA for assessing these body composition components.

Do vertical whole-body BIA analyzers accurately estimate body composition?

Tanita, Omron, and Biospace have models that combine upper and lower body BIA technology to provide varying levels of whole-body assessments. The Omron HBF 359 is an eight-electrode multiple-frequency analyzer (50 kHz and 500 μA) that estimates skeletal muscle mass and visceral fat in addition to %BF. Wang and colleagues (2013) investigated the predictive accuracy of the Omron HBF 359 compared with DXA for %BF and with MRI for skeletal muscle mass and visceral fat in a sample of Chinese adults (100 men and 100 women). The correlations between the two methods of estimating %BF ranged from $r =$ .80 (men) to $r =$ .86 (women). On average, Omron %BF significantly underestimated the DXA reference measure by 5.8% BF (men) and 9.6% BF (women) (Wang et al. 2013). MRI skeletal muscle percentage was significantly overestimated by 1.9% for the men but not for the women, although the correlations ($r =$ .72 and .71, respectively) were significant. MRI visceral fat was overestimated by 13.3% for the men ($r =$ .82) but underestimated by 8.5% for the women ($r =$ .85). Consequently, Wang

and associates (2013) concluded that, for their sample of Chinese adults, the HBF 359 accurately and reliably estimated skeletal muscle percentage, but there was room for improvement in estimating %BF and visceral fat. Additional research on other racial population subgroups is recommended.

The Tanita MC-180MA is a multifrequency body composition analyzer. It was compared against a Lunar iDXA in order to determine how closely the two methods estimated the total body and regional fat mass of more than 400 Irish adults ranging in age from 18 to 29 yr (Leahy et al. 2012). The Tanita underestimated overall %BF from DXA, with the difference between methods being most notable for the women and as levels of body fatness increased. Fat in the trunk region was significantly overestimated by the Tanita for the men, but the methods produced similar trunk region values for the women. Leahy and colleagues reported that the Tanita accurately estimates FFM in the arms and legs compared with the iDXA. Although they reported that the two methods were interchangeable for men with body fat levels lower than 25%, they did not support using the Tanita to estimate body composition in the trunk region.

The Tanita BC-418 is a single-frequency (50 kHz) analyzer. Compared with the Lunar Prodigy Primo DXA reference, it underestimates FM (kg) while overestimating FFM (kg) of postmenopausal women (Gába et al. 2015). Similar to the results of Leahy and colleagues (2012), as the women's body fat levels increase, so do the FM differences between methods.

Hurst and colleagues (2016) compared the dual-frequency InBody230 to both DXA (QDR Discovery A) and ADP for adults spanning the age and BMI ranges. For the sample, %BF from the InBody was significantly lower (~2% BF) compared with both DXA and ADP, but more closely aligned with the DXA %BF. Limits of agreement between the InBody and both references were large. The authors suggested the underlying cause of the large limits of agreement with the InBody and DXA is most likely the DXA results at the extremes of the distribution and not the InBody (Hurst et al. 2016).

How does my client's hydration level affect the accuracy of bioimpedance measures?

A major source of error with the BIA method is intra-individual variability in whole-body resistance due to factors that alter the client's hydration. Between

3.1% and 3.9% of the variance in resistance may be attributed to day-to-day fluctuations in body water (Jackson et al. 1988). Factors such as eating, drinking, dehydrating, and exercising alter the hydration state, thereby affecting total body resistance and the estimate of FFM. Measuring resistance 2 to 4 hr after a meal decreases R as much as 17 Ω and likely overestimates the FFM of your client by almost 1.5 kg (Deurenberg et al. 1988). Likewise, Gallagher, Walker, and O'Dea (1998) found a significant decrease in impedance (Z) 2 hr following breakfast, and this effect lasted for 5 hr after consumption. In contrast to these studies, at only 1 hr postmeal, there appear to be greater individual variability and smaller changes in R (Fogelholm et al. 1993). Kushner, Gudivaka, and Schoeller (1996) concluded that eating or drinking minimally influences whole-body Z within 1 hr following consumption but is likely to decrease Z (<3%) at 2 to 4 hr. Dehydration has the opposite effect: R increases (~40 Ω), leading to a 5.0 kg underestimation of FFM (Lukaski 1986).

Androutsos and associates (2015) investigated the influence of a drink- or food-based intervention (2 days each) on impedance as monitored through foot-to-foot bioimpedance analysis (Tanita TBF-300). The drink intervention group consumed 750 ml of mineral water one day and an equal volume of a sport electrolyte drink the second day. The food-based group consumed a high-carbohydrate meal and a high-fat meal on days 1 and 2, respectively. Preingestion and immediate postingestion BIA (time 0) assessments were performed. Additional assessments at 30 min intervals for a 2 hr postingestion follow-up were undertaken. Impedance (Z) significantly increased at all time points for the two drinks as compared with baseline. However, %BF increased with respect to baseline only for the time 0 water consumers. Ingesting the sport electrolyte beverage caused increases in %BF relative to baseline at every time point postingestion.

The two meal interventions increased Z every 30 min beginning with the 30 min postingestion assessment, also as compared with baseline. The high-fat meal also increased Z at time 0. The increase in %BF with meal ingestion followed the same pattern as did the change in Z. Beginning at the 90 min mark, the relative changes in Z and %BF of the food-based group were significantly different from those of the water consumers at those time points. Consequently it is logical to expect that body composition assessments with bioelectrical impedance will be affected if beverages or food are consumed within the 2 hr preceding the assessment (Androutsos et al. 2015). That effect may last even beyond that demarcation.

How does exercise affect bioimpedance measures?

Kushner and colleagues (1996) suggested three ways in which exercise may influence BIA measurements:

- Increased blood flow and warming of skeletal muscle tissue reduce Z and the specific resistivity (ρ) of muscle.
- Increased cutaneous blood flow, skin temperature, and sweating lower Z.
- Fluid loss due to exercise increases Z.

The effect of aerobic exercise on resistance measurements partially depends on exercise intensity and duration. Jogging and cycling at moderate intensities (~70% $\dot{V}O_2max$) for 90 to 120 min substantially decreased R (by 50-70 Ω), resulting in a large overestimation of FFM (~12 kg) (Khaled et al. 1988; Lukaski 1986). In contrast, cycling at lower intensities (100 and 175 W) for 90 min had a much smaller effect on R (1-9 Ω) (Deurenberg et al. 1988). Liang and Norris (1993) reported a decrease in R of about 3% immediately after 30 min of moderate-intensity exercise, but R returned to normal 1 hr postexercise with water *ad libitum*. The decrease in R following strenuous exercise most likely reflects a relatively greater loss of body water in the sweat and expired air than the loss of electrolytes. This difference leads to a higher electrolyte concentration in the body's fluids, thereby lowering R (Deurenberg et al. 1988).

The BIA method was found to adequately predict changes in TBW after heat-induced dehydration and glycerol-induced hyperhydration but not after exercise-induced dehydration; thus, factors other than just total fluid volume affect BIA measures following exercise (Koulmann et al. 2000). Researchers hypothesized that the redistribution of body fluids to active muscles during exercise, which relatively increases hydration in these segments (legs), might partially conceal the decreased fluid volumes in less active segments (trunk and arms).

Can I measure bioimpedance at any time during a client's menstrual cycle?

Although the menstrual cycle alters TBW, the ratio of extracellular to intracellular water, and body weight, researchers found only small differences in bioimpedance measures (Z and R) between the follicular and premenstrual stages (~5-8 Ω) and between menses and the follicular stage (~7 Ω) (Deurenberg et al. 1988; Gleichauf and Rose 1989). However, the average body weight of the women studied was stable (<0.2 kg difference) during the menstrual cycle. In women experiencing relatively large body weight gains (2-4 kg or 4.4-8.8 lb) during the menstrual cycle, a large part of the gain is due to an increase (1.5 kg or 3.3 lb on average) in TBW (Bunt et al. 1989). Until there are more conclusive data on this issue, you should take BIA measurements at a time during the menstrual cycle when the client perceives she is not experiencing a large weight gain. This practice should minimize error and more accurately estimate FFM for your clients.

Is there high agreement between bioimpedance values measured by two different technicians?

Technician skill is not a major source of BIA measurement error. There is virtually no difference in R measurements taken by different technicians, provided that standardized procedures for electrode placement and client positioning are closely followed (Jackson et al. 1988). The proximal electrodes in particular need to be correctly positioned at the wrist and ankle, as a 1 cm (0.4 in.) displacement may result in a 2% error in R (Elsen et al. 1987). Lukaski (1986) reported a 16% increase in R (~79 Ω) due to improper electrode placement.

How does body position affect bioimpedance measures?

Proper positioning of the client is important for an accurate measurement. As a standard practice, whole-body resistance is measured with the client lying in a supine position. Changes in body position alter Z values as much as 12% (Lozano, Rosell, and Pallas-Areny 1995); moving from a standing to supine position immediately increases Z by about 3% because of fluid shifts (Kushner et al. 1996). Also, the amount of time the client lies supine before Z is recorded needs to be standardized; in the supine position, Z gradually increases over several hours (Kushner et al. 1996). Experts recommend having your client lie supine for at least 10 min before BIA measurement (Ellis et al. 1999). Subsequent analyses are equivocal in their recommendations regarding fluid equilibration time. One research team indicates that 5 min in a supine position is sufficient to allow TBW to stabilize; ICW and ECW need more time (Gibson et al. 2015). A more conservative TBW and ECW equilibration of "within a 15 min time period" is recommended by Thurlow's group (2017). In addition, make sure the client's arms are abducted (30°-45°) from the trunk and that the thighs are not touching each other. Crossing the limbs short-circuits the electrical path, dramatically affecting bioimpedance values. For bioimpedance analysis with the client in an upright position, have the client stand for 5 min before taking the measurement (Gibson et al. 2015).

Should I measure whole-body bioimpedance on the right or left side of the body?

The standard practice is to measure whole-body bioimpedance on the right side of the body. The differences between R measurements using ipsilateral (right arm–right leg or left arm–left leg) and contralateral (right arm–left leg or left arm–right leg) electrode placements are generally small (Graves et al. 1989; Lukaski et al. 1985).

How does temperature affect bioimpedance?

Bioimpedance measurements should be made with the client lying supine on a nonconductive surface (e.g., stretcher bed or mat) in a room at normal ambient temperature (25 °C [77 °F]). Researchers have demonstrated that ambient temperature affects skin temperature, and R varies inversely with skin temperature (Caton et al. 1988; Gudivaka, Schoeller, and Kushner 1996; Liang, Su, and Lee 2000). Cool ambient temperatures (~14 °C) drop skin temperature (24 °C compared with 33 °C under normal conditions), significantly increasing total body R (by 35 Ω, on average) and decreasing estimated FFM (by ~2.2 kg) (Caton et al. 1988). Liang and colleagues (2000) reported a slightly greater difference in R (46 Ω) between cold (17 °C ambient temperature and 28.7 °C skin temperature) and hot (35 °C ambient and 35.8 °C skin temperature) conditions.

OTHER ANTHROPOMETRIC METHODS

Anthropometry refers to the measurement of the size and proportion of the human body. Body weight and stature (standing height) are measures of body

ANTHROPOMETRIC ASSESSMENTS CONDUCTED WITH A MOBILE APP

LeanScreen, an Apple mobile app, uses three photos (two frontal views and one sagittal view) taken in accordance with app guidelines; sex and height must be key-entered. The user digitally identifies widths and depths on the photos. This requires some knowledge of anatomical landmarks, as the demarcations are interpreted by the app as being circumferences of the neck, waist, abdomen, and hips. The software does the rest of the work to estimate %BF.

To date, two research teams have investigated the app in relation to known methods. For a small sample of adults, there were no significant differences in %BF estimations between LeanScreen, SKF, and BIA (Shaw, Robinson, and Peart 2017). Compared with DXA and manually measured circumferences for a sizeable sample of weight-stable adults, there were significant underestimations of %BF. Less than 45% of the %BF estimates were within ±4% of those measured by DXA (MacDonald et al. 2017). Both research teams reported that the reliability of the app is high ($r > .97$). However, the large intraindividual variability between the app and other methods currently limits its use for purposes beyond general knowledge.

---

size, whereas ratios of weight to height represent body proportion. Circumferences, SKF thicknesses, skeletal diameters, and segment lengths may be used to assess the sizes and proportions of body segments. A **circumference (C)** is a measure of the girth of a body segment such as the arm, thigh, waist, or hip. A **skeletal diameter (D)** is a measure of bony width or breadth (e.g., of the knee, ankle, or wrist).

Anthropometric measures such as circumferences, SKFs, and skeletal diameters have been used to assess total and regional body composition. Also, anthropometric indices such as body mass index (BMI), waist-to-hip circumference ratio (WHR), waist circumference, and sagittal abdominal diameter (SAD) are used to identify individuals at risk for disease. Compared with SKFs, other anthropometric measures are relatively simple and inexpensive, and they do not require a high degree of technical skill and training. They are well suited for large epidemiological surveys and for clinical purposes.

The basic principles underlying the use of anthropometric measures such as circumference, skeletal diameter, and BMI to estimate body composition are as follows:

• *Circumferences are affected by fat mass, muscle mass, and skeletal size; therefore, they are related to fat mass and lean body mass.* Jackson and Pollock (1976) reported that circumference and bony diameter are markers of lean body mass (muscle mass and skeletal size); however, some circumferences are also highly associated with body fat. These findings confirm that circumferences reflect both fat and fat-free components of body composition.

• *Skeletal size directly relates to lean body mass.* Behnke (1961) proposed that lean body mass could be accurately estimated from skeletal diameters and developed equations for doing so. Cross-validation of these equations yielded a moderately high ($r = .80$) relationship and closely estimated average lean body mass values obtained from hydrodensitometry (Wilmore and Behnke 1969, 1970). Behnke's hypothesis was also supported by the observation that skeletal diameters, along with circumferences, are strong markers of lean body mass (Jackson and Pollock 1976).

• *To estimate total body fat from weight-to-height indices, the index should be highly related to body fat but independent of height.* On the basis of data from two large-scale epidemiological surveys (National Health and Nutrition Examination Surveys I and II), Micozzi and colleagues (1986) reported that BMI (body weight divided by height squared) is not significantly related to the height of men ($r = -.06$) and women ($r = -.16$). However, BMI is not totally independent of height, especially in younger children (<15 yr). When the analysis is controlled for age and adiposity, BMI is independent of height (Heymsfield et al. 2016). Although BMI was directly related to SKF thickness and the estimated fat area of the arm ($r = .72-.80$) (Micozzi et al. 1986), the relationship of BMI to body fat varies with age, gender, and ethnicity (Deurenberg and Deurenberg-Yap 2001; Deurenberg, Yap, and van Staveren 1998; Gallagher et al. 1996; Rush et al. 1997; Wang et al. 1994).

Using the Anthropometric Method to Estimate Body Composition

Although some anthropometric prediction models use SKFs, circumferences, and skeletal diameters to estimate body composition, only those equations using circumferences and diameters are addressed in this chapter, for the following reasons:

- The predictive accuracy of anthropometric (circumference and diameter) equations is not greatly improved by the addition of SKF measures.

- Anthropometric equations using only circumferences estimate the body fatness of obese individuals more accurately than SKF prediction equations (Seip and Weltman 1991).

- Compared with SKFs, circumferences and skeletal diameters can be measured with less error (Bray and Gray 1988a).

- Some practitioners may not have access to SKF calipers.

Anthropometric prediction equations estimate total body density (Db), relative body fat (%BF), and fat-free mass (FFM) from combinations of body weight, height, skeletal diameters, and circumferences. Generally, equations using only skeletal measures have larger prediction errors than those using both circumferences and bony diameters. Like SKF and BIA equations, anthropometric equations are based on either population-specific or generalized models.

Population-specific anthropometric equations are valid only for individuals whose physical characteristics (age, gender, ethnicity, and level of body fatness) are similar to those of the specific population. For example, anthropometric equations developed to estimate the body composition of obese individuals (Weltman et al. 1988; Weltman et al. 1987) should not be applied to nonobese individuals.

On the other hand, generalized equations, applicable to individuals of various age and body fatness, have been developed for heterogeneous populations of women (15-79 yr; 13%-63% BF) and men (20-78 yr; 2%-49% BF) (Tran and Weltman 1988, 1989). The predictive accuracy of these generalized equations for estimating the %BF of obese men and women was similar to that of fatness-specific (obese) equations (Seip and Weltman 1991). Typically, generalized equations include body weight or height, along with two or three circumferences, as predictors of Db or %BF. As in generalized SKF models, the relationship between some circumference measures and Db is curvilinear (Tran and Weltman 1988, 1989). Also, age has been shown to be an independent predictor of Db for women (Tran and Weltman 1989). Table 8.6 provides anthropometric prediction equations for various population subgroups.

Using Anthropometric Indices to Classify Disease Risk

Anthropometric measures have other uses besides estimating body composition. In large-scale epidemiological surveys and clinical settings, indirect anthropometric indices such as BMI, WHR, waist circumference, and SAD are used to assess regional fat distribution (upper and lower body fat) and to identify at-risk individuals.

Body Mass Index

The **body mass index (BMI)** is used to classify individuals as obese, overweight, and underweight; to identify individuals at risk for obesity-related diseases; and to monitor changes in the body fatness of clinical populations (Roger et al. 2012; U.S. Department of Health and Human Services 2000b; World Health Organization 1998). Body mass index is a significant predictor of body fat levels, cardiovascular disease, and type 2 diabetes (Ehrampoush et al. 2016; Freedman et al. 2012). Low BMI values have also been associated with poor outcome and survival in clinical clients prone to protein-energy wasting (Leal et al. 2012). Because of this association and the fact that BMI is easily calculated (BMI = body weight / height squared), BMI is widely used in population-based and prospective studies to identify at-risk individuals.

Body mass index, however, is limited as an index of obesity (body fatness) because it does not account for the whole-body or regional composition of and contribution to body weight. In addition, factors such as age, ethnicity, body build, physical activity level, and frame size affect the relationship between BMI and %BF. Thus, using BMI as an index of obesity may result in misclassifications of underweight,

Table 8.6 Circumference Prediction Equations

Population subgroup	Equation	Reference
White women, 15-79 yr	Db (g·cc^{-1})[a] = 1.168297 − 0.002824(abdom C[b]) + 0.0000122098(abdom C[b])^2 − 0.000733128(hip C) + 0.000510477(ht) − 0.00021616(age)	Tran and Weltman (1989)
White men, 15-78 yr	%BF = −47.371817 + 0.57914807(abdom C[b]) + 0.25189114(hip C) + 0.21366088(iliac C) − 0.35595404(BM)	Tran and Weltman (1988)
White, obese women, 20-60 yr	%BF = 0.11077(abdom C[b]) − 0.17666(ht) + 0.14354(BM) + 51.033	Weltman et al. (1988)
White, obese men, 24-68 yr	%BF = 0.31457(abdom C[b]) − 0.10969(BM) + 10.834	Weltman et al. (1987)

Db = body density; %BF = percent body fat; BM = body mass (kg); ht = height (cm).

[a]Use population-specific conversion formula to calculate %BF from Db.

[b]Abdom C (cm) is the average abdominal circumference measured at two sites: (1) anteriorly midway between the xiphoid process of sternum and the umbilicus and laterally between the lower end of the rib cage and iliac crests; (2) at the umbilicus level.

overweight, and obese. Also, because BMI is a better measure of nonabdominal and abdominal subcutaneous fat than of visceral fat (Camhi et al. 2011), other anthropometric indices need to be used to assess fat distribution.

Body mass index (BMI) is the ratio of body weight to height squared: BMI (in kg·m^{-2}) = wt (in kilograms) / ht^2 (in meters). To calculate BMI, measure the body weight in kilograms and convert the height from centimeters to meters (m = cm / 100). Alternatively, you can use a nomogram (see figure 8.15) to calculate a client's BMI (Bray 1978). To use this nomogram, plot the client's height and body weight in the appropriate columns, and connect the two points with a ruler. Read the corresponding BMI at the point where the connecting line intersects the BMI column.

Table 8.7 describes current standards for classifying BMI values. The World Health Organization (1998) defines obesity as a BMI of 30 kg·m^{-2} or more, overweight as a BMI between 25 and 29.9 kg·m^{-2}, and underweight as a BMI of less than 18.5 kg·m^{-2}. These suggested cutoffs are based on the relationship between BMI and morbidity and mortality reported in observational studies in Europe and the United States. There is a J-shaped curve associated with years of life lost and BMI at ages 30, 50, and 70 that indicates a level of minimal likelihood of early mortality for those with BMIs in the normal weight range. For a given BMI greater than 30 kg·m^{-2}, the expected number of years of life lost is greatest for the 30 and 50 yr olds. When the BMI is in the overweight category men are at an increasingly higher risk of early death than are women (Ashwell et al. 2014).

The use of BMI in health risk appraisals assumes that people who are disproportionately heavy are so because of excess fat mass. However, controversy exists concerning the most appropriate cutoff for designating obesity (Deurenberg 2001) and whether or not the cutoff points used for Western and European populations are appropriate for use with Asian populations (Wang et al. 2012). Caution is also urged when using BMI values to identify employees for whom health insurance costs will rise for failure to meet a specific BMI target. An evaluation of adult data in the NHANES 2005-2012 database and BMI's ability to correctly identify their cardiometabolic profile indicates that approximately 75 million American adults will be misclassified based on BMI (Tomiyama et al. 2016).

The relationship between BMI and %BF is affected by age, gender, ethnicity, and body build (Camhi et al. 2011; Deurenberg et al. 1998; Snijder, Kuyf, and Deurenberg 1999). For a given BMI value, older individuals have a greater %BF compared with their younger counterparts, and young adult males have a lesser %BF than young adult females. Also, for a given %BF, age- and gender-matched whites have a higher BMI (1.3-4.6 kg·m^{-2}) compared with other ethnic groups (e.g., African-Americans, Chinese, Indonesians, Ethiopians, and Polynesians) (Camhi et al. 2011; Deurenberg et al. 1998). These findings suggest that using a universal BMI cutoff to define obesity (≥30 kg·m^{-2}) may not be appropriate. Ethnic-specific cutoff values need to be established that account for the relationship between BMI and %BF and for the morbidity and mortality risks in relation to BMI for specific ethnic groups (Antoine-Jonville, Sinnapah, and Hue 2012; Deurenberg 2001; Wang et al. 2012). On the other hand, some researchers believe new ethnic-specific

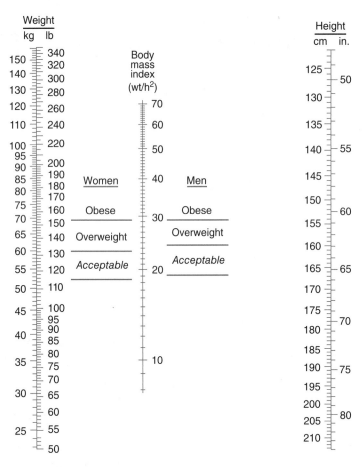

FIGURE 8.15 Nomogram for body mass index.

Reprinted by permission from Macmillan Publishers Ltd. *International Journal of Obesity,* G.A. Bray, "Definition, Measurement, and Classification of the Syndromes of Obesity, 2 no. 2 (1978): 99-112. Copyright 1978.

BMI cut points are not needed. Rather, they suggest that more effort be focused on understanding how the body shape, composition, and segmental proportions underlying BMI relate to health risks and

Table 8.7 Classification of Overweight and Obesity Based on Body Mass Index (BMI)

Classification	BMI value
Underweight	<18.5
Normal weight	18.5-24.9
Overweight	25.0-29.9
Obesity	
Class I	30.0-34.9
Class II	35.0-39.9
Class III	≥40.0

Data from World Health Organization 1998.

outcomes as well as significant clinical conditions (Heymsfield et al. 2016).

Waist Circumference

Waist circumference is recognized as a useful measure of regional adiposity (i.e., abdominal obesity) and as a predictor of obesity-related cardiometabolic disease (Ehrampoush et al. 2016; Moore 2009; Yoon and Oh 2014). It also appears useful in estimating health-related differences in cardiorespiratory fitness in adults 20 to 85 yr of age (Drystad et al. 2017). Waist circumference as a proxy for abdominal fat is reported to have a greater impact on overall adiposity for women compared with men (Ehrampoush et al. 2016). Coupled with BMI, waist circumference predicts musculoskeletal injury risk (Nye et al. 2014) and health risk better than BMI alone (Ardern, Katzmarzyk, and Ross 2003; Zhu et al. 2004). Freedman and Ford (2015) suggest that trends in obesity might be underestimated, especially for women, if obesity is defined by BMI alone. However, waist circumference and its use in various anthropometric indices are considered to be more universally informative than BMI for some racial and ethnic minorities (Tarleton et al. 2015). Yoon and Oh (2014) identified waist circumference cutoff values (men: 85 cm or 33.5 in.; women: 80 cm or 31.5 in.) that may be beneficial for predicting a variety of chronic conditions associated with abdominal obesity in a sample of Korean adults. The National Cholesterol Education Program (NCEP; 2001) recommends using waist circumference cutoffs of >102 cm (40 in.) for men and >88 cm (34.6 in.) for women to evaluate obesity as a risk factor for cardiovascular and metabolic diseases. The International Diabetes Foundation (2006) identified more conservative waist circumference values for Europids (people from North America and Europe); they also identified maximal values for South Asian, Chinese, Japanese, Ethnic South and Central American, Sub-Saharan African, and Eastern Mediterranean and Middle Eastern populations.

Selection of the most appropriate waist circumference cut-points is complex given that age, sex, race, ethnicity, and BMI influence these values; optimum waist circumference cut-points vary according to health outcomes and the population studied (Klein et al. 2007). For example, Kim and associates (2011) identified waist circumference cutoff values for Korean men and women, respectively, that are more conservative than those proposed by Zhu and colleagues (2005) and the NCEP (2001). Likewise, the cutoff points were identified as being 87 cm (34 in.) and 85 cm (33.5 in.), respectively, for elderly (≥65 yr) Korean men and women (Lim et al. 2012). Furthermore, waist circumference measured midway between the iliac crest and the lowest ribs is reported to be superior to waist circumference measured at the superior border of the iliac crest in a sample of Taiwanese adults; the midpoint waist circumference is more highly correlated to visceral fat area, blood pressure, HbA1C, blood glucose, triglycerides, HDL-C, and C-reactive protein compared with the waist circumference measured at the iliac crest for that population subgroup (Ma et al. 2012).

Waist-to-Hip Ratio

The **waist-to-hip ratio (WHR)** is an indirect measure of lower and upper body fat distribution.

Upper body obesity, or central adiposity, measured by the WHR moderately relates ($r = .48-.61$) to risk factors associated with cardiovascular and metabolic diseases in men and women (Ohrvall, Berglund, and Vessby 2000). Young adults with WHR values in excess of 0.94 for men and 0.82 for women are at high risk for adverse health consequences (Bray and Gray 1988b). The optimal WHR for Korean men and women (30-80 yr) is <0.90. A WHR above 0.90 has good sensitivity (men: 82.9%; women 65.3%) and specificity (men: 55.6%; women: 70.9%) for detecting two or more factors (beyond waist circumference) associated with metabolic syndrome in this population subgroup (Kim et al. 2011).

Although the WHR has been used as an anthropometric measure of central adiposity and visceral fat, it has certain limitations:

- The WHR of women is affected by menopausal status (Kim et al. 2011; Svendsen et al. 1992; Weits et al. 1988). Postmenopausal women show more of a male pattern of fat distribution than do premenopausal women (Ferland et al. 1989).

- The WHR is not valid for evaluating fat distribution in prepubertal children (Peters et al. 1992).

- The accuracy of the WHR in assessing visceral fat decreases with increasing fatness.

- Hip circumference is influenced only by subcutaneous fat deposition; waist circumference is affected by both visceral fat and subcutaneous fat depositions. Thus, the WHR may not accurately detect changes in visceral fat accumulation (Goran, Allison, and Poehlman 1995; van der Kooy et al. 1993). Large WHR values have been associated with an increased risk of first stroke (Oliveira, Avezum, and Roever 2015).

To calculate the waist-to-hip ratio (WHR), divide waist circumference (in centimeters) by hip circumference (in centimeters). The measurement site for waist circumference, however, has not been universally standardized. The World Health Organization (1998) recommends measuring waist circumference midway between the lower rib margin and the iliac crest and measuring hip circumference at the widest point over the greater trochanters. In contrast, the *Anthropometric Standardization Reference Manual*

(Callaway et al. 1988) recommends measuring the waist circumference at the narrowest part of the torso and the hip circumference at the level of the maximum extension of the buttocks. The WHR norms (table 8.8) were established using the measurement procedures described in the *Anthropometric Standardization Reference Manual*. Instead of calculating the WHR by hand, you can use the WHR nomogram (figure 8.16) to obtain values for your clients. Plot the client's waist and hip circumferences in the corresponding columns of the nomogram and connect these points with a straight line. Read the WHR at the point where this line intersects the WHR column.

Waist-to-Height Ratio

The **waist-to-height ratio (WHTR)** (i.e., waist circumference / standing height) has been suggested as a better indicator of adiposity and health risks than waist circumference alone (Ashwell, Gunn and Gibson 2011; Ashwell and Hsieh 2005; Hsieh, Yoshinaga, and Muto 2003). To minimize years of life lost because of obesity-related factors and maximize life expectancy, an optimal WHTR of 0.50 (men) and 0.46 (women) in conjunction with sex-specific adult BMIs of 24 and 26 kg·m^{-2}, respectively, is recommended (Ashwell et al. 2014). As a rule, waist circumference should be less than half the height. The risk of premature mortality increases for both men and women, even in their younger years, if their WHTR is in the "consider action" category (WHTR = 0.5 to 0.6). This risk increases dramati-

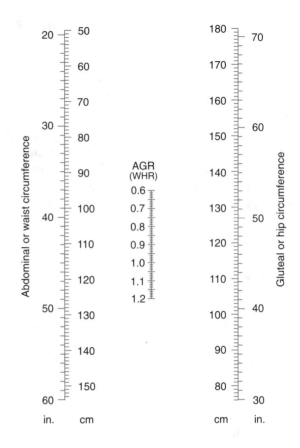

FIGURE 8.16 Nomogram for waist-to-hip ratio (WHR).

Reprinted from G.A. Bray and D.S. Gray, "Obesity: Part I - Pathogenesis," *The Western Journal of Medicine* 149 (1988): 429-441, by permission of BMJ Publishing Group.

Table 8.8 Waist-to-Hip Circumference Ratio Norms for Men and Women

		RISK			
	Age	Low	Moderate	High	Very high
Men	20-29	<0.83	0.83-0.88	0.89-0.94	>0.94
	30-39	<0.84	0.84-0.91	0.92-0.96	>0.96
	40-49	<0.88	0.88-0.95	0.96-1.00	>1.00
	50-59	<0.90	0.90-0.96	0.97-1.02	>1.02
	60-69	<0.91	0.91-0.98	0.99-1.03	>1.03
Women	20-29	<0.71	0.71-0.77	0.78-0.82	>0.82
	30-39	<0.72	0.72-0.78	0.79-0.84	>0.84
	40-49	<0.73	0.73-0.79	0.80-0.87	>0.87
	50-59	<0.74	0.74-0.81	0.82-0.88	>0.88
	60-69	<0.76	0.76-0.83	0.84-0.90	>0.90

Adapted from Bray and Gray 1988.

cally if the WHTR exceeds 0.6, as that places them in the "take action" category. To see the J-shaped relationship between years of life lost and WHTR for 30, 50, and 70 yr olds, see the work of Ashwell and associates (2014).

Flegal and colleagues (2009) reported that WHTR, waist circumference, and BMI were highly related (r = .85-.97) across age groups and genders. Although all three of these anthropometric indices performed similarly as indicators of body fatness, the relationship of WHTR with %BF was slightly higher (r = .66-.87). WHTR was found to be consistently superior to both BMI and waist circumference in terms of serving as an indicator of disease outcome or risk factors for cardiovascular diseases, diabetes mellitus, metabolic syndrome, hypertension, and dyslipidemia (Ashwell, Gunn, and Gibson 2011).

The Ashwell Body Shape Chart can be used to identify a client's health risk based on body shape (see appendix D.6). To use this chart, measure the client's standing height and waist circumference at the umbilical level. Find the point corresponding to the height (y-axis of chart) and waist circumference (x-axis). This chart is applicable to adults from all racial and ethnic groups, as well as children 5 yr of age or older.

Sagittal Abdominal Diameter

The **sagittal abdominal diameter (SAD)** is a measure of the anteroposterior thickness of the abdomen at the umbilical level. It is also a simple indicator of the amount of dysfunctional visceral adipose tissue in the body, known to lead to aberrations in blood glucose level, insulin resistance, and increased risk for developing type 2 diabetes mellitus (Kahn et al. 2014). The SAD is strongly related to visceral adipose tissue in men (r =.82) and women (r = .76), even after adjusting for BMI (r = .66 and .63, respectively, for men and women) (Zamboni et al. 1998). However, this relationship is stronger in lean or moderately overweight individuals than in obese individuals. Compared with waist circumference, WHR, and BMI, SAD is more strongly related to risk factors for cardiovascular and metabolic diseases in women and men (Ohrvall et al. 2000). In support of Ohrvall's findings, Kahn and colleagues (2014) found a greater association between SAD and disease-causing blood glucose abnormalities independent of BMI, age, and waist circumference.

At age 60, men's SAD value is strongly correlated to waist circumference, BMI, and WHR; whereas, for women, the only strong correlations are between SAD with waist circumference and BMI. Sex-specific SAD cutoff values of 22 cm and 20 cm, respectively, have been identified for men and women. Beyond these values, cardiometabolic risk scores increase (Risérus et al. 2010).

According to an 8 yr longitudinal study of 5,168 Finnish adults, the relative risk of developing diabetes between the lowest and highest quartiles was similar for SAD (14.7) and BMI (15.0); the relative risk from waist circumference (11.4) and WHR (12.5) were lower. The combination of high SAD and high BMI formed the most powerful predictor of incident diabetes (Pajunen et al. 2013). The SAD is also associated with cardiovascular disease risk factors in older women (67-78 yr) (Turcato et al. 2000); likewise, SAD was directly correlated with triglyceride and blood glucose levels and inversely related with HDL-C in a sample of overweight Brazilian adults with an average age and BMI of 54 yr and 30.5 kg·m^{-2}, respectively (Pimentel et al. 2011).

The procedures for measuring SAD have not been standardized. In most studies, SAD was measured while the client was lying supine, legs extended, on an examination table. A sliding-beam anthropometer is used to measure the vertical distance (to the nearest 0.1 cm) between the top of the table and the abdomen at the level of the umbilicus or iliac crests. In some studies, SAD was measured with the hips and legs flexed or with the client standing instead of lying supine.

Using Anthropometric Measures to Classify Frame Size

Skeletal diameters are used to classify frame size in order to improve the validity of height-weight tables for evaluating body weight. The rationale for including frame size is that skeletal breadths are important estimators of the bone and muscle components of fat-free mass. Estimating frame size allows you to differentiate between those who weigh more because of a large musculoskeletal mass and those who weigh more because of a large fat mass (Himes and Frisancho 1988). Since there are health implications for individuals who are overweight, a critical evaluation of body weight is important. You can approximate frame size using reference data for elbow width. For men, elbow width ≤6.7 cm is small and ≥8.1 cm is large. Values ≤5.7 cm and ≥7.2 cm are classified, respectively, as small and large frame size for women (Frisancho 1984). The anatomical landmarks for measurement are described in appendix D.5, Standardized Sites for Bony Breadth Measurements.

Anthropometric Techniques

You must practice in order to become proficient in measuring skeletal diameters and circumferences. Following the standardized procedures (see Standardized Procedures for Anthropometric Measurements) will increase the accuracy and reliability of your measurements (Callaway et al. 1988; Wilmore et al. 1988).

Sources of Measurement Error

The accuracy and reliability of anthropometric measures are potentially affected by equipment, technician skill, and client factors (Bray 1978; Callaway et al. 1988). The following questions and responses concern these sources of measurement error.

What equipment will I need to measure bony widths?

Use skeletal anthropometers and sliding or spreading calipers to measure bony widths and body breadths (see figure 8.17). The precision characteristics (0.05-0.50 cm) and range of measurement (0-210 cm) depend on the type of skeletal anthropometer or caliper you are using (Wilmore et al. 1988). The instruments must be carefully maintained and must be calibrated periodically so that their accuracy can be checked and restored.

Can I use any type of tape measure to measure body circumferences?

Use an anthropometric tape measure to measure circumferences (see figure 8.17). The tape measure should be made from a flexible material that does not stretch with use. You can use a plastic-coated tape measure if an anthropometric tape measure is not available. Some anthropometric tapes have a spring-loaded handle (i.e., Gulick handle) that allows a constant tension to be applied to the end of the tape during the measurement.

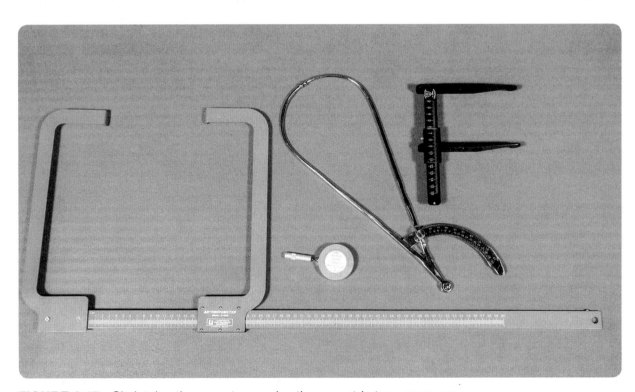

FIGURE 8.17 Skeletal anthropometers and anthropometric tape measure.

Standardized Procedures for Anthropometric Measurements

1. Take all circumference and bony diameter measurements of the limbs on the right side of the body.

2. Carefully identify and measure the anthropometric site. Be meticulous about locating anatomical landmarks used to identify the measurement site (see appendix D.4, Standardized Sites for Circumference Measurements, and appendix D.5, Standardized Sites for Bony Breadth Measurements), and instruct your clients to relax their muscles during the measurement.

3. Take a minimum of three measurements at each site in rotational order.

4. To measure the breadth of smaller segments, like the elbow or wrist, use small sliding calipers (range of 30 cm or 11.8 in.) with greater scale precision instead of larger skeletal anthropometers (range of 60-80 cm or 23.6-31.5 in.).

5. Hold the skeletal anthropometer or caliper in both hands so the tips of the index fingers are adjacent to the tips of the caliper.

6. Place the caliper on the bony landmarks and apply firm pressure to compress the underlying muscle, fat, and skin. Apply pressure to a point where the measurement no longer continues to decrease.

7. Use an anthropometric tape to measure circumferences. Hold the zero end of the tape in your left hand, positioned below the other part of the tape that is held in your right hand.

8. Apply tension to the tape so that it fits snugly around the body part but does not indent the skin or compress the subcutaneous tissue.

9. For some circumferences (e.g., waist, hip, and thigh), you should align the tape in a horizontal plane, parallel to the floor.

How much skill and practice are required to ensure accurate circumference and skeletal diameter measurements?

Technician skill is not a major source of measurement error for these methods compared with the SKF and ultrasound methods. However, you need to practice in order to perfect the identification of the measurement sites and your measurement technique. Experts recommend practicing on at least 50 people and taking a minimum of three measurements for each site in rotational order (Callaway et al. 1988). Closely follow standardized testing procedures for locating measurement sites, positioning the anthropometer or tape measure, and applying tension during the measurement. Appendix D.4 (Standardized Sites for Circumference Measurements) and appendix D.5 (Standardized Sites for Bony Breadth Measurements) describe some of the most commonly used circumference and skeletal diameter sites.

Is there good agreement in circumference and skeletal diameter values when the measurements are taken by two different technicians?

Variability in circumference measurements taken by different technicians is relatively small (0.2-1.0 cm), with some sites differing more than others (Callaway et al. 1988). Skilled technicians can obtain similar values even when measuring circumferences of obese individuals (Bray and Gray 1988a).

Are the circumferences of obese clients more easily measured than SKFs?

As with the SKF method, it is more difficult to obtain consistent measurements of circumference for obese compared with lean individuals (Bray and Gray 1988a). However, circumferences are preferable to SKFs for measuring obese clients, for several reasons:

- You can measure circumferences of obese individuals regardless of their size, whereas the maximum aperture of the SKF caliper may not be large enough to allow measurement.
- Measurement of circumferences requires less technician skill.
- Differences between technicians are smaller for circumferences than for SKF measurements (Bray and Gray 1988a).

Is it possible to accurately measure bony widths of heavily muscled and obese clients?

Accurate measurement of bony diameters in heavily muscled or obese individuals may be difficult because the underlying muscle and fat tissues must be firmly compressed. It may be difficult to identify and palpate bony anatomical landmarks, leading to error in locating the measurement site.

Key Points

▶ Body composition is a key component of health and physical fitness; total body fat and fat distribution are related to disease risk.

▶ Standards for percent body fat can be used to classify body composition.

▶ Average %BF and standards for obesity vary according to age, gender, and physical activity levels.

▶ Hydrostatic weighing is a valid and reliable reference method for assessing body composition.

▶ Air displacement plethysmography is an alternative to hydrostatic weighing for measuring body volume and deriving body density.

▶ Dual-energy X-ray absorptiometry is increasingly recognized as a reference method for assessing body composition.

▶ The absolute values of body composition variables determined by different DXA scanners are difficult to compare because of differences in manufacturers and software versions.

▶ Population-specific conversion formulas, based on multicomponent models of body composition, should be used to convert Db into percent body fat.

▶ The SKF method is widely used in field and clinical settings.

▶ Generalized SKF equations for the prediction of Db are reliable and valid for a wide range of individuals.

▶ The ultrasound method is gaining recognition as a viable noninvasive alternative to the SKF method.

▶ Bioelectrical impedance analysis is a viable alternative for assessing body composition of diverse population subgroups.

▶ Circumferences and skeletal diameters can be used to estimate body composition.

▶ Body mass index is a crude index of total body fatness.

▶ Waist-to-hip ratio, waist circumference, WHTR, and SAD are acceptable indices for identifying at-risk clients.

Key Terms

Learn the definition for each of the following key terms. Definitions of terms can be found in the glossary.

air displacement plethysmography (ADP)

anthropometry

Archimedes' principle

attenuation

bioelectrical impedance analysis (BIA)

bioimpedance spectroscopy (BIS)

body density (Db)

body mass index (BMI)

body surface area

body volume (BV)

Boyle's law

circumference (C)

damping technique

densitometry

dual-energy X-ray absorptiometry (DXA)

fat-free body (FFB)

fat-free mass (FFM)

fat mass (FM)

hemiscan procedure

hydrodensitometry

hydrostatic weighing (HW)

impedance (Z)

multicomponent model

percent body fat (%BF)

reactance (X_c)

relative body fat (%BF)

residual volume (RV)

resistance (R)

resistance index (ht^2 / R)

sagittal abdominal diameter (SAD)

skeletal diameter (D)

skinfold (SKF)

tare weight

thoracic gas volume (TGV)

two-component model

ultrasound

underwater weight (UWW)

waist-to-height ratio (WHTR)

waist-to-hip ratio (WHR)

Review Questions

In addition to being able to define each of the key terms, test your knowledge and understanding of the material by answering the following review questions.

1. Why is it important to assess the body composition of your clients?

2. What are the standards for classifying obesity and minimal levels of body fat for men and women?

3. Explain why many researchers are calling for BMI and anthropometric cutoff points that are specific for the client's ethnicity.

4. Explain musculoskeletal changes and differences associated with gender, age, and physical activity that make BMI better than adiposity for explaining body shape.

5. What are the assumptions of the two-component model of body composition? Identify two commonly used two-component model equations for converting Db into %BF.

6. Explain how gender, ethnicity, and age affect FFB density and, therefore, two-component model estimates of %BF.

7. Name three methods you can use to obtain reference measures of body composition. Which method is best? Explain your choice.

8. Identify two ways to measure (not estimate) a client's Db.

9. Distinguish between total Db and FFB density.

10. Describe how the HW method could be modified to test clients who are unable to be weighed under water at RV.

11. Identify potential sources of measurement error for the SKF and ultrasound methods.

12. Explain the differences between A- and B-mode ultrasound result displays.

13. In lay terms, explain the basic theory underlying the use of BIA.

14. To obtain accurate estimates of body composition using the BIA method, your client must adhere to pretesting guidelines. Identify these client guidelines.

15. Explain how BMI, WHR, WHTR, and waist circumference may be used to identify clients at risk due to obesity.

16. Identify suitable field methods and prediction equations (i.e., SKF, BIA, or other anthropometric methods) to estimate body composition for each of the following subgroups of the population: older adults, children, obese individuals, and athletes.

CHAPTER 9

Designing Weight Management and Body Composition Programs

KEY QUESTIONS

▶ What is obesity and how prevalent is it world-wide?

▶ What are the health risks associated with having high or low levels of body fat?

▶ What are the primary causes of overweight and obesity?

▶ How is healthy body weight determined?

▶ What steps should I follow in planning a weight management program?

▶ What are the recommended guidelines for weight loss and weight gain programs?

▶ Why is exercise important for weight management?

▶ What types of exercise are best for weight loss?

▶ Does exercising without dieting improve body composition?

Health and longevity are threatened when a person is either overweight or underweight. Overweight and obesity increase the risk of developing serious cardiovascular, pulmonary, and metabolic diseases and disorders. Likewise, individuals who are underweight may have a higher risk than others of cardiac, musculoskeletal, and reproductive disorders. Thus, healthy weight is key to a healthy and longer life.

As a health and fitness professional, you have an enormous challenge and responsibility to help determine a healthy body weight for your clients and to provide scientifically sound weight management programs for them. This chapter presents guidelines and techniques for determining healthy body weight. You will learn about weight control principles and practices, as well as guidelines for designing exercise programs for weight loss, weight gain, and body composition change.

OBESITY, OVERWEIGHT, AND UNDERWEIGHT: DEFINITIONS AND TRENDS

Individuals with body fat levels falling at or near the extremes of the body fat continuum are likely to have serious health problems that reduce life expectancy and threaten their quality of life. Obese individuals have a higher relative risk of cardiovascular ischemic heart disease (2.0×), stroke (1.55×), dyslipidemia, hypertension, glucose intolerance, insulin resistance, diabetes mellitus (6.0×), obstructive pulmonary disease, gallbladder disease, osteoarthritis, and cancers of the colon (1.2×), esophagus (2.3×), gallbladder (1.5×), and endometrium (2.5×)

(U.S. Department of Health and Human Services 2000b; International Association for the Study of Obesity 2012). The prevalence of diabetes is highest among obese (18.5%) followed by overweight (8.2%) and normal weight (5.4%) individuals, and this same pattern exists for hypertension (35.7%, 26.4%, and 19.8%, respectively) and dyslipidemia (49.7%, 44.2%, and 28.6%, respectively) (Saydah et al. 2014). Obesity is independently associated with coronary heart disease (CHD), heart failure, cardiac arrhythmia, stroke, and menstrual irregularities (Pi-Sunyer 1999).

At the opposite extreme, underweight individuals with too little body fat tend to be malnourished. These people have a relatively higher risk of fluid-electrolyte imbalances, osteoporosis and osteopenia, bone fractures, muscle wasting, cardiac arrhythmias and sudden death, peripheral edema, and renal and reproductive disorders (Fohlin 1977; Mazess, Barden, and Ohlrich 1990; Vaisman, Corey, et al. 1988). One disease associated with extremely low body fat levels is anorexia nervosa. **Anorexia nervosa,** an eating disorder found primarily in females, is characterized by excessive weight loss. It afflicts approximately 1% of the female population in the United States (Hudson et al. 2007). Compared with normal-weight women, those with anorexia have extremely low body fat (8%-13% body fat), signs of muscle wasting, and less bone mineral content and bone density (Mazess, Barden, and Ohlrich 1990; Vaisman, Rossi, et al. 1988).

DEFINITIONS OF OBESITY, OVERWEIGHT, AND UNDERWEIGHT

Obesity is an excessive amount of body fat relative to body weight. The term is not synonymous with overweight. In many epidemiological studies, **overweight** is defined as a body mass index (BMI) between 25 and 29.9 kg/m^2, obesity is defined as a BMI of 30 kg/m^2 or more, and **underweight** is defined by a BMI of less than 18.5 kg/m^2 (U.S. Department of Health and Human Services 2000b). To identify children and adolescents who are overweight, the 85th and 95th percentile cutoffs for age and sex developed from the Centers for Disease Control and Prevention growth charts are commonly used in the United States. Children with a BMI

greater than or equal to the 95th percentile for their age and sex are categorized as obese; those with BMI values between the 85th and 94th percentiles are categorized as overweight. However, these definitions are not universally accepted. Pooled international data for BMI have been used to develop international standards for evaluating childhood overweight and obesity. These standards are based on growth curves that relate the cutoff points for BMI of different age-gender groups (2-18 yr) to the adult categories for overweight (BMI ≥25 kg/m^2) and obesity (BMI ≥30 kg/m^2) (see Cole et al. 2000).

Because these criteria do not take into account the composition of an individual's body weight, they are limited as indexes of obesity and may result in misclassifications of underweight, overweight, and obesity. Considerable variability in body composition exists for any given BMI. Some individuals with low BMIs may have as much relative body fat as those with higher BMIs. Older people have more relative body fat at any given BMI than younger people (Baumgartner, Heymsfield, and Roche 1995). Thus, the prevalence of obesity could be worse than currently thought.

TRENDS IN OVERWEIGHT AND OBESITY

Globally, the prevalence of overweight and obesity has reached pandemic proportions. The prevalence of obesity in the world more than doubled between 1980 and 2014 (World Health Organization 2016c). Worldwide, more than 1.9 billion adults are overweight; of these, over 600 million are obese (World Health Organization 2016c) when using the previously stated BMI criteria. Thus, approximately 13% of the world's population is obese. Some researchers have projected that the prevalence of obesity will continue upward, with 20% of the world's population reaching obese status by the year 2030 (Smith and Smith 2016). However, some studies suggest that the increases in prevalence of obesity for adults and children in some countries may be slowing or leveling off (Flegal et al. 2012; Ogden et al. 2014; Rokholm, Baker, and Sorensen 2010; Townsend, Rutter and Foster 2012). For example, in the United States, 36.5% of adults are obese (BMI >30 kg/m^2), and 17.0% of youth are obese (BMI ≥95th percentile) (Ogden et al. 2015). Obesity prevalence has not changed significantly in either of these groups since 2003-2004; however, the increase in obesity is significant dating back to 1999-2000. These data further document that the rate at which obesity is increasing in the United States might be slowing, but it is not declining. Additionally, the proportion of Americans who are severely obese (≥ 40 kg/m^2) continues to increase, from 3.9% in 2000 to 6.6% in 2010. The trend of severe (morbid) obesity varies by gender and ethnicity; the prevalence among women is about 50% higher than among men, and about twice as high among blacks when compared with Hispanics or whites (Sturm and Hattori 2012).

The prevalence of overweight and obesity in adults varies among countries, depending in part on the nation's level of industrialization. For example, the United States, Canada, Australia, and nearly all of Europe have an overweight prevalence >60%. In contrast, the prevalence of overweight in India, Afghanistan, Indonesia, and most of the countries in Africa is <20%. For an interactive world map of individual country statistics on BMI and prevalence of overweight and obesity, search the Global Health Observatory data of the World Health Organization (WHO) (www.who.int/gho/ncd/risk_factors/overweight/en).

Over the past 30 yr, the prevalence of overweight and obesity in children has increased substantially. Globally, 170 million children (2-18 yr) are estimated to be overweight (World Health Organization 2012a). Ahluwalia and colleagues (2015) reported that overweight prevalence in 11, 13, and 15 yr olds did not change from 2002 to 2010 in the majority of countries included in their study, but it did increase in many Eastern European countries. The prevalence of children and adolescents (6-19 yr) who are overweight or obese (BMI $\geq$85th percentile) in the United States is about 34% (Ogden et al. 2014). The combined prevalence of overweight and obesity is also 34% in Greek children (Kotanidou et al. 2013). In comparison, researchers recently reported that the prevalence of overweight and obese children in Australia varied from 12.4% to 30.2% depending on the territory (Ho et al. 2017). Prevalence values ranged from 18.6% to 29.9% and 14.7% to 19.0% for South Korean boys and girls (10-19 yr), respectively, depending on the criteria used to define overweight (Bahk and Khang 2016).

Collectively, there appears to have been an increase in overweight prevalence among youth worldwide up to about 2003, with a stabilization occurring over the next decade (Bahk and Khang 2016; Ho et al. 2017; Kotanidou et al. 2013; Ogden et al. 2014). Also, it is alarming that there are an estimated 41 million children under the age of 5 yr who are overweight or obese (World Health Organization 2016c). According to this WHO report, the problem of infant obesity, once considered unique to high-income nations, is an increasing problem in low- and middle-income countries. However, in the United States, there was actually a significant decrease in obesity among preschool children (2-5 yr); prevalence dropped from 13.9% in 2003-2004 to 8.4% in 2011-2012 (Ogden et al. 2014).

Because of the health risks and medical costs associated with obesity, the goal of the U.S. surgeon general is to reduce the prevalence of overweight in children and obesity in adults to no more than 14.6% and 30.6%, respectively, by the year 2020 (U.S. Department of Health and Human Services 2012).

OBESITY: TYPES AND CAUSES

Combating obesity is not an easy task. Many overweight and obese individuals have incorporated patterns of overeating and physical inactivity into their lifestyles, while others have developed eating disorders, exercise addictions, or both. In an effort to lose weight quickly and to prevent weight gain, many are lured by fad diets and exercise gimmicks; some resort to extreme behaviors, such as avoiding food, bingeing and purging, and exercising compulsively. Nicklas and colleagues (2012) reported that obese adults who lost at least 5% of body weight achieved meaningful weight loss if they ate less fat, exercised more, used prescription weight loss medications, or participated in commercial weight loss programs.

In a survey of weight control practices of adults in the United States, Weiss and colleagues (2006) reported that 48% of women and 34% of men were trying to lose weight by means of such practices as eating less food, eating less fat, choosing low-calorie foods, and exercising. Less common practices included drinking water, skipping meals, eating diet foods, taking special supplements or diet pills, joining weight loss programs, taking prescription diet pills, and taking laxatives. Only one-third of those trying to lose weight reported using the recommended method of restricting caloric intake and increasing physical activity to at least 150 min/wk; less than 25% combined caloric restriction with higher levels of physical activity (>300 min/wk).

In a report on leisure-time physical activity among overweight adults in the United States (Prevalence of Leisure-Time Physical Activity 2000), two-thirds of overweight adults reported that they engaged in physical activity to try to lose weight; however, only 20% exercised at least 30 min a day at a moderate intensity on most days of the week. Although most of these individuals exercised 30 min or longer per session, only a minority exercised at least five times per week. Similarly, Kruger, Yore, and Kohl (2007) reported in their study of leisure-time physical activity patterns that fewer than half of people trying to lose or maintain weight were *regularly* active. Therefore, low frequency of physical activity was the main reason the physical activity recommendation was not met.

TYPES OF OBESITY

How fat is distributed in the body may be more important than total body fat for determining one's risk of disease. The waist-to-hip ratio (WHR) is strongly associated with **visceral adipose tissue (VAT)**, and the impact of regional fat distribution on health is related to the amount of VAT located in the abdominal cavity. Abdominal fat is strongly associated with diseases such as CHD, diabetes, hypertension, and hyperlipidemia (Bjorntorp 1988; Blair et al. 1984; Ducimetier, Richard, and Cambien 1989).

The terms **android obesity** and **gynoid obesity** refer to the localization of excess body fat mainly in the upper body (android) or lower body (gynoid). Android obesity (apple shaped) is more typical of males; gynoid obesity (pear shaped) is more characteristic of females. However, some men may have gynoid obesity, and some women may have android obesity. Other terms are also used to describe types of obesity and regional fat distribution. Android obesity is frequently simply called **upper body obesity**, and gynoid obesity is often described as **lower body obesity**.

In field settings, you can assess regional fat distribution using the WHR. Chapter 8 presents measurement procedures (see Waist-to-Hip Ratio) and WHR norms (see table 8.8). Generally, young adults with WHR values in excess of 0.94 for men and 0.82 for women are at very high risk for adverse health consequences (Bray and Gray 1988b).

CAUSES OF OVERWEIGHT AND OBESITY

Many questions may arise in regard to overweight and obesity. This section addresses common questions relating to their causes.

Why do people gain or lose weight?

An energy imbalance in the body results in a weight gain or loss. Energy is balanced when the caloric intake equals the caloric expenditure. A **positive energy balance** is created when the input (food intake) exceeds the expenditure (resting metabolism plus activity level). For every 3,500 kcal of excess energy accumulated, 1 lb (0.45 kg) of fat is stored in the body. A **negative energy balance** is produced when the energy expenditure exceeds the energy input. People can accomplish this by reducing the food intake or increasing the physical activity level. A caloric deficit of approximately 3,500 kcal produces a loss of 1 lb of fat.

How are energy needs and energy expenditure measured?

Energy need and expenditure are measured in kilocalories (kcal). A **kilocalorie** is defined as the amount of heat needed to raise the temperature of 1 kg (2.2 lb) of water 1 °C. Direct calorimetry is used to measure the energy yield and caloric equivalent of various foods. These foods are burned in a closed chamber in the presence of oxygen, and the amount of heat liberated is measured precisely in kilocalories. Table 9.1 gives the energy yield and caloric equivalents for carbohydrate, protein, and fat.

The energy, or caloric, need is a function of an individual's metabolic rate and physical activity level. The **basal metabolic rate (BMR)** is a measure of the minimal amount of energy (kcal) needed to maintain basic and essential physiological functions such as breathing, blood circulation, and temperature regulation. Basal metabolic rate varies according to age, gender, body size, and body composition. For assessment of BMR, the individual needs to be rested and fasted and should be in a controlled environment. Since this is not always practical, we use the term **resting metabolic rate (RMR)**, or **resting energy expenditure (REE)**, to indicate the energy required to maintain essential physiological processes in a relaxed, awake, and reclined state. The RMR is approximately 10% higher than the BMR.

Total energy expenditure (TEE) is the sum of the energy expended for BMR or RMR, **dietary thermogenesis** (i.e., energy needed for digesting, absorbing, transporting, and metabolizing foods), and physical activity. Some experts have further divided the physical activity portion into **exercise activity thermogenesis (EAT)** and **non-exercise activity thermogenesis (NEAT)** (i.e., energy expenditure of occupation, leisure, activities of daily living, and unconscious or spontaneous motion such as fidgeting) (Aragon et al. 2017). It is estimated that BMR makes up 60% to 70% of TEE; dietary thermogenesis is 8% to 15%, and EAT and NEAT are 15% to 30% and 15% to 50%, respectively (Aragon et al. 2017). The gold standard for measuring TEE is the doubly labeled water (with deuterium and oxygen-18) method. This method is expensive and requires considerable expertise as well as specialized equipment. Therefore, age- and gender-specific prediction equations have been developed to estimate TEE (see table 9.2 and Steps for Estimating TEE later in the chapter).

Table 9.1 Energy Yield and Caloric Equivalents for Macronutrients

Nutrient	Energy yield (kcal·g^{-1})	Caloric equivalents (kcal·L^{-1} O$_2$)
Carbohydrate	4.1	5.1
Protein	4.3	4.4
Fat	9.3	4.7

Table 9.2 Prediction Equations for Estimating TEE (kcal·day^{-1}) of Children and Adults

Gender and age	Equation	Physical activity coefficient (PA)
Male 3-18 yr	TEE = 88.5 − (61.9 × age) + PA [(26.7 × wt) + (903 × ht)]	1.00, if PAL is ≥1.0 and <1.4 (sedentary)
		1.13, if PAL is ≥1.4 and <1.6 (low)
		1.26, if PAL is ≥1.6 and <1.9 (active)
		1.42, if PAL is ≥1.9 and <2.5 (very active)
Male ≥19 yr	TEE = 662 − (9.53 × age) + PA [(15.9 × wt) + (540 × ht)]	1.00, if PAL is ≥1.0 and <1.4 (sedentary)
		1.11, if PAL is ≥1.4 and <1.6 (low)
		1.25, if PAL is ≥1.6 and <1.9 (active)
		1.48, if PAL is ≥1.9 and <2.5 (very active)
Female 3-18 yr	TEE = 135.3 − (30.8 × age) + PA [(10.0 × wt) + (934 × ht)]	1.00, if PAL is ≥1.0 and <1.4 (sedentary)
		1.16, if PAL is ≥1.4 and <1.6 (low)
		1.31, if PAL is ≥1.6 and <1.9 (active)
		1.56, if PAL is ≥1.9 and <2.5 (very active)
Female ≥19 yr	TEE = 354 − (6.91 × age) + PA [(9.36 × wt) + (726 × ht)]	1.00, if PAL is ≥1.0 and <1.4 (sedentary)
		1.12, if PAL is ≥1.4 and <1.6 (low)
		1.27, if PAL is ≥1.6 and <1.9 (active)
		1.45, if PAL is ≥1.9 and <2.5 (very active)

TEE = total energy expenditure in kcal·day^{-1}; PA = physical activity coefficient; wt = body weight in kilograms; ht = height in meters; PAL = physical activity level.

From Institute of Medicine 2002/2005.

Alternatively, energy expenditure during basal, resting, or activity states can be measured in laboratory settings through indirect calorimetry. In this case, the body's energy expenditure is estimated from oxygen utilization. Every liter of oxygen consumed per minute yields approximately 5 kcal (see

ACTIVITY TRACKERS: ARE THEY ACCURATE FOR ESTIMATING ENERGY EXPENDITURE?

Being able to track energy (caloric) expenditure is of great importance for those pursuing weight loss and weight maintenance goals. But the technology to track energy expenditure (EE) with a high degree of accuracy is still lacking. Research results are mixed on the ability of activity trackers to accurately compute TEE in controlled laboratory settings, during semi-structured activities, and in free-living environments. Although the correlation between activity tracking accelerometers is reported to be moderate to strong, significant underestimations of the reference values are common. Accelerometers, categorized as research-grade (ActiGraph GT3X+, BodyMedia Core, Body Media SenseWear), underestimate energy expenditure in comparison to the gold standard, indirect calorimetry (Bai et al. 2016; Ferguson et al. 2015; Imboden et al. 2017; Kim and Welk 2015).

Consumer-targeted devices worn during a variety of activities produce large differences and variable estimates of EE and tend to underestimate reference values of EE (Bai et al 2016; Ferguson et al. 2015; Imboden et al. 2017; Kim and Welk 2015; Price et al. 2017; Sasaki et al. 2015). Typically, the proprietary algorithms developed by the manufacturers account for differences between devices. Although some accelerometers perform better during moderate- to fast-paced activities (ActiGraph GT3X+, BodyMedia SenseWear, Core Armband), others perform better during slow-paced activities (activPAL). Lyden and associates (2017) reported that the activPAL accurately categorizes sedentary behaviors as well as light-intensity and MVPA exercise compared with direct observation. Triaxial and multisensory devices tend to provide more accurate estimates of TEE than uniaxial devices (Van Remoortel et al. 2012).

table 9.1). For specific physical activities, energy expenditure is typically expressed in METs (see chapter 4 and appendix E.3) as a multiple of the RMR. One MET equals the assumed relative rate of oxygen consumption of 3.5 ml·min^{-1} for each kilogram of body weight (3.5 ml·kg^{-1}·min^{-1}) or the relative rate of energy expenditure of 1 kcal·hr^{-1} for each kilogram of body weight (1 kcal·hr^{-1}·kg^{-1}).

How is RMR regulated?

Thyroxine is extremely important in regulating RMR. Thyroid tumors or lack of iodine in the diet can result in inadequate production of this hormone. Underproduction of thyroxine can reduce RMR 30% to 50%. If energy input and expenditure are not adjusted accordingly, the positive energy balance that is created results in a weight gain.

Growth hormone, epinephrine, norepinephrine, and various sex hormones may elevate RMR as much as 20%. These hormones increase during exercise and may be responsible for the elevation in RMR after cessation of exercise.

Does weight gain increase both the number and size of fat cells?

Obesity is associated with increases in both the number (hyperplasia) and size (hypertrophy) of fat cells. A normal-weight individual has 25 to 30 billion fat cells, whereas an obese person may have as many as 42 to 106 billion fat cells. Also, the adipose cell size of obese individuals is on the average 40% larger than that of nonobese persons (Hirsh 1971). Caloric restriction and exercise are effective in reducing fat cell size but not the number of fat cells in adults (Hirsh 1971; Spalding et al. 2008).

Traditional thought is that the number of fat cells is set during childhood and adolescence, and this number remains constant in both lean and obese adults, even if substantial weight changes occur (Spalding et al. 2008). In other words, adipocytes experience hypertrophy and atrophy with weight gain and loss, respectively, but the number of cells does not change throughout adulthood. Epidemiological studies suggest that weight gain in the first 6 mo of life is primarily a gain in fat and that this time period is critical for development of obesity and cardiometabolic problems in adulthood (Gillman 2008). This has led some to speculate that the key to preventing obesity is to closely monitor dietary intake and energy expenditure during the adolescent growth spurt and puberty, as this could potentially retard the development of new fat cells. However, this traditional thought has been challenged. Tchoukalova and colleagues (2010) induced a body fat gain of about 4 kg in normal-weight adult men and women. They observed that adipocytes experienced hypertrophy in the upper body but hyperplasia in the lower body. They theorized that forming new fat cells in the lower body might actually be a protective mechanism against accumulating more fat in the upper body in response to overfeeding. Whatever the reason, it appears that differences in preadipocyte cell dynamics may allow for regional hyperplasia in response to overfeeding. In a recent review, Cuthbertson and colleagues (2017) seem to confirm this new theory. They claim that **subcutaneous adipose tissue (SAT)** remodels itself to adapt to overfeeding, and this remodeling can occur by either hypertrophy or hyperplasia.

What is the relative importance of genetics and environment in developing obesity?

Scientists have debated the relative contributions of genetics and environment to obesity. Mayer (1968) observed that only 10% of children who had normal-weight parents were obese. Overweight adolescents have a 70% chance of becoming overweight adults; this probability increases to 80% if one parent or both parents are overweight or obese (U.S. Department of Health and Human Services 2007). Deficiencies in a few genes, most notably melanocortin-4 receptor and leptin, have been associated with obesity (Selassie and Sinha 2011). Although these data suggest a genetic influence, they do not rule out environmental influences such as individual choices about eating and exercising. Bray (2004) described a useful way to think about the relationship of genes to obesity when he wrote "the genetic background loads the gun, but the environment pulls the trigger."

In a controlled study of long-term (100 days) overfeeding in identical twins, Bouchard and colleagues (1990) observed large individual differences in the tendency toward obesity and distribution of body fat, even within each pair of twins. Changes in body weight due to overfeeding of the twins were moderately correlated ($r = .55$). Overall, increases in body weight, fat mass, trunk fat, and VAT were three times greater in high weight gainers compared with low weight gainers. These data suggest that genotype explains some, but not all, of a person's adaptation to a sustained energy surplus. Approximately 25% of the variability among individuals in absolute and relative body fat is attributed to genetic factors, and 30% is associated with cultural (environmental) factors (Bouchard et al. 1988). Although the identification of genes related to obesity is highly researched, studies to identify common nucleotide polymorphisms associated with BMI have not been able to explain more than 2% of the variability in BMI. Much of the interindividual variability in body weight is attributable to the interactions between genes and environment or genes and behavior (Bouchard 2008).

Recent research indicates that genes influence not only weight gain but also how and where excess body fat is deposited, and this can affect one's health. For example, some individuals have a normal BMI yet they have a metabolically obese phenotype, characterized by increased VAT relative to SAT, putting them at risk for metabolic and cardiovascular disease. In other words, when these individuals overeat, they have a tendency to store excess fat viscerally rather than subcutaneously. The opposite is also true; some people have a higher BMI yet a lower risk for metabolic disease because they have a higher SAT:VAT ratio, or a higher SAT capacity (Cuthbertson et al. 2017). Thus, with overfeeding, genetic and epigenetic factors are at play to determine the distribution of adipose tissue.

Hill and Melanson (1999) suggested that the major cause of obesity in the United States is environment. Over the past 30 yr, the U.S. population has been exposed to an environment that strongly promotes the consumption of high-fat, energy-dense foods (increased energy intake) as well as reliance on technology that discourages physical activity and reduces the amount of physical activity (decreased energy expenditure) needed for daily living. Similarly, Swinburn and associates (2011) and Selassie and Sinha (2011) addressed the interactions between environmental and individual factors, including genetic makeup. Selassie and Sinha (2011) identified increased portion sizes and consumption of high-fructose corn syrup and sweetened beverages along with more sedentary careers and more leisure time spent on computers rather than in physical activity as contributing behavioral factors to obesity. Swinburn and colleagues (2011) concluded that changes in the food supply and marketing environments that promote high energy intake, along with increased mechanization and the subsequent reduction in physical activity, are key factors associated with the obesity epidemic.

WEIGHT MANAGEMENT PRINCIPLES AND PRACTICES

Proper nutrition (eating a well-balanced diet) and daily physical activity are key components of a weight management program. In weight management programs, most clients are interested in losing body weight and body fat, but some need to gain body weight. The basic principle underlying safe and effective weight loss programs is that weight can be lost only through a negative energy balance, which is produced when the caloric expenditure exceeds the caloric intake. The most effective way of creating a caloric deficit is through a combination of diet (restricting caloric intake) and exercise (increasing caloric expenditure). On the other hand, for weight gain programs, the caloric intake must exceed the caloric expenditure in order to create a positive energy balance. Weight Management Principles summarizes principles and practices underlying the design of weight management programs.

People can win the battle of controlling body weight and obesity not only by understanding why they eat and monitoring their food intake closely but also by incorporating more physical activity into their lifestyles. The physically active lifestyle is characterized by

- daily aerobic exercise;
- strength and flexibility exercises;
- increased participation in recreational activities such as bowling, golf, tennis, and dancing; and
- increased physical activity in the daily routine at home and work through restricting use of labor-saving devices such as escalators, power tools, automobiles, and home and garden appliances.

DESIGNING WEIGHT MANAGEMENT PROGRAMS: PRELIMINARY STEPS

In designing weight management programs for weight loss or weight gain, you need to set body weight goals and assess the calorie intake and expenditure for your clients.

SETTING BODY WEIGHT GOALS

To set healthy body weight goals for your clients, you must first assess their present body weight, BMI, or body fat levels. You can easily measure a client's body weight by using a calibrated bathroom or physician's scale. Clients should wear indoor clothing but not shoes.

TELEMONITORING SCALES: ELIMINATING SELF-REPORTED WEIGHT ERRORS

Self-reported weight is often inaccurate, and the errors are more common in overweight individuals (Rowland 1990). Telemonitoring scales allow for the immediate transmission of a client's weight to a remote site, thereby eliminating any self-report inaccuracies. These scales have been used in several weight loss intervention studies. In a study by VanWormer and colleagues (2009), obese participants' weights were automatically transmitted to counselors who could provide customized feedback. They found that study participants who self-weighed at least once per week were 11 times more likely to lose at least 5% of their prestudy body weight after 6 mo. Bluetooth-connected weighing scales allowing study participants to self-weigh at home and have their data automatically transmitted to investigators at remote sites are being used in studies of people who have type 2 diabetes (Wild et al. 2013) and weight gain during pregnancy (Bogaerts et al 2017).

WEIGHT MANAGEMENT PRINCIPLES

Weight loss	Weight gain	Exercise
• A well-balanced diet for good nutrition contains carbohydrate, protein, fat, vitamins, minerals, and water.	• The dietary protein intake should be increased to 1.2-1.6 g·kg⁻¹ body weight.	• The major cause of obesity is lack of physical activity, not overeating.
• The weight loss should be gradual—no more than 2 lb (1 kg) a week.	• The weight gain should be gradual—no more than 2 lb a week.	• For fat-weight loss, aerobic exercise should be performed daily or twice daily.
• The caloric intake should be at least 1,200 kcal·day⁻¹, and the caloric deficit should not exceed 1,000 kcal·day⁻¹.	• The daily caloric intake should exceed caloric needs by 400-500 kcal·day⁻¹.	• Resistance exercise training is excellent for maintaining fat-free mass (for weight loss) and increasing FFM (for weight gain).
• A caloric deficit of 3,500 kcal is needed to lose 1 lb (0.5 kg) of fat.	• A positive energy balance of 2,800-3,500 kcal is needed to gain 1 lb of muscle tissue.	• For weight loss, exercise helps create a caloric deficit by increasing caloric expenditure.
• Weight loss should be due to fat loss rather than lean body tissue.	• Weight gain should be due to increased fat-free mass (FFM) rather than fat mass.	• Exercise is better than dieting for maximizing fat loss and minimizing lean tissue loss.
• On the same diet, a taller, heavier person will lose weight at a faster rate than a shorter, lighter person because of a higher RMR.	• The individual should eat three meals and two or three healthy snacks per day (e.g., dried fruits, nuts, seeds, and some liquid meals).	• Compared with fat, muscle tissue is more metabolically active and uses more calories at rest.
• Weight loss rate decreases over time because the difference between the caloric intake and caloric needs gets smaller as one loses weight.	• Protein powders are no more effective than natural protein sources (e.g., lean meats, skim milk, and egg whites).	• Low-intensity, longer-duration exercise maximizes total energy expenditure better than high-intensity, shorter-duration exercise.
• Men lose weight faster than women because of a higher RMR.	• Amino acid supplements may promote muscle growth if taken immediately before or after exercise.	• RMR remains elevated 30 min or longer after vigorous exercise.
• The individual should eat at least three meals a day.	• Vitamin B₁₂, boron, and chromium supplements do not increase fat-free mass.	• At a given heart rate, the more physically fit individual expends calories at a faster rate than the less fit individual.
• Quick weight loss diets, diet pills, and appetite suppressants should be avoided.		• Exercise does not increase appetite.
• Carnitine supplementation does not promote body fat loss.		• Passive exercise devices (e.g., vibrators and sauna belts) do not massage away excess fat.
• Compulsive eating behaviors should be identified and modified.		• Spot reduction exercises do not preferentially mobilize subcutaneous fat stored near the exercising muscles.
		• To increase caloric expenditure, avoid using labor-saving devices at home and work.

When you are evaluating a client's body weight, you should not use height-weight tables established by insurance companies. These tables are limited for two reasons:

- The values represent height and weight with shoes and clothing. Whether individuals were measured with shoes and clothing was not standardized.

- Data were obtained from individuals who could afford life insurance; the data represent predominantly young to middle-aged white males and females and therefore are not representative of other population groups.

Individuals with a BMI from 18.5 up to 25 are considered to be at a **healthy body weight** by many health standards. However, determining a healthy body weight from either BMI or any height-weight table alone may lead to invalid conclusions regarding a client's level of body fatness and health risk. These methods do not take into account the body composition of the individual. For example, with the use of BMI or height-weight tables, many mesomorphs having a large fat-free mass are classified as overweight, yet their body fat content may be lower than average. Similarly, individuals may be overfat or obese even though they are underweight according to the BMI and height-weight tables. Therefore, you should use the body composition technique to estimate a healthy body weight and body fat level for your clients.

When you use the body composition technique for estimating healthy body weight and body fat levels, assess the fat-free mass (FFM) and percent fat (%BF) using one of the methods described in chapter 8. A healthy body weight is based on the client's present FFM and %BF goal. Because some fat is needed for good health and nutrition, individuals should attempt to achieve a %BF somewhere between the low and upper values recommended in table 8.1. Remember, minimal %BF depends on age and is estimated to be 5% to 10% for males and 12% to 15% for females. Cutoff values for obesity are also age dependent, ranging from >22% to >31% BF for males and >35% to >38% BF for females. For an example of how to calculate healthy body weight using the body composition technique, see Sample Calculation of Healthy Body Weight.

With aging, there is a tendency to accumulate body weight and excess fat. Typically, adults may expect to gain 15 lb (9 kg) of fat weight and lose 5 lb (2.3 kg) of lean body mass per decade of life (Evans and Rosenberg 1992; Forbes 1976). This weight gain is primarily characterized by an increase in body fat and a decrease in muscle mass and is associated with declining physical activity levels with age. Each individual should attempt to maintain body weight and fatness at healthy levels.

ASSESSING CALORIE INTAKE AND ENERGY EXPENDITURE

The second step in planning weight management programs is to assess the client's energy (calorie) intake and expenditure. You will use these baseline data to estimate the rate of weight loss or weight gain and the amount of time needed to achieve long-term goals of body composition and body weight.

Energy Intake

A food record (see appendix E.1, Food Record and RDA Profile) is used to determine an individual's daily caloric intake. The client keeps a record of the type and quantity of foods eaten each day for 3 to 7 days. Make certain the client records all foods consumed; underreporting of food intake ranges from 10% to 45%. Use computer software to assess the average daily caloric intake and to compare average nutrient intakes against recommended amounts for each nutrient. Several dietary analysis programs are

---

SAMPLE CALCULATION OF HEALTHY BODY WEIGHT

Demographic Data

Client: 31 yr old male

Current body composition:

Body weight = 185 lb (84.1 kg)

Body fat = 20% BF

Fat-free mass (FFM) = 148 lb (67.3 kg)

Goals: 12% BF and 88% FFM

Steps

1. Determine the client's present %BF using one of the body composition methods (see chapter 8).

2. Calculate the client's present FFM (in pounds): 185 lb × 0.80 (current %FFM) = 148 lb (67.3 kg).

3. Set reasonable body composition goals for client: 12% BF and 88% FFM.

4. Divide the present FFM (in pounds) by the %FFM goal to obtain target body weight: 148 lb / 0.88 = 168 lb (76.4 kg).

5. Calculate weight loss by subtracting target body weight from present body weight: 185 − 168 = 17 lb (7.7 kg). Assuming that FFM is maintained, this client must lose 17 lb of fat to achieve his target body weight and body fat level.

available online. The food record can also help you analyze dietary patterns such as types of foods consumed, frequency of eating, and the caloric content of each meal. For a ranking of smartphone apps for tracking food intake, see Patel and colleagues (2015).

Energy Expenditure

You can use either the factorial method or the TEE method to assess the energy needs of your clients. For the **factorial method**, RMR or REE and the additional calories expended during work, household chores, personal daily activities, and exercise are estimated. Various methods used to estimate RMR and the additional energy requirements for occupational and physical activities are presented in this section. Although the factorial approach may reasonably estimate your clients' energy expenditure, it is limited in that the equations used to estimate RMR have prediction errors. Also, it is neither feasible nor

practical to measure the wide range of activities performed throughout a normal day. Therefore, the TEE method for estimating total energy expenditure has been endorsed by the Institute of Medicine (2005). For the **total energy expenditure (TEE) method**, the individual's TEE is predicted using equations derived from doubly labeled water measures of TEE in free-living individuals (see table 9.2).

Factorial Method: Estimation of Resting Energy Expenditure

Indirect calorimetry can be used to obtain reference measures of RMR or REE. Prediction equations are an inexpensive alternative to indirect calorimetry (see Methods of Estimating Resting Metabolic Rate). You can estimate body surface area (BSA) from height and weight using the nomogram in figure 9.1.

The average male or female between 20 and 40 yr of age burns 38 kcal·hr⁻¹ and 35 kcal·hr⁻¹, respectively, for each square meter of BSA. For example,

METHODS OF ESTIMATING RESTING METABOLIC RATE

Method	Equation
I. BODY SURFACE AREA (BSA)[a]	
Men	RMR = BSA × 38 kcal·hr⁻¹ × 24 hr
Women	RMR = BSA × 35 kcal·hr⁻¹ × 24 hr
II.A. HARRIS-BENEDICT EQUATIONS[b]	
Men	RMR = 66.473 + 13.751(BM) + 5.0033(ht) − 6.755(age)
Women	RMR = 655.0955 + 9.463(BM) + 1.8496(ht) − 4.6756(age)
II.B. MIFFLIN ET AL. EQUATIONS[b]	
Men	RMR = 9.99(BM) + 6.25(ht) − 4.92(age) + 5.0
Women	RMR = 9.99(BM) + 6.25(ht) − 4.92(age) − 161
II.C. MOLNAR ET AL. (1995) EQUATION	
Boys (10-16 yr)	RMR = 50.9 (BM) + 25.3 (ht) − 50.3 (age) + 26.9
Girls (10-16 yr)	RMR = 51.2 (BM) + 24.5 (ht) − 207.5 (age) + 1629.8
III. FAT-FREE MASS (FFM)	
Men and women	RMR = 500 + 22 (FFM in kg)
IV. QUICK ESTIMATE (FROM BODY MASS)	
Men	RMR = BM (in lb) × 11 kcal·lb⁻¹
	RMR = BM (in kg) × 24.2 kcal·kg⁻¹
Women	RMR = BM (in lb) × 10 kcal·lb⁻¹
	RMR = BM (in kg) × 22.0 kcal·kg⁻¹

[a]Adjust RMR for age. RMR decreases 2% to 5% per decade after age 40.

[b]BM in kilograms; ht in centimeters; age in years.

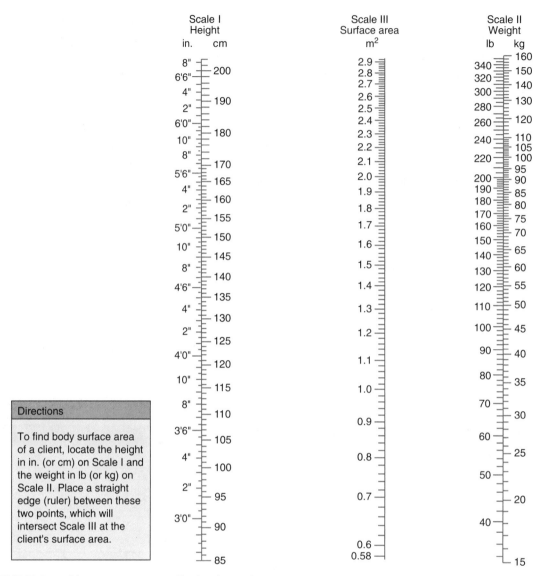

FIGURE 9.1 Nomogram to predict body surface area.

Reprinted by permission from W.E. Collins, *Clinical Spirometry* (Braintree, MA: Warren E. Collins, 1967), 33. Copyright Warren E. Collins.

according to method I for estimating RMR, a 5 ft 2 in. (157.5 cm), 120 lb (54.5 kg) female has a BSA of 1.54 m^2 and a daily resting metabolic need of 1,294 kcal (1.54 m^2 × 35 kcal·hr^{-1} × 24 hr).

You can obtain a quicker but less accurate estimate of REE by multiplying the body weight (BW) by a factor of 10 (for BW measured in pounds) or 22 (for BW measured in kilograms) for women and by a factor of 11 (for BW in pounds) or 24.2 (for BW in kilograms) for men (see method IV). With this method, the REE for the woman in our example is 1,200 kcal (120 lb × 10).

Resting energy expenditure gradually decreases with age because the number of metabolically active cells is reduced. The REE declines 2% to 5% during each decade of life after age 25 (Sharkey and Gaskill 2007). To prevent gradual weight gain with aging, people must reduce caloric intake or increase physical activity level. In the past, the Harris-Benedict (1919) equations (method II.A) were widely used to estimate REE of adults. However, the American Dietetic Association (2003) recommends using the equations of Mifflin and colleagues (1990) to estimate the REE of healthy individuals (see method II.B). Both equations (Harris-Benedict and Mifflin) are gender specific and take into account not only height and weight but also age. Roza and Shizgal (1984) cross-validated the original Harris-Benedict equations, developed new equations using data from a large number of subjects, and concluded that the original equations published in 1919 yielded identical estimates of REE. Also, the Harris-Benedict equations accurately estimated the REE of a large sample ($N = 2,528$) of normal-weight, overweight, and obese individuals, but these equations tended to overestimate REE in underweight persons (Muller et al. 2004; O'Riordan et al. 2010). In contrast, the American Dietetic Association (2003) reported that the Harris-Benedict equations generally overestimated REE but that the equations of Mifflin and colleagues accurately estimated (within ±10%) the REE for 80% of their sample. The Mifflin equation is also the most accurate for adults with BMIs of 25 to 40 kg/m^2 (Weijs 2008).

Indirect calorimetry is the method of choice for measuring REE, especially in obese populations where prediction equations tend to systematically underestimate REE of these clients (Wilms et al. 2010). The Harris-Benedict equations and the equations of Mifflin and colleagues, however, may provide a practical alternative for estimating REE when planning weight management programs for overweight or obese individuals. For children (10-16 yr), the gender-specific prediction equations (method II.C) provide a reasonably accurate estimate of REE (Hofsteenge et al. 2010; Molnar et al. 1995).

In addition to body size and age, REE is influenced by body composition. Muscular individuals have a higher REE than fatter individuals of the same body weight because fat tissue is less metabolically active than muscle tissue. The RMRs of women are 5% to 10% lower than those of men (McArdle, Katch, and Katch 1996). This lower rate may be attributable to a greater relative fat content and lower FFM for women. To use method III (see Methods of Estimating Resting Metabolic Rate), you must measure the FFM of your client using one of the body composition methods suggested in chapter 8.

Factorial Method: Estimation of Additional Caloric Requirements

Resting energy expenditure accounts for 50% to 70% of total daily caloric needs, but this value depends on the activity level and occupation of the person. The percentage is greater for less active individuals, who require fewer calories above the resting level. For example, if a sedentary male office worker has a resting metabolic need of 1,680 kcal, the additional caloric need as a consequence of the nature of his work is approximately 40% above resting level, or 672 kcal. Provided he performs no additional physical activities, his total daily caloric need is 2,352 kcal. In this case, REE accounts for 71% of his total daily caloric requirements. Table 9.3 presents additional caloric requirements for selected occupational activity levels.

Table 9.3 Additional Energy Requirements for Selected Activity Levels

Occupational activity level*	PERCENTAGE ABOVE BASAL METABOLISM	
	Men	Women
Sedentary	15	15
Lightly active	40	35
Moderately active	50	45
Very active	85	70
Exceptionally active	110	100

*Examples for each occupational activity level are as follows:

Sedentary = inactive.

Lightly active = most professionals, office workers, shop workers, teachers, homemakers.

Moderately active = workers in light industry, most farm workers, active students, department store workers, soldiers not in active service, commercial fishing workers.

Very active = full-time athletes and dancers, unskilled laborers, forestry workers, military recruits and soldiers in active service, mine workers, steel workers.

Exceptionally active = lumberjacks, blacksmiths, female construction workers.

After determining the daily energy needs of the client from his REE and occupation, you can estimate his additional calorie expenditure due to physical activity and exercise by using a physical activity log (appendix E.2, Physical Activity Log). The individual records every activity performed and the total amount of time spent in each activity. The estimated energy expenditure for a variety of activities is listed in appendix E.3, Gross Energy Expenditure for Conditioning Exercises, Sports, and Recreational Activities. You can calculate the total caloric expenditure for each activity by converting the METs to kcal·kg^{-1}·hr^{-1} (1 MET = 1 kcal·kg^{-1}·hr^{-1}) and multiplying this value by the client's body weight (kg). This yields the total number of kilocalories the client expends per hour of that activity. You can determine the kcal·min^{-1} expenditure by dividing the kcal·hr^{-1} by 60 min. Calculate the total caloric energy expenditure of the activity by multiplying the kcal·min^{-1} by the duration of the activity.

Keeping a physical activity log is a very time-consuming process for both you and your clients, and it may not increase the accuracy of your estimate of additional caloric expenditure because many clients tend to overestimate the actual duration of their physical activity. It may be best to just ask your clients to list the frequency, intensity, and average time for the physical activities and sports they perform on a regular basis; you can then determine their calorie expenditure for each activity as just described. Add these values to the daily caloric need estimated for their RMR and occupation, and advise clients that on days they are active they can increase their calorie intake accordingly.

Total Energy Expenditure Method

For this method, the age- and gender-specific equations in table 9.2 are used to estimate your clients' TEE. These equations predict TEE from age, body weight, height, and physical activity coefficient. The physical activity coefficient depends on your clients' **physical activity level (PAL)**; given that energy expenditure is highly dependent on physical activity, PAL is commonly described as the ratio of TEE to BMR (PAL = TEE / BMR). The PAL categories were developed from doubly labeled water measures of TEE and BMR in normal, healthy individuals. Data from elite athletes and extremely active individuals

(i.e., military personnel and astronauts) were not included (Brooks et al. 2004). Physical activity levels are classified as sedentary (1.0 to <1.4), low (1.4 to <1.6), active (1.6 to <1.9), and very active (1.9 to <2.5). To obtain a fairly good estimate of your clients' PAL, you can use various tools such as self-reported physical activity questionnaires, physical activity diaries, pedometers, accelerometers, heart rate monitors, and other wearable technology (Keim, Blanton, and Kretsch 2004). For information about the validity and reliability of pedometers and accelerometers for monitoring physical activity levels, see chapter 3. Steps for Estimating TEE illustrates how you can use the TEE equations to estimate your clients' daily energy expenditure.

DESIGNING WEIGHT LOSS PROGRAMS

When the caloric expenditure exceeds the caloric intake, a negative energy balance, or caloric deficit, is created. The most effective way of producing this deficit is to use a combination of caloric restriction and exercise. Because a deficit of 3,500 kcal is needed to lose 1 lb (0.45 kg) of fat, you can easily calculate the daily caloric deficit that is needed to result in the target weekly weight loss you set for your client. An average deficit of 500 kcal will produce a weekly weight loss of approximately 1 lb (0.45 kg), given that 500 kcal × 7 days = 3,500 calories. An average deficit of 1,000 will produce a weight loss of 2 lb (0.90 kg) a week (1,000 kcal × 7 days, or 2 lb). The daily caloric deficit should not exceed 1,000 kcal per day.

It is important to note that the relationship of 3,500 kcal to 1 lb (0.45 kg) of fat is mathematical; however, in reality this weight loss rule is overly simplistic (Cuthbertson et al. 2017; Hall et al. 2011). This relationship assumes that body weight changes reflect changes in adipose tissue without regard to changes in FFM. An increase in lean mass as a result of resistance training, for example, would increase RMR and alter this relationship. Conversely, losses of FFM reduce RMR, making it more difficult to lose weight. Hall and colleagues (2011) at the National Institutes of Health (NIH) considered all these variables in creating a web-based simulator for predicting weight change over time by using a mathematical modeling approach. The Body Weight Planner is available on the NIH website at www.niddk.nih.gov/health-information/weight-management/body-weight-planner. Additionally, the Body Weight Planner is linked to the U.S. Department of Agriculture's SuperTracker (www.supertracker.usda.gov), another web-based program that provides a personalized meal plan based on a person's goals and results from the Body Weight Planner.

To ensure that the weight loss is a result of the loss of body fat rather than lean body tissue, you should do the following:

- Use the body composition method to estimate the client's healthy body weight and fat loss.

- Encourage daily participation in aerobic exercise and resistance training programs to enhance the loss of fat and to conserve FFM.

- Work with a nutritionist to plan a diet that restricts calorie intake but contains adequate amounts of good sources of carbohydrate, protein, and fat. The diet should contain at least 130 g of carbohydrate per day and 0.8 g of protein per kilogram of body weight per day.

When you design the weight loss program of diet and exercise, use descriptive data to help set reasonable goals for your clients. These data include age, gender, height, body weight, relative body fat (%BF), %BF goal, average calorie intake, cardiorespiratory fitness level, and occupation. See Steps for Designing a Weight Loss Program.

EXERCISE PRESCRIPTION FOR WEIGHT LOSS

Exercise alone—without dieting—has only a modest effect on weight loss. The most successful weight loss programs, therefore, use a combination of dieting and exercising to optimize the energy deficit and to maintain weight loss. The options for weight loss diet plans can be overwhelming. For a comprehensive review of major diet archetypes and their effects on body composition, see the recent position stand by the International Society of Sports Nutrition (Aragon et al. 2017). We suggest that you work closely with a nutrition professional when designing weight management programs for your clients. This is particularly important if a client has any metabolic complications (e.g., diabetes, dyslipidemia, hyper- or hypothyroidism). In the same way anyone can dispense personal training information without the appropriate educational training or certification

STEPS FOR ESTIMATING TEE

To estimate a client's total energy expenditure (TEE) from age- and gender-specific TEE equations, follow these steps:

- Step 1: Determine the client's gender and age (50 yr old male).

- Step 2: Measure the client's body weight and height (BW = 180 lb; ht = 70 in.). Convert body weight in pounds to body weight in kilograms: 180 lb / 2.204 = 81.7 kg. Convert height in inches to height in meters: 70 in × 0.0254 = 1.78 m.

- Step 3: Estimate your client's PAL (1.70, or active, from physical activity log).

- Step 4: Select the appropriate age- and gender-specific TEE prediction equation from table 9.2: for males ≥19 yr.

$$\text{TEE (kcal·day}^{-1}) = 662 - (9.53 \times \text{age}) + \text{PA} [(15.9 \times \text{wt}) + (540 \times \text{ht})]$$

- Step 5: Determine the physical activity coefficient corresponding to your client's PAL (1.25 for PAL = 1.70).

- Step 6: Substitute the values for age, body weight, physical activity, and height into the equation:

$$\text{TEE (kcal·day}^{-1}) = 662 - (9.53 \times 50 \text{ yr}) + 1.25 [(15.9 \times 81.7 \text{ kg}) + (540 \times 1.78 \text{ m})]$$

- Step 7: Calculate the estimated TEE (kcal·day^{-1}):

$$\text{TEE (kcal·day}^{-1}) = 662 - (9.53 \times 50 \text{ yr}) + 1.25 [(15.9 \times 81.7 \text{ kg}) + (540 \times 1.78 \text{ m})]$$

$$= 662 - (476.5) + [1.25 \times (1299 + 961)]$$

$$= 185.5 + 2,260$$

$$\text{TEE} = 2,445.7, \text{ or } 2,446 \text{ kcal·day}^{-1}$$

STEPS FOR DESIGNING A WEIGHT LOSS PROGRAM

Summary of Client's Demographic Data

1. *Client's age and gender:* 35 yr old female
2. *Height:* 62 in. or 157.5 cm
3. *Body weight:* 131 lb or 59.55 kg
4. *Percent fat:* 26% BF; *relative FFM:* 74%
5. *Percent fat goal:* 20% BF; *relative FFM goal:* 80%
6. *Average daily calorie intake:* 2,000 kcal
7. *Cardiorespiratory fitness level:* Below average
8. *Occupation:* Secretary

Steps

1. Assess the body weight and body composition of the client.
2. Assess the daily calorie intake of the subject (use 3- or 7-day food records).
3. Estimate a healthy target body weight based on the client's percent fat goal.

    Present FFM = 96.9 lb (131 lb × 0.74) (relative FFM)

    Target body weight = 121 lb (96.9 lb / 0.80) (relative FFM goal)

4. Calculate the weight loss and total calorie deficit needed to achieve that weight loss.

    a. Weight loss = 10 lb (131 lb − 121 lb)

    b. Caloric deficit = 35,000 kcal (10 lb × 3,500 kcal·lb^{-1})

5. Estimate the daily energy expenditure of the client from the following equation: energy expenditure = RMR + daily activity level.

    a. RMR = 655.0955 + 9.463(59.55 kg) + 1.8496(157.5 cm) − 4.6756(35 yr) = 1,346 kcal

    b. Daily occupational activity level: lightly active 35% above basal level (see table 9.3).

    Additional kcal = 1,346 × 0.35 = 471 kcal

    c. Total energy expenditure = 1,346 + 471 = 1,817 kcal

6. Plan to produce a calorie deficit of 700 to 800 kcal per day by reducing the calorie intake by 500 kcal per day and increasing the calorie expenditure by 200 to 300 kcal per day through exercise. To calculate caloric expenditure during exercise, refer to appendix E.3. Multiply the calories burned per minute per kilogram of body weight by the duration of the activity and the client's body weight. Continue this program until the total calorie deficit of 35,000 kcal is reached. In a little over 7 wk the client will lose approximately 10 lb (4.5 kg). This is a gradual average weight loss of 1 1/2 lb (0.7 kg) per week. Reassess the body composition to see if the percent fat goal was reached.

7. Put the client on a maintenance diet and exercise program.

    a. Calculate the total energy expenditure using an estimate of RMR based on the new body weight.

    RMR + activity level + exercise = total energy expenditure, where

    RMR = 1,303 kcal (use Harris-Benedict formula substituting a body weight of 55 kg)

    Occupational activity level = 456 kcal (1,303 × 0.35)

    Exercise = 300 kcal

    Total energy expenditure = 1,303 + 456 + 300 = 2,059 kcal

    b. Advise the client that if she continues to exercise daily, expending approximately 300 kcal per workout, she may increase her calorie intake to 2,060 kcal per day. However, for days when she cannot exercise, the calorie intake must be restricted to 1,760 kcal.

Week 1	Exercise = 100 kcal·day^{-1} × 7 days		=	700 kcal
	Diet = 500 kcal·day^{-1} × 7 days	Subtotal	=	3,500 kcal
			=	4,200 kcal
Week 2	Exercise = 150 kcal·day^{-1} × 7 days		=	1,050 kcal
	Diet = 500 kcal·day^{-1} × 7 days	Subtotal	=	3,500 kcal
			=	4,550 kcal
Weeks 3-4	Exercise = 200 kcal·day^{-1} × 14 days		=	2,800 kcal
	Diet = 500 kcal·day^{-1} × 14 days	Subtotal	=	7,000 kcal
			=	9,800 kcal
Weeks 5-6	Exercise = 250 kcal·day^{-1} × 14 days		=	3,500 kcal
	Diet = 500 kcal·day^{-1} × 14 days	Subtotal	=	7,000 kcal
			=	10,500 kcal
Week 7	Exercise = 300 kcal·day^{-1} × 7 days		=	2,100 kcal
	Diet = 500 kcal·day^{-1} × 7 days	Subtotal	=	3,500 kcal
		Total weeks 1-7	=	5,600 kcal
			=	34,650 kcal

(see the preface), anyone can give nutrition advice. However, there are restrictions on who can use the title dietitian or nutritionist. Table 9.4 is a summary of the statutory provision regarding professional regulation of dietitians and nutritionists in each state of the United States.

The amount of physical activity and exercise needed to benefit health, prevent overweight and obesity, or maintain weight loss differs (see table 9.5). For health benefits, the ACSM and AHA recommend at least 30 min of moderate-intensity (3-6 METs) physical activity on a minimum of 5 days/wk or 20 min of vigorous-intensity (>6.0 METs) activity on a minimum of 3 days/wk (American College of Sports Medicine 2009). Likewise, the Physical Activity Guidelines for Americans (Howley 2008) recommend 150 to 300 min/wk of moderate intensity (3-6 METs) or 75 to 150 min/wk of vigorous intensity or both (≥6.0 METs).

To prevent weight gain, the ACSM (2009) recommends moderate-intensity physical activity between 150 and 250 min/wk. However, the International Association for the Study of Obesity (IASO) consensus statement suggests that 30 min of daily physical activity (210 min/wk) may be insufficient for preventing weight gain or regain after weight loss (Saris et al. 2003). To maintain weight and to prevent unhealthy weight gain and transition to overweight or obesity in adults, 45 to 60 min of

moderate-to-vigorous activity (PAL = 1.7) on most, preferably all, days is recommended (Institute of Medicine 2005; U.S. Department of Health and Human Services 2005; Saris et al. 2003). For children and adolescents, at least 60 min of moderate to vigorous physical activity daily is recommended to maintain healthy body weight as well as good health and fitness (U.S. Department of Health and Human Services 2007).

The optimal physical activity level (PAL) for preventing weight gain differs from that for creating a negative energy balance for weight loss and maintenance of weight loss. For a modest weight loss (i.e., 2-3 kg or 4.4-6.6 lb), the ACSM (2009) recommends moderate-intensity physical activity between 150 and 250 min/wk; however, there is a dose effect for physical activity and weight loss, with >250 min/wk of physical activity associated with clinically significant (3% or greater) weight loss (American College of Sports Medicine 2009).

The ACSM (2009) acknowledges that physical activity is necessary to prevent regaining weight after weight loss. Although the specific amount of physical activity needed to prevent weight regain is uncertain at this time, some studies suggest that weight maintenance after weight loss is improved by engaging in more than 250 min/wk of physical activity. The ACSM (2009) noted that 60 min/day of walking at a moderate intensity is associated with

Table 9.4 Statutes Regarding Professional Regulation of Dietitians and Nutritionists in the United States

State	Statute	State	Statute
Alabama	Licensure of dietitian, nutritionist	Montana	Licensure of nutritionist; title protection for dietitian
Alaska	Licensure of dietitian, nutritionist	Nebraska	Licensure of medical nutrition therapist
Arizona	No statute	Nevada	Licensure for dietitian, LD, and RD
Arkansas	Licensure of dietitian	New Hampshire	Licensure of dietitian
California	Title protection for dietitian, RD, and NDTR	New Jersey	No statute
Colorado	No statute	New Mexico	Licensure of dietitian, nutritionist, nutrition associate
Connecticut	Certification of dietitian	New York	Certification of dietitian, nutritionist
Delaware	Licensure of dietitian, nutritionist	North Carolina	Licensure of dietitian, nutritionist
District of Columbia	Licensure of dietitian, nutritionist	North Dakota	Licensure of dietitian, nutritionist, RD
Florida	Licensure of dietitian, nutritionist, nutrition counselor	Ohio	Licensure of dietitian
Georgia	Licensure of dietitian	Oklahoma	Licensure of dietitian
Hawaii	Licensure of dietitian	Oregon	Licensure of dietitian
Idaho	Licensure of dietitian	Pennsylvania	Licensure of dietitian-nutritionist
Illinois	Licensure of dietitian, nutritionist	Puerto Rico	Licensure of dietitian, nutritionist
Indiana	Certification of dietitian	Rhode Island	Licensure of dietitian, nutritionist
Iowa	Licensure of dietitian	South Carolina	Licensure of dietitian
Kansas	Licensure of dietitian	South Dakota	Licensure of dietitian, nutritionist
Kentucky	Licensure of dietitian; certification of nutritionist	Tennessee	Licensure of dietitian, nutritionist
Louisiana	Licensure of dietitian	Texas	Title protection for dietitian
Maine	Licensure of dietitian, NDTR	Utah	Certification of dietitian
Maryland	Licensure of dietitian, nutritionist	Vermont	Certification of dietitian
Massachusetts	Licensure of dietitian, nutritionist	Virginia	Title protection for dietitian, nutritionist
Michigan	Pending status: licensure of dietitian, nutritionist	Washington	Certification of dietitian, nutritionist
Minnesota	Licensure of dietitian, nutritionist	West Virginia	Licensure of dietitian
Mississippi	Licensure of dietitian; title protection for nutritionist	Wisconsin	Certification of dietitian
Missouri	Licensure of dietitian	Wyoming	Licensure of dietitian

RD = registered dietitian; NDTR = nutrition and dietetics technician, registered; LD = licensed dietitian.

© 2018 Academy of Nutrition and Dietetics, Eatright.org [January 17, 2018]. Adapted and reprinted with permission.

weight maintenance. To maintain weight loss and to prevent weight regain in formerly obese adults, the IASO consensus statement (see Saris et al. 2003) recommends a minimum of 60 min, but preferably 80 to 90 min, of moderate-intensity (2.8-4.3 METs) physical activity and exercise (e.g., walking or cycling) per day. This intensity and duration of physical activity approximately equals 35 min of vigorous activity (6-10 METs or PAL = 1.9-2.5).

Table 9.5 summarizes physical activity recommendations for health benefits, healthy weight loss, and weight management. The exercise prescription for weight loss and weight management will differ depending on the client's goal. You can use the infor-

Table 9.5 Physical Activity and Exercise Recommendations for Health Benefits, Healthy Weight Loss, and Weight Management

Goal	Intensity	Duration	Frequency (days/wk)	Source
Health benefit	Moderate[a] Vigorous Moderate Vigorous	At least 30 min 20 min 150-300 min/wk 75-150 min/wk	5 minimum 3 minimum	ACSM and AHA USDHHS
Weight loss	Moderate	150-250 min/wk[c]		ACSM
Weight maintenance and prevention of weight gain	Moderate[a] (PAL ~1.7) to vigorous[b] (PAL ~1.9-2.5) Moderate	45-60 min 150-250 min/wk	5-7	IASO, IOM, and USDHHS ACSM
Prevention of weight regain	Moderate Moderate Vigorous Moderate	60-90 min At least 60 but preferably 80-90 min At least 35 min >250 min/wk	7 7 7	USDHHS IASO IASO ACSM

ACSM = American College of Sports Medicine; AHA = American Heart Association; IASO = International Association for the Study of Obesity; IOM = Institute of Medicine (United States); USDHHS = U.S. Department of Health and Human Services; PAL = physical activity level.

[a]Moderate intensity ≅ 2.8 to 4.3 METs; PAL ≅ 1.7.

[b]Vigorous intensity ≅ 6 to 10 METs; PAL ≅ 1.9 to 2.5.

[c]Accumulate a total duration of activity of 150 min/wk, progressing to 200 to 250 min/wk; total weekly exercise energy expenditure ≥ 2,000 kcal·wk⁻¹.

mation in table 9.5 to develop exercise prescriptions for weight loss, weight maintenance, and prevention of weight gain or regain.

Benefits of Exercise

The section highlights some common questions about the benefits of exercise in a weight loss program.

Why is physical activity an essential part of weight loss programs?

It is important that you present realistic expectations to your clients and let them know that exercise alone—without diet modification—results in only modest weight loss. Individual weight loss from exercise alone is highly variable, but when performed at recommended levels for general health benefits (i.e., 150 min/wk), losses often amount to only 2 kg or less in studies lasting 4 to 6 mo (Swift et al. 2014). With high-volume exercise (>500 kcal per session), substantial weight loss occurs (7%-8% of mass in 12-14 wk), but this volume of training is not sustainable or practical for many people (Swift et al. 2014). So why prescribe exercise for weight loss? Even without weight loss, exercise confers numerous health benefits (see chapter 1). For example, in a review of studies specific to children and adolescents, both diet only and diet plus exercise resulted in similar weight loss; however, the addition of exercise led to greater

improvements in HDL, fasting glucose, and fasting insulin levels (Ho et al. 2013). Furthermore, exercise improves body composition even in the absence of weight loss. Exercise maintains or slows down the loss of FFM that occurs with dieting only and is important for maintaining weight loss after dieting.

A recent study by Drenowatz and colleagues (2017) highlights the importance of physical activity for maintaining body weight over time. These researchers tracked 195 young adults who had no intention for weight change over a 2 yr period. Body composition and energy expenditure measurements were collected every 3 mo. After 2 yr, 57% of the participants had maintained their weight (<5% weight change), while 14% lost weight (–6.9 kg) and 29% gained weight (7.1 kg). The average total daily energy expenditure and total daily energy intake remained stable in all three groups. However, moderate to vigorous physical activity increased by about 35 min/day in the participants who lost weight and decreased by the same amount in the participants who gained weight. Further demonstrating the importance of exercise for maintaining a healthy body weight, Catenacci and colleagues (2011) used triaxial accelerometers to track the moderate to vigorous physical activity of successful weight loss maintainers and overweight participants. The weight loss maintainers engaged in about 290 min/wk of sustained physical activity compared with just 134 min/wk for the overweight group.

Several studies demonstrate that body composition (and consequently long-term health) improves by adding exercise to the weight loss program even if exercise does not substantially increase the amount of weight lost. Maintaining FFM is particularly important in older adults at risk for sarcopenia. Weinheimer, Sands, and Campbellnure (2010) reviewed weight loss studies of middle-aged and older adults. When diet alone was the strategy for weight loss, a substantial amount of the weight lost (≥15%) was in the form of FFM in 81% of the study groups. In contrast, when exercise was included only 39% of the study groups demonstrated substantial losses in FFM.

Pavlou and colleagues (1985) studied the contribution of exercise to the preservation of FFM in mildly obese males on a rapid weight loss diet. The exercise group dieted and participated in an 8 wk walking-jogging program, 3 days/wk. The nonexercising group dieted only. Although the total weight loss of the exercise group (−11.8 kg) and nonexercise group (−9.2 kg) was similar, the composition of the weight loss differed significantly. The exercise group maintained FFM (−0.6 kg), while the nonexercise group lost a significant amount of FFM (−3.3 kg). Also, the exercise group lost more fat (11.2 kg) than the nonexercise group (5.9 kg). In other words, for the nonexercising subjects, only 64% of the total weight loss was fat weight compared with 95% for the exercising subjects. The researchers concluded that the addition of aerobic exercise to the dietary regimen preserves existing FFM and increases fat utilization for energy production, and it is more effective in reducing fat stores than diet alone.

Similarly, Kraemer, Volek, and colleagues (1999) compared the effects of a weight loss dietary regimen with and without exercise in overweight men. The diet-only group did not exercise; the exercise groups participated in either an aerobic exercise program or a combined aerobic and resistance training exercise program, 3 days/wk for 12 wk. By the end of the program, all three groups lost a similar amount of body weight (~9-10 kg), but the composition of the weight loss differed significantly. For the diet-only group, only 69% of the total weight loss was fat weight compared with 78% for the diet plus aerobic exercise group and 97% for the diet and exercise (aerobic + resistance training) group. These results suggest that using a combination of aerobic and resistance training exercises in conjunction with dieting is more effective than dieting alone for preserving FFM and maximizing fat loss.

How does exercise promote fat loss and the preservation of lean body mass?

In response to aerobic and resistance training exercise, levels of growth hormone, epinephrine, and norepinephrine increase. These hormones stimulate the mobilization of fat from storage and activate the enzyme lipase, which breaks down triglycerides into free fatty acids. Free fatty acids are then metabolized, and they serve as an important energy source, especially during aerobic exercise. Heavy resistance training exercise also stimulates the release of anabolic hormones such as testosterone and growth hormone, resulting in increased protein synthesis, muscle growth, and FFM (Kraemer et al. 1991).

How does improved cardiorespiratory fitness help control body weight?

As an individual's cardiorespiratory fitness level increases through training, the amount of work the person can accomplish at a given submaximal heart rate increases. Thus, the more-fit individual expends calories faster than the less-fit individual at a given exercise heart rate. For example, at a heart rate of 150 bpm, the rate of energy expenditure is approximately 10 and 15 $kcal \cdot min^{-1}$ for fair and superior fitness levels, respectively.

During high-intensity aerobic exercise, lactate production increases and inhibits fatty acid metabolism. However, endurance training increases the lactate threshold (point at which lactate accumulates significantly in the blood). In aerobically trained individuals, the percentage of the energy derived from the oxidation of free fatty acids during submaximal exercise is greater than that derived from glucose oxidation (Coyle 1995; Mole, Oscai, and Holloszy 1971). The reduction in muscle glycogen utilization is also associated with a greater rate of oxidation of intramuscular triglyceride (Coyle 1995).

To expend the amount of energy recommended to prevent weight regain after weight loss, cardiorespiratory fitness ($\dot{V}O_2$max) needs to increase. Therefore, weight reduction programs should increase cardiorespiratory fitness so that participants are able to reach this physical activity goal within a reasonable amount of time (Saris et al. 2003).

What effect does exercise have on the REE?

Another reason for including exercise in the weight loss program is its positive effect on REE. Research indicates that exercise may counter the reduction in RMR that usually occurs as a result of dieting (Thompson, Manore, and Thomas 1996). It is well known that the rate of weight loss declines in the later stages of dieting because of a decrease in REE. The lowered REE is an energy-conserving metabolic adaptation to prolonged periods of caloric restriction (Donahue et al. 1984). In a study of 12 overweight females, Donahue and colleagues (1984) reported that diet alone caused a 4.4% reduction in the relative REE (REE / BW). After the addition of 8 wk of aerobic exercise to the program, the relative REE increased by 5%. The net effect of exercise was to offset the diet-induced metabolic adaptation and return the REE to the normal, prediet level.

Exercise may also facilitate weight loss by causing an increase in postexercise REE. Moderate- to high-intensity aerobic exercise increases the postexercise REE by 5% to 16%, and the elevated REE may persist for 12 to 39 hr postexercise (Bahr et al. 1987; Bielinski, Schultz, and Jequier 1985; Sjodin et al. 1996). The postexercise elevation in REE appears to be related to the exercise intensity and duration (Brehm 1988). Cycling at 70% $\dot{V}O_2$max for 20 min produced a 5% to 14% elevation in REE for 12 hr in young, healthy men (Bahr et al. 1987). Although it is tempting to apply these findings to clients who are elderly or obese, it is not known whether the postexercise metabolic response of these individuals is similar to that of young men.

Are wearable activity monitors helpful for losing weight?

Self-monitoring increases awareness of energy balance. Real-time continuous feedback might motivate some clients to make better dietary and physical activity choices. In a recent systematic review, Goode and colleagues (2017) concluded that wearable monitors such as accelerometers have a small positive effect on physical activity and weight loss. They noted that these effects are diminished when compared against other robust weight loss interventions rather than just inactive controls. Also, the duration of most of the studies reviewed was 24 wk or less, making it difficult to assess long-term effectiveness. They suggested that future studies investigate integrating wearables with other weight loss strategies. That is what Shuger and colleagues (2011) did. They placed 197 overweight or obese adults who were under the 150 min/wk recommendation of moderate to vigorous physical activity into one of four groups: self-directed weight loss, group-based behavioral weight loss program, wearing an activity monitor, or the group-based program plus the activity monitor. Those in the group-based program who were wearing the activity monitors lost the most weight at the end of the 9 mo intervention. All groups reduced waist circumference, but no group lost significantly more girth than others.

Recently, Jakicic and colleagues (2016) conducted a randomized controlled trial that spanned 2 yr with 471 adults. For the first 6 mo, both groups received a behavioral weight loss intervention (low-calorie diet, physical activity, and group counseling), after which participants were randomized into a standard intervention group that self-monitored diet and physical activity using a website and an enhanced intervention group that used a wearable tracker with web interface to monitor diet and activity. At the end of 24 mo, the standard intervention group actually lost more weight (–5.9 kg) than the group that used wearable technology (–3.5 kg). Both groups had similar improvements in body composition, fitness, physical activity, and diet. Taken together, these studies suggest that wearable technology might provide a modest improvement in physical activity and weight loss in the short term, but these devices do not seem to offer any benefit over traditional weight loss interventions over the long term.

Types of Exercise

This section addresses common concerns regarding the types of exercise suitable for weight loss programs.

Is aerobic exercise better than resistance exercise for weight loss?

Most weight loss programs recommend energy restriction (diet) and increased physical activity to create an energy deficit. Evidence suggests a dose-response relationship for weight loss; individuals performing the greatest amount of physical activity achieve greater weight loss. Aerobic exercise (e.g., walking) is effective for weight loss, fat loss, and long-term weight control (Gordon-Larsen et al. 2009; Nelson and Folta 2009).

Although resistance training increases muscle mass and REE, this mode of training does not produce a clinically significant weight loss (~3% of body weight) and does not increase weight loss when combined with calorie restriction. Resistance training, however, may increase the loss of fat mass when combined with aerobic exercise (American College of Sports Medicine 2009). Also, the combination of aerobic and resistance training has been shown to have a positive effect on preventing weight gain and on regaining harmful VAT following a diet-induced weight loss (Hunter et al. 2010).

Although aerobic exercise is more effective than resistance training for reducing body weight and fat mass, resistance training plays an important role in preserving FFM and increasing REE, especially for overweight older adults on a weight loss diet (Avila et al. 2010). Combining these two modes of training may be the most effective way to maximize fat loss while maintaining metabolically active FFM.

Is high-intensity exercise better than light- to moderate-intensity exercise for weight loss?

An important reason for including exercise as part of a weight loss program is to maximize energy expenditure, thereby creating a larger negative energy balance. Weight loss and loss of fat mass are positively related to weekly energy expenditure (Ross and Janssen 2001). When the same amount of energy is expended, total fat oxidation is higher during low-intensity exercise than during high-intensity exercise. Close examination of energy expenditure during selected physical activities (appendix E.3, Gross Energy Expenditure for Conditioning Exercises, Sports, and Recreational Activities) reveals that increases in speed (intensity) of exercise produce only small increases in the rate of energy expenditure (METs).

For example, if a 123 lb (56 kg) woman increases the speed of running from a slow speed (5.0 mph or 12 min·mi^{-1}) to a faster speed (7.0 mph or 8.5 min·mi^{-1}), the rate of expenditure increases only 3.2 kcal·min^{-1}. At the 8.5 min·mi^{-1} pace, the woman expends 11.5 METs (11.5 kcal·kg^{-1}·min^{-1} or 10.7 kcal·min^{-1}) and is able to run a maximum distance of 3 mi (4.8 km). The duration of the workout is 25.5 min (8.5 min·mi^{-1} × 3 mi), and the total caloric expenditure is 274 kcal (25.5 min × 10.7 kcal·min^{-1}). When she reduces the exercise intensity by decreasing her speed to a pace of 12 min·mi^{-1}, her relative energy expenditure decreases (8 METs or 8 kcal·kg^{-1}·min^{-1} or 7.5 kcal·min^{-1}), but she is able to run a distance of 4 mi (6.4 km). The duration of the workout increases to 48 min (12 min·mi^{-1} × 4 mi), and the total caloric expenditure is increased (48 min × 7.5 kcal·min^{-1} = 360 kcal). Thus, the duration of the exercise and total distance may be somewhat more important than the speed (intensity) of exercise for maximizing the energy expenditure.

In 2009, Nicklas and colleagues reported that vigorous aerobic exercise (70%-75% heart rate reserve [HRR]) and moderate-intensity aerobic exercise (45%-50% HRR), combined with caloric restriction, produced similar amounts of weight loss and abdominal fat loss in overweight and obese women. Given that most obese individuals prefer to exercise at a slower pace and at low to moderate intensity, it probably is not necessary to prescribe vigorous-intensity exercise as part of a weight loss program.

What aerobic exercise mode is best to maximize fat loss?

In a meta-analysis of 53 studies dealing with the effects of exercise on body weight and composition, Ballor and Keesey (1991) reported that fat loss for males participating in aerobic exercise training was, on average, 1.9 kg for cycling (0.11 kg·wk^{-1}) and 1.6 kg for running and walking (0.12 kg·wk^{-1}). For resistance training, body weight increased an average of 1.2 kg, but fat mass was reduced by 1.0 kg. For females, fat mass decreased significantly (1.3 kg) for running and walking but not cycling. These studies suggest that in terms of fat loss, aerobic exercise modes are equally effective for men, but running and walking may be better than cycling for women.

Are spot-reduction exercises effective for decreasing body fat in localized regions of the body?

Specific spot-reduction exercises are no more effective than general aerobic exercise for changing limb and body girth measurements or for altering total body composition (Carns et al. 1960; Noland and Kearney 1978; Roby 1962; Schade et al. 1962). Katch and colleagues (1984) assessed changes in the diameter of adipose cells from the abdomen and gluteal and subscapular sites resulting from a 27-day training program in which each subject performed 5,004 sit-ups. Although the training significantly reduced fat cell diameter, the effect was similar at all three sites: abdomen, −6.4%; gluteal, −5.0%; and subscapular, −3.7%. It appears that a sit-up exercise program does not preferentially reduce the fat in the abdominal region.

Despres and colleagues (1985) reported that a 20 wk cycling program significantly reduced %BF and body weight. Cycling affected trunk skinfolds (SKFs) (–22%) more than extremity SKFs (–12.5%). If fat was mobilized preferentially from subcutaneous stores near the exercising muscle mass, one would expect the lower extremity SKFs to be more affected by cycling than the trunk SKFs. Yet Despres and colleagues (1985) noted an 18% reduction in the suprailiac SKF and a 13% reduction in the thigh SKF. This suggests that SAT in the abdomen is more sensitive to the lipolytic effect of catecholamines than SAT in the thighs (Smith et al. 1979).

The enzyme lipoprotein-lipase is responsible for lipid accumulation. In women, lipoprotein-lipase activity is higher in the gluteofemoral region than in the abdominal region (Litchell and Boberg 1978). Estrogen and progesterone appear to enhance lipoprotein-lipase activity in women. Also, the lipolytic response to catecholamines is lower in the femoral than in the abdominal depots for both men and women (Rebuffe-Scrive 1985).

Thus, the regional distribution and mobilization of adipose tissue appear to follow a biologically selective pattern regardless of type of exercise. Even with weight reduction, the relative fat distribution remains stable as measured by the WHR; however, the waist-to-thigh ratio decreases, suggesting that the thigh region is slightly more resistant to fat mobilization in women (Ashwell et al. 1985).

In addition, upper body resistance training does not appear to preferentially reduce SAT in the upper arm. Kostek and colleagues (2007) reported that subcutaneous fat changes, measured by magnetic resonance imaging (MRI), in trained and untrained arms did not differ significantly following 12 wk of resistance training. These findings suggest that resistance training exercise does not result in spot reduction.

DESIGNING WEIGHT GAIN PROGRAMS

Because genetics plays an important role in weight gain, some clients may have difficulty gaining weight, especially if they have inherited a high RMR. Before prescribing weight gain programs, you should rule out the possibility that diseases and psychological disorders associated with malnutrition (e.g., anorexia nervosa) are not causing your client to be underweight. For athletes who are competing in weight classes, Macedonio and Dunford (2009) provide detailed information and suggestions for making weight.

The number of additional calories needed in order for a person to gain 1 lb (0.45 kg) of muscle tissue has not yet been firmly established. However, research suggests that an excess of 2,800 to 3,500 kcal is required. As with weight loss, the 3,500 kcal rule is theoretical. For a more accurate and individualized estimate of number of additional calories needed to gain a specific amount of weight over a certain time period, use the NIH's Body Weight Planner (see Designing Weight Loss Programs section). Adding 500 to 1,000 kcal·day^{-1} to the diet promotes weight gain; however, only 30% to 50% of the weight gain is muscle. Given that the remaining amount of the weight gain is fat, the International Society of Sports Nutrition does not recommend ingesting a high-calorie diet to build muscle mass (Kreider et al. 2010).

As with weight loss programs, the diet portion of the plan is just as important as the exercise portion for gaining weight. The emphasis should be on increasing lean mass rather than body fat. The International Society of Sports Nutrition recommends a daily protein intake of 1.4 to 2.0 g·kg^{-1} of body weight, in doses of 0.25 g·kg^{-1}, evenly distributed every 3 to 4 hr throughout the day for building muscle mass (Jäger et al. 2017). Again, it is highly recommended that you consult a trained nutrition professional when planning weight gain diets. When comparing your clients' typical nutrient intakes against recommended dietary intakes, you should focus on the same questions as outlined for weight loss programs (see the Exercise Prescription for Weight Loss section). Specifically,

- use the body composition method to estimate a healthy target weight and the amount of FFM to be gained;
- work closely with a nutrition professional to make sure your clients consume an adequate amount of high-quality protein;
- prescribe resistance training as outlined in the next section;
- track changes in FM and FFM throughout the weight gain program using the body composition assessment methods described in chapter 8.

Guidelines for Exercise Prescription for Weight Gain

- **Mode:** Resistance training
- **Intensity:** 70% to 75% 1-RM or 10-RM to 12-RM
- **Sets:** Three for novices; more than three for advanced weightlifters
- **Number of exercises:** One or two per muscle group for novices; three or four per muscle group for advanced weightlifters
- **Duration:** 60 min or longer
- **Frequency:** 3 days/wk for novices; 5 or 6 days/wk for advanced weightlifters
- **Length of program:** Dependent on desired weight gain
- **Rest:** 2 min between sets

EXERCISE PRESCRIPTION FOR WEIGHT GAIN

As part of the weight gain program, you should prescribe resistance training to increase muscle size. A high-volume resistance training program is the best approach for maximizing the development of muscle size. Because some clients may not be able to tolerate this volume of training at first, novice weightlifters should start slowly by performing only three sets of each exercise at the prescribed intensity and by reducing the number of exercises for each muscle group. Depending on the client's goal, this may be sufficient to increase FFM. For some clients, however, you may need to progressively increase the training volume in order to elicit further improvements in muscle size and FFM. See Guidelines for Exercise Prescription for Weight Gain for resistance training recommendations.

DESIGNING PROGRAMS TO IMPROVE BODY COMPOSITION

Some clients may wish to improve their body composition without changing their body weight. For these individuals, you can design exercise programs to decrease body fat, increase FFM, or both. Research has shown that regular participation in an exercise program may alter an individual's body composition. Aerobic exercise and resistance training are effective modes for decreasing SKF thicknesses, fat weight, and %BF of both women and men.

QUESTIONS ABOUT EXERCISE AND BODY COMPOSITION CHANGES

This section addresses commonly asked questions about what role exercise plays in altering body composition.

What is the effect of aerobic exercise training on body fat?

Numerous studies have been conducted to determine the effect of aerobic exercise training on body composition. The modes of exercise include cycling, walking, jogging, running, and swimming. Wilmore and colleagues (1970) reported that a 10 wk jogging program (3 days/wk) produced a significant increase in body density of sedentary men. Because total body weight decreased and FFM remained stable, the increase in body density was attributed almost entirely to fat loss. Pollock and colleagues (1971) also noted that a 20 wk walking program (4 days/wk) produced a decrease in %BF and total body weight of men.

In addition to total fat loss, aerobic exercise is critical for inducing loss of VAT. As mentioned previously, VAT is of greater importance than total fat with regard to adverse health effects. It was determined through meta-analysis that aerobic exercise is effective at reducing VAT, but resistance exercise is not (Ismail et al. 2012).

Which aerobic exercise mode is best for maximizing fat loss?

One study compared cycling, running, and walking of equal frequency, duration, and intensity (Pollock, Miller, et al. 1975). All three programs produced significant reductions in %BF and body weight. Also, Despres and colleagues (1985) reported that a 20 wk cycling program (4 or 5 days/wk) resulted in significant reductions in body weight, %BF, and fat cell weight in a group of sedentary men. In contrast, a major finding in a recent meta-analysis of high-intensity interval training (HIT) was that running was effective at reducing the fat mass of overweight and obese people but cycling was not (Wewege et al. 2017). The authors had no clear explanation for why the different exercise modalities produced different results, but they theorized that more muscle recruitment during running for a given submaximal workload could lead to greater energy expenditure. Nevertheless, the high impact of running might produce more injuries, and that should also be a consideration for your overweight and obese clients.

How many times a week should I exercise to maximize the loss of body fat?

The frequency of the training program may affect the magnitude of the changes in body composition. Pollock, Miller, and colleagues (1975) compared aerobic exercise programs consisting of 2, 3, or 4 days/wk. Even though the total mileage and caloric expenditure were the same, exercising 2 days/wk was not sufficient to produce significant alterations in body composition. The authors concluded that a program of 3 or 4 days/wk produces significant body composition changes, with 4 days/wk being superior to 3 days/wk.

Does the intensity of aerobic exercise affect body composition changes?

Irving and colleagues (2008) compared the effects of low-intensity (RPE ~10-11) and high-intensity (RPE ~12-15) exercise training on VAT and body composition of obese women with metabolic syndrome. Using computerized technology, they noted that high-intensity training produced significantly larger reductions in SAT and VAT in the abdomen compared with low-intensity training. Similarly, a large effect size (.7) was reported for decreased android fat mass in a group that performed cycle ergometry intervals (1:2 min ratio of 90% and 30%

$\dot{V}O_2$peak), but there was no effect for a group that maintained 50% $\dot{V}O_2$peak; training groups were matched for total energy expenditure (Wallman et al. 2009). Also, reductions in total fat, subcutaneous leg and trunk fat, and insulin resistance in young women were greater for a group that performed HIT 3 days/wk for 15 wk compared with the same frequency for a steady-state exercise group (Trapp et al. 2008). In a recent review and meta-analysis of this topic, Wewege and colleagues (2017) determined that both HIT and moderate-intensity continuous training are effective at reducing FM and waist circumference, but neither is more effective than the other. However, HIT requires about 40% less training time.

What effect does resistance training have on body fat and FFM?

Although resistance training may increase body weight, it positively affects fat mass, %BF, and FFM (Ballor and Keesey 1991). Cullinen and Caldwell (1998) found that normal-weight women (19-44 yr) participating in a moderate-intensity resistance training program (2 days/wk for 12 wk) significantly increased FFM (~4.5%) and decreased %BF (~8.7%). In Wilmore's study (1974), subjects trained 2 days/wk for 10 wk. At each training session, they performed two sets of 7-RM to 9-RM for eight different weight training exercises. Men and women exhibited similar alterations in body composition. Although the total body weight remained stable, the FFM increased significantly for both sexes. As a result of resistance training, the relative body fat decreased 9.6% and 10.0% for women and men, respectively. Velthuis and colleagues (2009) reported that a 12 mo program of moderate to vigorous exercise combining aerobic and resistance training did not produce significant changes in body weight of sedentary postmenopausal women. However, body composition was affected positively, with the exercise group showing significant improvements in FM, %BF, FFM, and waist circumference. The loss of lean mass can be attenuated during periods of energy deficit with resistance training and a high protein intake (1.8-3.0 g·kg^{-1}·day^{-1}) (Churchward-Venne et al. 2013).

Conventional thought is that resistance training improves FFM, but aerobic exercise is necessary for loss of FM. However, the results of several recent studies suggest that adding resistance training to aerobic exercise augments the FM loss. In a randomized intervention study, sedentary overweight and obese adults were placed into either an aerobic exercise group or a combined aerobic-resistance exercise group (Sanal, Ardic, and Kirac 2013). Not surprisingly, the FFM increase was greater in the combined exercise group than the aerobic-only exercise group after 12 wk. But adding resistance exercise to aerobic exercise also enhanced the reduction of FM in the legs for women. Drenowatz and colleagues (2015) tracked 348 young adults with BMIs between 20 and 35 kg/m² over a year. In addition to monitoring TEE with a wearable device, participants self-reported the type of activity they were doing and had their body composition measured every 3 mo. Similar to the results of Sanal, Ardic, and Kirac (2013), resistance training had a positive effect on both lean mass and FM, whereas aerobic exercise affected FM only. Furthermore, in the subset of overweight and obese participants, resistance exercise actually had a greater effect on FM than did aerobic exercise.

How does exercise promote body composition changes?

The significant loss of fat weight and %BF with aerobic exercise and resistance training is a function of hormonal responses to the exercise. Exercise increases the circulatory levels of growth hormone (GH), and the levels remain elevated for 1 to 2 hr after exercise (Hartley et al. 1972; Hartley 1975). Exercise also stimulates the release of catecholamines from the adrenal medulla. Both GH and catecholamines increase the mobilization of free fatty acids from storage (Hartley 1975). Eventually, the muscle may metabolize these free fatty acids during rest and low-intensity exercise.

The increase in FFM with resistance training may be due to muscle hypertrophy, increased protein content in the muscle, or increased bone density. Muscle hypertrophy and increased protein are mediated by changes in serum testosterone and GH levels in response to weightlifting. Immediately following heavy resistance weightlifting, serum testosterone levels are significantly elevated for men but not for women (Fahey et al. 1976; Weiss, Cureton, and Thompson 1983). Growth hormone levels in men are increased significantly for 15 min following a 21 min bout of high-intensity (85% of 1-RM) leg press exercises. However, low-intensity, high-repetition (28% of 1-RM, 21 reps per set) leg presses produced no significant change in GH even though the total

amount of work and duration of exercise were equal. Thus, the intensity and number of repetitions play a role in GH release in response to weightlifting exercise (Vanhelder, Radomski, and Goode 1984).

In addition, resistance training has an effect on the hormonal profiles of younger (30 yr) and older (62 yr) men (Kraemer, Häkkinen, et al. 1999). Following a 10 wk periodized strength-power training program, young men had significant increases in free testosterone at rest and in response to weightlifting exercise. Younger men also showed increases in resting levels of IGF (insulin-like growth factor) binding protein-3 after training. For the older men, training produced a significant increase in total testosterone in response to weightlifting exercise, as well as a significant reduction in resting cortisol levels.

Are exercise-induced changes in body composition influenced by genotype?

Raue and colleagues (2012) identified and compared gene sets responsible for eliciting a growth response to resistance training in young (24 yr) and old (84 yr) adults. They noted that age affects the genetic response of skeletal muscle to resistance exercise and that these genes are correlated with gains in muscle size and strength. These findings may explain, in part, interindividual variations in muscle hypertrophy and changes in FFM in response to resistance training.

Research has demonstrated that genotype and alleles are associated with risk of obesity. An **allele** is defined as one member of a pair or series of genes that occupy a specific position on a specific chromosome. Individuals with the obesity-associated genotype (FTO) and the risk allele (A/A) are 1.67 times more at risk for obesity than those without the A/A allele. Rankinen and colleagues (2010) reported that the FTO genotype is related to body fat responses to aerobic exercise training. Individuals with the obesity risk allele (A/A) were more resistant to changes in adiposity; the loss of FM and %BF was three times less than that of individuals with the C allele. This finding may represent one mechanism by which the FTO allele promotes overweight and obesity. Recently, Leonska-Duniec and colleagues (2017) confirmed the relationship between FTO and increased BMI. However, despite changes in BMI, BMR, FM, FFM, HDL, and glucose following a 12 wk training program, there was no interaction between the FTO gene with the risk allele and physical activity on any of these variables. Contrary to the research of Rankinen and colleagues (2010), this finding suggests that even in those with a genetic predisposition to obesity, physical activity is still effective at modifying body composition and obesity-related traits.

EXERCISE PRESCRIPTION FOR BODY COMPOSITION CHANGE

It is clear that both aerobic exercise and resistance training contribute to body composition change. Combining these two types of exercise may be the most effective way to alter body composition of nondieting individuals (Dolezal and Potteiger 1998). When designing exercise programs to promote changes in body composition, adhere to the guidelines for exercise prescription for fat loss and for fat-free mass gain. Prescribe aerobic exercise to reduce body fat and resistance training exercise to increase FFM. See Guidelines for Exercise Prescription for Fat Loss and Guidelines for Exercise Prescription for Fat-Free Mass Gain.

Guidelines for Exercise Prescription for Fat Loss

- **Goal:** Fat loss
- **Mode:** Type A and B aerobic activities (see Classification of Aerobic Exercise Modalities in chapter 5)
- **Intensity:** Moderate to high (RPE 10-15) or HIT
- **Duration:** 30 to 45 min
- **Frequency:** Minimum of 3 days/wk
- **Length:** Minimum of 8 wk

Guidelines for Exercise Prescription for Fat-Free Mass Gain

- **Goal:** Increase FFM and reduce body fat
- **Mode:** Dynamic resistance training
- **Intensity:** 70% to 85% 1-RM
- **Repetitions:** 6 to 12
- **Sets:** Three
- **Frequency:** Minimum of 3 days/wk
- **Length:** Minimum of 8 wk

Key Points

▶ Obesity is an excess of body fat that increases health risks.

▶ Two types of obesity are upper body (android) and lower body (gynoid) obesity.

▶ The number of fat cells in the body is determined primarily during childhood and adolescence; however, recent research suggests that adults can experience hyperplasia in certain areas of the body with overfeeding.

▶ Physical inactivity contributes to the cause of obesity.

▶ The body composition method provides a useful estimate of a healthy body weight.

▶ Fitness professionals should consult with nutrition professionals when designing weight loss and weight gain plans.

▶ Effective weight loss programs create a negative energy balance by restricting caloric intake and increasing physical activity and exercise; weight gain programs create a positive energy balance by increasing caloric intake.

▶ For weight loss programs, the combined daily caloric deficit due to calorie restriction and extra exercise should not exceed 1,000 kcal; for weight gain programs, the daily caloric intake should exceed the energy need by no more than 500 kcal.

▶ Adding a combination of aerobic and resistance training exercises to the dieting regimen is an effective way to maximize fat loss and preserve FFM during weight loss.

▶ The optimal amount of physical activity for preventing weight gain differs from that needed to create a negative energy balance for weight loss and for maintenance of weight loss.

▶ For weight gain programs, resistance training will ensure that most of the weight gain is due to increases in lean body tissues.

▶ Aerobic exercise and resistance training are effective ways to improve body composition without changing body weight.

Key Terms

Learn the definition for each of the following key terms. Definitions of terms can be found in the glossary.

allele

android obesity

anorexia nervosa

basal metabolic rate (BMR)

dietary thermogenesis

exercise activity thermogenesis (EAT)

factorial method

gynoid obesity

healthy body weight

hyperplasia

hypertrophy

kilocalorie (kcal)

lower body obesity

negative energy balance

non-exercise activity thermogenesis (NEAT)

obesity

overweight

physical activity level (PAL)

positive energy balance

resting energy expenditure (REE)

resting metabolic rate (RMR)

subcutaneous adipose tissue (SAT)

total energy expenditure (TEE)

total energy expenditure (TEE) method

underweight

upper body obesity

visceral adipose tissue (VAT)

Review Questions

In addition to being able to define each of the key terms, test your knowledge and understanding of the material by answering the following review questions.

1. Using BMI, what are the cutoff values for classification of obesity, overweight, healthy body weight, and underweight?

2. Describe how you can determine a healthy body weight for a client.

3. For typical weight loss programs, identify the minimal caloric intake per day and maximal caloric deficit (i.e., negative energy balance) per day. What is the best way to create this daily caloric deficit?

4. Explain why a taller, heavier person will lose weight at a faster rate than a shorter, lighter person when the two individuals are on the same diet.

5. Explain why exercise is an important component of weight loss and weight gain programs.

6. Describe two methods you can use to estimate the energy needs of your clients.

7. Describe the optimal amount of physical activity (intensity, duration, and frequency) for health benefits, weight loss, weight maintenance, and prevention of weight regain.

8. Estimate the daily caloric intake for a 50 yr old, 150 lb (68 kg) female professor who is 5 ft 5 in. and who bikes a total of 60 min, 5 days/wk, to and from the university.

9. Describe the basic exercise prescriptions for weight loss and weight gain programs.

CHAPTER 10

Assessing Flexibility

KEY QUESTIONS

▶ What is the difference between static and dynamic flexibility?

▶ What factors affect flexibility? How is flexibility assessed?

▶ Are indirect measures of flexibility valid and reliable?

▶ What are the general guidelines for flexibility testing?

▶ What test can I use to assess the flexibility of older adults?

▶ How can I test the lumbar stability of my clients?

Flexibility is an important, yet often neglected, component of health-related fitness. Adequate levels of flexibility are needed for maintenance of functional independence and performance of activities of daily living (ADLs) such as bending to pick up a newspaper or getting out of the backseat of a two-door car. Over the years, flexibility tests have been included in most health-related fitness test batteries, since it has been long thought that lack of flexibility is associated with musculoskeletal injuries and low back pain. However, compared with research on other physical fitness components, not many studies substantiate the importance of flexibility to health-related fitness.

Research suggests that individuals with too little flexibility (**ankylosis**) or too much (**hypermobility**) are at higher risk than others for musculoskeletal injuries (Jones and Knapik 1999), but there is limited evidence that a greater than normal amount of flexibility actually decreases injury risk (Knudson, Magnusson, and McHugh 2000). Also, research fails to support an association between lumbar or hamstring flexibility and the occurrence of low back pain (Jackson et al. 1998; Kuukkanen and Malkia 2000; Stutchfield and Coleman 2006). Still, flexibility should be included in health-related fitness test batteries to identify individuals at the extremes who may have a higher risk of musculotendinous injury.

This chapter describes direct and indirect methods for assessing flexibility. It presents guidelines for flexibility testing as well as norms for commonly used flexibility tests.

BASICS OF FLEXIBILITY

Flexibility and joint stability are highly dependent on the joint structure, as well as on the strength and number of ligaments and muscles spanning the joint. To fully appreciate the complexity of flexibility, you should review the anatomy of joints and muscles. This section deals with the definitions and nature of flexibility and also presents factors influencing joint mobility.

DEFINITIONS AND NATURE OF FLEXIBILITY

Flexibility is the ability of a joint, or series of joints, to move through a full **range of motion (ROM)** without injury. **Static flexibility** is a measure of the total ROM at the joint; it is limited by the extensibility of the musculotendinous unit. **Dynamic flexibility** is a measure of the rate of torque or resistance developed during stretching throughout the ROM. Although dynamic flexibility accounts for 44% to 66% of the variance in static flexibility (Magnusson et al. 1997; McHugh et al. 1998), more research is needed to firmly establish the relationship between static and dynamic flexibility and to determine whether these two types of flexibility are distinct entities or two aspects of the same flexibility component (Knudson et al. 2000).

The ROM is highly specific to the joint (i.e., specificity principle) and depends on morphological factors such as the joint geometry and the joint capsule, ligaments, tendons, and muscles spanning the joint. The joint structure determines the planes of motion and may limit the ROM at a given joint. **Triaxial joints** (e.g., ball-and-socket joints of the hip and shoulder) afford a greater degree of movement in more directions than **nonaxial, uniaxial,** or **biaxial joints** (see table 10.1).

The tightness of soft tissue structures such as muscle, tendons, and ligaments is a major limitation to both static and dynamic flexibility. Johns and Wright (1962) determined the relative contribution of soft tissues to the total resistance encountered by the joint during movement:

- Joint capsule—47%
- Muscle and its fascia—41%
- Tendons and ligaments—10%
- Skin—2%

The joint capsule and ligaments consist predominantly of collagen, a nonelastic connective tissue. The muscle and its fascia, however, have elastic connective tissue; therefore, they are the most important structures in terms of reducing resistance to movement and increasing dynamic flexibility.

The tension within the muscle-tendon unit affects both static flexibility (ROM) and dynamic flexibility (stiffness or resistance to movement). The tension within this unit is attributed to the **viscoelastic properties** of connective tissues, as well as to the degree of muscular contraction resulting from the stretch reflex (McHugh et al. 1992). Individuals with less flexibility and tighter muscles and tendons have a greater contractile response during stretching exercises and a greater resistance to stretching. The **elastic deformation** of the muscle-tendon unit during stretching is proportional to the load or tension applied, whereas the **viscous deformation** is proportional to the speed at which the tension is applied. When the muscle and tendon are stretched and held at a fixed length (e.g., during **static stretching**), the tension within the unit, or tensile stress, decreases over time (McHugh et al. 1992). This is called **stress relaxation**. A single static stretch sustained for 90 sec produces a 30% increase in viscoelastic stress relaxation and decreases muscle stiffness for up to 1 hr (Magnusson 1998).

Studies examining the viscoelastic effects of stretching have clearly demonstrated that increases in joint ROM are associated with decreases in passive resistance to stretch (McHugh and Cosgrave 2010). The immediate and prolonged effects of static stretching, however, depend on total duration of stretching. A stretch duration of 2 min or less has no prolonged effect on muscle stiffness; 50% of the effect of a 4 min stretch duration on passive resistance is lost in 10 min; 50% of the effect of an 8 min stretch is lost within 30 min (McHugh and Cosgrave 2010). Nakamura and associates (2011) reported that 5 min of static stretching decreased stiffness of the muscle and the muscle-tendon unit, and this effect lasted for at least 10 min following static stretching. Herda and colleagues (2011) noted that the type of static stretching affects muscle-tendon stiffness; constant-tension static stretching is more effective than constant-angle static stretching in decreasing muscle-tendon stiffness. Both forms of static stretching, however, produced similar improvements in ROM and similar decrements in strength.

Table 10.1 Joint Classification by Structure and Function

Type of joint	Axes of rotation	Movements	Examples
Gliding	Nonaxial	Gliding, sliding, twisting	Intercarpal, intertarsal, tarsometatarsal
Hinge	Uniaxial	Flexion, extension	Knee, elbow, ankle, interphalangeal
Pivot	Uniaxial	Medial and lateral rotation	Proximal radioulnar, atlantoaxial
Condyloid and saddle	Biaxial	Flexion, extension, abduction, adduction, circumduction	Wrist, atlanto-occipital, metacarpophalangeal, first carpometacarpal
Ball and socket	Triaxial	Flexion, extension, abduction, adduction, circumduction, rotation	Hip, shoulder

To date, a handful of studies have considered the acute effects of dynamic stretching on passive muscle stiffness (Chen et al. 2015; Herda et al. 2013; Mizuno and Umemura 2016; Samukawa et al. 2011). All found that ROM increased after dynamic stretching, but there is some debate as to how this increase in ROM occurs. Samukawa and colleagues (2011) reported that dynamic stretching lengthened the displacement of the musculotendinous junction. In contrast, Mizuno and Umemura (2016) reported no displacement of the musculotendinous junction with increased ankle ROM, and the passive mechanical properties (such as stiffness) of the musculotendinous unit remained unchanged. They theorized that the increased ROM that accompanies dynamic stretching might be due to enhanced stretch tolerance. However, Herda and colleagues (2013) reported a decrease in passive resistive torque and passive stiffness following 2 min of dynamic stretching of the knee flexors. Chen and associates (2015) also reported that muscle stiffness of the hamstrings decreased significantly more in a dynamic stretching group compared with static stretching and control groups in their sample of young men with limited passive straight leg elevation.

Additionally, Mahieu and associates (2007) reported that 6 wk static and ballistic stretching programs had different effects on passive resistive torque and tendon stiffness. Both forms of stretching increased ankle dorsiflexion ROM. Static stretching significantly reduced passive resistive torque of the calf muscles but had no effect on Achilles tendon stiffness, whereas ballistic stretching had the reverse effect—Achilles tendon stiffness decreased, but passive resistive torque of the plantar flexors was unchanged.

FACTORS AFFECTING FLEXIBILITY

Flexibility is related to body type, age, gender, and physical activity level. This section addresses some commonly asked questions about flexibility.

Does body type limit flexibility?

Individuals with large hypertrophied muscles or excessive amounts of subcutaneous fat may score poorly on ROM tests because adjacent body segments in these people contact each other sooner than in those with smaller limb and trunk girths. However, this does not necessarily mean that all heavily muscled or obese individuals have poor flexibility. Many bodybuilders and obese individuals who routinely stretch their muscles have adequate levels of flexibility.

Why do older individuals tend to be less flexible than younger people?

Inflexible and older individuals have increased muscle stiffness and a lower stretch tolerance compared with younger individuals with normal flexibility (Magnusson 1998). As muscle stiffness increases, static flexibility progressively decreases with aging (Brown and Miller 1998; Gajdosik, Vander Linden, and Williams 1999). A decline in physical activity and development of arthritic conditions, rather than a specific effect of aging, are the primary causes for the loss of flexibility as one grows older. Still, flexibility training can help counteract age-related decreases in ROM. Girouard and Hurley (1995) reported significant improvements in shoulder and hip ROM of older men (50-69 yr) following 10 wk of flexibility training. Thus, older persons can benefit from flexibility training and should be encouraged to perform stretching exercises at least two times a week to counteract age-related decreases in ROM (Garber et al. 2011; Tremblay et al. 2011).

Are females more flexible than males?

Some evidence suggests that females are generally more flexible than males at all ages (Alter 2004; Payne et al. 2000). The greater flexibility of women is usually attributed to gender differences in pelvic structure and hormones that may affect connective tissue laxity (Alter 2004). Allison and colleagues (2015) recently compared musculoskeletal, biomechanical, and physiological gender differences in United States military personnel. Female soldiers demonstrated significantly greater ROM for shoulder extension, abduction, and external rotation, as well as hip extension and knee flexion, than their male counterparts. It was also noted that the females had better hamstring flexibility and less posterior shoulder tightness than the males. There were no significant gender differences for shoulder flexion and internal rotation, hip flexion, torso rotation, and calf flexibility.

How do physical activity and inactivity affect flexibility?

Habitual movement patterns and physical activity levels apparently are more important determinants of flexibility than gender, age, and body type (Harris 1969; Kirby et al. 1981). Lack of physical activity is a major cause of inflexibility. It is well documented that inactive persons tend to be less flexible than active persons (McCue 1953) and that exercise increases flexibility (Chapman, deVries, and Swezey 1972; deVries 1962; Hartley-O'Brien 1980). Disuse, due to lack of physical activity or immobilization, produces shortening of the muscles (i.e., **contracture**) and connective tissues, which in turn restricts joint mobility.

Moving the joints and muscles in a repetitive pattern or maintaining habitual body postures may restrict ROM because of the tightening and shortening of the muscle tissue. For example, joggers and people who sit behind a desk for long periods need to stretch the hamstrings and low back muscles to counteract the tautness developed in these muscle groups.

Does warming up affect flexibility?

Although active warm-up exercises such as walking, jogging, and stair climbing increase muscle temperature and decrease muscle stiffness, warming up alone does not increase ROM (deWeijer, Gorniak, and Shamus 2003; Shrier and Gossal 2000). Female taekwondo athletes who underwent active and passive warm-up protocols did not increase ROM of the plantar flexors, but those in the static stretching group did (Nuri, Ghotbi, and Faghihzadeh 2013). The effect of combining stretching and active warm-up on passive resistance to stretch has not been studied extensively. Some studies, however, have shown that active warm-up combined with either static or dynamic stretching is more effective than stretching alone in increasing the length of the hamstring muscles (deWeijer, Gorniak, and Shamus 2003), in improving ROM (Murphy et al. 2010; Perrier, Pavol, and Hoffman 2011; Shrier and Gossal 2000), and in decreasing passive resistance (Magnusson et al. 2000). In fact, Murphy and associates (2010) reported that 5 min of running before and after static stretching resulted in greater increases in hip flexor ROM than did static stretching alone or 10 min of running prior to static stretching. The improvement in ROM lasted for 30 min.

Can you develop too much flexibility?

It is important to recognize that excessive amounts of stretching and flexibility training may result

in hypermobility, or an increased ROM of joints beyond normal, acceptable values. Hypermobility leads to **joint laxity** (looseness or instability) and may increase one's risk of musculoskeletal injuries. For example, it is not uncommon for gymnasts and swimmers to experience shoulder dislocations because of joint laxity and hypermobility. As an exercise specialist, you need to be able to accurately assess ROM and to design stretching programs that improve your clients' flexibility without compromising joint stability.

ASSESSMENT OF FLEXIBILITY

Field and clinical tests are available for assessing static flexibility. Although ROM data are important, measures of dynamic flexibility (i.e., joint stiffness and resistance to movement) may be more meaningful in terms of physical performance. Dynamic flexibility tests measure the increase in resistance during muscle elongation; several studies have shown that less stiff muscles use elastic energy more effectively during movements involving the stretch-shortening cycle (Kubo et al. 2000; Kubo, Kawakami, and Fukunaga 1999). However, dynamic flexibility testing is limited to the research setting because the equipment is expensive. Typically, static flexibility is assessed in field and clinical settings by direct or indirect measurement of the ROM.

DIRECT METHODS OF MEASURING STATIC FLEXIBILITY

To assess static flexibility directly, measure the amount of joint rotation in degrees using a goniometer, electrogoniometer, flexometer, or inclinometer. The following sections describe the procedures for these tests.

Universal Goniometer and Digital Goniometer Test Procedures

The universal **goniometer** is a protractor-like device with two steel or plastic arms that measure the joint angle at the extremes of the ROM (see figure 10.1). The stationary arm of the goniometer is attached at

General Guidelines for Flexibility Testing

To assess a client's flexibility, you should select a number of test items because of the highly specific nature of flexibility (Dickinson 1968; Harris 1969). Direct tests that measure the range of joint rotation in degrees are usually more useful than indirect tests that measure static flexibility in linear units. When administering these tests,

- have the client perform a general warm-up followed by static stretching prior to the test,

avoiding fast, jerky movements and stretching beyond the pain-free range of joint motion;

- administer three trials of each test item;
- compare the client's best score against norms in order to obtain a flexibility rating for each test item; and
- use the test results to identify joints and muscle groups in need of improvement.

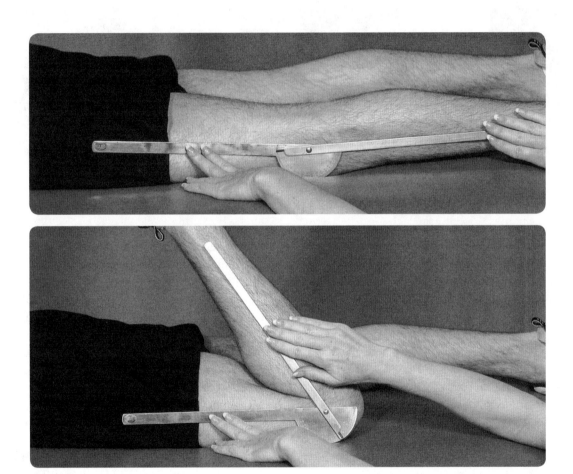

FIGURE 10.1 Measuring range of motion at the knee joint using a universal goniometer.

the zero line of the protractor, and the other arm is movable. To use the goniometer, place the center of the instrument so it coincides with the fulcrum, or axis of rotation, of the joint. Align the arms of the goniometer with bony landmarks along the longitudinal axis of each moving body segment. Measure the ROM as the difference between the joint angles

(degrees) at the extremes of the movement.

Inexpensive digital goniometers are now readily available (see figure 10.2). The testing procedure is identical to that of the universal goniometer, but the device provides a digital ROM value rather than requiring the practitioner to read the result from the protractor-like dial. No significant differences were

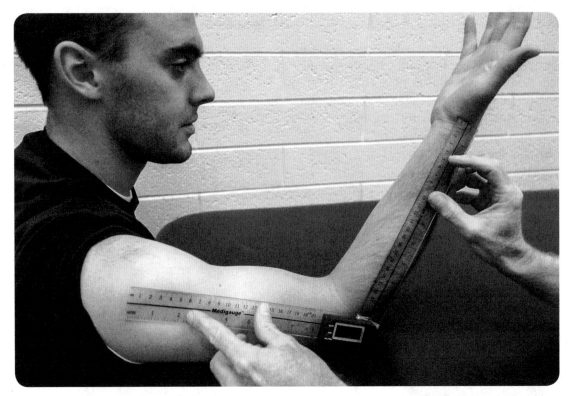

FIGURE 10.2 Measuring range of motion at the elbow joint using a digital goniometer.
Dale R. Wagner.

found between universal and digital goniometers when five therapists measured five joint motions on each of six patient models (Carey et al. 2010). They concluded that digital goniometers have acceptable criterion-related validity for measuring joint ROM, and the inter- and intrarater reliability is equivalent to the universal goniometer. Furthermore, the digital display might reduce reading errors.

Table 10.2 summarizes procedures for measuring ROM for various joints using a universal goniometer. The American College of Sports Medicine (ACSM; 2018) recommends using goniometers to obtain precise measurement of joint ROM. For more detailed descriptions of these procedures, see Greene and Heckman 1994 and Norkin and White 1995. Table 10.3 presents average ROM values for healthy adults.

Electrogoniometer Test Procedures

An **electrogoniometer** consists of one or two flexible potentiometers, or strain gauges, between two end-blocks. One block is placed on the stationary body segment while the other is designed for the movable segment. The blocks are affixed to the skin with double-sided tape. The center of the flexible cable housing the potentiometers should be placed over the center of the joint (see figure 10.3). Once in place, the client simply moves the limb, and the voltage output from the potentiometer varies depending on the joint angle. Electrogoniometers are available in different sizes to accommodate the size of the person and joint to be tested.

Electrogoniometers offer several advantages over universal goniometers and digital goniometers. First, they are flexible, not rigid like universal and digital devices. Second, they are much easier to use because the technician's hands are free. Third, with a two-channel electrogoniometer, measurements can be made in two planes simultaneously. For example, wrist flexion and extension can be measured at the same time as radial and ulnar deviation. Several researchers have evaluated electrogoniometers against motion analysis and have concluded that they provide a high degree of reliability and validity for measuring joint ROM (Bronner, Agraharasamakulam, and Ojofeitimi 2010; Urwin et al. 2013).

Table 10.2 Universal Goniometer Measurement Procedures

Video 10.1

Joint	Body position	Axis of rotation	Stationary arm	Moving arm	Stabilization	Special considerations
SHOULDER						
Extension	Prone	Acromion process	Midaxillary line	Lateral epicondyle of humerus	Scapula and thorax	Elbow is slightly flexed and palm of hand faces body.
Flexion	Supine	Same as extension	Same as extension	Same as extension	Scapula and thorax	Palm of hand faces body.
Abduction	Supine	Anterior axis of acromion process	Midline of anterior aspect of sternum	Medial midline of humerus	Scapula and thorax	Palm of hand faces anteriorly; humerus is laterally rotated; elbow is extended.
Medial/lateral rotation	Supine	Olecranon process	Perpendicular to floor	Styloid process of ulna	Distal end of humerus and scapula	Arm is abducted 90°; forearm is perpendicular to supporting surface in mid-pronated-supinated position; humerus rests on pad so that it is level with acromion process.
ELBOW						
Flexion	Supine	Lateral epicondyle of humerus	Lateral midline of humerus	Lateral midline of radial head and styloid process	Distal end of humerus	Arm is close to body; pad is placed under distal end of humerus; forearm is fully supinated.
FOREARM						
Pronation	Sitting	Lateral to ulna styloid process	Parallel to anterior midline of humerus	Lies across dorsal aspect of forearm, just proximal to styloid processes of radius and ulna	Distal end of humerus	Arm is close to body, elbow flexed 90°; forearm is midway between supination and pronation (thumb toward ceiling).
Supination	Sitting	Medial to ulna styloid process	Parallel to anterior midline of humerus	Lies across ventral aspect of forearm, just proximal to styloid processes of radius and ulna	Distal end of humerus	Testing position is same as for pronation of forearm.
WRIST						
Flexion and extension	Sitting	Lateral aspect of wrist over the triquetrum	Lateral midline of ulna, using olecranon and ulnar styloid processes for reference	Lateral midline of fifth metacarpal	Radius and ulna	Client sits next to supporting surface, abducts shoulder 90°, and flexes elbow 90°; forearm is in mid-supinated-pronated position; palm of hand faces ground; forearm rests on supporting surface; hand is free to move.
Radial or ulnar deviation	Sitting	Middle of dorsal aspect of wrist over capitate	Dorsal midline of forearm, using lateral humeral epicondyle for reference	Dorsal midline of third metacarpal	Distal ends of radius and ulna	Same as for wrist flexion.

(continued)

315

Table 10.2 (continued)

Joint	Body position	Axis of rotation	Stationary arm	Moving arm	Stabilization	Special considerations
HIP						
Flexion and extension	Supine; prone	Lateral aspect of hip joint, using greater trochanter for reference	Lateral midline of pelvis	Lateral midline of femur, using lateral epicondyle for reference	Pelvis	Knee is allowed to flex as range of hip flexion is completed; knee is flexed during hip extension.
Abduction and adduction	Supine	Centered over anterior superior iliac spine	Horizontally align arm with imaginary line between anterior superior iliac spines	Anterior midline of femur, using midline of patella for reference	Pelvis	Knee is extended during abduction.
Medial/lateral rotation	Sitting	Centered over anterior aspect of patella	Perpendicular to floor	Anterior midline of lower leg, using crest of tibia and point midway between malleoli for reference	Distal end of femur; avoid rotation and lateral tilt of pelvis	Client sits on supporting surface, knees flexed 90°; place towel roll under distal end of femur; contralateral knee may need to be flexed so that hip being measured can complete full range of lateral rotation.
KNEE						
Flexion	Supine	Over the lateral epicondyle of femur	Lateral midline of femur, using greater trochanter for reference	Lateral midline of fibula, using lateral malleolus and fibular head for reference	Femur to prevent rotation, abduction, and adduction	As knee flexes, the hip also flexes.
ANKLE						
Dorsiflexion and plantar flexion	Sitting	Over the lateral aspect of lateral malleolus	Lateral midline of fibula, using head of fibula for reference	Parallel to lateral aspect of fifth metatarsal	Tibia and fibula	Client sits on end of table with knee flexed and ankle positioned at 90°.
SUBTALAR						
Inversion and eversion	Sitting	Centered over anterior aspect of ankle midway between malleoli	Anterior midline of lower leg, using the tibial tuberosity for reference	Anterior midline of second metatarsal	Tibia and fibula	Client sits with knee flexed 90° and lower leg over edge of supporting surface.
LUMBAR SPINE						
Lateral flexion	Standing	Centered over posterior aspect of spinous process of S1	Perpendicular to the ground	Posterior aspect of spinous process of C7	Pelvis to prevent lateral tilt	Client stands erect with 0° of spinal flexion, extension, and rotation.
Rotation	Sitting	Centered over superior aspect of client's head	Parallel to imaginary line between tubercles of iliac crests	Imaginary line between two acromion processes	Pelvis to prevent rotation	Client keeps feet flat on floor to stabilize pelvis.

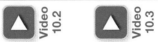

Video 10.2

Video 10.3

Table 10.3 Average Range of Motion (ROM) Values for Healthy Adults

Joint	ROM (degrees)	Joint	ROM (degrees)
SHOULDER		**THORACIC-LUMBAR SPINE**	
Flexion	150-180	Flexion	60-80
Extension	50-60	Extension	20-30
Abduction	180	Abduction	25-35
Medial rotation	70-90	Rotation	30-45
Lateral rotation	90	**HIP**	
ELBOW		Flexion	100-120
Flexion	140-150	Extension	30
Extension	0	Abduction	40-45
RADIOULNAR		Adduction	20-30
Pronation	80	Medial rotation	40-45
Supination	80	Lateral rotation	45-50
WRIST		**KNEE**	
Flexion	60-80	Flexion	135-150
Extension	60-80	Extension	0-10
Radial deviation	20	**ANKLE**	
Ulnar deviation	30	Dorsiflexion	20
CERVICAL SPINE		Plantar flexion	40-45
Flexion	45-60	**SUBTALAR**	
Extension	45-75	Inversion	30-35
Lateral flexion	45	Eversion	15-20
Rotation	60-80		

Data from Greene and Heckman 1994; American Medical Association 1988.

Researchers are experimenting with wearable goniometers so that joint angles can be measured in real time while clients are performing daily tasks. Tognetti and colleagues (2014, 2015) described a textile-based goniometer with an electrically insulated layer sandwiched between two layers of knitted piezoresistive fabrics. The resistance difference between the two layers is measured. When the sensor is flat, the resistance difference is zero, but when the sensor is flexed the resistance difference is proportional to the angle it is being bent. Output from the textile goniometer and a triaxial accelerometer are fused to provide ambulatory ROM data (Tognetti et al. 2015).

Flexometer Test Procedures

Another tool you can use to measure ROM is the Leighton **flexometer** (see figure 10.4). This device consists of a weighted 360° dial and weighted pointer. The ROM is measured in relation to the downward pull of gravity on the dial and pointer. To use this device, strap the instrument to the body segment, and lock the dial at 0° at one extreme of the ROM. After the client executes the movement, lock the pointer at the other extreme of the ROM. The degree of arc through which the movement takes place is read directly from the dial. Tests have been devised to measure the ROM at the neck, trunk, shoulder, elbow, radioulnar, wrist, hip, knee, and ankle joints using the Leighton flexometer (Hubley-Kozey 1991; Leighton 1955).

Inclinometer Test Procedures

The **inclinometer** is another type of gravity-dependent goniometer (see figure 10.5). To use this device,

Video
10.4

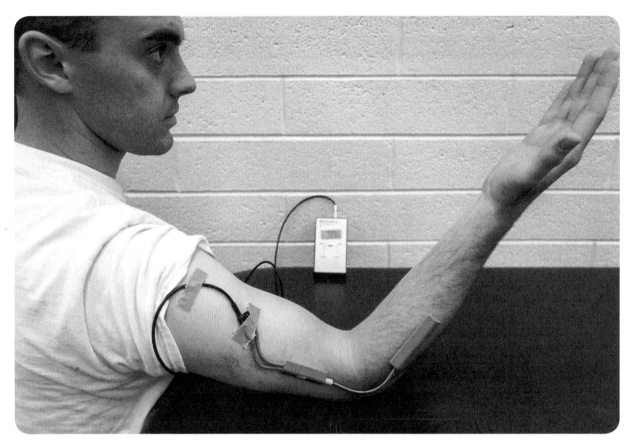

FIGURE 10.3 Measuring range of motion at the elbow joint using an electrogoniometer.
Dale R. Wagner.

hold it on the distal end of the body segment. The inclinometer measures the angle between the long axis of the moving segment and the line of gravity. This device is easier to use than the flexometer and universal goniometer because it is held by hand on the moving body segment during the measurement and does not have to be aligned with specific bony landmarks. The American Medical Association (1988) recommends the double-inclinometer technique, using two inclinometers, to measure spinal mobility (see figure 10.5).

As is the case with goniometers, digital inclinometers are now commonly available and might reduce reading error.

Validity and Reliability of Direct Measures

The validity and reliability of these devices for directly measuring ROM are highly dependent on the joint being measured and technician skill. Radiography is considered to be the best reference method for establishing validity of goniometric measurements. Research shows high agreement between ROM measured by radiographs and universal goniometers for the hip and knee joints (Ahlback and Lindahl 1964; Enwemeka 1986). Mayer, Tencer, and Kristoferson (1984) reported no difference between radiography and the double-inclinometer technique for assessing spinal ROM of patients with low back pain.

The intratester and intertester reliabilities of goniometric measurements are affected by difficulty in identifying the axis of rotation and palpating bony landmarks. Measurements of upper extremity joints are generally more reliable than ROM measurements of the lower extremity joints (Norkin and White 1995). Generally, the inclinometer reliably measures ROM at most joints; however, the intertester reliability of inclinometer measurements is variable and joint specific. Studies have reported reliability coefficients ranging from .48 for lumbar extension (Williams, Binkley, et al. 1993) to .96 for subtalar joint position (Sell et al. 1994). Also, the intrarater reliabilities for inclinometer measurements of the flexibility of the

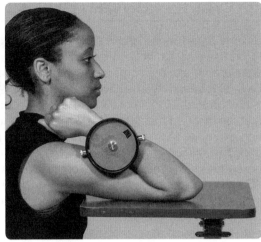
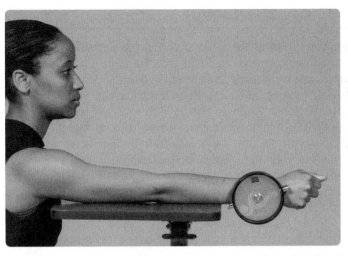

FIGURE 10.4 Measuring range of motion at the elbow joint using a Leighton flexometer.

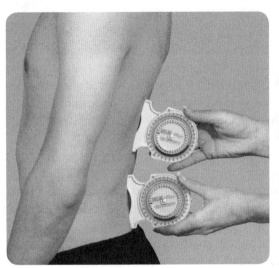
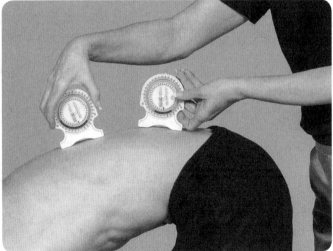

FIGURE 10.5 Measuring lumbosacral flexion using the double-inclinometer technique.

iliotibial band (hip adduction) and for ROM measurements of the lumbar spine and lordosis generally exceed .90 (Ng et al. 2001; Reese and Bandy 2003). To obtain accurate and reliable ROM measurements, you need a thorough knowledge of anatomy and of standardized testing procedures, as well as training and practice to develop your measurement techniques.

INDIRECT METHODS OF MEASURING STATIC FLEXIBILITY

Because of the belief that lack of flexibility is associated with low back pain and musculoskeletal injuries, most health-related fitness test batteries include a sit-and-reach test to evaluate the static flexibility of the lower back and hamstring muscles (Payne et al. 2000). The sit-and-reach test provides an indirect linear measurement of the ROM. Several sit-and-reach protocols have been developed using either a yardstick (meter stick) or a box, or both, to measure flexibility in inches or centimeters.

Although some fitness professionals assume the sit-and-reach is a valid measure of low back and hamstring flexibility, research has shown these tests to be moderately related to hamstring flexibility (r = .39-.89) but poorly related to low back flexibility (r = .10-.59) in children (Patterson at al. 1996), adults (Hui et al. 1999; Hui and Yuen 2000; Jackson and Langford 1989; Martin et al. 1998; Minkler and

SMARTPHONE AS AN INCLINOMETER

Several smartphone applications (apps) are available, free or for a nominal charge, allowing the phone to be used as an inclinometer. Many of the apps used to measure ROM use the smartphone's built-in accelerometers, but some also use magnetometers and others are photographic based (Milani et al. 2014). Several research teams have investigated the reliability and validity of these apps, with promising results (Charlton et al. 2015; Vohralik et al. 2015; Wellmon et al. 2016). Wellmon and colleagues (2016) demonstrated that the inherent measurement error (independent of client factors) due to the smartphone, installed apps, and examiner skill is <2° of measurement variability. Vohralik and associates (2015) compared an app to a digital inclinometer and found it to be a reliable and valid measure of ankle dorsiflexion. Charlton and colleagues (2015) created a custom app and evaluated it against a bubble inclinometer and a nine-camera 3D motion analysis system. The reliability and validity of the smartphone app was comparable to the bubble inclinometer, and the validity compared to the motion analysis was excellent (*ICCs* >.88) for six of seven hip movements. The consensus is that bubble and digital inclinometers are preferable if available, but if not, smartphone apps provide a reliable and valid method of assessing ROM. Search for "goniometer" or "inclinometer" on iTunes or Google Play for an app that meets your needs.

Patterson 1994), and older adults (Jones et al. 1998). Moreover, in a prospective study of adults, Jackson and colleagues (1998) reported that the sit-and-reach test has poor criterion-related validity and is unrelated to self-reported low back pain. Likewise, Grenier, Russell, and McGill (2003) noted that sit-and-reach test scores do not relate to a history of low back pain or discomfort in industrial workers. Although sit-and-reach scores were moderately related (*r* = .42) to lumbar ROM in the sagittal plane, the sit-and-reach test could not distinguish between workers who had low back discomfort and workers who did not. The researchers concluded that standard fitness test batteries should include measures of lumbar ROM instead of the sit-and-reach test to assess low back fitness. Lumbar ROM in the sagittal plane can be measured directly with an inclinometer (double-inclinometer technique, see figure 10.5) or indirectly with the skin distraction test. (See the Skin Distraction Test section later in this chapter.)

Although research affirms that the sit-and-reach test does not validly measure low back flexibility, it may still be used to provide an indirect measure of hamstring length. Davis and colleagues (2008) reported that sit-and-reach scores were moderately related to other measures of hamstring length such as sacral angle (*r* = .65), knee extension angle (*r* = .57), and straight leg raise (*r* = .65). However, in a study of 141 young male athletes, Muyor and colleagues (2014) found that the sit-and-reach test had only low to moderate validity as a measure of hamstring flexibility. In fact, pelvic tilt and lumbar flexibility

explained the greatest amount of variability in sit-and-reach scores, and hamstring extensibility had very little influence. Sit-and-reach tests should be limited to identifying individuals at the extremes who may have a higher risk of muscle injury because of hypermobility or lack of flexibility in the hamstring muscles.

The following sections describe the protocols for various types of sit-and-reach tests as well as the skin distraction test. Before clients take any of these tests, have them perform a general warm-up to increase muscle temperature, as well as stretching exercises for the muscle groups to be tested. When monitoring your clients' progress using these tests, be certain to record and to standardize the time of testing. Time of day may affect modified sit-and-reach test performance, with higher scores achieved later in the day (Guariglia et al. 2011). Unless otherwise stated, have your clients remove their shoes for all sit-and-reach test protocols.

Standard Sit-and-Reach Test

The ACSM (2018) and the Canadian Society for Exercise Physiology (2013) recommend using the standard sit-and-reach test to assess hip and hamstring flexibility. This test uses a sit-and-reach box with a zero point at 26 cm. Have clients sit on the floor with their knees extended and the soles of their feet against the edge of the box. The inner edges of the soles of the feet must be 6 in. (15.2 cm) apart. Instruct clients to keep their knees fully extended, arms evenly stretched, and hands parallel with the

Table 10.4 Age-Gender Norms for Standard Sit-and-Reach Test

	AGE (YR)					
	15-19 yr	**20-29 yr**	**30-39 yr**	**40-49 yr**	**50-59 yr**	**60-69 yr**
MEN						
Excellent	≥39	≥40	≥38	≥35	≥35	≥33
Very good	34-38	34-39	33-37	29-34	28-34	25-32
Good	29-33	30-33	28-32	24-28	24-27	20-24
Fair	24-28	25-29	23-27	18-23	16-23	15-19
Needs improvement	≤23	≥24	≥22	≥17	≥15	≥14
WOMEN						
Excellent	≥43	≥41	≥41	≥38	≥39	≥35
Very good	38-42	37-40	36-40	34-37	33-38	31-34
Good	34-37	33-36	32-35	30-33	30-32	27-30
Fair	29-33	28-32	27-31	25-29	25-29	23-26
Needs improvement	≥28	≥27	≥26	≥24	≥24	≥22

Note: Distance is measured in centimeters using a sit-and-reach box with the zero point at 26 cm. If using a box with the zero point at 23 cm, subtract 3 cm from each value in this table.

Source: Canadian Physical Activity Training for Health (CSEP-PATH®). 2013. Used with permission of the Canadian Society for Exercise Physiology.

palms down (fingertips may overlap) as they slowly reach forward as far as possible along the top of the box. Have clients hold this position for ~2 sec. Advise your clients that lowering the head maximizes the distance reached. The client's score is the most distant point along the top of the box that the fingertips contact. If the client's knees are flexed or motion is jerky or bouncing, do not count the score. Administer two trials and record the maximum score to the nearest 0.5 cm. Table 10.4 presents age-gender norms for this test.

V Sit-and-Reach Test

The V sit-and-reach, also known as the YMCA sit-and-reach test, uses a yardstick instead of a box. Secure the yardstick to the floor by placing tape (12 in. long) at a right angle to the 15 in. (38 cm) mark on the yardstick. The client sits, straddling the yardstick, with the knees extended (but not locked) and feet spread 12 in. (30.5 cm) apart. The heels of the feet touch the tape at the 15 in. mark. Instruct the client to reach forward slowly and as far as possible along the yardstick while keeping the two hands parallel (fingertips may overlap) and to hold this position momentarily (~2 sec). Make certain the knees do not flex and that the client does not lead

with one hand. The score (in centimeters or inches) is the most distant point on the yardstick contacted by the fingertips. Table 10.5 presents percentile ranks for the V sit-and-reach test.

Modified Sit-and-Reach Test

Video 10.5

To account for a potential bias due to limb-length differences (i.e., individuals who have short legs relative to the trunk and arms may have an advantage when performing the standard sit-and-reach test), Hoeger (1989) developed a modified sit-and-reach test that takes into account the distance between the end of the fingers and the sit-and-reach box and uses the finger-to-box distance as the relative zero point. This test uses a 12 in. (30.5 cm) sit-and-reach box (see figure 10.6). The client sits on the floor with buttocks, shoulders, and head in contact with the wall; extends the knees; and places the soles of the feet against the box. A yardstick is placed on top of the box with the zero end toward the client. Keeping the head and shoulders in contact with the wall, the client reaches forward with one hand on top of the other, and the yardstick is positioned so that it touches the fingertips. This procedure establishes the relative zero point for each client. As you firmly hold the yardstick in place, the client reaches

Table 10.5 Percentile Ranks for the V Sit-and-Reach Test

	AGE (YR)											
	18-25 yr		26-35 yr		36-45 yr		46-55 yr		56-65 yr		>65 yr	
PERCENTILE RANK	**M**	**F**	**M**	**F**	**M**	**F**	**M**	**F**	**M**	**F**	**M**	**F**
90	22	24	21	23	21	22	19	21	17	20	17	20
80	20	22	19	21	19	21	17	20	15	19	15	18
70	19	21	17	20	17	19	15	18	13	17	13	17
60	18	20	17	20	16	18	14	17	13	16	12	17
50	17	19	15	19	15	17	13	16	11	15	10	15
40	15	18	14	17	13	16	11	14	9	14	9	14
30	14	17	13	16	13	15	10	14	9	13	8	13
20	13	16	11	15	11	14	9	12	7	11	7	11
10	11	14	9	13	7	12	6	10	5	9	4	9

F = females; M = males.

Note: Score is measured in inches. To convert inches to centimeters, multiply value in table by 2.54.

Data from YMCA of the USA 2000.

forward slowly, sliding the fingers along the top of the yardstick. The score (in inches) is the most distant point on the yardstick contacted by the fingertips. Table 10.6 provides age-gender percentile norms for the modified sit-and-reach test.

Research comparing the standard and modified sit-and-reach test scores indicated that individuals with proportionally longer arms than legs (lower finger-to-box distance) had significantly better scores on the standard sit-and-reach test than those with moderate or high finger-to-box distances; in contrast, the modified sit-and-reach test scores did not differ significantly among the three groups (Hoeger et al. 1990; Hoeger and Hopkins 1992). Similar to the traditional sit-and-reach test, the modified sit-and-reach test was only moderately related to criterion measures of hamstring flexibility and poorly related to low back flexibility (Hui et al. 1999; Minkler and Patterson 1994). Consequently, it appears that the validity of the modified sit-and-reach test is no better than that of the standard sit-and-reach test for assessing flexibility of the low back and hamstring muscle groups.

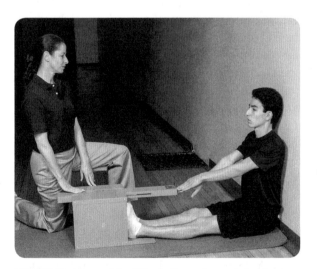 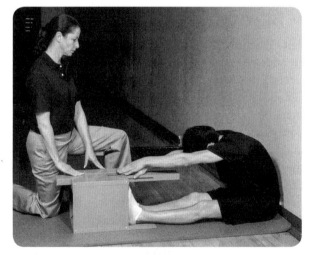

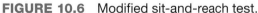

FIGURE 10.6 Modified sit-and-reach test.

Table 10.6 Percentile Ranks for the Modified Sit-and-Reach Test

Percentile rank	WOMEN			MEN		
	≤35 yr	36-49 yr	≥50 yr	≤35 yr	36-49 yr	≥50 yr
≥90: Well above average	≥17.9	≥17.4	≥15.0	≥17.2	≥16.1	≥15.0
70-89: Above average	16.2-17.8	15.2-17.3	13.6-14.9	15.8-17.1	13.9-16.0	12.3-14.9
30-69: Average	13.7-16.1	12.2-15.1	9.2-13.5	13.0-15.7	10.8-13.8	9.3-12.2
10-29: Below average	10.1-13.6	9.7-12.1	7.5-9.1	9.2-12.9	8.3-10.7	7.8-9.2
<10: Well below average	≤10.0	≤9.6	≤7.4	≤9.1	≤8.2	≤7.7

Note: Score is measured to the nearest 0.25 in. (0.6 cm). To convert inches to centimeters, multiply value in table by 2.54.

Adapted from W.W.K. Hoeger and S.A. Hoeger, *Lifetime Physical Fitness & Wellness: A Personalized Program,* 13th ed. (Stamford, CT: Cengage, 2015), 28, and W.C. Beam and G.A. Adams, *Exercise Physiology Laboratory Manual,* 6th ed. (New York: McGraw Hill, 2011), 249.

Back-Saver Sit-and-Reach Test

The standard, modified, and V sit-and-reach tests require the client to stretch the hamstring muscles of both legs simultaneously, causing some discomfort when the anterior portions of the vertebrae are compressed during the stretch. The back-saver sit-and-reach test was devised to relieve some of this discomfort by measuring the flexibility of the hamstring muscles one leg at a time. Instruct the client to place the sole of the foot of the extended (tested) leg against the edge of the sit-and-reach box and to

flex the untested leg, placing the sole of that foot flat on the floor 2 to 3 in. (5-8 cm) to the side of the extended (tested) knee (see figure 10.7). Then follow the instructions for the standard sit-and-reach test to determine the client's flexibility score for each leg.

Research suggests that the validity of this test (r = .39-.71) is similar to that of the standard sit-and-reach test (r = .46-.74) for assessing hamstring flexibility of men and women (Hui and Yuen 2000; Jones et al. 1998). Chillon and colleagues (2010) noted, however, that hip angle explained 42% of the variance in back-saver sit-and-reach test scores of adolescents. Lumbar angle and thoracic angle

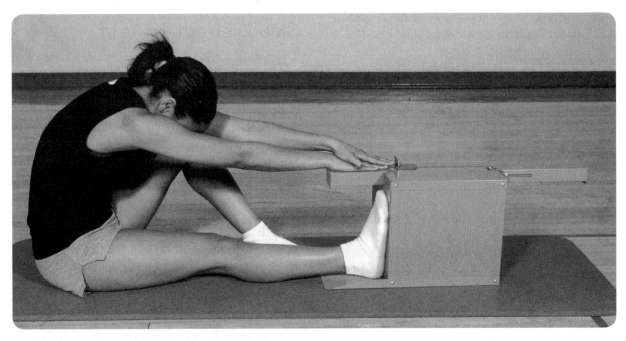

FIGURE 10.7 Back-saver sit-and-reach test.

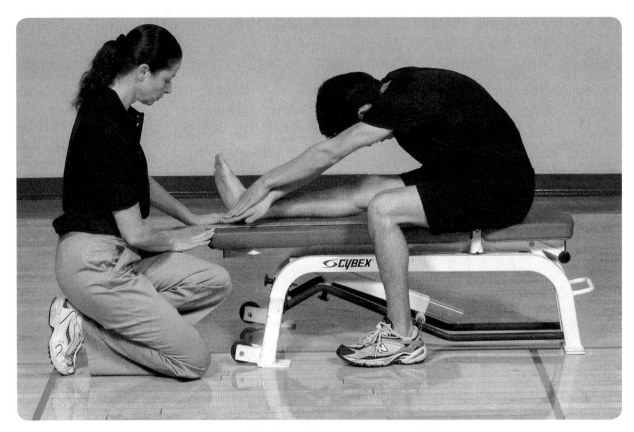

FIGURE 10.8 Modified back-saver sit-and-reach test.

explained an additional 30% and 4% of the variance, respectively. These findings suggest that, in adolescents, the back-saver sit-and-reach test may provide a valid measure of hip and low back flexibility. Norms for this test are available elsewhere (see Cooper Institute for Aerobics Research 1992).

Modified Back-Saver Sit-and-Reach Test

Video 10.6

While performing the back-saver sit-and-reach test, some participants may complain about the uncomfortable position of the untested leg. Hui and Yuen (2000), therefore, modified this test by having the client perform a single-leg sit-and-reach on a 12 in. (30.5 cm) bench (see figure 10.8). Instruct the client to place the untested leg on the floor with the knee flexed at a 90° angle. Align the sole of the foot of the tested leg with the 50 cm mark on the meter rule. Then follow the instructions for the standard sit-and-reach test to determine the client's hamstring flexibility for each leg. Hui and Yuen (2000) reported that the validity of this test ($r = .50$-.67) for assessing hamstring flexibility was similar to that of the standard ($r = .46$-.53) and V

($r = .44$-.63) sit-and-reach tests. The modified back-saver test, however, was rated as the most comfortable compared with the other test protocols. Norms for this test have not yet been established.

Skin Distraction Test

The modified Schober test (MacRae and Wright 1969) and the simplified skin distraction test (Van Adrichem and van der Korst 1973) are useful in assessing low back flexibility. These field tests are reliable and have good agreement with radiographic measurements of spinal flexion and extension (Williams, Binkley, et al. 1993). For the simplified skin distraction test, place a 0 cm mark on the midline of the lumbar spine at the intersection of a horizontal line connecting the left and right posterior superior iliac spines while the client is standing erect. Place a second mark 15 cm (5.9 in.) superior to the 0 cm mark (see figure 10.9). As the client flexes the lumbar spine, these marks move away from each other; use an anthropometric tape measure to measure the new distance between the two marks. The lumbar flexion score is the difference between this measurement and the initial length between the skin markings (15 cm). In a group of 15

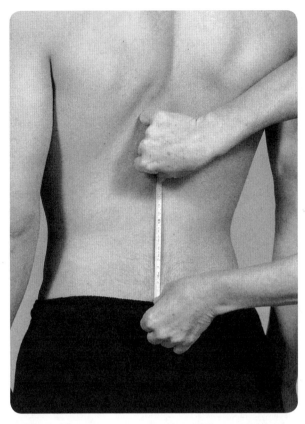 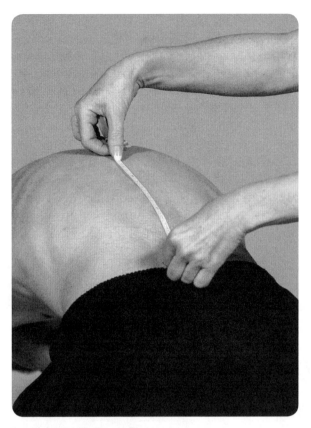

FIGURE 10.9 Measuring lumbosacral flexion using the simplified skin distraction test.

to 18 yr old subjects, the simplified skin distraction scores averaged 6.7 ± 1.0 cm in males and 5.8 ± 0.9 cm in females. However, normal values for other age groups are not yet available. You can also use this technique to measure lumbar spinal extension (simplified skin attraction test) by having the client extend backward and measuring the difference between the initial length and the new distance between the superior and inferior skin markings.

LUMBAR STABILITY TESTS

Lumbar instability increases the risk of developing low back pain. The primary muscle groups responsible for stabilizing the lumbar spine are the trunk extensors (erector spinae), trunk flexors (rectus abdominis and abdominal oblique muscles), and lateral flexors (quadratus lumborum). Research indicates that muscle endurance is more protective than muscle strength for reducing low back injury (McGill 2001). To evaluate the balance in the isometric endurance capabilities of these muscle groups in healthy individuals, McGill, Childs, and Liebenson (1999) used three tests: trunk extension,

trunk flexion, and side bridge.

To measure the isometric endurance of the trunk extensors, have your client lie prone with the lower body secured (use straps) to the test bed at the ankles, knees, and hips and with the upper body extended over the edge of the bed. The test bed should be approximately 25 cm (10 in.) above the surface of the floor. During the test, the client holds the upper arms across the chest, with the hands resting on the opposite shoulders. Instruct your client to assume and maintain a horizontal position above the floor for as long as possible. Use a stopwatch to record in seconds the time from which the client assumes the horizontal position until the upper body contacts the floor.

To measure the isometric endurance of the trunk flexors, have your client sit on a test bench with a movable back support set at a 60° angle. The client flexes the knees and hips to 90° and folds the arms across the chest. Use toe straps to secure the client's feet to the test bench. Instruct your client to maintain this body position for as long as possible after you lower or remove the back support. End the test when the client's trunk falls below the 60° angle. Use a stopwatch to record in seconds the elapsed time.

To measure the isometric endurance of the lateral flexors, use the side bridge. Ask your client to assume a side-lying position on a mat, with the legs extended. The top foot should be placed in front of the lower foot for support. Instruct your client to lift the hips off the mat while supporting the body in a straight line on one elbow and the feet for as long as possible. The client should hold the uninvolved arm across the chest. End the test when the client's hips return to the mat. Use a stopwatch to record in seconds the elapsed time. Administer this test for both the right and left sides of the body.

Refer to McGill, Childs, and Lieberson (1999) for gender-specific means for the isometric endurance of the trunk extensor, trunk flexor, and lateral flexor muscle groups. Additionally, refer to table 6.3 for normative data for forearm planks. You can use these reference values to evaluate lumbar stability and to set training goals for your clients.

FLEXIBILITY TESTING OF OLDER ADULTS

Flexibility is an important component of the functional fitness of older individuals. Older adults need to safely perform activities of daily living (ADLs) in order to maintain their functional independence as they age. Flexibility facilitates ADLs such as getting in and out of a car or chair, dressing, and bathing. The Senior Fitness Test, developed by Rikli and Jones (2013), includes two measures of flexibility for older adults—the chair sit-and-reach and the back scratch tests.

CHAIR SIT-AND-REACH TEST

Many older individuals have difficulty performing sit-and-reach tests because functional limitations (e.g., low back pain and poor ROM) prevent them from getting down to and up from the floor. Jones

Table 10.7 Chair Sit-and-Reach Test Norms

Percentile rank	60-64 YR F	60-64 YR M	65-69 YR F	65-69 YR M	70-74 YR F	70-74 YR M	75-79 YR F	75-79 YR M	80-84 YR F	80-84 YR M	85-89 YR F	85-89 YR M	90-94 YR F	90-94 YR M
95	8.7	8.5	7.9	7.5	7.5	7.5	7.4	6.6	6.6	6.2	6.0	4.5	4.9	3.5
90	7.2	6.7	6.6	5.9	6.1	5.8	6.1	4.9	5.2	4.4	4.6	3.0	3.4	1.9
85	6.3	5.6	5.7	4.8	5.2	4.7	5.2	3.8	4.3	3.2	3.7	2.0	2.5	0.9
80	5.5	4.6	5.0	3.9	4.5	3.8	4.4	2.8	3.6	2.2	3.0	1.1	1.7	0.0
75	4.8	3.8	4.4	3.1	3.9	3.0	3.7	2.0	3.0	1.4	2.4	0.4	1.0	−0.7
70	4.2	3.1	3.9	2.4	3.3	2.4	3.2	1.3	2.4	0.6	1.8	−0.2	0.4	−1.4
65	3.7	2.5	3.4	1.8	2.8	1.8	2.7	0.7	1.9	0.0	1.3	−0.8	−0.1	−1.9
60	3.1	1.8	2.9	1.1	2.3	1.1	2.1	0.1	1.4	−0.8	0.8	−1.3	−0.7	−2.5
55	2.6	1.2	2.5	0.6	1.9	0.6	1.7	−0.5	1.0	−1.4	0.4	−1.9	−1.2	−3.0
50	2.1	0.6	2.0	0.0	1.4	0.0	1.2	−1.1	0.5	−2.0	−0.1	−2.4	−1.7	−3.6
45	1.6	0.0	1.5	−0.6	0.9	−0.6	0.7	−1.7	0.0	−2.6	−0.6	−2.9	−2.2	−4.2
40	1.1	−0.6	1.1	−1.1	0.5	−1.2	0.2	−2.3	−0.4	−3.2	−1.0	−3.5	−2.7	−4.7
35	0.5	−1.3	0.6	−1.8	0.0	−1.8	−0.3	−2.9	−0.9	−4.0	−1.5	−4.0	−3.3	−5.3
30	0.0	−1.9	0.1	−2.4	−0.5	−2.4	−0.8	−3.5	−1.4	−4.6	−2.0	−4.6	−3.8	−5.8
25	−0.6	−2.6	−0.4	−3.1	−1.1	−3.1	−1.3	−4.2	−2.0	−5.3	−2.6	−5.3	−4.4	−6.5
20	−1.3	−3.4	−1.0	−3.9	−1.7	−3.9	−2.0	−5.0	−2.6	−6.2	−3.2	−5.9	−5.1	−7.2
15	−2.1	−4.4	−1.7	−4.8	−2.4	−4.8	−2.8	−6.0	−3.3	−7.2	−3.9	−6.8	−5.9	−8.1
10	−3.0	−5.5	−2.6	−5.9	−3.3	−5.9	−3.7	−7.1	−4.2	−8.4	−4.8	−7.8	−6.8	−9.1
5	−4.0	−7.3	−3.9	−7.5	−4.7	−7.6	−5.0	−8.8	−5.0	−10.2	−6.3	−9.3	−7.9	−10.7

F = females; M = males.

Note: Score is measured in inches. To convert inches to centimeters, multiply value in table by 2.54.

Adapted by permission from R. Rikli and C. Jones, *Senior Fitness Test Manual*, 2nd ed. (Champaign, IL: Human Kinetics, 2013), 158.

and colleagues (1998) devised a chair sit-and-reach test that is similar to the back-saver protocol (see figure 10.8) in that it tests only one leg, thereby reducing stress on the spine and lower back. Compared with standard ($r = .71$-$.74$) and back-saver ($r = .70$-$.71$) sit-and-reach protocols, the chair test yielded similar criterion-related validity coefficients ($r = .76$-$.81$) as a measure of hamstring flexibility in older (>60 yr) men and women. Table 10.7 presents age-gender norms for the chair sit-and-reach test.

Purpose: Assess lower body (hamstring) flexibility.

Application: A measure of the ability to perform ADLs such as climbing stairs and getting in and out of a car, chair, or bathtub.

Equipment: You will need a folding chair that has a seat height of 17 in. (43 cm) and that will not tip forward, as well as an 18 in. (46 cm or half a yardstick) ruler.

Test procedures: Place the folding chair against a wall for stability, and have your client sit on the front edge of the seat. The client extends the leg being tested in front of the hip, with the heel on the floor and the ankle dorsiflexed approximately 90°. The client flexes the untested leg so that the sole of the foot is flat on the floor about 6 to 12 in. (15-30.5 cm) to the side of the body's midline. With the extended leg as straight as possible and the hands on top of each other (palms down), the client slowly bends forward at the hip joint, keeping the spine as straight as possible and the head in normal alignment (not tucked) with the spine (see figure 10.10). The client reaches down the extended leg, trying to touch the toes, and holds this position for 2 sec. Place the ruler parallel to the client's lower leg, and administer two practice trials followed by two test trials.

Scoring: The middle of the big toe (medial aspect) at the end of the shoe represents a zero score. Reaches short of the toes are recorded as minus scores; reaches beyond the toes are recorded as plus scores. Record the best score to the nearest half inch and compare it against the norms in table 10.7.

BACK SCRATCH TEST

Limited ROM in the upper body, especially in the shoulder joints, may cause painful movement and

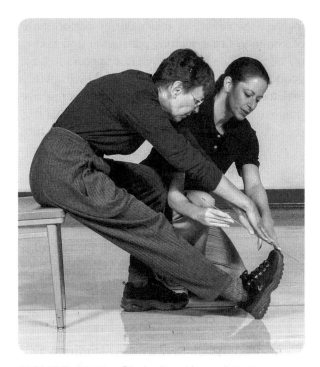

FIGURE 10.10 Chair sit-and-reach test.

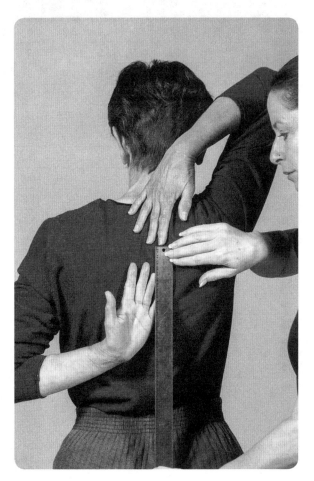

FIGURE 10.11 Back scratch test.

increase the chance of injury during performance of common tasks such as putting on and taking off clothes. The back scratch test appears to have good construct validity, as evidenced by its ability to detect declines in shoulder flexibility across age groups (60-90 yr) (Rikli and Jones 1999). Table 10.8 presents age-gender norms for the back scratch test.

Purpose: Assess upper body (shoulder joint) flexibility.

Application: A measure of the ability to perform ADLs such as combing hair, dressing, and reaching for a seat belt.

Equipment: You will need an 18 in. (46 cm) ruler.

Test procedures: Ask your client to reach, with the preferred hand (palm down and fingers extended), over the shoulder and down the back while reaching around and up the middle of the back with the other hand (palm up and fingers extended) (see figure 10.11). Allow the client to choose the best, or preferred, hand through trial and error. Administer two practice trials followed by two test trials.

Scoring: Use the ruler to measure the overlap (plus score) or gap (minus score) between the middle fingers of each hand. If the fingers just touch each other, record a zero. Record the best score to the nearest half inch, and compare this value against the norms in table 10.8.

Table 10.8 Back Scratch Test Norms

Percentile rank	60-64 YR F	60-64 YR M	65-69 YR F	65-69 YR M	70-74 YR F	70-74 YR M	75-79 YR F	75-79 YR M	80-84 YR F	80-84 YR M	85-89 YR F	85-89 YR M	90-94 YR F	90-94 YR M
95	5.0	4.5	4.9	3.9	4.5	3.5	4.5	2.8	4.3	3.2	3.5	1.7	3.9	0.7
90	3.8	2.7	3.5	2.2	3.2	1.8	3.1	0.9	2.8	1.2	1.9	−0.1	2.2	−1.1
85	2.9	1.6	2.6	1.0	2.3	0.6	2.2	−0.3	1.8	−0.1	0.8	−1.2	0.9	−2.2
80	2.2	0.6	1.9	0.0	1.5	−0.4	1.3	−1.3	0.9	−1.2	−0.1	−2.2	−0.1	−3.2
75	1.6	−0.2	1.3	−0.8	0.8	−1.2	0.6	−2.2	0.2	−2.1	−0.9	−3.0	−1.0	−4.0
70	1.1	−0.9	0.7	−1.6	0.3	−2.0	0.0	−2.9	−0.4	−2.9	−1.6	−3.7	−1.8	−4.7
65	0.7	−1.5	0.2	−2.2	−0.2	−2.6	−0.5	−3.6	−1.0	−3.6	−2.1	−4.3	−2.5	−5.3
60	0.2	−2.2	−0.3	−2.9	−0.8	−3.3	−1.1	−4.3	−1.6	−4.3	−2.8	−5.0	−3.2	−6.0
55	−0.2	−2.8	−0.7	−3.5	−1.2	−3.9	−1.6	−4.9	−2.1	−5.0	−3.3	−5.6	−3.8	−6.6
50	−0.7	−3.4	−1.2	−4.1	−1.7	−4.5	−2.1	−5.6	−2.6	−5.7	−3.9	−6.2	−4.5	−7.2
45	−1.2	−4.0	−1.7	−4.7	−2.2	−5.1	−2.6	−6.3	−3.1	−6.4	−4.5	−6.8	−5.2	−7.8
40	−1.6	−4.6	−2.1	−5.3	−2.6	−5.7	−3.1	−6.9	−3.7	−7.1	−5.0	−7.4	−5.8	−8.4
35	−2.1	−5.3	−2.6	−6.0	−3.2	−6.4	−3.7	−7.6	−4.2	−7.8	−5.7	−8.1	−6.5	−9.1
30	−2.5	−5.9	−3.1	−6.6	−3.7	−7.0	−4.2	−8.3	−4.8	−8.5	−6.2	−8.7	−7.2	−9.7
25	−3.0	−6.6	−3.7	−7.4	−4.2	−7.8	−4.8	−9.0	−5.4	−9.3	−6.9	−9.4	−8.0	−10.4
20	−3.6	−7.4	−4.3	−8.2	−4.9	−8.6	−5.5	−9.9	−6.1	−10.2	−7.7	−10.2	−8.9	−11.2
15	−4.3	−8.4	−5.0	−9.2	−5.7	−9.6	−6.4	−10.9	−7.0	−11.3	−8.6	−11.2	−9.9	−12.2
10	−5.2	−9.5	−5.9	−10.4	−6.6	−10.8	−7.3	−12.1	−8.0	−12.6	−9.7	−12.3	−11.2	−13.3
5	−6.4	−11.3	−7.3	−12.1	−7.9	−12.5	−8.8	−14.0	−9.5	−14.6	−11.3	−14.1	−13.0	−15.1

F = females; M = males.

Note: Score is measured in inches. To convert inches to centimeters, multiply value in table by 2.54.

Adapted by permission from R. Rikli and C. Jones, *Senior Fitness Test Manual*, 2nd ed. (Champaign, IL: Human Kinetics, 2013), 159.

Key Points

▶ Static flexibility is a measure of the total ROM at the joint.

▶ Dynamic flexibility is a measure of the rate of torque or resistance developed during movement through the ROM.

▶ Flexibility is highly joint specific, and the ROM depends, in part, on the structure of the joint.

▶ Lack of physical activity is a major cause of inflexibility.

▶ A universal goniometer, electrogoniometer, flexometer, or inclinometer can be used to obtain direct measures of ROM.

▶ A yardstick and anthropometric tape measure can be used to obtain indirect measures of ROM.

▶ Sit-and-reach tests are only moderately related to hamstring flexibility and poorly related to low back flexibility.

▶ The chair sit-and-reach and the back scratch tests can be used to assess flexibility of older adults.

▶ Lumbar instability increases risk of developing low back pain.

▶ Muscle endurance is more protective than muscle strength for reducing low back injury.

Key Terms

Learn the definition for each of the following key terms. Definitions of terms can be found in the glossary.

ankylosis

biaxial joint

contracture

dynamic flexibility

elastic deformation

electrogoniometer

flexibility

flexometer

goniometer

hypermobility

inclinometer

joint laxity

nonaxial joint

range of motion (ROM)

static flexibility

static stretching

stress relaxation

triaxial joint

uniaxial joint

viscoelastic properties

viscous deformation

Review Questions

In addition to being able to define each of the key terms, test your knowledge and understanding of the material by answering the following review questions.

1. Why are flexibility tests included in most health-related fitness test batteries?

2. Identify and explain how morphological factors affect range of joint motion.

3. How do age, gender, and physical activity (or lack thereof) affect flexibility?

4. Identify and briefly describe three direct methods for measuring static flexibility.

5. Do sit-and-reach tests yield valid measures of hamstring and low back flexibility? Explain.

6. Is the modified sit-and-reach test more valid than the standard sit-and-reach test for assessing hamstring and low back flexibility?

7. Describe three tests that can be used to evaluate lumbar stability.

8. Describe two tests that indirectly measure the flexibility of older adults.

CHAPTER 11

Designing Programs for Flexibility and Low Back Care

KEY QUESTIONS

▶ How do training principles apply to the design of flexibility training programs?

▶ Are all methods of stretching safe and effective for improving flexibility?

▶ What are the recommended guidelines for designing a stretching program?

▶ How do you individualize flexibility programs to meet the goals and abilities of each client?

▶ How often does a client need to exercise to improve flexibility?

▶ Is there an optimal combination of stretch duration and repetitions for improving range of motion?

▶ Can low back syndrome be prevented?

▶ What exercises are recommended for low back care?

Flexibility training is a systematic program of stretching exercises that progressively increases the range of motion (ROM) of joints over time. It is well documented that stretching improves flexibility and ROM. Generic exercise prescriptions for improving flexibility are not recommended; flexibility programs should be individualized to address the needs, abilities, and physical activity interests of each client. Your clients' flexibility assessments (see chapter 10) can help you focus on the joints and muscle groups needing improvement. Lifestyle assessments (see appendix A.5) can help identify muscle groups and body parts with limited joint mobility caused by habitual body postures (e.g., sitting at a desk for long times at work) or repetitive movement patterns during exercise (e.g., jogging).

This chapter presents guidelines for designing flexibility programs. Basic training principles are applied to developing flexibility programs. The chapter compares various methods of stretching and addresses questions about the flexibility exercise prescription. In addition, it presents approaches and recommendations for designing low back care programs.

TRAINING PRINCIPLES

The principles of overload, specificity, progression, and interindividual variability (see the Basic Principles for Exercise Program Design section in chapter 3) apply to flexibility programs. Flexibility is joint specific (Cotten 1972; Harris 1969; Munroe and Romance 1975); to increase the ROM of a particular joint, select exercises that stretch the appropriate muscle groups (i.e., apply the specificity principle). Review your anatomy and kinesiology, particularly muscle origins and insertions, joint structures and functions, and agonist-antagonist muscle pairs. For excellent anatomical illustrations of muscles stretched during the performance of a variety of flexibility exercises, see Nelson and Kokkonen (2014). To improve ROM at a joint, your clients must overload the muscle group by stretching the muscles beyond their normal resting length but not beyond the pain-free ROM. The pain-free ROM varies among individuals (interindividual variability principle), depending on their **stretch tolerance** (the amount of resistive force to stretch within target muscles that a person can tolerate before experiencing pain) and their perception of stretch and pain (Magnusson 1998; Shrier and Gossal 2000). Periodically your clients will need to increase the total time of stretching by increasing the duration or number of repetitions of each stretch in order to ensure the overload required for further ROM improvements (progression principle).

STRETCHING METHODS

Traditionally, four stretching methods have been used to improve ROM: ballistic, slow static, dynamic, and proprioceptive neuromuscular facilitation. **Ballistic stretching** uses jerky, bouncing movements to lengthen the target muscles, whereas **static stretching** uses slow, sustained muscle lengthening to increase ROM. **Dynamic stretching** is typically performed with slow movements that are repeated several times, producing an increased range of joint motion. Commonly used **proprioceptive neuromuscular facilitation (PNF)** stretching techniques involve maximal or submaximal contractions (isometric or dynamic) of target (agonist) and opposing (antagonist) muscle groups followed by passive stretching of the target muscles (Chalmers 2004).

Stretching techniques are classified as active, passive, or active-assisted. In **active stretching**, the client moves the body part without external assistance (i.e., voluntarily contracts the muscle). In **passive stretching**, the client relaxes the target muscle group as the body part is moved by an assistant (e.g., partner, personal trainer, physical therapist, or athletic trainer). In **active-assisted stretching**, the client moves the body part to the end of its active ROM and the assistant then moves the body part beyond its active ROM. Table 11.1 summarizes the advantages and disadvantages of stretching methods. The following questions address issues you should consider when selecting a stretching method for a client's flexibility program.

Which method of stretching is best for improving ROM?

All four stretching methods (ballistic, dynamic, slow static, and PNF) produce acute and chronic gains in flexibility and ROM at the knee, hip, trunk, shoulder, and ankle joints (Thacker et al. 2004; Mahieu et al. 2007). Although slow static stretching is considered safer than ballistic or PNF stretching and is easier to perform because it does not require special equipment or an assistant, each stretching method has its proponents. Proprioceptive neuromuscular facilitation stretching is frequently used in sport and rehabilitation settings, while ballistic and dynamic stretching are often preferred by those engaging in explosive activities.

Konrad, Stafilidis, and Tilp (2016) compared dorsiflexion ROM before and after four repetitions of 30 sec of either static, ballistic, or PNF stretching. All stretching groups increased ROM and decreased passive resistive torque, with no clinically relevant difference between stretching groups. Likewise, Maddigan, Peach, and Behm (2012) noted that static stretching, traditional assisted PNF, and unassisted PNF (using a stretch strap) produce similar gains in static (active and passive) ROM and dynamic ROM of the hip flexors. In an extensive review of static, dynamic, and PNF stretching research, Behm et al.

Table 11.1 Comparison of Stretching Techniques

Factor	Ballistic	Slow static	Dynamic	PNF
Risk of injury	High	Low	Medium	Medium
Degree of pain	Medium	Low	Medium	High
Resistance to stretch	High	Low	Medium	Medium
Practicality (time and assistance needed)	Good	Excellent	Excellent	Poor
Efficiency (energy consumption)	Poor	Excellent	Good	Poor
Effective for increasing ROM	Good	Good	Good	Excellent

PNF = proprioceptive neuromuscular facilitation; ROM = range of motion.

(2016) concluded it was not possible to rank one stretching method over another for increasing ROM. Furthermore, each stretching method has distinct loading characteristics that likely influence the specific mechanisms responsible for increasing ROM. These findings suggest that all types of stretching should be considered for training and rehabilitation programs. Therefore, choose a method that meets each client's specific abilities (e.g., stretch tolerance and pain threshold), needs, and long-term goals.

Video 11.1

What are some of the commonly used PNF stretching techniques, and how are they performed?

Various PNF techniques use different combinations of dynamic (concentric and eccentric) and isometric contraction of target and opposing muscle groups. The **contract-relax (CR)** and **contract-relax agonist contract (CRAC) techniques** are common PNF procedures. In the CR technique, the client first isometrically contracts the target muscle group; this is immediately followed by slow, passive stretching of the target muscle group. The first two steps of the CRAC and CR techniques are identical except the client assists the CRAC stretching phase by actively contracting the opposing muscle group. For example, to stretch the pectoral muscles, the client sits on the floor and extends the arms horizontally. The client isometrically contracts the pectoral muscles as the partner offers resistance to horizontal flexion. Following the isometric contraction, the partner slowly stretches the pectorals as the client actively contracts the horizontal extensors in the upper back (see figure 11.1). For detailed explanations and illustrations of PNF and facilitated stretching techniques, see Alter (2004) and McAtee and Charland (2007).

What are the general recommendations for performing PNF stretches?

The following steps are recommended for performing PNF stretches to increase ROM:

- Stretch the target muscle group by moving the joint to the end of its ROM.
- Isometrically contract the stretched muscle group against an immovable resistance (such as a partner or wall) for 5 to 10 sec.
- Relax the target muscle group as you stretch it actively or passively (with a partner) to a new point of limitation.

- For the CRAC technique, contract the opposing muscle group submaximally for 5 or 6 sec to facilitate further stretching of the target muscle group.

Which PNF technique is best?

Several researchers have reported that the CRAC technique is superior to the CR technique for increasing ROM (Alter 2004; Ferber, Osternig, and Gravelle 2002; Moore and Hutton 1980; Osternig et al. 1990). However, these investigators also noted that CRAC produced larger gains in electromyographic activity, meaning that the muscle was under more tension. Despite an increase in joint ROM, this technique may not induce muscular relaxation, and Ferber, Osternig, and Gravelle (2002) noted that extra care should be taken when applying this technique to older adults. Therefore, you need to consider the client's stretch tolerance when selecting a PNF stretching technique.

Kay, Dods, and Blazevich (2016) recently introduced a modified CR technique that reduces the pain and risk of PNF. Instead of performing the contraction while the muscle was stretched, the study participants returned to anatomical position for the contraction; thus, the contraction was performed "off stretch," resulting in a stretch-return-contract (SRC) sequence. Compared with CR, the SRC technique was equally effective at increasing dorsiflexion ROM and reducing both muscle and tendon stiffness, but the tensile loading of the tendon was 10.6% less during SRC. The practical application is a reduced risk of muscle damage and less pain with the SRC technique, yet it is equally effective as CR.

Are there any disadvantages to PNF stretching?

A major disadvantage of the PNF technique is that most of the exercises cannot be performed alone. An assistant is needed to resist movement during the isometric contraction phase and to apply external force during the stretching phase. Overstretching may cause injury, especially if the assistant has not been carefully trained in the correct PNF procedures. Assisted stretching procedures such as PNF should be carefully performed by trained clients or exercise professionals who understand the correct

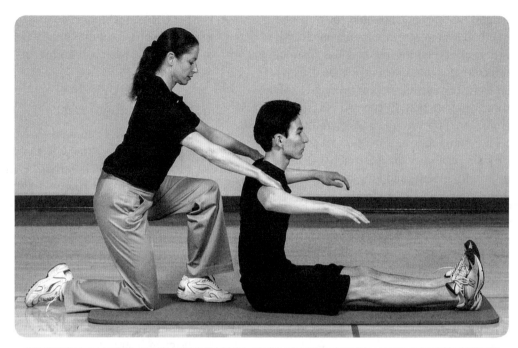

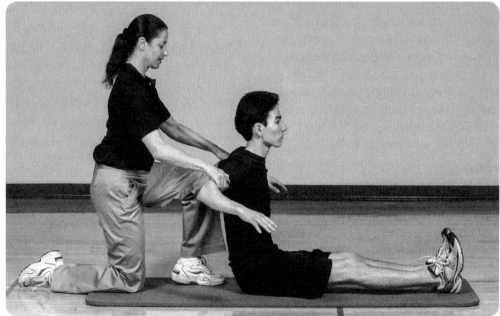

FIGURE 11.1 Contract-relax agonist contract (CRAC) proprioceptive neuromuscular facilitation stretching technique for the shoulder horizontal flexors.

procedures and the risks of incorrect stretching (Knudson, Magnusson, and McHugh 2000).

Why is slow static stretching safer than ballistic stretching?

Some exercise professionals recommend slow static stretching over ballistic stretching because there is less chance of injury and muscle soreness resulting from jerky, rapid movements. Mahieu and associates (2007) observed that a 6 wk slow static stretching program produced a significant increase in ankle dorsiflexion ROM resulting from a significant decrease in passive resistive torque of the calf muscles. Ballistic stretching, however, had no effect on passive resistance but produced a significant decrease in the stiffness of the Achilles tendon.

Ballistic stretching uses relatively fast bouncing motions to produce stretch. The momentum of the moving body segment rather than external force pushes the joint beyond its present ROM. This technique appears counterproductive for increasing muscle relaxation and stretch. During the movement, the muscle spindles signal changes in both muscle length and contraction speed. Because of a lower threshold, the spindle responds more to the speed of the movement than to the length or position of the muscle. In fact, muscle spindle activity is directly proportional to the speed of movement. Thus, ballistic stretching evokes the stretch reflex, producing more contraction and resistance to stretch in the target muscle group. Also, the muscle has viscous properties. The viscous material resists elongation more when the stretch is applied rapidly (Taylor et al. 1990). Therefore, ballistic stretching places greater strain on the muscle and may cause microscopic tearing of muscle fibers and connective tissues.

In slow static stretching, the client stretches the target muscle group when the joint is at the end of its ROM. While maintaining this lengthened position, the client slowly applies torque to the target muscle group to stretch it further. Because the dynamic portion of the muscle spindle rapidly adapts to the lengthened position, spindle discharge decreases. This decrease lessens the reflex contraction of the target muscle group and allows the muscle to relax and be stretched even further. The force needed to lengthen a muscle is affected by the rate of stretching and by the duration over which the target muscle group is held at a specific length (Taylor et al. 1990). Resistance to elongation is greater for rapid (e.g., ballistic) stretching than for slow static stretching. Also, the resistance produced by the viscous properties of the muscle decreases over time as the target muscle is held at its stretched length. The resulting **stress relaxation** allows further elongation of the target muscle group (Chalmers 2004).

How do constant-angle and constant-torque static stretching produce gains in flexibility?

The term *static stretching* implies that the joint angle does not change during the stretching exercise. With constant-angle stretching, the resistance to stretch in the muscle-tendon unit decreases as the joint is held at a constant angle. As mentioned earlier,

this is referred to as the stress relaxation response. With constant-torque stretching, the torque applied to the muscle decreases muscle stiffness, thereby improving ROM. During constant-torque stretching, technically the joint is not static; the joint angle increases because of the constant pressure applied to the muscle-tendon unit, causing it to elongate. This is known as **viscoelastic creep**.

In a study comparing the effects of constant-angle and constant-tension static stretching on passive torque, passive ROM, and muscle-tendon stiffness, Herda and coworkers (2011) reported that both forms of static stretching improve ROM; however, only constant-torque stretching decreases muscle-tendon stiffness. They concluded that constant-torque stretching changes both the viscosity and elasticity of the muscle-tendon unit, whereas constant-angle stretching affects only the viscosity. These findings suggest that constant-torque stretching may be better suited than constant-angle stretching for reducing risk of muscle strain when treating injuries such as Achilles tendonitis and plantar fasciitis. More research is warranted to fully understand the mechanisms underlying changes in muscle-tendon stiffness with different forms of stretching.

What are the physiological mechanisms underlying flexibility gains when stretching actively or passively?

The mechanisms responsible for flexibility gains differ for passive and active stretching. With passive stretching, the targeted muscle does not contract. Riley and Van Dyke (2012) discussed evidence suggesting that passive stretching produces transient reductions in muscle stiffness due to viscoelastic relaxation lasting about 24 hr. Passively stretching the hamstrings 1 min/day for 10 consecutive days using a Biodex dynamometer produced a progressive reduction in stiffness. To be effective, however, passive stretching needs to be performed daily because reversion to prestretch levels begins in 24 hr. Lengthening the muscle tissue during passive stretching affects fibroblasts in the mysium coverings wrapped around muscle fibers, the muscle fasciculi, tendons, and connective tissues surrounding nerve fibers. The fibroblasts respond to the mechanical stimuli of the stretch, producing changes in these connective tissues, thereby reducing muscle-tendon stiffness.

With active stretching, the lengthened muscle contracts during the stretching exercise. The actual length of the muscle may increase provided the muscle is stretched beyond its optimal length needed for maximum overlap of contractile filaments and crossbridge formation. This point in the range of joint motion at which optimal muscle length is achieved is limited by the individual's pain tolerance, and it depends on the optimal length of each targeted muscle (Riley and Van Dyke 2012). Active tension (stretching plus contractile activity) is needed to stimulate production of sarcomeres in series within the muscle fiber, thereby increasing the actual length of the targeted muscle. This process depends on calcium-dependent pathways (i.e., calcium from the sarcoplasmic reticulum) that regulate the number of series sarcomeres produced in response to stretching combined with muscle contractile activity.

These findings potentially affect exercise prescriptions for flexibility programs. When the goal of the program is to improve flexibility of clients with limited ROM due to injury, immobilization, reduced mobility, or habitual body postures, active stretching may be more beneficial than passive stretching to restore their muscle length and ROM. Flexibility programs using passive stretching exercises should be performed daily because muscle-tendon stiffness continuously adapts and adjusts day to day to the experienced ROM (Riley and Van Dyke 2012).

What are the physiological mechanisms underlying the increased ROM produced by the PNF method?

In reviews by Sharman, Cresswell, and Riek (2006) and Hindle and colleagues (2012), four theoretical mechanisms responsible for gains in ROM from PNF stretching were identified. These theories include autogenic inhibition, reciprocal inhibition, viscoelastic stress relaxation, and gate control theory of pain modulation. Unfortunately, there is little empirical evidence to support any of these mechanisms.

Autogenic inhibition refers to a reduction in the excitability of the targeted muscle because of inhibitory signals sent from the Golgi tendon organ, or GTO, during isometric contraction (i.e., greater GTO activation leads to reflex relaxation). Also, voluntary contraction of opposing muscle groups during CRAC stretching was simply explained by **reciprocal inhibition** (as the opposing muscle group

is voluntarily contracted, the target muscle group is reflexively inhibited). Traditionally, increases in ROM from PNF stretching were attributed to autogenic or reciprocal inhibition or both; however, these simple explanations are likely inadequate to explain the complex mechanisms underlying muscle stretch.

In contrast to the neurophysiological hypotheses of autogenic and reciprocal inhibition, more contemporary views of how PNF stretching improves ROM include the viscoelastic properties of stretched muscle (stress relaxation hypothesis) and the ability to tolerate stretching (gate control theory). Muscles and tendons have both elastic and viscous properties. The amount of tension needed to elongate the musculotendinous unit (MTU) is dictated by the elastic property of the MTU, while the viscous property resists the elongation of a rapid stretch. However, the viscous material loses its ability to resist the elongation force over time (stress relaxation), and the MTU will elongate if the tension is sustained. Although this seems like a plausible theory, the change in passive torque within the muscle that accompanies stress relaxation is short lived, lasting less than an hour after PNF stretching (Magnusson et al. 1996).

The gate control theory, explaining what occurs when two stimuli such as pain and stretch activate their respective receptors simultaneously, may help explain longer-term adaptations from PNF stretching. Stretching a muscle beyond its natural ROM and contracting it is seen as potentially damaging, resulting in activation of the GTOs to prevent injury. However, with a consistent and repeated PNF protocol, the GTOs adapt, becoming more accustomed to increased stretch and force applied to the muscle, and cause less inhibition (Hindle et al. 2012).

What is the recommended duration and intensity of the static contraction phase during PNF stretching to maximize long-term gains in ROM?

In a review of PNF stretching studies, Sharman, Cresswell, and Riek (2006) reported that the static contraction duration of the targeted muscle was between 3 and 15 sec. Although there is some evidence for a correlation between longer static contraction duration and increased ROM (Rowlands, Marginson, and Lee 2003), the ROM gains reported in the majority of reviewed studies were independent of the duration of the static contraction. Sharman,

Cresswell, and Riek (2006) recommended the shortest duration of 3 sec. There is some disagreement regarding the optimal intensity of the static contraction during PNF to optimize ROM gains. Feland and Marin (2004) found no significant difference in ROM improvements using 20%, 60%, and 100% of maximum voluntary contraction (MVC), so Sharman, Cresswell, and Riek (2006) recommended a low intensity of 20% MVC to minimize risk. Subsequent to this recommendation, other researchers have reported that static contractions of 60% to 65% MVC during PNF stretching produce the greatest improvement in ROM (Kwak and Ryu 2015; Sheard and Paine 2010). Regardless, all agree that 100% MVC is not necessary for increasing ROM with PNF stretching. The American College of Sports Medicine (ACSM) recommends 3 to 6 sec of 20% to 75% MVC followed by a 10 to 30 sec assisted stretch (2018).

DESIGNING FLEXIBILITY PROGRAMS: EXERCISE PRESCRIPTION

After assessing a client's flexibility, you must identify the joints and muscle groups needing improvement and select an appropriate stretching method and the specific exercises for the exercise prescription. Appendix F.1 illustrates flexibility exercises for various regions of the body. For additional stretching exercises, see Alter (2004), Frederick and Frederick (2017), McAtee and Charland (2014), and Nelson and Kokkonen (2014). Follow the guidelines (see Guidelines for Designing Flexibility Programs and Client Guidelines for Stretching Programs later in this chapter), and be sure to address the following questions regarding the client's exercise prescription.

How many exercises should be included in a flexibility program?

A well-rounded program includes at least one exercise for each of the major muscle groups of the body, including the neck, shoulders, upper and lower back, pelvis, hips, and legs. It is especially important to select exercises for problem areas such as the lower back, hips, and posterior thighs and legs. Use the results of the flexibility tests to identify specific muscle groups with relatively poor flexibility, and include more than one exercise for these muscle groups. The workout should take 15 to 30 min depending on the number of exercises to be performed.

Are some stretching exercises safer than others?

Some stretching exercises are not recommended for flexibility programs because they create excessive stress, thereby increasing the client's chance of musculoskeletal injuries—especially to the knee joints and low back region. Appendix F.2, Exercise Dos and Don'ts, illustrates exercises that are contraindicated for flexibility programs and suggests alternative exercises you can prescribe to increase the flexibility of specific muscle groups. For detailed analysis of risk factors and options for minimizing risk for certain stretching exercises, see Alter (2004).

What is a safe intensity for stretching exercises?

The intensity of slow static stretching and PNF stretching exercises should always be below the pain threshold of the individual. Some mild discomfort will occur, especially during PNF exercises when the target muscle is contracted isometrically. However, as stated previously, this contraction can be less than MVC (Kwak and Ryu 2015; Rowlands, Marginson, and Lee 2003; Sheard and Paine 2010), and the joint should not be stretched beyond its pain-free ROM (American College of Sports Medicine 2018).

How long does each stretch need to be held?

The ACSM (2018) recommends holding a stretched position for 10 to 30 sec for most adults and 30 to 60 sec for older adults. After a 5 wk program of static hamstring stretches for either 30, 60, 90, or 120 sec, similar benefits in passive knee extension ROM were achieved regardless of stretch duration (Ford, Mazzone, and Taylor 2005). This suggests that holding a stretch for 30 sec is just as effective as longer stretches at improving ROM. Depending on the objective, it may be important to consider the intensity of the stretch in conjunction with the duration. Freitas and colleagues (2015) had participants hold stretches for 90 sec at maximal tolerable intensity, 135 sec at 75% intensity, and 180 sec at 50%. They concluded that the higher-intensity stretch was best for achieving ROM gains, but the longer stretch duration potentiated passive torque decrease.

Research suggests that the total stretching time in a workout may be more important than the duration of each stretch (Cipriani, Abel, and Pirrwitz 2003; Johnson et al. 2014; Roberts and Wilson 1999; Zakas et al. 2005). This seems to be the case regardless of whether study participants had good ROM (Cipriani, Abel, and Pirrwitz 2003), had tight hamstrings (Johnson et al. 2014), were young athletes (Roberts and Wilson 1999), or were older adults (Zakas et al. 2005). Johnson and colleagues (2014) had participants perform either 10 sec stretches for nine repetitions or 30 sec stretches for three repetitions for a total stretching time of 90 sec, 6 days/wk for 6 wk. Both groups showed similar improvements in knee extension ROM. Zakas and associates (2005) compared a single stretch of 60 sec against two stretches of 30 sec and four stretches of 15 sec. The other research teams used different stretching durations (e.g., 5 sec × 9 reps vs. 15 sec × 3 reps for a total stretching time of 45 sec, or 10 sec × 6 reps vs. 30 sec × 2 reps for a total stretching time of 60 sec). All came to the same conclusion that similar ROM gains are achieved with multiple shorter-duration stretches or fewer longer-duration stretches.

The findings from these studies have implications for designing flexibility programs. For clients with a low stretch tolerance, you can prescribe shorter stretch duration (e.g., 10 sec) and more repetitions; for those who can tolerate longer stretch durations (30 sec or more), you can prescribe fewer repetitions.

In light of these findings, you should consider having your clients perform each stretching exercise for a total of 45 sec to 2 min. The combination of duration and repetitions used to reach this recommended total should be individualized to each client's tolerance for the sensation of stretching. For short durations, the stretch should be sustained at least 10 sec. As flexibility improves, you can progressively overload the target muscle groups by changing either the stretch duration (10-30 sec) or the number of repetitions so that the total time the stretched position is held gradually increases. As your clients' stretch tolerance improves, consider increasing the duration and decreasing the number of repetitions of each stretch. Remember that you must gradually increase the total stretching time for each exercise in order to ensure overload and further improvements in ROM.

How many repetitions of each exercise should be performed?

The ACSM (2018) recommends performing two to four repetitions of each stretching exercise and accumulating a stretching duration of 60 sec for each exercise. As flexibility improves during the training program, the number of repetitions of each flexibility exercise may be gradually increased to five or six to progressively overload the muscle group. However, recent research indicates that a single 30 sec static stretch to maximal tolerated discomfort is sufficient to reduce fascicle stiffness, and additional repetitions do not further affect mechanical properties of the muscle (Opplert, Gentry, and Babault 2016). The ACSM recommendation of 60 sec is within the 45 sec to 2 min range given in the previous paragraph. The Opplert et al. 2016 study contradicts this recommendation, but it is important to include this contradictory finding.

How often should flexibility exercises be performed?

The Physical Activity Guidelines for Americans states that all adults should stretch to maintain flexibility for physical activity and performance of activities for daily living (U.S. Department of Health and Human Services 2008). Flexibility exercises should be performed a minimum of 2 days/wk (American College of Sports Medicine 2018), but preferably daily (Knudson et al. 2000). Flexibility exercises should be performed after moderate or vigorous physical activity, and they are often an integral part of the cool-down segments of aerobic exercise and resistance training workouts.

Does stretching prior to physical activity prevent injury?

For years clinicians, coaches, and exercise practitioners have recommended stretching as part of the warm-up. Because an active warm-up prevents injury and because stretching is commonly included in the warm-up, one could easily, but mistakenly, conclude that stretching prevents injury. However, the evidence as to whether stretching before exercise can prevent injury is equivocal.

In a systematic review, Behm and colleagues (2016) identified 12 studies; 8 showed some effectiveness of stretching. However, they noted that it is difficult to confidently attribute injury reduction to preactivity stretching because the studies varied in design, stretch duration, type of activity, stretching with and without warm-up, and definition of injury. The type of activity and the joint studied might also influence the results. For example, a stretching program to improve shoulder rotation in high school pitchers resulted in significantly fewer shoulder injuries (as defined as inability to play for more than a week because of shoulder symptoms) for the stretching group compared with a control group (Shitara et al. 2017). In contrast, a review of the impact of stretching on injury prevention in endurance runners concluded that stretching has no clinical benefit on the risk reduction of chronic injuries in this population (Baxter et al. 2017). For more explosive activities such as sprinting, there may be an injury prevention benefit. Stojanovic and Ostojic (2011) surmised that increased flexibility likely decreases incidence of muscle strain injury in soccer players, but they cautioned that this assumption is based on indirect evidence. Randomized controlled investigations that support the argument that preactivity stretching prevents injury are lacking.

There is some evidence supporting the use of preparticipation stretching for reducing risk of muscle strains during or after performance (Chen et al. 2015; Chen et al. 2011; McHugh and Cosgrave 2010). Chen and colleagues (2015) reported that 15 sec of static stretching repeated six times was more effective than dynamic stretching or no stretching at reducing muscle soreness and biomarkers of muscle damage (creatine kinase and myoglobin) following maximal eccentric contractions. However, in several systematic reviews and meta-analyses of interventions to minimize exercise-induced muscle soreness, the authors concluded that stretching either before, after, or before and after exercise does not result in any clinically relevant reductions in delayed-onset muscle soreness (DOMS) (Herbert, de Noronha, and Kamper 2011; Torres et al. 2012). For more information about DOMS, refer to chapter 7.

Does stretching affect maximal muscle performance?

In the most extensive systematic review of this topic to date, Behm and colleagues (2016) evaluated 125 static stretching studies, 48 dynamic stretching studies, and 11 PNF stretching studies. Their analysis considered dose-response relationship, the perfor-

mance task (power-speed or strength), and contraction type (concentric, eccentric, or static). Overall, static stretching and PNF stretching reduced performance by 3.7% and 4.4%, respectively, but performance improved by 1.3% when dynamic stretching was performed before the activity. When the static stretch totaled ≥60 sec, the decrements in performance were greater (–4.6%) than when the total stretch duration was <60 sec (–1.1%), but there was no dose-response relationship for PNF or dynamic stretching. However, the authors noted that the lag time between stretching and the performance measurement was often short (3-5 min). A more realistic time gap between stretching and athletic performance is likely ≥10 min, and the influence stretching had on performance was trivial in studies with this lag time.

The Canadian Society for Exercise Physiology (www.csep.ca) created a position stand based on the review by Behm and colleagues (2016). They do not recommend prolonged (≥60 sec) static stretching if the activity will take place within 5 min of the stretch. However, they also claim there is likely a greater benefit than cost (in terms of performance, ROM, and injury prevention) when stretching is incorporated into an optimal preevent warm-up that includes aerobic and task-specific dynamic activities.

Can vibration-aided static stretching increase flexibility?

A review of the literature (Cochrane 2013) and a meta-analysis (Osawa and Oguma 2013) have been carried out on this topic. It is clear that adding vibration to the stretching exercise can enhance ROM beyond what is obtainable with static stretching alone, both acutely and over several sessions or weeks of training. The additive effects of vibration might be small but are nevertheless significant (Osawa and Oguma 2013). Furthermore, there does not appear to be any detrimental effect on muscle power, offering an added advantage over static stretching without vibration (Cochrane 2013). However, vibration training has little impact on sprint performance (Cochrane 2013).

There are still several unanswered questions regarding vibration training. First, the mechanisms by which vibration enhances flexibility are not fully understood. There are numerous theories, including increased stretch tolerance due to a decrease in pain sensation; increased blood flow, which increases muscle temperature; inhibition of the antagonist; decreased musculoskeletal stiffness; and suppression of the central nervous system (Cochrane 2013; Osawa and Oguma 2013). Second, researchers have used a variety of combinations of vibration devices, frequencies, amplitudes, volumes, and durations. Thus, the optimal vibration strategy to combine with stretching for increasing ROM is still unknown.

Does the flexibility exercise prescription need to be adapted for older individuals?

Range of motion decreases with age because of disuse, changes in tissue viscoelasticity, and diseases such as arthritis. There is little doubt that stretching improves ROM in older adults (Stathokostas et al. 2012). However, the results are mixed as to whether flexibility training improves functional outcomes that might help older adults maintain independence. In an extensive systematic review of this topic, Stathokostas and colleagues (2012) concluded that a relationship between improved flexibility and functional outcomes could not yet be established. Additionally, the results were too varied to make any clear exercise prescription recommendations for older adults regarding the optimal type of stretch, duration, and number of repetitions for improving flexibility or functional outcomes.

At this time, it is not possible to firmly recommend how to change program guidelines when designing flexibility programs for older adults. Regardless of the stretching method you use with older adults, take care not to exceed the stretch tolerance of your clients. Age-related changes in the viscoelastic properties of muscle and connective tissue reduce the stretch tolerance of older adults. Additionally, ordering prescribed stretches so that all floor-based stretches are grouped together, rather than placing them between standing stretches, is advisable in this population.

You can use the general guidelines presented in this section as a starting point for designing flexibility programs. You should individualize programs to take into account client factors such as tolerance to stretching and pain, needs, and long-range goals. For example, shorter-duration–higher-repetition static stretching may be more appropriate for clients with low stretch tolerance, whereas longer-duration PNF stretching may be more suitable for athletes or for clients in injury rehabilitation programs. Also, the optimal duration, frequency, and total time of stretching may vary among muscle groups because their viscoelastic properties and response to the stretch stimulus may differ (Shrier and Gossal 2000). See Sample Flexibility Program later in this chapter for a program designed for a 35 yr old woman who wants to improve her overall flexibility. Note that this program includes more than one exercise for muscle groups with poor to fair flexibility ratings.

Instruct clients who are engaging in stretching programs to adhere to the recommended guidelines (see Client Guidelines for Stretching Programs).

DESIGNING LOW BACK CARE EXERCISE PROGRAMS

Low back pain frequently causes activity restrictions for middle-aged and older adults, disabling 3 to 4 million people each year. Chronic low back pain is the number one cause of disability in the working population (Carpenter and Nelson 1999), and the lifetime prevalence might be as high as 84% (Almoallim et al. 2014). The safest and most effective way to prevent and rehabilitate low back injuries remains controversial. However, in a recent systematic review and meta-analysis, Steffens and colleagues (2016) concluded that exercise alone or in combination with education is effective for preventing low back pain, whereas other strategies such as shoe insoles, back belts, and education without exercise were not effective prevention methods. This section describes two exercise approaches for low back care programs as well as information about core stability and proper posture. The approach you select depends on the client's needs, health and fitness status, and training objective (e.g., reducing low back pain, lowering the risk of low back injury, or maximizing athletic performance).

Husu and Suni (2012) examined the relationship between health-related fitness (i.e., balance, flexibility, muscle endurance, and body mass index [BMI]) and low back pain in older adults. They reported that balance (measured by single-leg stand) and trunk flexibility (side-bending ROM) were the most pow-

Guidelines for Designing Flexibility Programs

- **Mode:** Static, dynamic, or PNF stretching for most clients; ballistic stretching may be useful for clients engaging in sports that involve ballistic movements
- **Number of exercises:** 10 to 12
- **Frequency:** Minimum of 2 days/wk, preferably daily
- **Intensity:** Slowly stretch the muscle to a position of mild discomfort
- **Duration of stretch:** 10 to 30 sec for static or dynamic stretching; 3 to 6 sec contraction followed by 10 to 30 sec of assisted stretching for PNF
- **Repetitions:** Two to four for each exercise so that the total duration of each stretching exercise is at least 60 sec
- **Volume:** 60 sec total stretching time for each flexibility exercise
- **Time:** 15 to 30 min per session

Based on Kravitz and Heyward 1995; American College of Sports Medicine 2018.

Client Guidelines for Stretching Programs

- Perform a general warm-up before stretching to increase body temperature and to warm the muscles to be stretched.
- Stretch all major muscle groups as well as opposing muscle groups.
- Focus on the target muscle involved in the stretch, relax the target muscle, and minimize the movement of other body parts.
- Hold the stretch for 10 to 30 sec; older individuals should hold the stretch 30 to 60 sec.
- Stretch to the limit (end point) of the movement, not to the point of pain.
- Keep breathing slowly and rhythmically while holding the stretch.
- Stretch the target muscle groups in different planes to improve overall ROM at the joint.
- Although stretching may not prevent injury or reduce muscle soreness, it is a reasonable practice to include stretching exercises after the active warm-up and cool-down phases of your exercise program (American College of Sports Medicine 2018).

erful predictors of low back pain. Poor fitness scores for dynamic trunk extension and BMI (≥ 27 kg/m^2) increased the risk of disability due to low back pain. Tests of trunk flexibility, trunk muscle endurance, balance, and BMI may be useful screening tools for identifying older clients with increased risk of low back pain and disorders.

TRADITIONAL APPROACH

Traditionally, low back care programs have been designed to correct improper alignment and support of the spinal column and pelvis. Generally, a combination of stretching and strengthening exercises is prescribed to increase (a) the ROM of the hip flexors, hamstrings, and low back extensor muscles and (b) the strength of the abdominal muscles.

Exercise professionals have focused primarily on strengthening the abdominal muscles in order to prevent low back pain and injury, giving little or no attention to the low back muscles. Research, however, suggests that low back strengthening programs are effective for relieving and preventing low back pain and injury (Carpenter and Nelson 1999). A current practice in some low back care programs is to include exercises to increase the strength and endurance of both the abdominal and low back extensor muscles.

SAMPLE FLEXIBILITY PROGRAM

Client Data

Age: 35 yr
Gender: Female
Body weight: 140 lb (63.6 kg)
Program goal: Improve overall flexibility
Time commitment: 20-30 min per workout
Number of exercises: 12
Method: Static stretching

Intensity: Just below pain threshold
Duration of stretch: 10 sec
Repetitions: 4-6 per exercise
Total stretch time: 50-120 sec per exercise
Frequency: Daily
Overload: Gradually increase stretch duration or repetitions up to a maximum of 2 min per exercise

Exercise[a]	Week	Duration (sec)	Reps	Total time (sec)	Muscle groups
Quad stretch (side lying)	1-3	10	5	50	Quadriceps femoris
	4-6	12	5	60	
	7-9	15	6	90	
Half-straddle stretch[b]	1-3	10	5	50	Hamstrings; trunk extensors (low back)
	4-6	12	5	60	
	7-9	15	6	90	
Double knee to chest (supine)[b]	1-3	10	6	60	Hamstrings; trunk extensors (low back)
	4-6	15	6	90	
	7-9	20	6	120	
Butterfly stretch (seated)	1-3	10	5	50	Hip adductors
	4-6	10	6	60	
	7-9	12	6	72	
Trunk flex (hands and knees)[b]	1-3	15	5	75	Trunk extensors (low back)
	4-6	20	5	100	
	7-9	20	6	120	
Crossed-leg trunk rotation	1-3	10	5	50	Hip abductors; trunk rotators
	4-6	15	5	75	
	7-9	15	6	90	
Achilles (calf) stretch	1-3	10	5	50	Ankle plantar flexors
	4-6	12	5	60	
	7-9	15	5	75	
Pelvic tilt	1-3	15	5	75	Abdominal muscles
	4-6	20	5	100	
	7-9	30	4	120	
Towel stretch (standing)	1-3	10	5	50	Shoulder extensors
	4-6	12	5	60	
	7-9	15	5	75	

Exercise[a]	Week	Duration (sec)	Reps	Total time (sec)	Muscle groups
Towel stretch (kneeling prone)	1-3	12	5	60	Shoulder flexors
	4-6	15	5	75	
	7-9	20	5	100	
Triceps stretch	1-3	10	5	50	Elbow extensors
	4-6	12	5	60	
	7-9	15	5	75	
Neck rotation	1-3	12	5	60	Neck flexors; neck lateral flexors; neck rotators
	4-6	12	6	72	
	7-9	15	5	75	

[a]For descriptions of exercises, see appendixes F.1 and F.3.

[b]Two or more exercises are included for the muscle groups with poor flexibility—the hamstrings and trunk extensors (low back).

To strengthen the low back (lumbar extensor) muscles, **pelvic stabilization** is a key requirement. If the pelvis is not stabilized during extension of the trunk, the hip extensor muscles rotate the pelvis (~110°), and the lumbar vertebrae maintain their relative position to each other (do not extend). On the other hand, when the pelvis is immobilized, the lumbar vertebrae extend (~72°) as the low back extensor muscles contract (Carpenter and Nelson 1999). Most calisthenic-type floor exercises do not isolate the low back muscles because the pelvis is free to move. Using a lumbar extension machine, with thigh and femur restraints to stabilize the pelvis, prevents hip extension and isolates the low back muscles during the movement. Exercising on a lumbar extension machine with a minimal training volume (one set of 8-15 reps of lumbar extension exercise to fatigue per week) significantly improves lumbar muscle strength and bone mineral density (Graves et al. 1994; Pollock, Garzarella, and Graves 1992) and reduces the incidence of back injuries (Mooney et al. 1995). Individuals with chronic low back pain who participate in this type of low back strengthening program can expect significant improvements in joint mobility and muscular strength and endurance as well as relief from pain (Carpenter and Nelson 1999).

To strengthen the abdominal muscles, select exercises that maximize the activation of the abdominal muscles but minimize the compression (load) of the lumbar vertebrae (i.e., a high challenge-to-compression ratio). Since the psoas muscle (prime mover for hip flexion) is a major source of spinal loading, choose exercises that minimize the activation of this muscle, such as bent-knee curl-ups (feet free or anchored), dynamic cross-knee curl-ups (curl-ups with a twist), isometric side support (side bridge), and dynamic sideward curl exercises (Axler and McGill 1997; Juker et al. 1998; Knudson 1999). The bent-knee curl-up exercise emphasizes the rectus abdominis, while the isometric side support emphasizes the abdominal oblique and quadratus lumborum muscles. Because of their low challenge-to-compression ratios, the following abdominal exercises are not recommended: straight leg or bent-knee sit-ups, supine straight leg raises, and hanging bent-knee raises (Axler and McGill 1997).

Using the traditional approach, the following exercises are recommended for low back care. Some of these exercises are described and illustrated in appendix F.3.

- Pelvic tilt (supine-lying position) to stretch the abdominal muscles
- Knee-to-chest (supine-lying position) to stretch the hamstring, buttock, and low back muscles
- Trunk flex (on hands and knees) to stretch the back, abdominal, and hamstring muscles

- Lumbar extension exercises with pelvic stabilization (on machine) to strengthen the low back extensors

- Curl-ups, dynamic cross-knee curl-ups, and isometric side-support exercises to strengthen the abdominal and quadratus lumborum muscles

- Single-leg extension (prone-lying position) to strengthen the hamstring and buttock muscles and to stretch the hip flexor muscles

ALTERNATIVE APPROACH

Studies suggest that the major cause of low back injury during exercise or performance of activities of daily living is lumbar instability rather than improper alignment of the spinal column and pelvis per se (McGill 2001). Research also indicates that muscle *endurance* is more protective than muscle *strength* for reducing low back injury, and that greater lumbar mobility (ROM) actually increases one's risk of low back injury (McGill 2001, 2016). Thus, sufficient stability of the lumbar spine (i.e., **lumbar stabilization**) is the major emphasis of this approach to low back care. To measure lumbar stability, see the Lumbar Stability Tests section in chapter 10. For detailed discussion and suggestions for applying the concept of lumbar stabilization to low back care programs, see Bracko (2004) and Norris (2000).

To develop and maintain lumbar stability, experts (McGill 2001) recommend the following:

- Bracing the lumbar spine during activity by isometrically cocontracting the abdominal wall and low back muscles

- Maintaining a neutral spine (i.e., the natural lordotic curve in the lumbar spine while standing upright) during activity

- Avoiding end ROM positions (fully flexed or extended) of the trunk while lifting or exercising

- Performing exercises that emphasize the development of muscle endurance rather than strength

The following sequence of exercises is specifically recommended for beginners who are starting a low back care program. These exercises are illustrated in appendix F.3.

- Cat-camel exercise to slowly and dynamically move through the full range of spinal flexion and extension, with emphasis on spinal mobility rather than pressing and holding the trunk position at the ends of the ROM (usually five or six cycles of this exercise are sufficient)

- Stretching exercises to increase mobility at the hip and knee joints

- Curl-ups with one leg flexed and hands placed underneath the lumbar spine to help in maintaining a neutral spine

- Isometric side-support (side bridge) exercises for the quadratus lumborum and abdominal oblique muscles

- Single-leg extension holds (modified bird dog exercises) while on hands and knees for the low back and hip extensor muscles

- Isometric stabilization exercises requiring simultaneous contraction of the abdominal muscles to generate an abdominal brace during performance of other exercises

- Dynamic hollowing, or drawing of the navel toward the spine, for the deeper abdominal wall muscles (i.e., transverse abdominis and internal obliques)

The North American Spine Society (2009) recommends stretching, core strengthening, and resistance training exercises to prevent back pain and to maintain a healthy back. To view images for each of these exercises, go online to www.spine.org/knowyourback and select the Prevention tab.

- Neck, inner thigh, and hamstring stretches
- Shoulder rolls and frontal core stretches
- Backward bending
- Standing thread the needle
- Doorway chest stretch
- Wall wash
- Transverse and sagittal core strengthening
- Abdominal crunch and other abdominal exercises
- Neck press
- Side bridge
- Prone bridge or plank

CORE STABILITY TESTING AND TRAINING FOR LOW BACK PAIN

There is no consensus on the definition of *core* and the measurement of **core stability** let alone whether or not it is an effective treatment or preventive strategy for low back pain. Willson and colleagues (2005) narrowly defined the core as the lumbopelvic hip complex. Akuthota and associates (2008) described the core as a muscular box bordered anteriorly by the abdominals, posteriorly by the paraspinals and gluteals, superiorly by the diaphragm, and inferiorly by the pelvic floor and hip girdle. Behm and colleagues (2010a, 2010b) used an even broader definition to include the entire axial skeleton and all soft tissue with a proximal attachment to the axial skeleton. The muscles that contribute to core stability are listed in Core Stability Muscles and Function in chapter 7. Additionally, core stability programs should consider the sensory and motor components related to these soft tissues (Akuthota et al. 2008). Kibler, Press, and Sciascia (2006) defined core stability as the "ability to control the position and motion of the trunk over the pelvis to allow optimum production, transfer and control of force and motion to the terminal segment in integrated athletic activities" (p. 189).

The Sahrmann Core Stability Test (Sahrmann 2002) described in chapter 6 is a commonly used assessment tool. Akuthota and colleagues (2008) suggested 10 exercises that place the body in all three planes to measure core stability, and Tidstrand and Horneij (2009) reported good interrater reliability for the single-leg stance and sitting on a balance ball with one leg lifted. However, all these assessments require some subjective clinical judgement. Kahraman and colleagues (2016) recently developed a core stability assessment battery that includes more objective measurements. They put 38 patients with nonspecific low back pain through 33 tests that might relate to core stability. The tests were categorized into five components of core stability: strength, endurance, flexibility, motor control, and function. They selected the tests with the highest interrater reliability in each category to create a reliable core stability test battery (*ICC* ≥.90). The

test battery proposed by Kahraman and colleagues (2016) includes the following:

- Partial curl-up test (strength)
- Side bridge (endurance)
- Trunk flexor test (endurance)
- Sit-and-reach test (flexibility)
- Single-leg hop (function)
- Lateral step-down (function)
- Unilateral stance test with eyes open (motor control)

Training strategies for developing core stability are as varied as the definition of the core. Behm and colleagues (2010a, 2010b) recommended using ground-based free weight lifts (e.g., squats, dead lifts) for training the core musculature but noted the benefit of resistance exercises on unstable surfaces and that this type of training might decrease the incidence of low back pain. Akuthota and colleagues (2008) proposed a core stability program that includes abdominal bracing from a variety of postures to isolate the transversus abdominis; quadruped arm and leg lifts (bird dog) for the paraspinals; side planks for the quadratus lumborum and obliques; and trunk curls for the rectus abdominis.

Although there is a strong theoretical basis that core stability training will aid in the prevention or treatment of low back pain, does it really work? After a systematic review of the literature, Stuber and colleagues (2014) were critical of the quantity and quality of the literature addressing this question. They noted there were very few randomized controlled trials, precluding any conclusions about whether core stability training was better than conventional treatment or training for reducing low back pain. Likewise, Davin and Callaghan (2016) determined that evidence is inconclusive that stabilization exercises are more effective than other forms of exercise for treating low back pain. In a meta-analysis with limited studies, Wang, Zheng, and associates (2012) concluded that core stability exercise is more effective than general exercise for reducing pain and disability in patients with chronic low back pain in the short term, but no longer-term (>6 mo) differences in reducing pain were observed between exercise strategies.

PILATES FOR LOW BACK PAIN

Pilates is a popular exercise method, particularly among women, that emphasizes precision of movement. Introduced in the 1920s by Joseph Pilates, it is a blend of Greek and Roman gymnastics, yoga, Zen meditation, and martial arts (Kloubec 2011). Pilates exercises emphasize stabilizing the core musculature and controlling breathing before going through a controlled ROM. The exercises can be performed on a mat or on a specialized sliding platform with springs and pulleys called a reformer.

There is strong evidence that Pilates develops abdominal muscular endurance and posterior trunk flexibility (Kibar et al. 2016; Sekendiz et al. 2007); thus, it is logical that Pilates training might be considered beneficial for treating low back pain. Considerable research exists on Pilates but of variable quality. Recently, Lin and associates (2016) conducted a systematic review of the effects of Pilates on patients with chronic nonspecific low back pain. They limited their review to only randomized controlled trials of high quality. They determined that 6 to 12 wk of Pilates training offers significant improvement in pain relief and functional capacity compared with usual or routine health care. However, other exercise treatment that includes waist or torso movement was just as effective as Pilates. Yamato and colleagues (2016) concurred, stating Pilates is more effective than minimal intervention for treating chronic low back pain but likely no better than other forms of exercise. In a recent study, men (40-55 yr) with chronic low back pain were randomly assigned to Pilates training, McKenzie back exercises, or a control group. Pain decreased and general health improved in both treatment groups, but there was no difference between Pilates and McKenzie exercises (Hasanpour-Dehkordi, Dehghani, and Solati 2017).

Key Points

▶ The specificity, overload, progression, and interindividual variability principles should be applied to designing flexibility programs.

▶ Four methods of stretching are static, dynamic, ballistic, and PNF.

▶ Some consider PNF superior to other stretching techniques for increasing ROM, but all methods (PNF, ballistic, dynamic, and static) effectively increase ROM.

▶ The contract-relax (CR) and contract-relax agonist contract (CRAC) are common PNF stretching techniques.

▶ Ballistic stretching is not generally recommended because of its high risk for injury and muscle soreness.

▶ For static stretching programs, gains in ROM are related to the total time the stretch is sustained; total time of stretching is a function of stretch duration and the number of repetitions of the exercise.

▶ A well-rounded flexibility program includes at least one exercise for each major muscle group.

▶ Muscle groups should not be stretched beyond the pain-free ROM.

▶ Typically, the duration of the stretch should be 10 to 15 sec for beginners and no more than 60 sec for more advanced clients.

▶ Beginners should start with two to four repetitions of each exercise.

▶ Flexibility exercises should be performed a minimum of 2 days/wk but preferably daily.

▶ To progressively overload the target muscle group, gradually increase the total time of the stretch (60-120 sec) by increasing the duration of stretch (10-60 sec) and the number of repetitions (4-6 reps).

▶ Stretching does not prevent overuse injuries or improve physical performance, but it may reduce the risk of muscle strains.

▶ Short-duration (<45 sec) static stretching is not detrimental to strength, power, and speed performances, and it may be included as part of the preparticipation warm-up routine.

▶ Lumbar instability is a major cause of low back problems.

▶ Exercises that develop and maintain lumbar stability are recommended for low back care programs.

▶ Exercises developing muscle endurance may be more effective than exercises developing muscle strength for the prevention and treatment of low back injuries.

▶ The Sahrmann Core Stability Test (Sahrmann 2002) is popular among clinicians, and the test battery by Kahraman and colleagues (2016) has excellent interrater reliability.

▶ It is questionable whether core stability training and Pilates are any more effective than conventional exercise training that includes the torso for reducing low back pain.

Key Terms

Learn the definition of each of the following key terms. Definition of terms can be found in the glossary.

active-assisted stretching

active stretching

autogenic inhibition

ballistic stretching

contract-relax agonist contract (CRAC) technique

contract-relax (CR) technique

core stability

dynamic stretching

flexibility training

lumbar stabilization

passive stretching

pelvic stabilization

Pilates

proprioceptive neuromuscular facilitation (PNF)

reciprocal inhibition

static stretching

stress relaxation

stretch tolerance

viscoelastic creep

Review Questions

In addition to being able to define each of the key terms, test your knowledge and understanding of the material by answering the following review questions.

1. Explain why ballistic stretching is not usually recommended for flexibility programs.

2. Identify two sensory receptors of the musculotendinous unit, and explain how each receptor is affected by slow static stretching.

3. What are the physiological mechanisms responsible for gains in ROM from PNF stretching?

4. Identify three high-risk flexibility exercises and suggest safe alternatives.

5. What are the advantages and disadvantages of slow static, dynamic, and PNF stretching?

6. Describe the basic guidelines for designing flexibility programs. Explain how the specificity and overload training principles apply.

7. Explain why stretching does not prevent injury.

8. Describe three abdominal exercises that have high challenge-to-compression ratios.

9. What are the similarities and differences between the traditional and alternative approaches to low back care programs?

10. Describe the recommended sequence of exercises for starting a low back care program.

CHAPTER 12

Assessing Balance and Designing Balance Programs

KEY QUESTIONS

▶ What are static and dynamic balance?

▶ What factors affect balance?

▶ How is balance assessed?

▶ What are general guidelines for balance testing?

▶ What is balance training?

▶ What types of exercise are best suited for improving balance?

▶ What are the general recommendations for designing balance training programs?

Although balance is not generally included in health-related physical fitness test batteries, it is gaining recognition as a key component of functional fitness. In the past, balance was viewed primarily as a performance-based measure, with balance training geared toward improving sport performance. In a worldwide survey of fitness trends for 2018, fitness programs for older adults and functional fitness ranked number 9 and 10, respectively (Thompson 2017).

Balance is an especially important component of functional fitness for older adults in terms of preventing falls, performing activities of daily living (ADLs), and maintaining functional independence. In the United States, more than one in four older adults (65 yr or older) fall each year; falling is the leading cause of injury deaths among older adults (Bergen, Stevens, and Burns 2016). Over the past decade, the rate of fall-related deaths rose steadily in this population (www.cdc.gov/injury/wisqars). To reduce the risk of falling, older adults are encouraged to exercise regularly and to engage in physical activity modes that improve strength, power, and balance. The most recent Physical Activity Guidelines for

Americans (U.S. Department of Health and Human Services 2008) and the Canadian Physical Activity Guidelines (Tremblay et al. 2011) recommend that older ($\geq$65 yr) adults with poor mobility participate in balance activities. Also, the American College of Sports Medicine position statements on exercise for older adults (Chodzko-Zajko et al. 2009) and the quality and quantity of exercise for developing and maintaining fitness (Garber et al. 2011) recommend balance and neuromotor training for older individuals with poor mobility or at risk for falls. **Neuromotor training** includes exercises to improve balance, agility, gait, coordination, and proprioception (American College of Sports Medicine 2018; Bushman 2011, 2012). This type of training is especially beneficial as part of comprehensive exercise programs for older adults.

This chapter presents definitions and theoretical frameworks for balance and describes tools and tests for its assessment. Guidelines for balance testing are presented along with norms for selected balance tests. Suggestions for designing training programs to improve balance are also provided.

DEFINITIONS AND NATURE OF BALANCE

Balance is the ability to keep the body's center of gravity within the base of support when one is maintaining a static position, performing voluntary movements, or reacting to external disturbances. Postural stability and equilibrium are terms often used to refer to the construct of balance. Clinically, balance is commonly thought of as static or dynamic. **Static balance** is the ability to maintain the center of gravity within the supporting base while standing or sitting, whereas **dynamic balance** refers to maintaining an upright position while the center of gravity and base of support are moving and the center of gravity is moving outside of the supporting base (e.g., walking). **Reactive balance** is the ability to compensate and recover from perturbations while standing or walking (e.g., maintaining balance after tripping over an obstacle). **Functional balance** refers to the ability to perform daily movement tasks requiring balance such as picking up an object from the floor, dressing, and turning to look at something behind you.

Balance is a complex construct involving multiple biomechanical, neurological, and environmental systems. Over the years, the theoretical frameworks dealing with balance have moved from reflex and hierarchical perspectives to a dynamic systems model that describes how these systems function and interact to achieve balance and postural control. The reflex model assumes that sensory input controls motor output; the hierarchical model is based on control of movement by higher brain centers (e.g., cortex and midbrain). The dynamic systems model describes balance control as adaptive and functional, providing multiple solutions for accomplishing a movement goal. In this model, the higher brain centers work in conjunction with lower centers rather than control them. The visual, somatosensory (proprioception), and vestibular (inner ear) systems interact to maintain balance. The visual system provides information about the body's location relative to its environment; the somatosensory system discerns position and movements of body parts; the vestibular system provides information about head position in relation to gravity and senses how fast and in what direction the head is accelerating.

In addition, internal factors such as muscle tone, strength, and range of motion, as well as environmental factors, contribute to balance.

FACTORS AFFECTING BALANCE AND RISK OF FALLING

Balance is related to age, gender, body size, and physical fitness level. This section addresses some commonly asked questions about balance and the risk of falling.

How does body size affect balance?

The height of the body's center of gravity relative to the supporting base affects balance. The higher the center of gravity is from the base of support, the lower the stability. Shorter individuals have a lower center of gravity and therefore potentially greater stability compared with taller individuals. Both height and body weight are predictors of postural sway.

Does foot size affect balance?

There is a direct relationship between the size of the supporting base and stability; the larger the supporting base, the greater the stability. A larger base of support allows the vertical projection of the body's center of gravity (i.e., **line of gravity**) to move a greater distance before falling outside of the supporting base and losing balance. This explains why it is more difficult to maintain your balance while standing on the tips of your toes than when standing on both feet. Foot size (length and width) may affect balance especially when one is performing tasks that require standing on one leg.

Do women have better static balance than men?

Gender differences in skeletal structure (e.g., shape of pelvis) and body shape (apple vs. pear shaped) affect the location of the center of gravity within the body. Typically in women, the relative height of the center of gravity from the supporting base during standing tends to be lower than that of men (~55% and 57% of standing height, respectively) because of the wider pelvic structure of women and their tendency to be pear shaped. Therefore, one might hypothesize that static balance ability of women may be somewhat better than that of men. However, research does not support this. There were no gender differences in unipedal (one-leg) stance performance with eyes open and closed for adults 18 to 99 yr of age (Springer et al. 2007) or for adolescent track and field athletes (Knight et al. 2016).

How does preactivity stretching affect balance performance?

Some research suggests that preactivity stretching impairs physical performance by decreasing muscular strength and power (see chapter 11). Since strength and power are related to balance, one might speculate that stretching may negatively affect balance performance. In fact, a couple of studies reported that acute static stretching (stretch duration of 45 sec) decreases balance (Hoshang Bakhtiary, Aminian-Far, and Hedayati 2013; Behm et al. 2004). Both anterior-posterior and medial-lateral dynamic balance decreased in females assigned to three sets of 45 sec static stretches (hamstrings, quadriceps, and gastrocnemius), but there was no balance deficit in a group that did only 15 sec stretches (Hoshang Bakhtiary, Aminian-Far, and Hedayati 2013). On the other hand, some studies reported that shorter-duration (≤15 sec) static stretching and PNF CRAC stretching (proprioceptive neuromuscular facilitation; contract-relax with agonist contraction) significantly improve postural stability and dynamic balance of healthy young women and men (Costa et al. 2009; Nelson et al. 2012; Ryan, Rossi, and Lopez 2010).

What factors contribute to the risk of falling?

In addition to extrinsic factors (e.g., poor lighting, loose rugs, and obstacles in walkways), intrinsic factors contribute to the risk of falling. Factors such as muscle weakness and gait and balance problems are the second most common cause for falls in older adults (Rubenstein and Josephson 2002). Additionally, the ability to produce force quickly (i.e., muscle power) declines more rapidly than strength with advancing age (Granacher, Gruber, and Gollhofer 2010). Muscle power may be more relevant than muscle strength for preventing falls. The inability to compensate for unexpected disturbances in stance and gait (i.e., reactive balance), as well as the inability to maintain balance while simultaneously performing cognitive or other motor functions, may increase a person's risk of falling.

To assess risk of falling, Granacher and colleagues (2012) recommend a test battery that measures muscle power, dynamic steady-state balance under multitask conditions, and reactive balance. Recently, Kim and associates (2017) found that the Short Physical Performance Battery developed by Guralnik and colleagues in 1994 is a suitable screening tool for risk of falls, as fallers had significantly lower scores on this test battery than nonfallers in their study of 307 older adults aged 65 to 92 yr. This test battery measures lower limb function. It involves an assessment of standing balance with progressively more challenging foot positions, a 4 m walking test to assess gait speed, and five repetitions of standing as fast as possible from a seated position. This test battery was more associated with fall history than the timed up-and-go test or the Berg Balance Scale (both described later in this chapter).

Does regular exercise reduce the risk of falling?

Regular exercise may be one way to prevent falls and fall-related fractures. Carter and associates (2001) reported that impairments in muscle and joint function, the vestibular system, vision, proprioception, cognition, static and dynamic balance, and gait predispose individuals to falls and fractures. Balance, resistance, and flexibility training programs were more effective than endurance training for reducing risk of falling (Province et al. 1995). In a position statement from Exercise and Sports Science Australia, the authors declared that exercise is an effective method of preventing falls, but they stressed that the exercise prescription should progressively challenge balance (Tiedemann et al. 2011). Similarly, Shubert (2011) commented that an exercise program to prevent falls should focus on at least two of the following three modes of balance exercises: (1) movement around the center of mass, (2) use of a narrow base of support, and (3) minimal upper extremity support. Furthermore, 50 hr of balance training is the minimal dose to offer a protective effect against falling for older adults (Shubert 2011). General recommendations for exercises that challenge balance and therefore reduce the risk of falling are presented later in this chapter.

If exercise is an effective means of preventing falls, it is logical that exercise would also reduce the fear of falling in older adults. However, research suggests that this reduction is only small to moderate immediately after the exercise intervention and may not last long term (Kendrick et al. 2014). The investigators noted that the quality of research on this topic is poor, and there is a need for well-designed randomized trials.

ASSESSMENT OF BALANCE

Direct measures of balance may be obtained using computerized force plate devices to assess the adaptive functioning of the sensory, motor, and biomechanical components in accordance with the dynamic systems model of balance. For those who do not have access to the advanced technology necessary to obtain direct measures, field and clinical tests are available for assessing static and dynamic balance, as are tests of functional balance using indirect measures. For detailed descriptions and illustrations for static and dynamic balance field tests, see Reiman and Manske (2009). Because balance is complex, most balance test batteries are comprehensive and include multiple test items to assess both static and dynamic balance. A single simple test such as the one-leg stance may be limited in that it measures only a few of the components of balance.

ASSESSING STATIC AND DYNAMIC BALANCE WITH DIRECT MEASURES

The application of technology to balance assessment has produced a number of excellent computerized systems to assess static and dynamic balance. Generally, the relatively high cost (some >$100,000 U.S.) of these computerized systems, however, precludes their usefulness in most field and clinical settings. These systems consist of a computerized force plate with three or more force transducers that quantify vertical pressures applied to the support platform. These vertical pressures are used to derive the anteroposterior and mediolateral coordinates of the **center of pressure**. The systems provide data about postural sway and steadiness while the client remains motion-

less, with weight distribution between the feet, the ability to move the center of vertical force (center of pressure) to maintain balance, and automatic motor responses to platform disturbances (Guskiewicz and Perrin 1996). Force platform balance tests provide valid information about postural control that can be used to predict risk of falling among older people with and without a history of balance problems or falling (Pajala et al. 2008).

Computerized dynamic posturography assesses the individual and composite functioning of sensory, motor, and biomechanical components of balance (e.g., NeuroCom Equitest; figure 12.1). The motor control tests provide data about the client's responses to sudden movements of the force plate that threaten

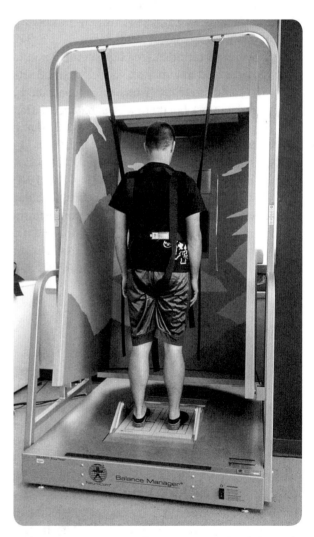

FIGURE 12.1 NeuroCom computerized dynamic posturography.

Dale R. Wagner.

USING NINTENDO WII TO ASSESS BALANCE

As a low-cost alternative to expensive force platforms and sophisticated, computerized posturography devices, the Nintendo Wii balance board has been successfully used to assess static and dynamic balance. When compared against laboratory tests, the Wii balance board yields valid and reliable measures of unidirectional and rotational displacement of the center of pressure for younger and older adults (Clark et al. 2010; Kalisch et al. 2011). The Wii balance board test was poorly correlated with functional mobility (timed up-and-go test and obstacle course) in a sample of seniors (Reed-Jones et al. 2012). However, the authors discovered a relationship between the Wii balance score and visual processing speed, suggesting that the Wii Fit balance test may provide supplemental information not obtained from standard functional mobility and balance tests. For the technical specifications of the Wii balance board (e.g., drift, hysteresis) for measuring center of pressure, see Weaver, Ma, and Laing (2017). For a review of the balance research that has been done using the Wii Fit, see Goble, Cone, and Fling (2014).

balance (i.e., reactive balance). The sensory organization tests examine the client's ability to maintain an upright posture when visual and proprioceptive sensory information is modified mechanically (Nashner 1997). This test has moderate to good validity and reliability for assessing the dynamic postural stability of physically active adults and older adults (Dickin and Clark 2007; Dickin 2010). The NeuroCom Balance Master can be used to assess functional tasks such as walking, turning, and changing posture (e.g., sitting to standing). It measures weight symmetry, weight shifts, and limits of stability.

The **limits of stability** test, a measure of the maximum excursion of the center of gravity, assesses the degree to which the individual is able to lean in several directions while maintaining balance over a fixed supporting base (Clark et al. 2005). Research shows this test provides reliable scores and predicts risk of falling (Clark, Rose, and Fujimoto 1997; Wallman 2001). The limits of stability in normal adults are 12° in the anteroposterior plane and 16° in the mediolateral direction.

The Biodex Stability System may be used to evaluate and train neuromuscular control by quantifying the ability to maintain dynamic postural stability on both stable and unstable surfaces. This system provides ongoing visual feedback to the individual while attempting to reproduce specified movement patterns of the center of gravity. Using the Biodex Stability System, one calculates the stability index by dividing the client's anteroposterior score (measured in degrees) by the normal value (12°) and multiplying by 100. Similarly, to calculate the mediolateral stability index, one divides the client's score by the normal value (16°) and multiplies by

100. Combined values less than 100% are indicative of balance problems (de Bruin et al. 2009).

In fitness, athletic, and rehabilitation settings, less expensive balance systems can be used to assess neuromuscular control, proprioception, and mechanoreceptor input (e.g., Biodex Stability System and Kinesthetic Ability Trainer). These systems, however, do not have the ability to quantify the vestibular and visual components of balance. Typically, they consist of a multiaxial platform positioned on a U-joint with eight movable springs, and they are used for balance training.

ASSESSING STATIC BALANCE WITH INDIRECT MEASURES

As early as the mid-1800s, Romberg developed tests to measure static balance with a narrowed base of support during standing. Steady-state static balance while standing can be assessed under single-task conditions (i.e., standing only) or multitask conditions (standing while performing other motor or cognitive tasks). To assess risk of falling, reactive balance should also be evaluated. This section describes the protocols for various types of static balance tests and reactive balance tests that may be easily used in field or clinical settings.

Romberg Tests

The Romberg tests measure static balance during standing with eyes open and eyes closed. For the original Romberg test, the client stands barefoot with arms folded across the chest and the feet close together in the frontal plane (Romberg test = feet side by side). For the modified Romberg test, also known as the sharpened Romberg test, the client stands barefoot using a tandem stance (feet positioned heel to toe) with eyes open and eyes closed. These tests are scored objectively; the number of seconds the client maintains a steady position without swaying, up to a maximum of 60 sec, is recorded.

The side-by-side and tandem stance tests were primarily developed to discriminate between poor and acceptable balance in elderly individuals. The test-retest reliability of the tandem stance test ranges from .76 (eyes closed) to .91 (eyes open) (Franchignoni et al. 1998). Shubert and colleagues (2006) reported that the tandem stance test is moderately related to walking speed ($r = .50$) and dynamic balance ($r = .46$) in older adults (65 yr and older) who are able to walk independently. Likewise, Gras and colleagues (2017) reported a moderate correlation between the modified Romberg test and a 10 m walk ($r = .45$) but strong correlations to the Berg Balance Scale ($r = .64$) and timed up-and-go test ($r = -.65$). Older adults who could maintain this tandem stance for 30 sec with eyes open scored better on the Berg and up-and-go tests than those who could not complete 30 sec of the modified Romberg test. Pajala and associates (2008) noted that the inability to complete the tandem stance is a significant predictor of fall risk. However, other researchers observed that the side-by-side and tandem stance tests have poor validity for predicting falls in older adults (Yim-Chiplis and Talbot 2000) and do not discriminate between individuals on the lower and higher ends of the balance spectrum (Curb et al. 2006).

Unipedal Stance Test

Video 12.1

The unipedal stance test, or timed one-leg stance test, also provides a simple measure of static balance performance. The validity of this test has been demonstrated by its relationship with gait performance, risk of falling, and ability to perform activities of daily living (ADLs) for older adults (Bohannon 2006a). The test-retest reliability of the one-leg stance ranges from .74 (eyes closed) to .91 (eyes open) (Whitney, Poole, and Cass 1998). This widely used test provides a reliable measure of static balance for children and adults (Emery 2003; Emery et al. 2005; Muehlbauer et al. 2011). The one-leg stance test makes up the balance assessment portion for a new field-based physical fitness test battery for preschool children (Ortega et al. 2015). At the opposite end of the age spectrum, poor one-leg stance performance is a powerful predictor of low back pain in older (70-85 yr) adults (Husu and Suni 2012).

For this test, the client stands on one leg with eyes open and closed. The test is scored as the number of seconds the client is able to maintain balance on the dominant leg. In a meta-analysis, Bohannon (2006b) reported that testing procedures for the one-leg stance test are not standardized. The following are some of the testing procedures that varied:

- Client was barefoot or wearing shoes.
- Dominant, nondominant, or both legs were tested.
- Maximum duration of the test varied between 5 and 60 sec.
- Number of trials varied from one to five.

Table 12.1 Age-Gender Norms for the Unipedal (One-Leg) Stance Test

| Age group (yr) | EYES OPEN (SEC) | | EYES CLOSED (SEC) | |
	Females	Males	Females	Males
18-39	45.1	44.4	13.1	16.9
40-49	42.1	41.6	13.5	12.0
50-59	40.9	41.5	7.9	8.6
60-69	30.4	33.8	3.6	5.1
70-79	16.7	25.9	3.7	2.6
80-99	10.6	8.7	2.1	1.8

Note: Maximum test duration is 45 sec. Use best of three trials.

Data from Springer et al. 2007.

TEST PROCEDURES FOR UNIPEDAL STANCE TEST

1. Determine clients' dominant leg by having them kick a ball.

2. Prior to raising one leg off the floor, clients fold their arms across the chest.

3. Clients stand barefoot on their dominant leg and raise the other foot near to but not touching the ankle of the stance limb. Start the stopwatch as soon as clients lift their foot off the floor.

4. For the eyes-open test, clients focus on a spot on the wall at eye level throughout the test.

5. Terminate the test when a client does any of the following:
   - Uncrosses or uses arms to maintain balance
   - Moves the raised foot away from the standing limb or touches the floor with the raised foot
   - Moves the weight-bearing foot to maintain balance
   - Exceeds maximum duration of 45 sec
   - Opens eyes during the eyes-closed one-leg stance test

6. Administer three trials and use the best score.

- Dependent measure was either best score or average of the trials.

The test duration most frequently reported in the 22 studies that Bohannon reviewed was 30 sec. The average one-leg stance (eyes open) time for apparently healthy older adults declined across age groups: 27.0 sec for 60 to 69 yr, 17.2 sec for 70 to 79 yr, and 8.5 sec for 80 to 99 yr. Springer and colleagues (2007) developed age-gender norms for the unipedal stance test (eyes open and closed) for adults 18 yr to 99 yr (see table 12.1). To use these norms, be certain to follow recommended testing procedures (see Test Procedures for Unipedal Stance Test).

Video 12.2

Balance Error Scoring System (BESS)

The Balance Error Scoring System (BESS), first described by Riemann, Guskiewicz, and Shields in 1999, is a field test of static balance that combines the Romberg tests and unipedal stance test. The BESS involves three stances: (1) feet side by side (Romberg), (2) standing on nondominant foot (unipedal) with contralateral limb in 20° to 30° of hip flexion and 40° to 50° of knee flexion, and (3) tandem with the heel of the dominant foot touching the toes of the nondominant foot. These three stances are performed twice, once on a firm surface (figure 12.2) and once on a medium-density foam pad (45 cm² × 13 cm thick, density 60 kg/m³; figure 12.3). Instruct clients to place

their hands on the iliac crest and close their eyes for each trial. Each stance is held for 20 sec.

The BESS is scored by summing 1 point for each error committed during each of the six 20-sec trials. If the client is unable to sustain the stance position for more than 5 sec, the trial is considered incomplete and is assigned a maximal error score of 10. The following are the errors to be scored in the BESS:

- Lifting hands off iliac crest
- Opening eyes
- Stepping, stumbling, or falling
- Moving hip into more than 30° of flexion or abduction
- Lifting forefoot or heel
- Remaining out of testing position for more than 5 sec

The BESS was originally validated against objective sway measures obtained by a NeuroCom (Riemann, Guskiewicz, and Shields 1999). The intraclass correlation coefficients for interrater reliability ranged from .78 to .96. In a review of the BESS, criterion-related validity was reported as moderate to high, and reliability ranged from moderate to good (Bell et al. 2011). Since very few errors occur during the double-leg stance on both firm and foam surfaces, Hunt and colleagues (2009) suggested eliminating this portion of the

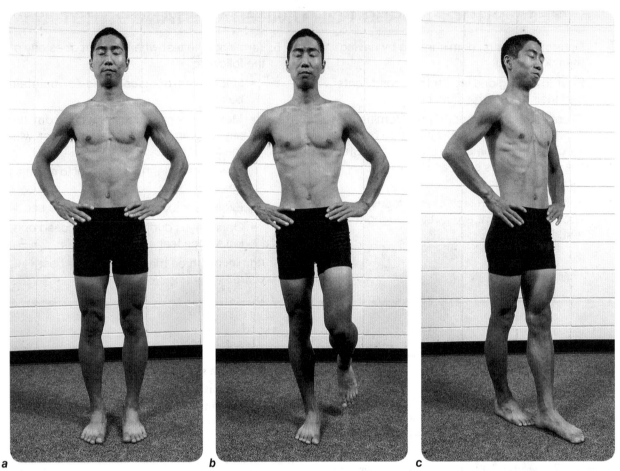

FIGURE 12.2 BESS test on firm surface: *(a)* feet side by side; *(b)* balanced on nondominant foot; *(c)* heel of dominant foot touching toes of nondominant foot.

test. With the double-leg stance condition removed, intraclass reliability increased. Hunt and colleagues (2009) suggested three trials of just four conditions (one-leg and tandem, both firm and foam), and this has become known as the modified BESS. Given that the BESS is an inexpensive, quick, and easy-to-administer field test, it is used in a variety of settings and populations, most commonly as a sideline assessment in the management of sport-related concussion (Guskiewicz 2011). The BESS can detect balance deficits in those who are concussed or fatigued, and BESS scores increase with ankle instability and age (Bell et al. 2011).

Reactive Balance Tests

Reactive balance tests assess the individual's ability to compensate and recover balance in response to unexpected external forces or perturbations.

Research suggests that tests of static, dynamic, and functional balance might be related, but reactive postural control is an independent domain of balance (Klein, Fiedler, and Rose 2011). The nudge test and postural stress test can be used to subjectively assess the reactive balance of your clients. For the nudge test, the examiner pushes against the sternum with light pressure while the client is standing with feet together. The response to this perturbation is graded on a scale of 0 to 2: 0 = client starts to fall and needs assistance to prevent falling; 1 = client maintains balance by moving the feet; and 2 = client remains stable throughout the test (Wild, Nayak, and Isaacs 1981). Given the subjective nature of this test, it may be best used as a quick and easy way to identify clients in need of a more sophisticated assessment of balance. The postural stress test measures the client's ability to recover standing balance in response

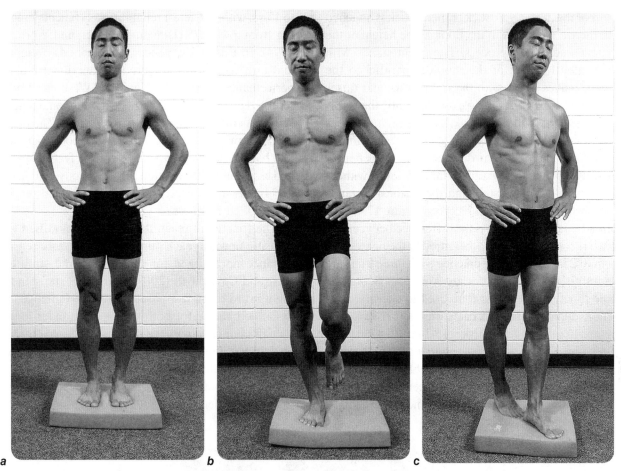

FIGURE 12.3 BESS test on balance pad: *(a)* feet side by side; *(b)* balanced on nondominant foot; *(c)* heel of dominant foot touching toes of nondominant foot.

to varying degrees of perturbations using a pulley weight system that displaces the center of gravity posteriorly. Three intensities of force relative to the client's body mass (i.e., 1.5%, 3%, and 4% of body mass) are applied to the client's waist. A 10-point scale is used to evaluate reactive balance, with a score of 0 indicating failure to remain upright and a score of 9 representing an efficient postural response to maintain a standing posture (Chandler, Duncan, and Studenski 1990).

ASSESSING DYNAMIC BALANCE WITH INDIRECT MEASURES

Dynamic balance is the ability to maintain postural stability while moving. Dynamic balance involves completing functional tasks without compromising

the base of support while moving; it is important for preventing falls, especially in older adults and children, and for preventing sport injuries in athletes and physically active individuals. This section describes field tests and clinical protocols for tests of dynamic balance of children, older adults, and athletes.

Functional Reach Tests

The functional reach test was developed to measure dynamic balance of adults by determining the maximum distance an individual can reach beyond arm's length without losing balance or moving the feet (Duncan et al. 1990). The validity of this test is good, with concurrent validity coefficients ranging between .64 (one-leg stance test) and .71 (center-of-pressure excursion). The test-retest reliability was .86 to .88 (Franchignoni et al. 1998; Whitney, Poole, and Cass 1998).

Video 12.3

For this test, a yardstick or meter stick is attached to the wall, parallel to the floor, at the height of the client's acromion process. The client stands with the lateral aspect of the shoulder parallel to the wall, makes a fist with the right hand, and raises the right arm with elbow extended until the fist is at the height of the yardstick. The initial measure is the point along the measuring stick corresponding to the distal end of the third metacarpal. The client is instructed to reach forward as far as possible without falling or taking a step, and the farthest distance reached along the stick is recorded (figure 12.4). The functional reach score is the difference between the two recorded distances, measured to the nearest 0.5 cm (0.25 in.). After one practice trial, three trials are administered, and scores are averaged. Scores on the functional reach test are used to classify older individuals into fall risk categories: low risk = >25.4 cm (>10 in.); moderate risk = 15.24 to 25.4 cm (6-10 in.); high risk = <15.24 cm (<6 in.); very high risk = unable to reach (Duncan et al. 1990, 1992).

The functional reach test has been used to assess the dynamic balance of children and adolescents, 5 to 15 yr, with test-retest reliability coefficients ranging from .64 to .75 (Donahue, Turner, and Worrell 1994). In this study, gender, height, body weight, and arm length did not predict functional reach performance. Conversely, Habib and Westcott (1998) reported that 17% of the variance in functional reach scores of children is attributed to age, and 15% of the variance may be attributed to height, body weight, and base of support (i.e., length of the feet). Norris and associates (2008) noted that only body weight (r = .34) was significantly related to functional reach scores of children 3 to 5 yr.

The functional reach test has been modified to measure upward reach during standing, with reach distance normalized for foot length and stature. Row and Cavanaugh (2007) stated that the standing upward reach test posed a greater challenge to dynamic balance for both younger and older individuals compared with the forward functional reach test. In addition, the reach strategy (i.e., whether or not the heels were raised from the floor during the test) accounted for differences in reach performances of older adults.

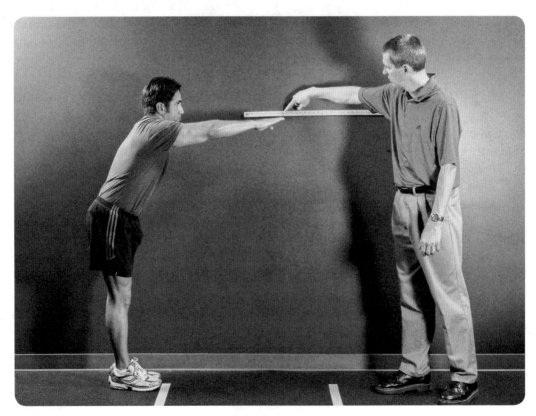

FIGURE 12.4 The functional reach balance test.

Thompson and Medley (2007) proposed a variation of the functional reach test to assess the forward and lateral reach of adults 21 to 97 yr while sitting in a chair. This modification of the functional reach test can be used to assess the dynamic balance and risk of falling for individuals who use wheelchairs or frail older adults who cannot perform the standing functional reach test. The researchers reported that sitting reach scores of older adults are significantly less than those of younger and middle-aged adults. In addition, length of the arms did not affect performance.

Timed Up-and-Go Tests

Video
12.4

Timed up-and-go tests are used to assess dynamic balance and agility. These performance attributes are related to functional abilities such as getting up from a seated position to answer the phone or doorbell in a timely manner; therefore, this test is typically included in balance test batteries for older adults. Podsiadlo and Richardson (1991) described the timed up-and-go test as the amount of time needed to rise from an armchair, walk to a line 3 m (10 ft) away, turn, and return to a seated position in the chair. The timed up-and-go test has excellent test-retest reliability ($r = .99$), and test scores are related to gait speed, stair climbing, risk of falling, postural stability, and cognitive ability (Bohannon 2006a; Herman, Giladi, and Hausdorff 2011; Oh

et al. 2011; Shumway-Cook, Brauer, and Woollacott 2000). Pondal and del Ser (2008) reported that approximately 26% of the variance in timed up-and-go scores of older adults (71-99 yr) without gait disturbances is explained by age, gender, body weight, nutrition status, and cognitive impairment.

The testing procedures used for the timed up-and-go test have varied. In some studies, chairs differ in terms of seat height (40-50 cm) and style (armchair or armless chair). Although almost all studies have the clients walking a distance of 10 ft (3 m), Rikli and Jones (2013) provide performance norms for an 8 ft (2.44 m) up-and-go test for older adults. Also, instructions for this test vary from walking at a normal pace to walking as quickly as possible. Usually more than one trial is administered (Bohannon 2006a). Each of these factors affects performance scores. Therefore, when using norms to evaluate your clients' performance on this test, make certain you administer the test in the same manner and with the same instructions used to develop the test norms.

On the basis of a meta-analysis of 21 studies that included 4,395 older adults (60-99 yr), Bohannon (2006a) concluded that timed up-and-go scores exceeding 9.0 sec for 60 to 69 yr, 10.2 sec for 70 to 79 yr, and 12.7 sec for 80 to 99 yr are considered to be worse than average for these age groups. Table 12.2 presents age-gender norms for older (>70 yr)

Table 12.2 Age-Gender Norms for the 3 m (10 ft) Timed Up-and-Go Test

| Percentile | AGE GROUP (YR) | | | | | | | |
| | 71-75 YR | | 76-80 YR | | 81-85 YR | | 86-99 YR | |
	M	F	M	F	M	F	M	F
95	13.3	15.0	14.3	18.6	19.5	20.0	21.0	22.0
90	11.0	14.0	13.6	15.2	14.0	17.6	18.2	19.6
80	10.0	13.0	11.0	13.0	13.0	15.0	13.8	16.0
70	9.0	12.0	10.0	12.0	12.0	14.2	12.0	15.0
60	9.0	11.0	10.0	11.0	10.0	12.0	11.2	13.8
50	8.0	10.0	9.0	10.0	9.0	12.0	11.0	12.0
40	8.0	10.0	8.0	9.4	8.0	11.0	10.6	12.0
30	7.0	9.0	7.0	9.0	8.0	10.0	8.1	10.4
20	7.0	9.0	7.0	8.0	8.0	10.0	7.4	9.8
10	6.4	7.5	7.0	6.6	7.0	8.0	6.7	9.0
5	5.7	7.0	6.0	5.8	6.0	8.0	6.0	9.0
1	5.0	6.0	5.0	5.0	5.0	8.0	6.0	9.0

M = males; F = females.

Note: Score is measured in seconds.

Data from Pondal and del Ser 2008.

adults (Pondal and del Ser 2008). For this variation of the timed up-and-go test, an armless chair with a 40 to 45 cm (about 16-18 in.) seat height was used. At the signal to go, subjects were instructed to stand up, walk toward the marker (10 ft or 3 m distance), turn around, walk back to the chair, and sit down again as quickly as possible.

As part of the Senior Fitness Test battery, Rikli and Jones (2013) suggest the 8 ft (2.44 m) timed up-and-go test for assessing the balance and agility of older adults. This test has excellent test-retest reliability ($r = .95$) and is able to categorize older adults according to functional independence. Table 12.3 presents age-gender norms for the 8 ft up-and-go test.

Purpose: Assess dynamic balance and agility.

Application: A measure of the ability to perform ADLs such as getting up quickly to answer the phone or go to the bathroom.

Equipment: You will need a folding chair that has a seat height of 17 in. (43 cm) and that will not tip forward, as well as a measuring tape and cone marker.

Test procedures: Place the folding chair against a wall for stability, and have your client sit in the middle of the chair, with hands on thighs, one leg slightly ahead of the other, and body leaning slightly forward. On the signal "go," have the client get up from the chair, walk as quickly as possible around a cone placed 8 ft

Table 12.3 Age-Gender Norms for 8 ft Timed Up-and-Go Test

Percentile rank	TIME (SEC)													
	60-64 YR		65-69 YR		70-74 YR		75-79 YR		80-84 YR		85-89 YR		90-94 YR	
	F	M	F	M	F	M	F	M	F	M	F	M	F	M
95	3.2	3.0	3.6	3.1	3.8	3.2	4.0	3.3	4.0	4.0	4.5	4.0	5.0	4.3
90	3.7	3.0	4.1	3.6	4.0	3.6	4.3	3.5	4.4	4.1	4.7	4.3	5.3	4.5
85	4.0	3.3	4.4	3.9	4.3	3.9	4.6	3.9	4.9	4.5	5.3	4.5	6.1	5.1
80	4.2	3.6	4.6	4.1	4.7	4.2	5.0	4.3	5.4	4.9	5.8	5.0	6.7	5.7
75	4.4	3.8	4.8	4.3	4.9	4.4	5.2	4.6	5.7	5.2	6.2	5.5	7.3	6.2
70	4.6	4.0	5.0	4.5	5.2	4.6	5.5	4.9	6.1	5.5	6.6	5.8	7.7	6.6
65	4.7	4.2	5.1	4.6	5.4	4.8	5.7	5.2	6.3	5.7	6.9	6.2	8.2	7.0
60	4.9	4.4	5.3	4.8	5.6	5.0	5.9	5.4	6.7	6.0	7.3	6.5	8.6	7.4
55	5.0	4.5	5.4	4.9	5.8	5.1	6.1	5.7	6.9	6.2	7.6	6.9	9.0	7.7
50	5.2	4.7	5.6	5.1	6.0	5.3	6.3	5.9	7.2	6.4	7.9	7.2	9.4	8.1
45	5.4	4.9	5.8	5.3	6.2	5.5	6.5	6.1	7.5	6.6	8.2	7.5	9.8	8.5
40	5.5	5.0	5.9	5.4	6.4	5.6	6.7	6.4	7.8	6.9	8.5	7.9	10.2	8.8
35	5.7	5.2	6.1	5.6	6.6	5.8	6.9	6.6	8.1	7.1	8.9	8.2	10.6	9.2
30	5.8	5.4	6.2	5.7	6.8	6.0	7.1	6.9	8.3	7.3	9.2	8.6	11.1	9.6
25	6.0	5.6	6.4	5.9	7.1	6.2	7.4	7.2	8.7	7.6	9.6	8.9	11.5	10.0
20	6.2	5.8	6.6	6.1	7.3	6.4	7.6	7.5	9.0	7.9	10.0	9.4	12.1	10.5
15	6.4	6.1	6.8	6.3	7.7	6.7	8.0	7.9	9.5	8.3	10.5	9.9	12.7	11.1
10	6.7	6.4	7.1	6.6	8.0	7.0	8.3	8.3	10.0	8.7	11.1	10.5	13.5	11.8
5	7.2	6.8	7.6	7.1	8.6	7.4	8.9	9.0	10.8	9.4	12.0	11.5	14.6	12.9

Note: Score is measured in seconds.

F = females; M = males.

Adapted by permission from R. Rikli and C. Jones, *Senior Fitness Test Manual*, 2nd ed. (Champaign, IL: Human Kinetics, 2013), 160.

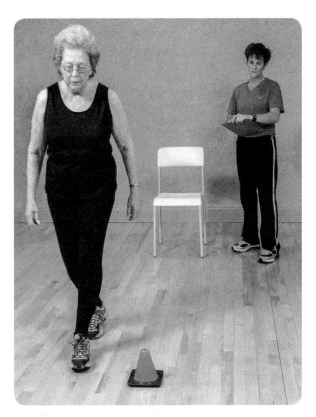

FIGURE 12.5 The 8 ft timed up-and-go test.

(2.44 m) away, and return to the chair (figure 12.5). Administer one practice trial followed by two test trials.

Scoring: Start the stopwatch exactly on the signal to go, and stop it at the exact time the client sits in the chair. Record the score to the nearest tenth of a second. Compare the best score of the two trials against the norms in table 12.3.

Star Excursion Balance Test and Y Balance Test

The star excursion balance test is a measure of dynamic balance that provides a significant challenge to athletes and physically active individuals. For this test, the individual must maintain a base of support on one leg while maximally reaching in different directions in a star pattern with the opposite leg. The goal of the test is to minimize displacement of the center of pressure and to maximize reach distance while maintaining unilateral support. The star excursion balance test is useful for screening deficits in dynamic postural control due to

musculoskeletal injuries (e.g., ankle instability) and during the rehabilitation of orthopedic injuries in otherwise healthy, physically active adults (Olmsted et al. 2002; Hegedus et al. 2015). For example, side-to-side asymmetry in the anterior direction may help identify athletes at risk for sustaining noncontact injuries to the lower limb (Stiffler et al. 2017). The reliability of this test ranges between .85 and .96 (Hertel, Miller, and Deneger 2000).

Although height and leg length were significantly related to excursion distance, foot type (pes planus, cavus, or rectus) and range of motion at the hip and ankle were not. Given that leg length accounted for 23% of variance in excursion distance, Gribble and Hertel (2003) recommend normalizing the test scores for leg length. To accomplish this, divide the excursion distance by the client's leg length and multiply by 100. Leg length is measured as the distance from the anterior superior iliac spine to the center of the medial malleolus with the client lying supine. Different foot alignments and hand positions also alter the reach distances, and maintaining the hands on the hips while changing the toe/heel position has been suggested for standardization (Cug 2017).

The star excursion balance test is performed with the client standing (preferably barefoot) in the middle of a grid formed by eight lines extending from the center at 45° from each other (see figure 12.6). The client is allowed six practice trials in each of the eight directions on each leg. Clients begin reaching in the anterior direction and progress clockwise around the grid. Three trials are administered in the eight directions for each limb. During the trials, the client reaches to the farthest point possible on the line with the most distal part of the reach foot, and the tester marks this point on the grid line. Between individual trials in each direction, the client is given a 10 sec rest. For each direction, the distance from the point of maximum excursion to the center of the grid is measured in centimeters using a standard tape measure. The average of the three trials is used to quantify reach distance in each direction. When both the dominant and nondominant limbs are tested, a 5 min rest is provided. Table 12.4 presents the average reach distances in the eight directions for young women and men (Gribble and Hertel 2003).

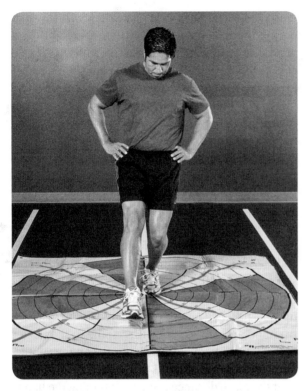

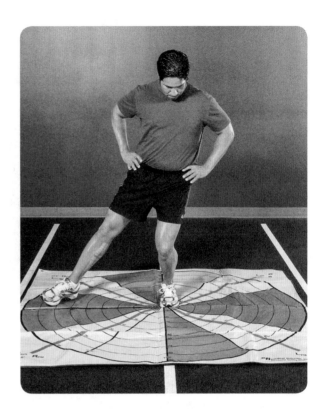

FIGURE 12.6 Star excursion balance test.

Table 12.4 **Average Normalized Distances (%) for Star Excursion Balance Test**

Reach direction	Male	Female
Anterior	79.2	76.9
Anterolateral	73.8	74.7
Lateral	80.0	79.8
Posterolateral	90.4	85.5
Posterior	93.9	85.3
Posteromedial	95.6	89.1
Medial	97.7	90.7
Anteromedial	85.2	83.1

Note: Normalized score (%) = excursion distance / leg length × 100. Distance and leg length are measured in cm.

One limitation of the star excursion balance test is the amount of time needed to administer 48 practice trials and 24 test trials for each leg. Robinson and Gribble (2008) reported that the number of practice trials may be reduced from six to four for each direction. Hertel and colleagues (2006) simplified the star excursion balance test using factor analysis. Results from the analysis showed that the posteromedial reach score is highly representative of all eight directions of the test. They recommend using just the anteromedial, medial, and posteromedial reach tasks to test for functional deficits caused by chronic ankle instability for young adults. Plisky and colleagues (2006; 2009) further modified the test by using only the anterior, posteromedial, and posterolateral directions (forming a "Y") in what has become known as the Y balance

Video
12.5

test. The Y balance test takes less time than the star excursion balance test and has superior test-retest and inter-rater reliability (Plisky et al. 2009). Despite the similarities in concept between the star excursion balance test and the Y balance test, differences exist. Reach distance is greater in the anterior direction during the star excursion test compared with the Y test (Coughlan et al. 2012; Fullam et al. 2014). Researchers theorized that different postural control strategies may be used for the two tests (Coughlan et al. 2012), and more hip flexion is involved during the Y balance test (Fullam et al. 2014); thus, the two tests are not interchangeable.

Gait Velocity Test

Gait velocity provides an indirect measure of dynamic balance while walking, and it may be useful for detecting mobility problems and assessing risk of falls for older adults. For gait velocity, the amount of time to walk a set distance is measured. The average gait velocity needed to safely cross a street during a green light is 122 cm·sec^{-1}; however, 96% of older ($\geq$65 yr) pedestrians walked with a gait velocity less than this value (Hoxie et al. 1994). Older individuals with a history of falling have slower gait velocities compared with those with no history of falls (Guimaraes and Isaacs 1980). Also, the risk of falls is significantly greater for individuals who stop walking when talking (Lundin-Olsson, Nyberg, and Gustafson 1997). However, adding a second task does not enhance the prediction of falls in older people; dual-task tests of gait speed are no more predictive of falls than simple gait velocity tests (Menant et al. 2014).

ASSESSING DYNAMIC BALANCE USING TEST BATTERIES

As mentioned earlier, balance is a complex construct. Most balance test batteries are comprehensive and include multiple test items to assess both static and dynamic balance. These test batteries require the client to perform a variety of functional tasks that mimic ADLs. The tasks usually include maintaining a fixed sitting or standing posture, walking, rising from a seated position, and transferring between chairs. This section presents commonly used balance test batteries.

Tinetti Performance-Oriented Mobility Assessment

The Performance-Oriented Mobility Assessment (POMA) is a test battery developed to assess balance and gait of older adults (Tinetti 1986). It contains 14 performance-based items that evaluate gait maneuvers and position changes encountered in normal daily activities, such as standing from a sitting position and stepping over an obstacle on an uneven surface. Each item is scored on a scale ranging from 0 (cannot perform) to 2 (normal performance); the maximum score is 28. This test battery provides a reliable and valid assessment of balance in elderly, community-dwelling populations, and scores are associated with risk of falling (Berg et al. 1992; Tinetti, Speechley, and Ginter 1988). Scores greater than 25 are indicative of good balance and lower fall risk (Mayson et al. 2008). For detailed instructions about the POMA, see Tinetti 1986 and Tinetti, Speechley, and Ginter 1988.

Berg Balance Scale

The Berg Balance Scale (BBS) is widely used to evaluate balance performance of nursing home residents and community-dwelling older adults. Inter- and intrarater reliability for this scale is extremely high ($r = .98$). The BBS has good concurrent validity: $r = .91$ with POMA test scores and $r = -.76$ with timed up-and-go scores (Podsiadlo and Richardson 1991; Tinetti 1986).

The BBS evaluates performance on 14 functional mobility tasks and takes about 15 min to administer. Participants are scored on a 5-point scale, with a score of 0 indicating that task could not be completed and a score of 4 indicating the task was performed independently (Berg et al. 1992). The maximum score is 56; a score of 45 or less used to identify individuals with greater risk for falls (Hawk et al. 2006). However, Muir and colleagues (2008) reported that the cutoff value of 45 has poor sensitivity (25%-42%) for predicting one or more falls in a community-dwelling older population. They concluded that multiple factors contribute to risk of falls in older people and that balance impairment alone does not adequately predict future risk. For complete instructions about scoring each item of the BBS, see Berg and colleagues 1992.

Dynamic Gait Index

The Dynamic Gait Index (DGI) provides a valid and reliable composite measure of a person's ability to adapt gait during movement-related tasks. This test battery consists of eight items that are scored on a scale of 0 (cannot perform) to 3 (normal performance), with a maximum score of 24. For some of the items, the task is supposed to be completed as quickly as possible. Also, some items require performing two tasks simultaneously, such as walking while turning the head and looking up on command. Mayson and colleagues (2008) reported a positive association between DGI scores and a measure of cognition. Performance on this test is dependent on balance, mobility, and cognitive function (Mayson et al. 2008). Scores >20 are associated with a lower incidence of falling (Riddle and Stratford 1999; Shumway-Cook et al. 1997). For detailed instructions and information about the DGI, see Shumway-Cook and Woollacott 1995.

DESIGNING BALANCE TRAINING PROGRAMS

The ACSM's 2008 Physical Activity Guidelines for Americans suggests balance training at least 3 days/wk for inactive and active older adults (≥65 yr). In a position statement on exercise for older adults (Chodzko-Zajko et al. 2009), the ACSM also recommended that older adults engage in balance activities at least twice a week. Subsequently, the ACSM expanded its position statement to include not only balance but also additional neuromotor skills—agility, gait, coordination, and proprioception (Garber et al. 2011). Neuromotor exercise training is specifically recommended for older adults who have poor mobility or who are at risk for falling. The ACSM (2018) makes no specific recommendations regarding the frequency, intensity, or type of exercise for neuromotor training; however, they commented that incorporating balance, agility, and proprioceptive exercise into a training program at least 2 days/wk is effective at reducing falls.

For older clients with balance and mobility disorders, participating in a balance training program may be beneficial for increasing mobility, performing ADLs safely, and preventing falls (Garber 2011). For younger and middle-aged adults, limited evidence supports definitive recommendations with regard to the benefits of neuromotor training, but there is substantial evidence that balance training and proprioceptive training reduce the risk of ankle sprains in athletes. In a systematic review of well-controlled studies, Hübscher and colleagues (2010) determined that balance training alone resulted in a significant 64% risk reduction of ankle sprains. In another study over 6 yr, researchers observed a significant 81% reduction in ankle sprains from the first 2 yr period to the third biennium in a team of professional basketball players taking part in a proprioceptive training program (Riva et al. 2016). Additionally, 6 wk of balance training after an acute ankle sprain substantially reduces the risk of a recurrent sprain (McKeon and Hertel 2008). When designing a balance program for your clients, follow the general recommendations of the ACSM (2018) (see Recommendations for Balance Training Programs).

BALANCE TRAINING EXERCISE PRESCRIPTION

Compared with the other physical fitness components, there is a lack of research on balance training for athletes, children, and middle-aged and older adults. It is difficult to compare studies examining the effects of exercise on balance because of diversity in the populations (e.g., young athletes to frail older adults), as well as the lack of standardization in balance outcome measures and training regimens. Also, there is no gold standard measure of balance. The following questions address issues you should consider when prescribing balance training for your clients.

What types of physical activities may be used to improve balance?

Given that balance performance is affected by muscle strength, power, and flexibility, resistance training and stretching programs may be useful for maintaining and improving balance. In addition to increasing strength and range of motion, Pilates, yoga, tai chi, dance, walking, and combinations of exercise modes may be suitable activities for improving balance. Balance discs, foam pads and rollers, balance boards including Nintendo Wii, stability balls, and computerized balance training systems are tools that may add variety and challenge to balance training programs.

Recommendations for Balance Training Programs

- Have clients engage in balance activities 2 or 3 days/wk.
- Progressively increase the difficulty of the balance exercises by using a narrower base of support such as two-leg stance, semitandem stance, tandem stance, and one-leg stance.
- Include dynamic movements that challenge the center of gravity such as tandem walking and circle turns.

- Displace the center of mass by stepping over obstacles and balancing on a rocker platform.
- Use exercises that stress postural muscles, such as heel stands and toe stands, and exercises that reduce visual or sensory input, such as standing with eyes closed or standing on a foam pad.
- Prescribe multifaceted activities such as tai chi and yoga.

In a review of exercise interventions to improve balance, Howe and colleagues (2007) analyzed results from 34 studies, with a total of 2,883 participants. Subsequently, this review was updated and expanded to include 60 additional studies involving 7,000 more participants (Howe et al. 2011). The researchers categorized the training interventions as follows: gait, balance, coordination, and functional tasks training; resistance training for strength and power; three-dimensional exercise including tai chi, yoga, dance, and qigong; general physical activity (walking or cycling); and computerized balance training, vibration platform training, and multimodal physical activity programs that used a combination of exercise modes. Table 12.5 summarizes the positive effects some of these interventions have on direct and indirect measures of balance. There was insufficient evidence that computerized balance training or vibration plate training improves balance.

What types of balance training activities can be used with older adults?

Numerous investigations have demonstrated that balance in older adults can be improved with exercise. However, Low, Walsh, and Arkesteijn (2017) recently set out to determine if postural control, as measured by center of pressure, can be improved in older adults, thereby identifying a mechanism to improve balance. They identified 22 randomized controlled trials that measured center of pressure in people >60 yr of age and involved either balance, resistance, or multicomponent exercise intervention. Balance exercise decreased total sway with eyes open and eyes closed, but neither resistance nor multicomponent training affected center-of-pressure

measurements. Thus, postural control is improved by balance training interventions but not resistance training or multicomponent training.

In contrast to postural control, studies that have evaluated balance in older adults overwhelmingly support a multicomponent strategy combining a variety of exercise modalities. In a systematic review of this topic, 7 of 10 trials reported that an exercise intervention enhanced balance and reduced the incidence of falls in physically frail older adults (Cadore et al. 2013). According to the authors, the best strategy seems to be training multiple components, such as balance, strength, and endurance. Of course, a multicomponent exercise plan has the added benefit of improving not only balance and functional performance but also cardiorespiratory fitness and metabolic health (Bouaziz et al. 2016). Granacher and colleagues (2013) suggested that core strength training, Pilates exercise, or both be included as an adjunct or even substitution to traditional balance and resistance training programs for older adults to improve balance and functional performance. In addition to traditional balance and resistance training programs, research supports group exercise programs such as tai chi, yoga, and Pilates (all discussed later in this chapter) for improving balance in the senior population. Additionally, 8 of 9 studies in a review of dance interventions to improve the health of older adults showed positive changes in balance; thus dance, regardless of style, is thought to improve balance and functional fitness in seniors (Woei-Ni Hwang and Braun 2015).

As mentioned previously in this text, exergaming (or virtual reality training) is popular among youth, but it is also being used to keep older adults active. In

Table 12.5 Positive Effects of Various Physical Activity Interventions on Balance

Type of training	Direct measures	Indirect measures
Gait, balance, coordination, functional tasks training	Static and dynamic stability with force platform Limits of stability	One-leg stance with eyes open Timed up-and-go Berg balance test Gait velocity
Resistance training	Omnidirectional tilt	Functional reach Timed up-and-go One-leg stance with eyes open and closed Tandem stance Gait velocity
Tai chi, yoga, dance, qigong training		Walking on balance beam One-leg stance with eyes open Timed up-and-go Gait velocity
General physical activity (walking)		Tandem walking Tandem stance Functional reach Walking on balance beam Timed up-and-go Walking speed
Multimodal training	Body sway Limits of stability	Functional reach Tandem stance Tandem walking Timed up-and-go One-leg stance with eyes open and closed Berg balance test

Note: Training significantly improved performance on the direct and indirect balance tests listed.

a recent meta-analysis, Donath, Rossler, and Faude (2016) evaluated the effectiveness of exergaming interventions on balance and functional mobility of people over 60 yr of age. Virtual reality training was superior to control groups for both standing balance and functional mobility, but slightly less effective than traditional balance training. The authors concluded that exergaming might serve as an attractive complement to other traditional exercise methods for improving balance and functional mobility for seniors.

Does resistance training improve balance?

Improved balance is often mentioned as one of the benefits of resistance training. Muscle weakness is one intrinsic factor related to balance disorders and risk of falling. Reduced muscle strength, especially in the lower extremities, affects a person's ability to perform ADLs such as stair climbing or standing

from a seated position. Orr, Raymond, and Singh (2008) published the first systematic review of studies that assessed the effect of progressive resistance exercise training on balance of older adults. They noted that only a small percentage of balance outcome measures were significantly improved by resistance training: static balance (26%), dynamic balance (14%), functional balance (57%), and computerized dynamic posturography (8%). Thus, resistance training as an isolated intervention does not consistently improve balance of older adults. In many of these studies, the researchers selected universal whole-body and lower body strength exercises for the resistance training programs instead of identifying key muscles used for balance, which may explain some of the discrepancy in results. Also, machine-based resistance training may not be as effective as free weight training for improving balance.

Recent randomized controlled trials further highlight the inconsistency in results dependent on the progressive resistance training program employed and the balance measure evaluated. Joshua and colleagues (2014) randomly assigned older adults (≥65 yr) to one of three groups: traditional balance training, progressive resistance training specific to the lower extremities, or a combination that received both treatments alternately. Over a 6 mo duration, all groups improved on the functional reach test; however, the resistance training group had significantly better change scores than the balance training group. In contrast, older adults who adhered to a multicomponent training protocol (aerobic, strength, and balance) for 16 wk improved their sit-to-stand and one-leg stance tests more than a resistance training group (total body on resistance machines) (Ansai et al. 2016).

Research suggests that strength alone is not the major underlying mechanism for poor balance. Muscle power (force × velocity) may also be a limiting factor in balance control. This is especially the case for reactive balance in which the act of stepping to catch one's balance requires muscle power and proprioception (Klein, Fiedler, and Rose 2011). Age-related decreases in neural processing may diminish the ability to develop force rapidly in response to postural challenges (Orr et al. 2008). In fact, power declines more rapidly than strength with advancing age (Granacher, Muehlbauer, and Gruber 2012). Mayson and colleagues (2008) reported that leg press velocity was positively related to dynamic balance performance (i.e., Berg Balance Scale, POMA, and Dynamic Gait Index), whereas greater leg strength was associated with better performance on static balance tests (e.g., unipedal stance test). In older men, power training with low loads (20% 1-RM) induced larger improvements in balance performance than did moderate (50% 1-RM) or heavy (80% 1-RM) loads (Orr et al. 2006). More research is needed to determine the most effective resistance training loads, modes, and volume for improving balance.

In future studies of progressive resistance training, it may be prudent to focus on the type of balance to be developed (i.e., static, dynamic, or functional) as well as specific muscle groups critical for balance such as the ankle dorsiflexors and plantar flexors, the knee extensors and flexors, and the hip abductors and adductors. Hess and Woollacott (2005) reported that a high-intensity strength training program targeting key lower extremity muscle groups (i.e., knee flexors and extensors and ankle plantar flexors and dorsiflexors) significantly improved postural control in balance-impaired older adults.

How effective is tai chi for improving balance and preventing falls in older adults?

Considerable research exists on the efficacy of tai chi for improving balance and preventing falls in older people. In a review that included seven randomized controlled trials, Huang and Liu (2015) reported that practicing tai chi significantly reduces the time to complete the up-and-go test in older adults. The one-leg stance and BBS are also improved. In a study that had older adults (60-80 yr) complete 15 min of tai chi, 15 min of balance exercises, 15 min of strength training, and 10 min of stretching, 3 days/wk for 12 wk, there were significant improvements over a control group (Zhuang et al. 2014). The improvements included 17.6% for the timed up-and-go test, 54.7% for the 30-sec chair stand test, and significant improvements in each direction of the star excursion balance test. In a review of 18 prospective studies, multiple studies reported improved static balance (posturography and one-leg stance) as well as dynamic and functional balance (posturography, functional reach, BBS, POMA, timed up-and-go) with tai chi training (Liu and Frank 2010). From this review, Liu and Frank (2010) determined that tai chi was more effective for balance improvement than routine daily activity but not significantly better than functional balance training or resistance training.

Systematic reviews from 2008 (Harmer and Li) and 2010 (Logghe et al.) evaluating the impact of tai chi on preventing falls were inconclusive. Despite fall reductions of 21% to 49%, Logghe and colleagues (2010) concluded that the evidence for the efficacy of tai chi was insufficient, and they thought a dose-effect relationship was likely. However, subsequent systematic reviews all indicated that practicing tai chi improves balance and reduces both fear of falling and the total number of falls (Lee and Ernst 2012; Liu and Frank 2010; Mat et al. 2015; Schleicher, Wedam, and Wu 2012). In a review of systematic reviews, Lee and Ernst (2012) stated that many of the health benefits attributed to tai chi are unsubstantiated, but the evidence is "convincingly positive" that tai chi is an effective fall prevention strategy. It is a better fall prevention strategy than education alone (Liu and Frank 2010). In a review limited to patients with osteoarthritis of the knee, Mat and colleagues (2015) concluded that tai chi, as well as strength training and aerobic exercise, but not water-based exercise, improved balance and fall risk in this population.

What is the optimal style of tai chi for improving balance?

Tai chi is practiced in a variety of styles (e.g., Yang, Wu, Chen, Sun, and Hao). The style and forms used are sometimes not indicated in the research, making it difficult to determine if one style is superior to another for improving balance. Schleicher, Wedam, and Wu (2012) noted that the styles identified in their review were the Yang, Sun, and Chen. Each style has its own movements and traditional length of practice. The most popular style practiced by older adults is Yang (Liu and Frank 2010), characterized by slow, large, graceful movements that blend from one pose to the next. A high stance position (knees bent <30°) and an upright posture add to its appeal with the older population. In contrast, the Chen style is more "martial" in appearance, with a lower stance plus stomping and explosive movements breaking up the slow movements. The Wu style is slow, and the Hao style requires a high stance position. In addition to the styles, there are a variety of forms (individual movements) within each style. Liu and Frank (2010) noted that the 24-form Yang style was the most frequently reported in their review of the literature, but shorter forms (e.g., 6-form Yang) are more appropriate for frail clients or those at low functional levels.

How many tai chi sessions are needed to show improvement in balance?

The research clearly shows that the number of tai chi sessions makes a difference in terms of training effects on balance. According to Schleicher, Wedam, and Wu (2012), in some cases balance improvements were observed with as little as 16 hr total of practice; however, there does appear to be a dose-effect relationship, with longer practice time leading to better balance and fall risk reduction. Generally, 40 or more sessions are needed to show significant improvements in balance performance. To reduce risk of falls, tai chi training programs should last at least 15 wk. Because of age-related declines in physical abilities, the duration and frequency of tai chi programs for older adults may need to be increased to derive the degree of improvement seen in younger adults. As with all training programs, the exercise prescription will vary depending on the client's ability and goals. There is no universally accepted exercise prescription for tai chi; however, Liu and Frank (2010) suggested the following for older people who are practicing tai chi to overcome balance deficits:

- Frequency: 2-3 days/wk
- Exercises: 12 or fewer forms
- Session time: At least 45 min
- Duration: At least 12 wk

Is yoga an effective exercise mode for improving balance?

Despite the popularity of yoga relative to tai chi, there are few yoga studies. In a systematic review of yoga for balance improvement in healthy individuals ranging from youth to older adults, 15 studies met the authors' inclusion criteria, but only 5 were randomized controlled trials (Jeter et al. 2014). As with tai chi, there are various styles of yoga, and the authors noted that the studies in their review varied by style, frequency, and duration. Nevertheless, there was at least one positive balance outcome in 11 of the 15 studies, indicating that yoga may have a beneficial effect on balance. In a meta-analysis limited to people >60 yr, Youkhana and colleagues (2016) determined that yoga practice leads to small improvements in balance and medium improvements in physical mobility. Nick and associates (2016) placed older adults (60-74 yr) who had poor balance scores (BBS <45) and a fear of falling (Modified Falls Efficacy Scale [MFES] <8) into either a control group or yoga group. Following 8 wk of yoga (two 1 hr sessions per week), the yoga group significantly improved their BBS and MFES scores, with no change for the control group.

In an interesting randomized controlled trial that compared yoga with tai chi and standard balance training, Ni and colleagues (2014) placed older adults with a history of falling into one of these three treatment groups for 12 wk. They observed improvements in field measures (8 ft up-and-go, one-leg stance, functional reach, and gait speed) as well as dynamic posturography scores in all three groups, but there were no differences between the groups. They suggest that yoga may be an alternative to tai chi and traditional balance training for improving postural stability. Similarly, Gothe and McAuley (2016) reported that yoga, performed 3 days/wk for 8 wk of a randomized controlled trial, was just as effective at improving the functional fitness of previously sedentary 55 to 79 yr olds as a stretching-strengthening program that followed the CDC and ACSM guidelines. These studies all suggest that yoga is at least as effective as other modes of exercise for improving balance and functional mobility.

Is Pilates an effective exercise mode for improving balance?

Much of the research on Pilates has focused on treating low back pain (see chapter 11); however, Pilates is also lauded by its practitioners as an excellent mode of exercise for improving balance. In a summary of systematic reviews based on randomized controlled trials, Kamioka and colleagues (2016) evaluated the effectiveness of Pilates exercise. In addition to providing short-term pain relief and functional improvement for chronic low back pain sufferers (see chapter 11), there is evidence of improved dynamic balance, flexibility, and muscular endurance in healthy people. After 16 Pilates sessions over 2 mo, older adults (61-87 yr) from a senior center improved their timed up-and-go and functional reach tests by 1.39 sec and 1.13 in., respectively (Pata, Lord, and Lamb 2014). They also decreased their fear of falling. In another study, participants significantly improved peak torque of the knee flexors and extensors and postural stability (measured with a Biodex Stability System) following 24 sessions of Pilates (1 hr sessions 3 days/wk for 8 wk) (Yu and Lee 2012).

In contrast to these positive results from studies with no control group or nonexercising controls, recent randomized controlled trials comparing Pilates with other exercise modes revealed no advantage of Pilates (Donath et al. 2016; Mesquita et al. 2015). Mesquita and colleagues (2015) placed 58 older women into one of three groups: PNF stretching, Pilates, or control. After 4 wk (three

50 min sessions per week), both treatment groups significantly improved in the timed up-and-go and functional reach tests, but there was no difference between PNF and Pilates. Donath and colleagues (2016) stratified 48 seniors to Pilates, traditional balance training, or control. Following 8 wk (two sessions per week), the traditional balance training group outperformed the Pilates group on the Y balance score and one-leg stance. Taken together, these results suggest that although Pilates improves balance, it is no more effective than other traditional exercise methods.

BALANCE TRAINING PROGRAMS

Balance training has been widely used in sports rehabilitation (injuries to ankle and knee joints) and in fall prevention programs for geriatric populations. Traditionally, these programs include static and dynamic exercises with eyes open and closed on stable and unstable surfaces. Although the training intensity, frequency, and volume vary greatly among studies using this approach, the results generally support traditional balance training for inducing short- and long-term improvements in balance and postural control (Granacher et al. 2011). Recently, perturbation-based balance training has been promoted to reduce risk of falling, given that slipping and tripping account for 30% to 50% of falls in older adults. Using this approach, perturbation exercises that mimic real-life conditions are included. Compared with the traditional approach, perturbation-based training appears to be more beneficial for improving reactive balance (i.e., recovery of equilibrium), demonstrating that the specificity principle also applies to balance training (Granacher et al. 2011).

Two recent reviews set out to define the dose-response relationships of balance training in young, healthy adults (Lesinski et al. 2015) and older adults (Granacher et al. 2017). The dose-response relationship and recommendations were similar for both groups. Both studies recommend a duration of 11 to 12 wk, with a frequency of three sessions a week, each exercise maintained for 21 to 40 sec. The duration of each training session is only 11 to 15 min for young adults (Lesinski et al. 2015) but 31 to 45 min for older adults (Granacher et al. 2017).

For young adults, the recommendation applies only to static balance; there is not yet enough research to make a recommendation for reactive balance. In contrast, for older adults, the effect size for this type of training was large on measures of reactive balance but only small to medium on static balance.

In light of the complex nature of balance, the current ACSM guidelines (2018) do not include a defined exercise prescription for balance. We recommend using the general guidelines presented in this section as a starting point. Individualize programs to take into account your clients' needs, goals, age, and physical activity status. Keep in mind that balance training is task specific. Task-specific exercises that target a single, specific balance or gait impairment are more effective than generalized exercise for

SAMPLE PROGRESSIVE BALANCE PROGRAM

Exercises	Basic	Moderate (motor[c] or cognitive[b] task)	Advanced (motor[c] and cognitive[b] task)
Sitting on a ball	• Sitting • Sitting in a circle, passing (rolling) a large ball • Sitting in a circle, kicking a ball • Sitting in a line, passing a ball • Sitting in a line, rolling a ball, slalom[c] • Sitting in pairs, hands together, pushing gently	• Sitting, adding a motor or cognitive task • Sitting in a circle, passing (rolling) a large ball, one foot on a cushion • Sitting in a circle, kicking a ball, feet or arms in different positions • Sitting in a line, passing a ball, one foot on a cushion • Sitting in a line, rolling a ball, slalom, one foot on a cushion • Sitting, parrying, a gentle push	• Sitting, adding both a motor and cognitive task • Sitting in a circle and passing (rolling) a large ball, both feet on a cushion • Sitting in a line, passing a ball, both feet on a cushion • Sitting in a line, rolling a large ball, slalom, both feet on a cushion
Standing	• Standing in a circle, chairs in between, passing (rolling) a large ball • Standing in a circle, passing around a big balloon • Standing in a line, passing a small balloon, slalom • Standing in a line, passing (rolling) a large ball, slalom • Tandem stance • Standing on one leg • Standing, one balance cushion under each foot • Standing, both feet on one balance cushion • Standing on soft foam mat • Standing in pairs, facing each other, both holding a ball; one leads and the other follows when moving the ball in the air • Standing in pairs, ball between chests, pushing gently	• Standing in a circle, hitting a balloon while doing a lunge • Standing in a circle, passing a ball, doing a lunge when passing • Standing in a circle, throwing a ball, doing a lunge when throwing • Standing in a circle, throwing a ball with different bases of support (e.g., vary feet position, cushions) • Standing in a circle, passing around a glass of water, one foot on balance cushion • Standing in a line, passing a small ball, slalom, with different bases of support • Standing in a line, passing (rolling) a large ball, slalom, with different bases of support • Standing with one hand on back of chair (support), one foot on balance cushion, doing lunges with other leg in different directions • Standing with different bases of support, adding a motor or cognitive task	• Adding a cognitive task to exercises in moderate level • Standing with different bases of support, adding both a motor and cognitive task

Exercises	Basic	Moderate (motor[a] or cognitive[b] task)	Advanced (motor[a] and cognitive[b] task)
Walking	• Slalom walking around four to seven balance cushions • Walking, stepping with one foot on balance cushions • Walking around a "messy" surrounding (e.g., chairs, balls, cones) • Walking forward at a fast speed and returning walking backward • Walking forward at a fast speed, finishing stepping up and down a two-step platform, returning at normal speed • Walking forward at a fast speed, finishing stepping up and down a two-step platform, returning walking backward • Semi-tandem or tandem walking	• Slalom walking, adding a motor or cognitive task • Walking, stepping on balance cushions, placed in a row wide apart • Walking around a "messy" surrounding, reciting or counting • Walking around, doing lunges on request (with left foot when tapped on left shoulder) • Walking forward at a fast speed and returning walking backward, adding a motor or cognitive task • Walking forward at a fast speed, finishing stepping up and down a two-step platform, returning at normal speed, adding a motor or cognitive task • Walking forward at a fast speed, finishing stepping up and down a two-step platform, returning walking backward, adding a motor or cognitive task • Walking on a soft foam mat, adding a motor or cognitive task • Tandem walking, adding a motor or cognitive task	• Slalom walking, adding both a motor and cognitive task • Walking, stepping on balance cushions placed in a row • Walking around buttoning and unbuttoning clothing or reciting or counting in a "messy" surrounding, doing lunges on request • Walking forward at a fast speed and returning walking backward, adding both a motor and cognitive task • Walking forward at a fast speed, finishing stepping up and down a two-step platform, returning at normal speed, adding both a motor and cognitive task • Walking forward at a fast speed, finishing stepping up and down a two-step platform, returning walking backward, adding both a motor and cognitive task • Walking on a soft foam mat, adding both a motor and cognitive task • Tandem walking, adding both a motor and cognitive task

[a]Motor tasks: moving arm, leg, head, or trunk (leaning, turning); buttoning and unbuttoning clothing; juggling a balloon; throwing and catching a ball; kicking a ball; carrying a glass of water; rolling a Ping-Pong ball on a tray; closing eyes.

[b]Cognitive tasks: counting (adding or subtracting by 3 or 7 from a given starting number); reading a newspaper; reciting categories of flowers, animals, cities, and so on.

[c]slalom: weaving or zigzag pattern around obstacles such as cones or cushions.

Adapted from A. Halvarsson, I-M Dohrn, and A. Stahle, "Taking Balance Training for Older Adults One Step Further: The Rationale for and Description of a Proven Balance Training Programme," *Clinical Rehabilitation* 29 (2015): 417-425. © The Authors, 2014. https://creativecommons.org/licenses/by/3.0/

improving balance. Techniques from a variety of exercise modalities can be combined to form a comprehensive balance program that challenges your clients. The Sample Progressive Balance Program illustrates how seated, standing, and movement balance activities may be adapted to increase the exercise challenge for further improvements in balance. In the Sample Multimodal Program, exercises from tai chi, Pilates, agility training, and lunges are used to improve balance and mobility of an older adult.

Many excellent resources are available for designing an individualized balance training program for your clients. *ABLE Bodies Balance Training* (see Scott 2008) presents a 16 wk exercise program that safely takes older adults through the exercise progressions for improving balance and mobility, flexibility, posture and core stability, strength, and cardiorespiratory endurance. Resources for developing safe exercise programs for improving balance and functional fitness of older adults are available (see Rose 2010; Scott 2008), and Granacher (2011) offers guidelines for designing programs for the older population (see Guidelines for Designing Balance Training Programs for Older Adults). For ideas about incorporating Pilates and yoga workouts into balance training programs, see Isacowitz (2014) and Shaw (2016).

SAMPLE MULTIMODAL BALANCE TRAINING PROGRAM

Client Data

Age: 65 yr

Gender: Female

Body weight: 145 lb

Program goal: Improve static and dynamic balance; prevent falls

Method: Tai chi, Pilates, lunges, and agility training

Frequency: 3 or more days/wk

Duration: 45 to 60 min per session

Exercise mode	Principles	Actions	Progressions
Tai chi	Increase limits of stability Improve rhythmic movements Increase ROM Control of center of gravity	Prayer wheel: slow, rhythmical weight shifts coordinated with large arm circles Cat walk: slow and purposeful steps, with diagonal weight shifts Cloud hands: slow lateral steps with trunk vertical Part the horse's mane: coordination of arms and legs while walking forward Repulsing the monkey: slow, backward walking with diagonal weight shifts	Learn one movement per week, starting with weight shift and leg placement, progressing to coordinated arm and torso movements.
Pilates	Improve postural control, functional transitions, and sequencing actions	Sit-to-stand maneuvers Floor transfers and bridging Rolling prone lying Bird dog, cat-camel Half-kneeling to stand	Gradually improve form and speed during the movements.
Lunges	Stepping for postural correction Increase limits of stability Quick change in direction	Postural correction: lean until center of mass is outside base of support, requiring a step; perform in all directions Multidirectional stepping in clockwise direction Dynamic lunge walking	Start with firm surface and progress to one foot on foam pad and then both feet on foam pad. Perform exercises in well-lit room, and progress to doing them while wearing sunglasses and then blindfolded. Use arms reciprocally while lunging, and then progress to lifting arms overhead while holding a ball.
Agility	Improve coordination Quick change in direction Increase mobility in tight spaces	High-knee stepping with hand slapping knees Lateral shuffle Tire course: wide-based quick, high steps and turns	Begin exercises at self-paced tempo and gradually increase speed. Progress to quick changes in direction and pace. Add dual tasks like counting aloud while moving.

Guidelines for Designing Balance Training Programs for Older Adults

- **Mode:** Tai chi; Pilates; yoga; static, dynamic, and reactive balance training exercises; resistance training for strength and power; or a combination of modes
- **Equipment:** Balance discs, foam pads and rollers, balance boards, stability balls, computerized balance systems, and force platforms to add variety and challenge to the program

- **Frequency:** Minimum of 2 days/wk
- **Sets and duration:** 3-8 sets; 20-40 sec each set
- **Time:** 20-30 min per session; 2 hr/wk
- **Length of program:** 3 to 6 mo depending on exercise mode

Key Points

▶ Balance is an important component of the functional fitness of older adults.

▶ To reduce risk of falling, older adults are encouraged to engage in balance activities at least 2 days/wk.

▶ Static balance is the ability to maintain the center of gravity within the supporting base during standing or sitting.

▶ Dynamic balance is the ability to maintain an upright position while the center of gravity and supporting base are moving.

▶ Reactive balance is the ability to compensate and recover from perturbations while standing or walking.

▶ Functional balance is the ability to perform daily movement tasks requiring balance.

▶ The dynamic systems model of balance describes balance control as adaptive and functional.

▶ Visual, somatosensory, and vestibular systems interact to maintain balance.

▶ Body size, foot size, gender, aging, and physical activity affect balance and risk of falling.

▶ Indirect measures of balance are valid and reliable and useful in field and clinical settings.

▶ Direct measures of balance can be used to assess static and dynamic balance and postural stability. Because the testing equipment is costly, these tests may be more suitable for research settings.

▶ Pilates, yoga, tai chi, dancing, walking, and resistance training are effective training modes for improving balance.

Key Terms

Learn the definition for each of the following key terms. Definitions of terms can be found in the glossary.

balance
center of pressure
computerized dynamic posturography
dynamic balance
functional balance
gait velocity
limits of stability

line of gravity
neuromotor training
reactive balance
static balance

Review Questions

In addition to being able to define each of the key terms, test your knowledge and understanding of the material by answering the following review questions.

1. Why is balance testing included in functional fitness test batteries?

2. Define neuromotor training.

3. Balance is a complex construct. Identify the biomechanical, neurological, and environmental systems that influence and control balance performance.

4. Define static, dynamic, and reactive balance, and give examples of tests that may be used to assess these types of balance.

5. Identify indirect balance tests that are typically used to assess functional balance in older adults and those that are typically used in clinical settings to assess balance in injured athletes.

6. Explain how the visual, proprioceptive, and vestibular systems interact to maintain and control balance.

7. Describe how aging affects balance.

8. Identify intrinsic factors that contribute to risk of falling in older adults.

9. Identify modes of exercise that can be used to improve balance.

10. What are the center of pressure and limits of stability, and how are these measures used to assess dynamic balance?

11. Briefly describe the generic exercise prescription for improving balance of older adults.

Health and Fitness Appraisal

This appendix includes questionnaires and forms you can duplicate and use for the pretest health screening of your clients. The PAR-Q+ (appendix A.1) is used to identify individuals who need medical clearance from their physicians before taking any physical fitness tests or starting an exercise program. The Medical History Questionnaire (appendix A.2) is used to obtain a personal and family health history for your clients. As part of the pretest health screening, ask your clients if they have any of the conditions or symptoms listed in Risk Factors, Signs, and Symptoms of Disease (appendix A.3).

The ePARmed-X+ (appendix A.4) may be used by physicians to assess and convey medical clearance for physical activity participation of your clients.

You can obtain a lifestyle profile for your clients by using either the Lifestyle Evaluation form (appendix A.5) or the Fantastic Lifestyle Checklist (appendix A.6). Be sure that each participant signs the Informed Consent (appendix A.7) before undergoing any physical fitness tests or engaging in an exercise program. Appendix A.8 includes websites for selected professional organizations and institutes.

Appendix A.1 Physical Activity Readiness Questionnaire for Everyone (PAR-Q+)

2018 PAR-Q+

The Physical Activity Readiness Questionnaire for Everyone

The health benefits of regular physical activity are clear; more people should engage in physical activity every day of the week. Participating in physical activity is very safe for MOST people. This questionnaire will tell you whether it is necessary for you to seek further advice from your doctor OR a qualified exercise professional before becoming more physically active.

GENERAL HEALTH QUESTIONS

Please read the 7 questions below carefully and answer each one honestly: check YES or NO.	YES	NO
1) Has your doctor ever said that you have a heart condition ☐ OR high blood pressure ☐?	☐	☐
2) Do you feel pain in your chest at rest, during your daily activities of living, **OR** when you do physical activity?	☐	☐
3) Do you lose balance because of dizziness **OR** have you lost consciousness in the last 12 months? Please answer **NO** if your dizziness was associated with over-breathing (including during vigorous exercise).	☐	☐
4) Have you ever been diagnosed with another chronic medical condition (other than heart disease or high blood pressure)? **PLEASE LIST CONDITION(S) HERE:** _____	☐	☐
5) Are you currently taking prescribed medications for a chronic medical condition? **PLEASE LIST CONDITION(S) AND MEDICATIONS HERE:** _____	☐	☐
6) Do you currently have (or have had within the past 12 months) a bone, joint, or soft tissue (muscle, ligament, or tendon) problem that could be made worse by becoming more physically active? Please answer **NO** if you had a problem in the past, but it *does not limit your current ability* to be physically active. **PLEASE LIST CONDITION(S) HERE:** _____	☐	☐
7) Has your doctor ever said that you should only do medically supervised physical activity?	☐	☐

☑ **If you answered NO to all of the questions above, you are cleared for physical activity.**
Please sign the PARTICIPANT DECLARATION. You do not need to complete Pages 2 and 3.

- ▶ Start becoming much more physically active – start slowly and build up gradually.
- ▶ Follow International Physical Activity Guidelines for your age (www.who.int/dietphysicalactivity/en/).
- ▶ You may take part in a health and fitness appraisal.
- ▶ If you are over the age of 45 yr and NOT accustomed to regular vigorous to maximal effort exercise, consult a qualified exercise professional before engaging in this intensity of exercise.
- ▶ If you have any further questions, contact a qualified exercise professional.

PARTICIPANT DECLARATION
If you are less than the legal age required for consent or require the assent of a care provider, your parent, guardian or care provider must also sign this form.

I, the undersigned, have read, understood to my full satisfaction and completed this questionnaire. I acknowledge that this physical activity clearance is valid for a maximum of 12 months from the date it is completed and becomes invalid if my condition changes. I also acknowledge that the community/fitness centre may retain a copy of this form for records. In these instances, it will maintain the confidentiality of the same, complying with applicable law.

NAME _____ DATE _____

SIGNATURE _____ WITNESS _____

SIGNATURE OF PARENT/GUARDIAN/CARE PROVIDER _____

⬤ **If you answered YES to one or more of the questions above, COMPLETE PAGES 2 AND 3.**

⚠ **Delay becoming more active if:**

- ✓ You have a temporary illness such as a cold or fever; it is best to wait until you feel better.
- ✓ You are pregnant - talk to your health care practitioner, your physician, a qualified exercise professional, and/or complete the ePARmed-X+ at **www.eparmedx.com** before becoming more physically active.
- ✓ Your health changes - answer the questions on Pages 2 and 3 of this document and/or talk to your doctor or a qualified exercise professional before continuing with any physical activity program.

2018 PAR-Q+

FOLLOW-UP QUESTIONS ABOUT YOUR MEDICAL CONDITION(S)

1.   **Do you have Arthritis, Osteoporosis, or Back Problems?**

If the above condition(s) is/are present, answer questions 1a-1c   If **NO** ☐ go to question 2

1a.	Do you have difficulty controlling your condition with medications or other physician-prescribed therapies? (Answer **NO** if you are not currently taking medications or other treatments)	YES ☐ NO ☐
1b.	Do you have joint problems causing pain, a recent fracture or fracture caused by osteoporosis or cancer, displaced vertebra (e.g., spondylolisthesis), and/or spondylolysis/pars defect (a crack in the bony ring on the back of the spinal column)?	YES ☐ NO ☐
1c.	Have you had steroid injections or taken steroid tablets regularly for more than 3 months?	YES ☐ NO ☐

2.   **Do you currently have Cancer of any kind?**

If the above condition(s) is/are present, answer questions 2a-2b   If **NO** ☐ go to question 3

2a.	Does your cancer diagnosis include any of the following types: lung/bronchogenic, multiple myeloma (cancer of plasma cells), head, and/or neck?	YES ☐ NO ☐
2b.	Are you currently receiving cancer therapy (such as chemotheraphy or radiotherapy)?	YES ☐ NO ☐

3.   **Do you have a Heart or Cardiovascular Condition?** *This includes Coronary Artery Disease, Heart Failure, Diagnosed Abnormality of Heart Rhythm*

If the above condition(s) is/are present, answer questions 3a-3d   If **NO** ☐ go to question 4

3a.	Do you have difficulty controlling your condition with medications or other physician-prescribed therapies? (Answer **NO** if you are not currently taking medications or other treatments)	YES ☐ NO ☐
3b.	Do you have an irregular heart beat that requires medical management? (e.g., atrial fibrillation, premature ventricular contraction)	YES ☐ NO ☐
3c.	Do you have chronic heart failure?	YES ☐ NO ☐
3d.	Do you have diagnosed coronary artery (cardiovascular) disease and have not participated in regular physical activity in the last 2 months?	YES ☐ NO ☐

4.   **Do you have High Blood Pressure?**

If the above condition(s) is/are present, answer questions 4a-4b   If **NO** ☐ go to question 5

4a.	Do you have difficulty controlling your condition with medications or other physician-prescribed therapies? (Answer **NO** if you are not currently taking medications or other treatments)	YES ☐ NO ☐
4b.	Do you have a resting blood pressure equal to or greater than 160/90 mmHg with or without medication? (Answer **YES** if you do not know your resting blood pressure)	YES ☐ NO ☐

5.   **Do you have any Metabolic Conditions?** *This includes Type 1 Diabetes, Type 2 Diabetes, Pre-Diabetes*

If the above condition(s) is/are present, answer questions 5a-5e   If **NO** ☐ go to question 6

5a.	Do you often have difficulty controlling your blood sugar levels with foods, medications, or other physician-prescribed therapies?	YES ☐ NO ☐
5b.	Do you often suffer from signs and symptoms of low blood sugar (hypoglycemia) following exercise and/or during activities of daily living? Signs of hypoglycemia may include shakiness, nervousness, unusual irritability, abnormal sweating, dizziness or light-headedness, mental confusion, difficulty speaking, weakness, or sleepiness.	YES ☐ NO ☐
5c.	Do you have any signs or symptoms of diabetes complications such as heart or vascular disease and/or complications affecting your eyes, kidneys, **OR** the sensation in your toes and feet?	YES ☐ NO ☐
5d.	Do you have other metabolic conditions (such as current pregnancy-related diabetes, chronic kidney disease, or liver problems)?	YES ☐ NO ☐
5e.	Are you planning to engage in what for you is unusually high (or vigorous) intensity exercise in the near future?	YES ☐ NO ☐

(continued)

2018 PAR-Q+

6. Do you have any Mental Health Problems or Learning Difficulties? *This includes Alzheimer's, Dementia, Depression, Anxiety Disorder, Eating Disorder, Psychotic Disorder, Intellectual Disability, Down Syndrome*

If the above condition(s) is/are present, answer questions 6a-6b   If **NO** ☐ go to question 7

6a.	Do you have difficulty controlling your condition with medications or other physician-prescribed therapies? (Answer **NO** if you are not currently taking medications or other treatments)	YES ☐	NO ☐
6b.	Do you have Down Syndrome **AND** back problems affecting nerves or muscles?	YES ☐	NO ☐

7. Do you have a Respiratory Disease? *This includes Chronic Obstructive Pulmonary Disease, Asthma, Pulmonary High Blood Pressure*

If the above condition(s) is/are present, answer questions 7a-7d   If **NO** ☐ go to question 8

7a.	Do you have difficulty controlling your condition with medications or other physician-prescribed therapies? (Answer **NO** if you are not currently taking medications or other treatments)	YES ☐	NO ☐
7b.	Has your doctor ever said your blood oxygen level is low at rest or during exercise and/or that you require supplemental oxygen therapy?	YES ☐	NO ☐
7c.	If asthmatic, do you currently have symptoms of chest tightness, wheezing, laboured breathing, consistent cough (more than 2 days/week), or have you used your rescue medication more than twice in the last week?	YES ☐	NO ☐
7d.	Has your doctor ever said you have high blood pressure in the blood vessels of your lungs?	YES ☐	NO ☐

8. Do you have a Spinal Cord Injury? *This includes Tetraplegia and Paraplegia*

If the above condition(s) is/are present, answer questions 8a-8c   If **NO** ☐ go to question 9

8a.	Do you have difficulty controlling your condition with medications or other physician-prescribed therapies? (Answer **NO** if you are not currently taking medications or other treatments)	YES ☐	NO ☐
8b.	Do you commonly exhibit low resting blood pressure significant enough to cause dizziness, light-headedness, and/or fainting?	YES ☐	NO ☐
8c.	Has your physician indicated that you exhibit sudden bouts of high blood pressure (known as Autonomic Dysreflexia)?	YES ☐	NO ☐

9. Have you had a Stroke? *This includes Transient Ischemic Attack (TIA) or Cerebrovascular Event*

If the above condition(s) is/are present, answer questions 9a-9c   If **NO** ☐ go to question 10

9a.	Do you have difficulty controlling your condition with medications or other physician-prescribed therapies? (Answer **NO** if you are not currently taking medications or other treatments)	YES ☐	NO ☐
9b.	Do you have any impairment in walking or mobility?	YES ☐	NO ☐
9c.	Have you experienced a stroke or impairment in nerves or muscles in the past 6 months?	YES ☐	NO ☐

10. Do you have any other medical condition not listed above or do you have two or more medical conditions?

If you have other medical conditions, answer questions 10a-10c   If **NO** ☐ read the Page 4 recommendations

10a.	Have you experienced a blackout, fainted, or lost consciousness as a result of a head injury within the last 12 months **OR** have you had a diagnosed concussion within the last 12 months?	YES ☐	NO ☐
10b.	Do you have a medical condition that is not listed (such as epilepsy, neurological conditions, kidney problems)?	YES ☐	NO ☐
10c.	Do you currently live with two or more medical conditions?	YES ☐	NO ☐

**PLEASE LIST YOUR MEDICAL CONDITION(S)
AND ANY RELATED MEDICATIONS HERE:** _____

_____

GO to Page 4 for recommendations about your current medical condition(s) and sign the PARTICIPANT DECLARATION.

Reprinted with permission from the PAR-Q+ Collaboration and the authors of the PAR-Q+ (Dr. Darren Warburton, Dr. Norman Gledhill, Dr. Veronica Jamnik, and Dr. Shannon Bredin).

2018 PAR-Q+

☑ **If you answered NO to all of the FOLLOW-UP questions (pgs. 2-3) about your medical condition, you are ready to become more physically active - sign the PARTICIPANT DECLARATION below:**

▶ It is advised that you consult a qualified exercise professional to help you develop a safe and effective physical activity plan to meet your health needs.

▶ You are encouraged to start slowly and build up gradually - 20 to 60 minutes of low to moderate intensity exercise, 3-5 days per week including aerobic and muscle strengthening exercises.

▶ As you progress, you should aim to accumulate 150 minutes or more of moderate intensity physical activity per week.

▶ If you are over the age of 45 yr and **NOT** accustomed to regular vigorous to maximal effort exercise, consult a qualified exercise professional before engaging in this intensity of exercise.

⬤ **If you answered YES to one or more of the follow-up questions about your medical condition:**

You should seek further information before becoming more physically active or engaging in a fitness appraisal. You should complete the specially designed online screening and exercise recommendations program - the **ePARmed-X+ at www.eparmedx.com** and/or visit a qualified exercise professional to work through the ePARmed-X+ and for further information.

⚠ **Delay becoming more active if:**

✓ You have a temporary illness such as a cold or fever; it is best to wait until you feel better.

✓ You are pregnant - talk to your health care practitioner, your physician, a qualified exercise professional, and/or complete the ePARmed-X+ **at www.eparmedx.com** before becoming more physically active.

✓ Your health changes - talk to your doctor or qualified exercise professional before continuing with any physical activity program.

⬤ You are encouraged to photocopy the PAR-Q+. You must use the entire questionnaire and NO changes are permitted.
⬤ The authors, the PAR-Q+ Collaboration, partner organizations, and their agents assume no liability for persons who undertake physical activity and/or make use of the PAR-Q+ or ePARmed-X+. If in doubt after completing the questionnaire, consult your doctor prior to physical activity.

PARTICIPANT DECLARATION

⬤ All persons who have completed the PAR-Q+ please read and sign the declaration below.

⬤ If you are less than the legal age required for consent or require the assent of a care provider, your parent, guardian or care provider must also sign this form.

I, the undersigned, have read, understood to my full satisfaction and completed this questionnaire. I acknowledge that this physical activity clearance is valid for a maximum of 12 months from the date it is completed and becomes invalid if my condition changes. I also acknowledge that the community/fitness center may retain a copy of this form for records. In these instances, it will maintain the confidentiality of the same, complying with applicable law.

NAME _____   DATE _____

SIGNATURE _____   WITNESS _____

SIGNATURE OF PARENT/GUARDIAN/CARE PROVIDER _____

——— **For more information, please contact** ———
www.eparmedx.com
Email: eparmedx@gmail.com

Citation for PAR-Q+
Warburton DER, Jamnik VK, Bredin SSD, and Gledhill N on behalf of the PAR-Q+ Collaboration.
The Physical Activity Readiness Questionnaire for Everyone (PAR-Q+) and Electronic Physical Activity Readiness Medical Examination (ePARmed-X+). Health & Fitness Journal of Canada 4(2):3-23, 2011.
Key References
1. Jamnik VK, Warburton DER, Makarski J, McKenzie DC, Shephard RJ, Stone J, and Gledhill N. Enhancing the effectiveness of clearance for physical activity participation; background and overall process. APNM 36(S1):S3-S13, 2011.
2. Warburton DER, Gledhill N, Jamnik VK, Bredin SSD, McKenzie DC, Stone J, Charlesworth S, and Shephard RJ. Evidence-based risk assessment and recommendations for physical activity clearance; Consensus Document. APNM 36(S1):S266-s298, 2011.
3. Chisholm DM, Collis ML, Kulak LL, Davenport W, and Gruber N. Physical activity readiness. British Columbia Medical Journal. 1975;17:375-378.
4. Thomas S, Reading J, and Shephard RJ. Revision of the Physical Activity Readiness Questionnaire (PAR-Q). Canadian Journal of Sport Science 1992;17:4 338-345.

The PAR-Q+ was created using the evidence-based AGREE process (1) by the PAR-Q+ Collaboration chaired by Dr. Darren E. R. Warburton with Dr. Norman Gledhill, Dr. Veronica Jamnik, and Dr. Donald C. McKenzie (2). Production of this document has been made possible through financial contributions from the Public Health Agency of Canada and the BC Ministry of Health Services. The views expressed herein do not necessarily represent the views of the Public Health Agency of Canada or the BC Ministry of Health Services.

Reprinted with permission from the PAR-Q+ Collaboration and the authors of the PAR-Q+ (Dr. Darren Warburton, Dr. Norman Gledhill, Dr. Veronica Jamnik, and Dr. Shannon Bredin).

Appendix A.2 Medical History Questionnaire

Demographic Information

Last name	First name	Middle initial
Date of birth	Sex	Home phone
Address	City, State	Zip code
Work phone	Family physician	

Section A

1. When was the last time you had a physical examination?

2. If you are allergic to any medications, foods, or other substances, please name them.

3. If you have been told that you have any chronic or serious illnesses, please list them.

4. Give the following information pertaining to the last three times you have been hospitalized. *Note:* Women, do not list normal pregnancies.

	Hospitalization 1	Hospitalization 2	Hospitalization 3
Reason for hospitalization	_____	_____	_____
Month and year of hospitalization	_____	_____	_____
Hospital	_____	_____	_____
City and state	_____	_____	_____

Section B

During the past 12 months

1. Has a physician prescribed any form of medication for you?	❐ Yes	❐ No
2. Has your weight fluctuated more than a few pounds?	❐ Yes	❐ No
3. Did you attempt to bring about this weight change through diet or exercise?	❐ Yes	❐ No
4. Have you experienced any faintness, light-headedness, or blackouts?	❐ Yes	❐ No
5. Have you occasionally had trouble sleeping?	❐ Yes	❐ No
6. Have you experienced any blurred vision?	❐ Yes	❐ No
7. Have you had any severe headaches?	❐ Yes	❐ No
8. Have you experienced chronic morning cough?	❐ Yes	❐ No
9. Have you experienced any temporary change in your speech pattern, such as slurring or loss of speech?	❐ Yes	❐ No
10. Have you felt unusually nervous or anxious for no apparent reason?	❐ Yes	❐ No
11. Have you experienced unusual heartbeats such as skipped beats or palpitations?	❐ Yes	❐ No
12. Have you experienced periods in which your heart felt as though it were racing for no apparent reason?	❐ Yes	❐ No

From A.L. Gibson, D.R. Wagner, and V.H. Heyward, *Advanced Fitness Assessment and Exercise Prescription,* 8th ed. (Champaign, IL: Human Kinetics, 2019).

At present

1. Do you experience shortness or loss of breath while walking with others your own age? ☐ Yes ☐ No

2. Do you experience sudden tingling, numbness, or loss of feeling in your arms, hands, legs, feet, or face? ☐ Yes ☐ No

3. Have you ever noticed that your hands or feet sometimes feel cooler than other parts of your body? ☐ Yes ☐ No

4. Do you experience swelling of your feet and ankles? ☐ Yes ☐ No

5. Do you get pains or cramps in your legs? ☐ Yes ☐ No

6. Do you experience any pain or discomfort in your chest? ☐ Yes ☐ No

7. Do you experience any pressure or heaviness in your chest? ☐ Yes ☐ No

8. Have you ever been told that your blood pressure was abnormal? ☐ Yes ☐ No

9. Have you ever been told that your serum cholesterol or triglyceride level was high? ☐ Yes ☐ No

10. Do you have diabetes? ☐ Yes ☐ No

    If yes, how is it controlled?

    ☐ Dietary means   ☐ Insulin injection

    ☐ Oral medication   ☐ Uncontrolled

11. How often would you characterize your stress level as being high?

    ☐ Occasionally   ☐ Frequently   ☐ Constantly

12. Have you ever been told that you have any of the following illnesses? ☐ Yes ☐ No

    ☐ Myocardial infarction   ☐ Arteriosclerosis   ☐ Heart disease   ☐ Thyroid disease

    ☐ Coronary thrombosis   ☐ Rheumatic heart   ☐ Heart attack   ☐ Heart valve disease

    ☐ Coronary occlusion   ☐ Heart failure   ☐ Heart murmur

    ☐ Heart block   ☐ Aneurysm   ☐ Angina

13. Have you ever had any of the following medical procedures? ☐ Yes ☐ No

    ☐ Heart surgery   ☐ Pacemaker implant

    ☐ Cardiac catheterization   ☐ Defibrillator

    ☐ Coronary angioplasty   ☐ Heart transplantation

Section C

Has any member of your immediate family been treated for or suspected to have had any of these conditions? Please identify their relationship to you (father, mother, sister, brother, etc.).

A. Diabetes

B. Heart disease

C. Stroke

D. High blood pressure

From A.L. Gibson, D.R. Wagner, and V.H. Heyward, *Advanced Fitness Assessment and Exercise Prescription,* 8th ed. (Champaign, IL: Human Kinetics, 2019).

Appendix A.3 Risk Factors, Signs, and Symptoms of Disease

Instructions: Ask your clients if they have any of the following conditions and risk factors. If so, refer them to their physicians to obtain a signed medical clearance prior to any exercise testing or participation. See the glossary for definitions of terms.

Client's name: _____ Date: _____

Risk Factors, Signs, and Symptoms of Disease

Condition	Yes	No	Comments
RISK FACTORS			
Male older than 45 yr			
Female older than 55 yr, or had hysterectomy, or is postmenopausal			
Smoking or quit smoking within previous 6 mo			
Blood pressure ≥ 130/90 mmHg			
Does not know blood pressure			
Taking blood pressure medication			
Blood cholesterol > 200 mg·dl^{-1}			
Does not know cholesterol level			
Has close relative who had heart attack or heart surgery before age 55 (father or brother) or age 65 (mother or sister)			
Physically inactive (<30 min of physical activity more than 4 days/wk)			
Overweight by more than 20 lb (9 kg)			
CARDIOVASCULAR*			
Hypertension			
Hypercholesterolemia			
Heart murmurs			
Myocardial infarction (heart attack)			
Fainting or dizziness			
Claudication			
Chest pain			
Palpitations			
Ischemia			
Tachycardia (rhythm disturbances)			
Ankle edema			
Stroke			

From A.L. Gibson, D.R. Wagner, and V.H. Heyward, *Advanced Fitness Assessment and Exercise Prescription,* 8th ed. (Champaign, IL: Human Kinetics, 2019).

Condition	Yes	No	Comments
PULMONARY			
Asthma			
Bronchitis			
Emphysema			
Nocturnal dyspnea			
Coughing up blood			
Exercise-induced asthma			
Breathlessness during or after mild exertion			
METABOLIC*			
Diabetes			
Obesity			
Glucose intolerance			
McArdle's syndrome			
Hypoglycemia			
Thyroid disease			
Cirrhosis			
MUSCULOSKELETAL			
Osteoporosis			
Osteoarthritis			
Low back pain			
Prosthesis			
Muscular atrophy			
Swollen joints			
Orthopedic pain			
Artificial joints			
RENAL*			
Abnormal protein level in urine			
Low glomerular filtration rate			
Changes in urination frequency, color, appearance, difficulty			
Anemia (fatigue, chills, shortness of breath, dizziness, weakness)			
Edema or fluid retention in periphery (one or both sides), face, hands			
Metallic taste in mouth			
Chronic itchiness			
Dialysis			

*Clients with a known cardiovascular, metabolic, or renal disease (or symptomology of these three disease classifications), should consult a physician before engaging in exercise.

From A.L. Gibson, D.R. Wagner, and V.H. Heyward, *Advanced Fitness Assessment and Exercise Prescription,* 8th ed. (Champaign, IL: Human Kinetics, 2019).

Appendix A.4 Electronic Physical Activity Readiness Medical Examination (ePARmed-X+)

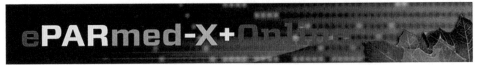

ePARmed-X+ Physician Clearance Follow-Up

This form is separated into three main sections:

A) Background information regarding the PAR-Q+ and ePARmed-X+ clearance process,
B) A brief history and demographic information regarding the participant, and
C) The physician's recommendations regarding the participant becoming more physically active.

At the end of this process, the participant is recommended to take this signed clearance form to a qualified exercise professional or other healthcare professional (as recommended in the ePARmed-X+) before becoming <u>more</u> physically active or engaging in a fitness appraisal.

A BACKGROUND INFORMATION REGARDING THE PAR-Q+ AND ePARmed-X+ CLEARANCE PROCESS

The ePARmed-X+ is an easy to follow interactive program (www.eparmedx.com) that can be used to determine an individual's readiness for increased physical activity participation or a fitness appraisal. The ePARmed-X+ supplements the paper and online versions of the new Physical Activity Readiness Questionnaire for Everyone (PAR-Q+).

Individuals who use the ePARmed-X+ have had a positive response to the PAR-Q+, or have been directed to the online program by a qualified exercise professional or another healthcare professional, owing to his/her current medical condition. At the end of the ePARmed-X+, it is possible that the participant is advised to consult a physician to discuss the various options regarding becoming <u>more</u> physically active. In this instance, the participant will be required to receive medical clearance for physical activity from a physician. Until this medical clearance is received, the participant is restricted to low intensity physical activity participation.

This document serves to assist both the participant and physician in the physical activity clearance process.

B PERSONAL INFORMATION

NAME: _____   SEX: ☐ M or ☐ F

ADDRESS: _____   BIRTHDATE (mm/dd/yy): _____
_____
_____

TELEPHONE: _____   HEALTH/MEDICAL NUMBER: _____

REASON FOR REFERRAL (SELECT ALL THAT APPLY):

☐ QUALIFIED EXERCISE PROFESSIONAL REFERRAL
☐ HEALTH CARE PROFESSIONAL REFERRAL
☐ ePARmed-X+ RECOMMENDATION

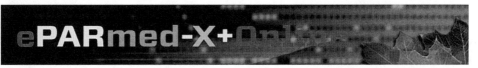

C ePARmed-X+ PHYSICAL ACTIVITY READINESS PHYSICIAN REFERRAL FORM

Based on the current review of the health status of _____ (name)
I recommend the following course of action:

☐ The participant should avoid engaging in physical activity at this time.

☐ The participant should engage in only a medically supervised physical activity/exercise program involving the supervision of a qualified exercise professional (or other appropriately trained health care professional) and overseen by a physician.

☐ The participant is cleared for intensity and mode appropriate physical activity/exercise training under the supervision of a qualified exercise professional.

☐ The participant is cleared for intensity and mode appropriate physical activity/exercise training with limited supervision (i.e., unrestricted physical activity).

The following precautions should be taken when prescribing exercise for the aforementioned participant:

o With the avoidance of: _____
_____
_____
_____

o With the inclusion of: _____
_____
_____
_____

NAME OF PHYSICIAN: _____

ADDRESS: _____

TELEPHONE: _____

Date of Medical Clearance (mm/dd/yy): _____

PHYSICIAN/CLINIC STAMP AND SIGNATURE	NOTE: This physical activity/exercise clearance is valid for a period of six months from the date it is completed and becomes invalid if the medical condition of the above named participant changes/worsens.

Version: September 7, 2014   Page 2 of 2   Copyright © PAR-Q+ Collaboration, 2014

Appendix A.5 Lifestyle Evaluation

Smoking habits

1. Have you ever smoked cigarettes, cigars, or a pipe? ❐ Yes ❐ No
2. Do you smoke presently? ❐ Yes ❐ No

    Cigarettes _____a day

    Cigars _____a day

    Pipefuls _____a day

3. At what age did you start smoking? _____years
4. If you have quit smoking, when did you quit?

Drinking habits

1. During the past month, how many days did you drink alcoholic beverages?
2. During the past month, how many times did you have five or more drinks per occasion?
3. On average, how many glasses of beer, wine, or highballs do you consume a week?

    Beer _____ glasses or cans

    Wine _____ glasses

    Highballs _____ glasses

    Other _____ glasses

Exercise habits

1. Do you exercise vigorously on a regular basis? ❐ Yes ❐ No
2. What activities do you engage in on a regular basis?

3. If you walk, run, or jog, what is the average number of miles you cover each workout?

    _____ miles

4. How many minutes on the average is each of your exercise workouts? _____minutes
5. How many workouts a week do you participate in on average? _____workouts
6. Is your occupation?

    _____ Inactive (e.g., desk job)

    _____ Light work (e.g., housework, light carpentry)

    _____ Heavy work (e.g., heavy carpentry, lifting)

7. Check those activities you would prefer in a regular exercise program for yourself:

    ❐ Walking, running, or jogging   ❐ Handball, racquetball, or squash

    ❐ Stationary running   ❐ Basketball

    ❐ Jumping rope   ❐ Swimming

    ❐ Bicycling   ❐ Tennis

    ❐ Stationary cycling   ❐ Aerobic dance

    ❐ Step aerobics   ❐ Stair-climbing

                                                                ❐ Other (specify)

From A.L. Gibson, D.R. Wagner, and V.H. Heyward, *Advanced Fitness Assessment and Exercise Prescription*, 8th ed. (Champaign, IL: Human Kinetics, 2019).

Dietary habits

1. What is your current weight? _____ lb _____ kg   height? _____ in. _____ cm

2. What would you like to weigh? _____ lb _____ kg

3. What is the most you ever weighed as an adult? _____ lb _____ kg

4. What is the least you ever weighed as an adult? _____ lb _____ kg

5. What weight-loss methods have you tried?

6. Which do you eat regularly?

   ❑ Breakfast   ❑ Midafternoon snack

   ❑ Midmorning snack   ❑ Dinner

   ❑ Lunch   ❑ After-dinner snack

7. How often do you eat out each week? _____ times

8. What size portions do you normally have?

   ❑ Small   ❑ Moderate   ❑ Large   ❑ Extra large   ❑ Uncertain

9. How often do you eat more than one serving?

   ❑ Always   ❑ Usually   ❑ Sometimes   ❑ Never

10. How long does it usually take you to eat a meal? _____ minutes

11. Do you eat while doing other activities (e.g., watching TV, reading, working)? _____

12. When you snack, how many times a week do you eat the following?

Cookies, cake, pie _____	Candy _____	Diet soda _____
Soft drinks _____	Doughnuts _____	Fruit _____
Milk or milk beverage _____	Potato chips, pretzels, etc. _____	
Peanuts or other nuts _____	Ice cream _____	
Cheese and crackers _____	Other _____	

13. How often do you eat dessert? _____ times a day _____ times a week

14. What dessert do you eat most often? _____

15. How often do you eat fried foods? _____ times a week

16. Do you salt your food at the table?   ❑ Yes   ❑ No

    ❑ Before tasting it   ❑ After tasting it

From A.L. Gibson, D.R. Wagner, and V.H. Heyward, *Advanced Fitness Assessment and Exercise Prescription*, 8th ed. (Champaign, IL: Human Kinetics, 2019).

Appendix A.6 Fantastic Lifestyle Checklist

INSTRUCTIONS: Unless otherwise specified, place an 'X' beside the box which best describes your behaviour or situation in the past month. Explanations of questions and scoring are provided on the next page.

FAMILY FRIENDS	I have someone to talk to about things that are important to me	almost never	seldom	some of the time	fairly often	almost always
	I give and receive affection	almost never	seldom	some of the time	fairly often	almost always
ACTIVITY	I am vigorously active for at least 30 minutes per day e.g., running, cycling, etc.	less than once/week	1-2 times/week	3 times/week	4 times/week	5 or more times/week
	I am moderately active (gardening, climbing stairs, walking, housework)	less than once/week	1-2 times/week	3 times/week	4 times/week	5 or more times/week
NUTRITION	I eat a balanced diet (see explanation)	almost never	seldom	some of the time	fairly often	almost always
	I often eat excess 1) sugar, or 2) salt, or 3) animal fats, or 4) junk foods.	four of these	three of these	two of these	one of these	none of these
	I am within ____kg of my healthy weight	not within 8 kg (20 lbs)	8 kg (20 lbs)	6 kg (15 lbs)	4 kg (10 lbs)	2 kg (5 lbs)
TOBACCO TOXICS	I smoke tobacco	more than 10 times/week	1 - 10 times/week	none in the past 6 months	none in the past year	none in the past 5 years
	I use drugs such as marijuana, cocaine	sometimes				never
	I overuse prescribed or 'over the counter' drugs	almost daily	fairly often	only occasionally	almost never	never
	I drink caffeine-containing coffee, tea, or cola	more than 10/day	7-10/day	3-6/day	1-2/day	never
ALCOHOL	My average alcohol intake per week is____ (see explanation)	more than 20 drinks	13-20 drinks	11-12 drinks	8-10 drinks	0-7 drinks
	I drink more than four drinks on an occasion	almost daily	fairly often	only occasionally	almost never	never
	I drive after drinking	sometimes				never
SLEEP SEATBELTS STRESS SAFE SEX	I sleep well and feel rested	almost never	seldom	some of the time	fairly often	almost always
	I use seatbelts	never	seldom	some of the time	most of the time	always
	I am able to cope with the stresses in my life	almost never	seldom	some of the time	fairly often	almost always
	I relax and enjoy leisure time	almost never	seldom	some of the time	fairly often	almost always
	I practice safe sex (see explanation)	almost never	seldom	some of the time	fairly often	always
TYPE of behaviour	I seem to be in a hurry	almost always	fairly often	some of the time	seldom	almost never
	I feel angry or hostile	almost always	fairly often	some of the time	seldom	almost never
INSIGHT	I am a positve or optimistic thinker	almost never	seldom	some of the time	fairly often	almost always
	I feel tense or uptight	almost always	fairly often	some of the time	seldom	almost never
	I feel sad or depressed	almost always	fairly often	some of the time	seldom	almost never
CAREER	I am satisfied with my job or role	almost never	seldom	some of the time	fairly often	almost always

STEP 1 Total the X's in each column → ☐ ☐ ☐ ☐ ☐

STEP 2 Multiply the totals by the numbers indicated (write your answer in the box below) → 0   x 1   x 2   x 3   x 4

STEP 3 Add your scores across the bottom for your grand total → ☐ + ☐ + ☐ + ☐ = ☐

Grand total (see explantion)

Appendix A.7 Informed Consent

In order to assess cardiorespiratory function, body composition, and other physical fitness components, the undersigned hereby voluntarily consents to engage in one or more of the following tests (check the appropriate boxes):

❒ Graded exercise stress test
❒ Body composition tests
❒ Muscle fitness tests
❒ Flexibility tests
❒ Balance tests

Explanation of the Tests

The graded exercise test is performed on a cycle ergometer or motor-driven treadmill. The workload is increased every few minutes until exhaustion or until other symptoms dictate that we terminate the test. You may stop the test at any time because of fatigue or discomfort.

The underwater weighing procedure involves being completely submerged in a tank or tub after fully exhaling the air from your lungs. You will be submerged for 3 to 5 seconds while we measure your underwater weight. This test provides an accurate assessment of your body composition.

For muscle fitness testing, you lift weights for a number of repetitions using barbells or exercise machines. These tests assess the strength and endurance of the major muscle groups in the body.

For evaluation of flexibility, you perform a number of tests. During these tests, we measure the range of motion in your joints.

For balance tests, we will be measuring the amount of time you can maintain certain stances or the distance you are able to reach without losing balance.

Risks and Discomforts

During the graded exercise test, certain changes may occur. These changes include abnormal blood pressure responses, fainting, irregularities in heartbeat, and heart attack. Every effort is made to minimize these occurrences. Emergency equipment and trained personnel are available to deal with these situations if they occur.

You may experience some discomfort during the underwater weighing, especially after you expire all the air from your lungs. However, this discomfort is momentary, lasting only 3 to 5 seconds. If this test causes you too much discomfort, an alternative procedure (e.g., skinfold or bioelectrical impedance test) can be used to estimate your body composition.

There is a slight possibility of pulling a muscle or spraining a ligament during the muscle fitness and flexibility testing. In addition, you may experience muscle soreness 24 or 48 hours after testing. These risks can be minimized by performing warm-up exercises prior to taking the tests. If muscle soreness occurs, appropriate stretching exercises to relieve this soreness will be demonstrated.

Expected Benefits From Testing

These tests allow us to assess your physical working capacity and to appraise your physical fitness status. The results are used to prescribe a safe, sound exercise program for you. Records are kept strictly confidential unless you consent to release this information.

Inquiries

Questions about the procedures used in the physical fitness tests are encouraged. If you have any questions or need additional information, please ask us to explain further.

From A.L. Gibson, D.R. Wagner, and V.H. Heyward, *Advanced Fitness Assessment and Exercise Prescription*, 8th ed. (Champaign, IL: Human Kinetics, 2019).

(continued)

Freedom of Consent

Your permission to perform these physical fitness tests is strictly voluntary. You are free to stop the tests at any point, if you so desire.

I have read this form carefully, and I fully understand the test procedures I will perform and the risks and discomforts. Knowing these risks and having had the opportunity to ask questions that have been answered to my satisfaction, I consent to participate in these tests.

_____   _____
Date   Signature of patient

_____   _____
Date   Signature of witness

_____   _____
Date   Signature of supervisor

From A.L. Gibson, D.R. Wagner, and V.H. Heyward, *Advanced Fitness Assessment and Exercise Prescription*, 8th ed. (Champaign, IL: Human Kinetics, 2019).

Appendix A.8 Websites for Selected Professional Organizations and Institutes

Name	Website address
American Association of Cardiovascular and Pulmonary Rehabilitation (AACPR)	www.aacvpr.org
American College of Sports Medicine (ACSM)	www.acsm.org
American Council on Exercise (ACE)	www.acefitness.org
American Fitness Professionals and Associates (AFPA)	www.afpafitness.com
American Society of Exercise Physiologists (ASEP)	www.asep.org
Athletics and Fitness Association of America (AFAA)	www.afaa.com
Australian Association for Exercise and Sports Science (AAESS)	www.aaess.com.au
Canadian Academy of Sport and Exercise Medicine (CASEM)	www.casem-acmse.org
Canadian Society for Exercise Physiology (CSEP)	www.csep.ca
Cooper Institute	www.cooperinst.org
Gatorade Sport Science Institute (GSSI)	www.gssiweb.com
IDEA Health and Fitness Association	www.ideafit.com
Institute for Credentialing Excellence	www.credentialingexcellence.org
International Association of Fitness Sciences	www.iafscertification.com
International Federation of Sports Medicine (FIMS)	www.fims.org
International Fitness Professionals Association (IFPA)	www.ifpa-fitness.com
International Health, Racquet, & Sportsclub Association	www.ihrsa.org
International Coalition for Aging and Physical Activity (ICAPA)	www.humankinetics.com/icapa
National Athletic Trainers Association (NATA)	www.nata.org
National Board of Fitness Examiners	www.nbfe.org
National Commission for Certifying Agencies (NCCA)	www.credentialingexcellence.org/ncca
National Strength and Conditioning Association (NSCA)	www.nsca-lift.org
North American Society for Pediatric Exercise Medicine (NASPEM)	www.naspem.org
SHAPE America	www.shapeamerica.org
Sports Medicine Australia	www.sma.org.au
Sports Medicine New Zealand	www.sportsmedicine.co.nz

Note: Organizations and institutes dealing with exercise physiology, sports medicine, or physical fitness.

From A.L. Gibson, D.R. Wagner, and V.H. Heyward, *Advanced Fitness Assessment and Exercise Prescription,* 8th ed. (Champaign, IL: Human Kinetics, 2019).

Cardiorespiratory Assessments

Appendix B.1 is a summary of GXT and cardiorespiratory field test protocols that are presented in more detail in chapter 4. This appendix summarizes popular maximal and submaximal protocols for treadmill, cycle ergometer, bench-stepping, stair-climbing, recumbent stepper, rowing ergometer, and distance run/walk tests, as well as methods you can use to obtain an estimate of your clients' $\dot{V}O_2$max for each protocol.

Appendix B.2, the Rockport Fitness Charts, provides age-gender norms for the Rockport walking test. These charts may be used to classify your clients' aerobic capacity.

Appendix B.3 presents a variety of step test protocols. Testing and scoring procedures are included for each protocol. For some protocols, prediction equations are available to estimate your clients' $\dot{V}O_2$max.

Appendix B.4 presents OMNI RPE and facial expression RPE scales for children and adults engaging in running and walking, stepping, elliptical training, and resistance exercise. Instructions for administering these scales are provided.

Appendix B.5 provides the answers to questions posed in the sample case study presented in chapter 5.

Appendix B.1 Summary of Graded Exercise Test and Cardiorespiratory Field Test Protocols

Test mode/protocol	Population	Type	Method to estimate $\dot{V}O_2$max	Description (page)
TREADMILL				
Balke	Active and sedentary men and women	Max or submax	Prediction equation Multistage equation/graphing	92
Modified Balke	Children	Max or submax	ACSM equations (walk/run) Multistage equations/graphing	116
Bruce	Active and sedentary men and women	Max or submax	Prediction equation Multistage equation/graphing	92
	Elderly	Max or submax	Prediction equation Multistage equation/graphing	
	Cardiac patients	Max or submax	Prediction equation Multistage equation/graphing	
Modified Bruce	High-risk and elderly	Max or submax	ACSM walking equation Multistage equation/graphing	93
Ebbeling (single-stage walking)	Healthy adults (20-59 yr)	Submax	Prediction equation	103
George (single-stage jogging)	Healthy adults (18-28 yr)	Submax	Prediction equation	103
Naughton	Male cardiac patients	Max or submax	Prediction equation Multistage equation/graphing	91
Perceptually regulated exercise test (PRET)	Active and sedentary adults (18-72 yr)	Max or submax	Multistage graphing	101
CYCLE ERGOMETER				
Åstrand	Healthy adults	Max	ACSM leg ergometry equation	98
Åstrand-Ryhming	Healthy adults	Submax	Nomogram	104
Bongers	Children Adolescents	Max	Prediction equation	116
Fox	Healthy adults	Max or submax	ACSM leg ergometry equation Prediction equation	98 or 108
YMCA	Healthy adults	Submax	Multistage equation/graphing	105
McMaster	Children	Max or submax	ACSM leg ergometry equation Multistage equation/graphing	116
Swain	Healthy adults	Submax	ACSM leg ergometry equation	107
BENCH STEPPING				
Åstrand-Ryhming	Healthy adults	Submax	Nomogram	108
Nagle	Healthy adults	Max	ACSM stepping equation	99
Queens College	Healthy adults (college age)	Submax	Prediction equation	108

From A.L. Gibson, D.R. Wagner, and V.H. Heyward, *Advanced Fitness Assessment and Exercise Prescription,* 8th ed. (Champaign, IL: Human Kinetics, 2019).

Test mode/protocol	Population	Type	Method to estimate $\dot{V}O_2max$	Description (page)
BENCH STEPPING				
STEP Tool	Adults (18-85 yr)	Submax	Prediction equation	108
Webb	Healthy adults (college age)	Submax	Prediction equation	109
Petrella et al.	Older adults	Submax	Prediction equation	109
Kasch Pulse Recovery	Children (6-12 yr)	Submax	Normative values for heart rate	118
STAIR CLIMBING				
Howley	Healthy adults	Submax	Multistage equation/graphing	110
StairMaster 4000PT	Active and sedentary women (20-25 yr)	Submax	Multistage equation/graphing	110
RECUMBENT STEPPER				
Billinger	Healthy adults	Max	Multistage equation	111
ROWING ERGOMETER				
Hagerman	Noncompetitive and unskilled rowers	Submax	Nomogram	111
ELLIPTICAL CROSS-TRAINER				
Dalleck et al.	Healthy young adults	Submax	Prediction equation	111
DISTANCE RUN/WALK				
1.0 mi run/walk	Children (8-17 yr)	Submax	Prediction equation	113
1.0 mi steady-state jog	Healthy adults (college age)	Submax	Prediction equation	113
1.5 mi run/walk	Healthy adults	Submax	Prediction equation	113
1.5 mi steady-state run	Healthy adults	Submax	Prediction equation	113
1.0 mi walk	Healthy adults	Submax	Prediction equation	114
9 min run	Healthy adults	Submax	Prediction equation	113
12 min run	Healthy adults	Submax	Prediction equation	113
20 m shuttle run	Children (8-19 yr)	Submax	Prediction equation	114
YYIR1C 16 m shuttle run	Children (6-10 yr)	Submax	Prediction equation	118

From A.L. Gibson, D.R. Wagner, and V.H. Heyward, *Advanced Fitness Assessment and Exercise Prescription,* 8th ed. (Champaign, IL: Human Kinetics, 2019).

Appendix B.2 Rockport Fitness Charts

Age-Gender Norms for the Rockport Walking Test

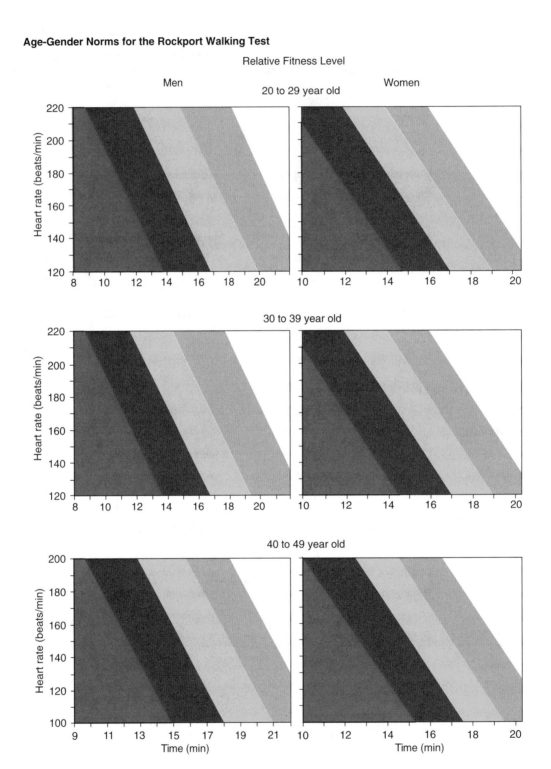

Reprinted with permission of The Rockport Company, Inc.

Age-Gender Norms for the Rockport Walking Test

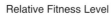

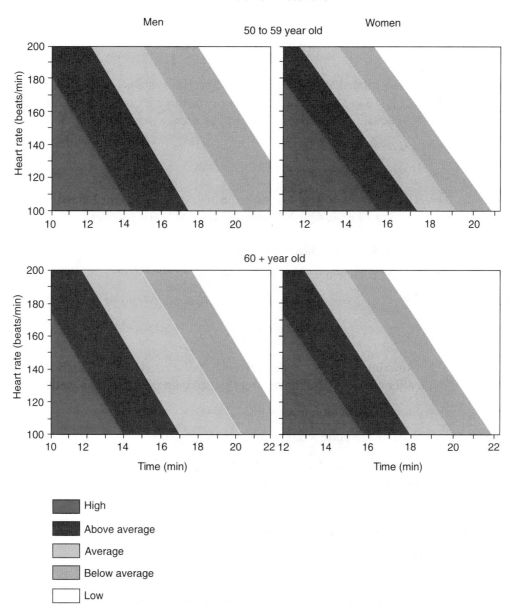

Appendix B.3 Step Test Protocols

Harvard Step Test (Brouha 1943)

Age and sex: Young men

Stepping rate: 30 steps·min^{-1}

Bench height: 20 in.

Duration of exercise: 5 min

Scoring procedures: Sit down immediately after exercise. The pulse rate is counted in 1/2 min counts, from 1 to 1 1/2, 2 to 2 1/2, and 3 to 3 1/2 min after exercise. The three 1/2 min pulse counts are summed and used in the following equation to determine physical efficiency index (PEI):

$$PEI = \frac{\text{duration of exercise (sec)} \times 100}{2 \times \text{sum of recovery HRs}}$$

You can evaluate the performance of college-age males using the following PEI classifications: <55 = poor, 55 to 64 = low average, 65 to 79 = average, 80 to 89 = good, and ≥90 = excellent.

Three-Minute Step Test (Hodgkins and Skubic 1963)

Age and sex: High school- and college-age women

Stepping rate: 24 steps·min^{-1}

Bench height: 18 in.

Duration of exercise: 3 min

Scoring procedures: Sit down immediately after exercise. The pulse rate is counted for 30 sec after 1 min of rest (1 to 1 1/2 min after exercise). Use the recovery pulse count in the following equation:

$$CV \text{ efficiency} = \frac{\text{duration of exercise (sec)} \times 100}{\text{recovery pulse} \times 5.6}$$

You can evaluate the performance of college-age women using the following classifications for cardiovascular (CV) efficiency: 0 to 27 = very poor, 28 to 38 = poor, 39 to 48 = fair, 49 to 59 = good, 60 to 70 = very good, and 71 to 100 = excellent.

OSU Step Test (Kurucz, Fox, and Mathews 1969)

Age and sex: Men 19 to 56 yr

Stepping rate: 24 to 30 steps·min^{-1}

Bench height: Split-level bench 15 and 20 in. high with an adjustable hand bar

Duration of exercise: 18 innings, 50 sec each

Phase I: 6 innings, 24 steps·min^{-1}, 15 in. bench

Phase II: 6 innings, 30 steps·min^{-1}, 15 in. bench

Phase III: 6 innings, 30 steps·min^{-1}, 20 in. bench

(Each inning consists of 30 sec of stepping and 20 sec of rest.)

Scoring procedures: Exactly 5 sec into each rest period, take a 10 sec pulse count. Terminate the test when the heart rate reaches 150 bpm (25 counts × 6). The score is the inning during which the heart rate reaches 150 bpm.

Eastern Michigan University Step Test (Witten 1973)

Age and sex: College-age women

Stepping rate: 24 to 30 steps·min^{-1}

Bench height: Tri-level bench 14 to 20 in.

Duration of exercise: 20 innings, 50 sec each

Phase I: 5 innings, 24 steps·min^{-1}, 14 in. bench

Phase II: 5 innings, 30 steps·min^{-1}, 14 in. bench

Phase III: 5 innings, 30 steps·min^{-1}, 17 in. bench

Phase IV: 5 innings, 30 steps·min^{-1}, 20 in. bench

(Each inning consists of 30 sec of stepping and 20 sec of rest.)

Scoring procedures: Exactly 5 sec into each rest period, take a 10 sec pulse count. Terminate the test when the heart rate reaches 168 bpm (28 counts × 6). The score is the inning during which the heart rate reaches 168 bpm.

Cotten Revision of OSU Step Test (Cotten 1971)

Age and sex: High school- and college-age men

Stepping rate: 24 to 36 steps·min^{-1}

Bench height: 17 in.

Duration of exercise: 18 innings, 50 sec each

Phase I: 6 innings, 24 steps·min^{-1}, 17 in. bench

Phase II: 6 innings, 30 steps·min^{-1}, 17 in. bench

Phase III: 6 innings, 36 steps·min^{-1}, 17 in. bench

(Each inning consists of 30 sec of stepping and 20 sec of rest.)

Scoring procedures: As with the OSU step test, the score is the inning during which the heart rate reaches 150 bpm (25 counts in 10 sec). $\dot{V}O_2$max in ml·kg^{-1}·min^{-1} can be estimated using the following equation:

$$\dot{V}O_2\text{max} = (1.69978 \times \text{step test score}) - (0.06252 \times \text{body weight in lb}) + 47.12525$$

Queens College Step Test (McArdle et al. 1972)

Age and sex: College-age women and men

Stepping rate: 22 steps·min^{-1} for women; 24 steps·min^{-1} for men

Bench height: 16 1/4 in.

Duration of exercise: 3 min

Scoring procedures: Remain standing after exercise. Beginning 5 sec after the cessation of exercise, take a 15 sec pulse count. Multiply the 15 sec count by 4 to express the score in beats per minute (bpm). $\dot{V}O_2$max in ml·kg^{-1}·min^{-1} can be estimated using the following equations:

Women: $\dot{V}O_2\text{max} = 65.81 - (0.1847 \times \text{HR})$

Men: $\dot{V}O_2\text{max} = 111.33 - (0.42 \times \text{HR})$

Appendix B.4 OMNI Rating of Perceived Exertion Scales

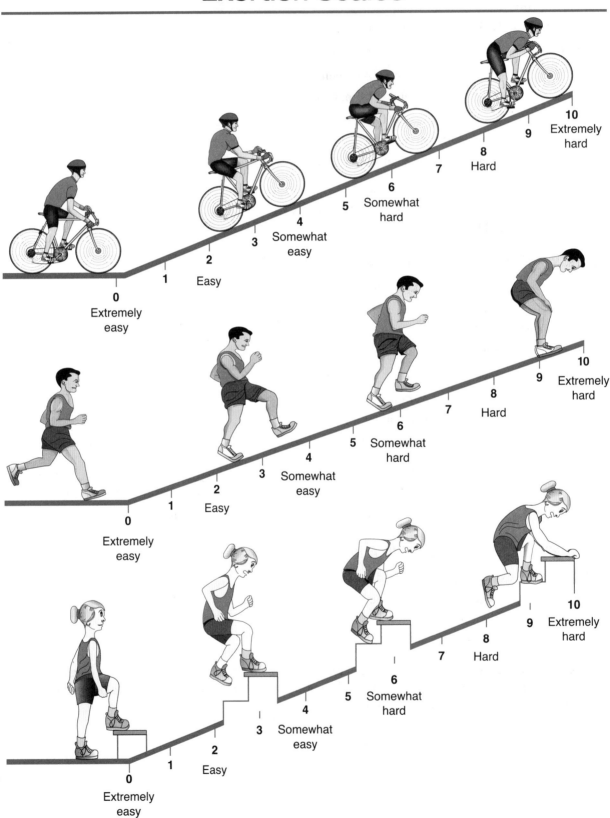

Reprinted, by permission, from R.J. Robertson, *Perceived Exertion for Practitioners: Rating Effort With the OMNI Picture System* (Champaign, IL: Human Kinetics, 2004), 141.

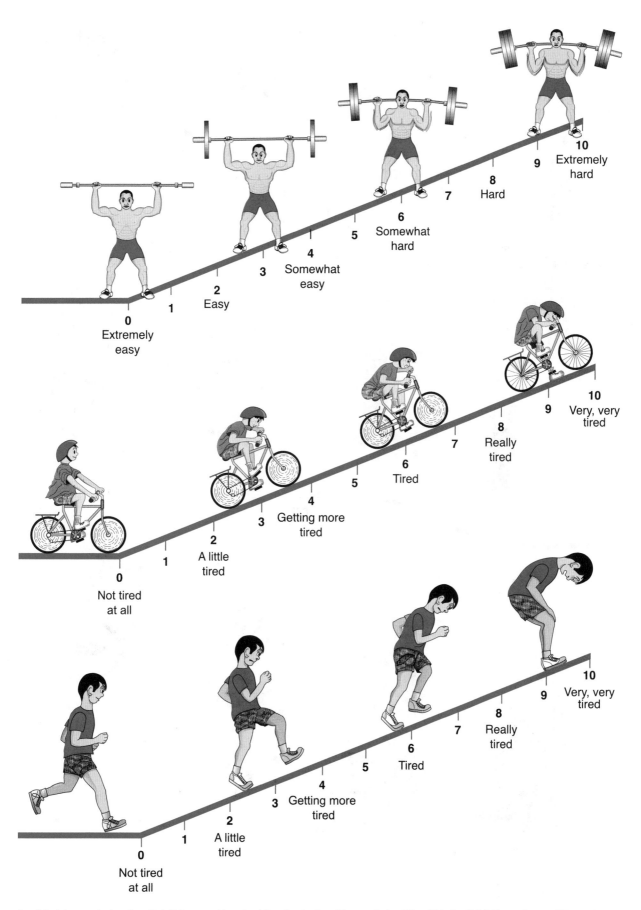

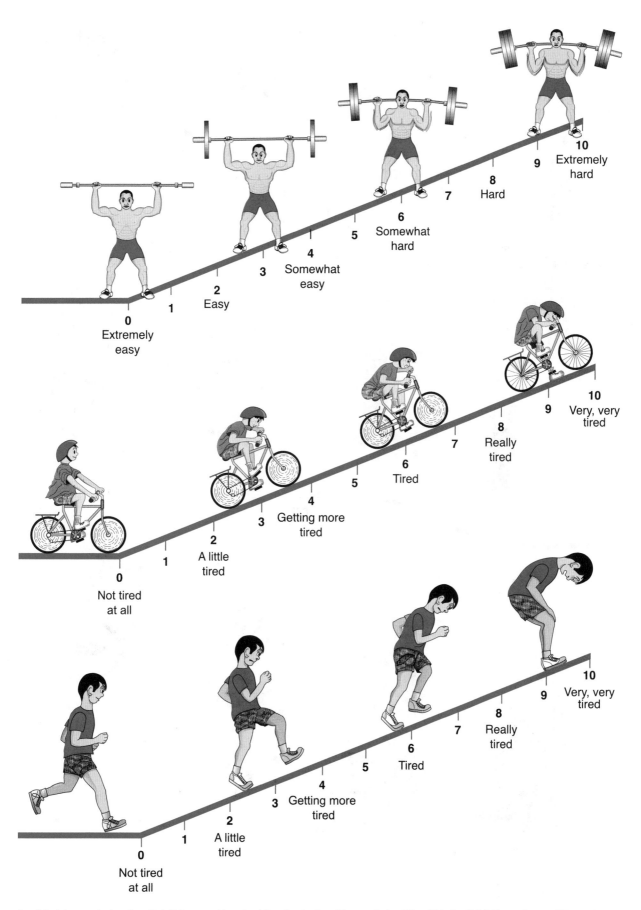

Reprinted, by permission, from R.J. Robertson, *Perceived Exertion for Practitioners: Rating Effort With the OMNI Picture System* (Champaign, IL: Human Kinetics, 2004), 141.

(continued)

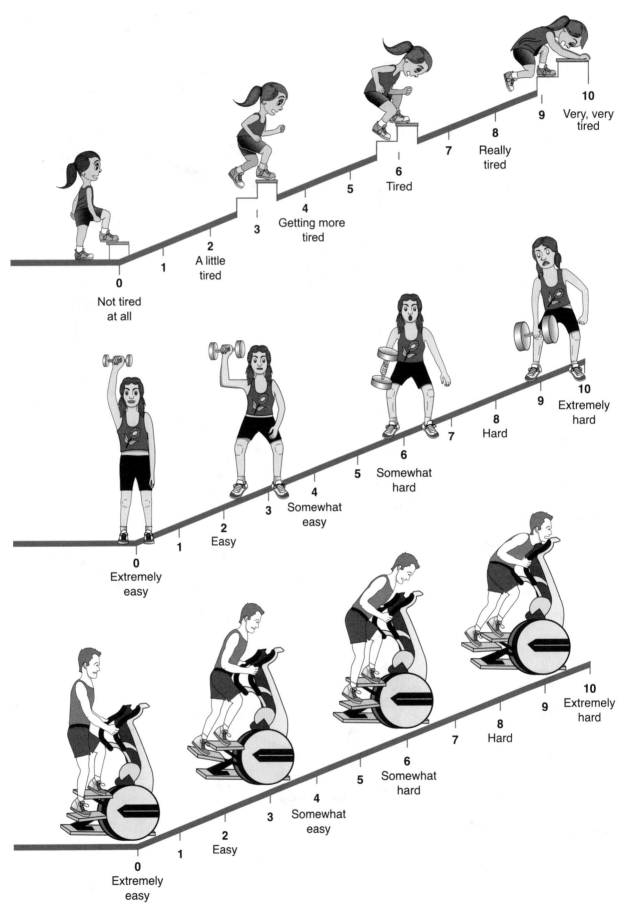

Reprinted, by permission, from R.J. Robertson, *Perceived Exertion for Practitioners: Rating Effort With the OMNI Picture System* (Champaign, IL: Human Kinetics, 2004), 141.

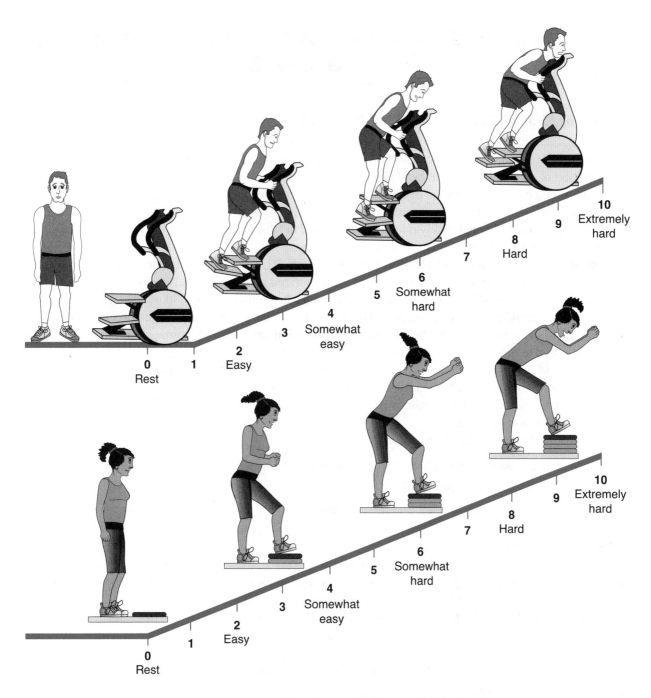

10 Extremely hard
9
8 Hard
7
6 Somewhat hard
5
4 Somewhat easy
3
2 Easy
1
0 Rest

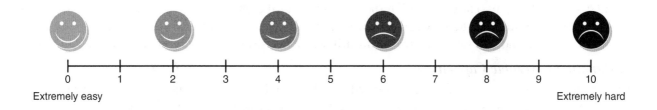

0   1   2   3   4   5   6   7   8   9   10

Extremely easy   Extremely hard

Appendix B.5 Analysis of Sample Case Study in Chapter 5

1. Need for Medical Clearance and CHD Risk Profile

This client has not participated in structured, moderate-intensity physical activity ≥30 min on ≥3 d·wk^{-1} for the past 3 mo. Her health history does not reveal any cardiovascular, metabolic, or renal disease. However, the sensation of dizziness and light-headedness while in a resting state may be considered a positive sign or symptom suggestive of one of the disease states of concern. Given her failure to meet the requirement of regular exercise and a positive symptomology, this client should obtain medical clearance prior to starting an exercise program. Although likely due to job stress, the headaches and discomfort in her neck should be brought to the physician's attention during that appointment.

This client has risk factors for CHD. Her total cholesterol (TC; 220 mg·dl^{-1}) is borderline high (200-230 mg·dl^{-1}), and her blood pressure (140/82 mmHg) is categorized as stage 2 hypertension (140-159 mm Hg). Also, her HDL-C (37 mg·dl^{-1}) and TC/HDL ratio (5.9) place her at higher risk (<40 mg·dl^{-1} and >5.0, respectively). She quit smoking cigarettes (one pack a day) 3 yr ago, which is a step in the right direction. Following the National Cholesterol Education Program's recommendation, you should encourage this client to have her LDL-C assessed to determine if she needs a cholesterol treatment program. Engaging in an aerobic exercise program should lower her systolic blood pressure. Her triglycerides and blood glucose levels are normal. Encourage her to dine out less frequently and to eat three well-balanced meals a day. When dining out, she should select foods that are low in saturated fat, cholesterol, and sodium. This may help lower her blood cholesterol and blood pressure.

The client is also at greater risk because of

- the high stress associated with her job (police officer) and lifestyle (divorced parent raising two children),
- family history of cardiovascular disease, and
- physical inactivity (she does not exercise regularly outside of work-related physical activity).

2. Special Considerations

The client has not exercised aerobically for the past 6 yr, and she has gained 15 lb during that time. It is likely that she will experience some discomfort when she starts her aerobic exercise program. Thus, it is important to initially prescribe low-intensity exercise to minimize her physical discomfort.

You also need to consider her busy schedule to find a convenient time for her to exercise. She reports feeling dizzy after eating. Although it is not your diagnosis to make, the likely reason is that she is eating only one meal a day, and the insulin surge after eating is lowering her blood glucose level. It is important to convince this client to start eating at least three meals a day to avoid this problem.

3. HR, BP, and RPE Responses to Graded Exercise Test

The client's HR response to the graded exercise test was normal. The exercise HR increased during each stage of the exercise test. The maximal heart rate (190 bpm) was very close to her age-predicted maximal HR (220 – 28 = 192 bpm). The client's BP response to the graded exercise test was normal. The diastolic BP remained fairly constant (78-82 mmHg), and the systolic BP increased with each stage of the exercise test. The RPEs were normal. The ratings increased linearly with exercise intensity, culminating with an RPE = 18.

4. Functional Aerobic Capacity

Being cleared by the physician, the client performed a graded exercise test and voluntarily terminated it because of fatigue. This was most likely a maximal-effort exercise test as indicated by the RPE (18) and the exercise heart rate (190 bpm) during the last stage of the graded exercise test. The treadmill speed and grade during the last stage of the protocol was 2.5 mph and 12%, respectively. This corresponds to a functional aerobic capacity of 7.0 METs or 24.5 ml·kg^{-1}·min^{-1}. According to the norms, this client's cardiorespiratory fitness level is *poor* for her age.

5. & 6. Training HRs

The graph of the client's HR and RPE responses to the graded exercise test is presented in figure B.5.

Given the client's poor cardiorespiratory fitness level and her lack of regular aerobic exercise, the initial minimal training intensity will be 50% $\dot{V}O_2R$ (4.0 METs), gradually increasing to a maximum intensity of 75% $\dot{V}O_2R$ (5.5 METs). The corresponding training HRs, extrapolated from figure B.4, are 152 bpm (50% $\dot{V}O_2R$ or 4.0 METs) and 174 bpm (75% $\dot{V}O_2R$ or 5.5 METs). The HRs and RPEs corresponding to the relative exercise intensities in the following chart were extrapolated from the graph.

%$\dot{V}O_2R$	METs	HR (bpm)	RPE
50%	4.0	152	12
60%	4.6	165	14
70%	5.2	170	15
75%	5.5	174	16

7. Speed Calculations (ACSM Formula for Walking on Level Course)

To calculate walking speed corresponding to 60% of the client's $\dot{V}O_2R$ [$0.60 \times (7 - 1) + 1$] = 4.6 METs):

a. Convert METs into ml·kg^{-1}·min^{-1}.

$$4.6 \text{ METs} \times 3.5 \text{ ml·kg}^{-1}\text{·min}^{-1} = 16.1 \text{ ml·kg}^{-1}\text{·min}^{-1}$$

b. Substitute into ACSM walking equation and solve for speed (m·min^{-1}).

$$\dot{V}O_2 = [\text{speed} \times 0.1] + [1.8 \times \text{speed} \times \text{grade}] + \text{resting } \dot{V}O_2$$

$$16.1 \text{ ml·kg}^{-1}\text{·min}^{-1} = [\text{speed} \times 0.1] + [1.8 \times \text{speed} \times 0\% \text{ grade}] + 3.5 \text{ ml·kg}^{-1}\text{·min}^{-1}$$

$$12.6 \text{ ml·kg}^{-1}\text{·min}^{-1} = \text{m·min}^{-1} \times 0.1$$

$$126 \text{ m·min}^{-1} = \text{speed}$$

c. Convert speed (m·min^{-1}) into miles per hour (26.8 m·min^{-1} = 1 mph).

$$126 \text{ m·min}^{-1}/26.8 \text{ m·min}^{-1} = 4.7 \text{ mph}$$

d. Convert miles per hour into minutes per mile walking pace.

$$60 \text{ min·hr}^{-1} / 4.7 \text{ mph} = 12.8 \text{ min·mile}^{-1}, \text{ or } 12:48 \text{ (12 min, 48 sec per mile)}$$

Follow these same steps to calculate the walking speed corresponding to 70% $\dot{V}O_2R$ and 75% $\dot{V}O_2R$.

(Answers: 70% $\dot{V}O_2R$ = 5.5 mph; 75% $\dot{V}O_2R$ = 5.9 mph)

8. Lifestyle Modifications

- Eat three well-balanced meals a day.
- Avoid fried foods high in saturated fats, cholesterol, and sodium.
- Dine out less frequently, and select restaurants offering healthy food choices (e.g., salad bar, grilled skinless chicken, or fish).
- Exercise aerobically at least 3 days a week.
- Try using relaxation techniques (e.g., stretching, progressive relaxation, mental imagery) to relax in the evening instead of drinking wine.

(continued)

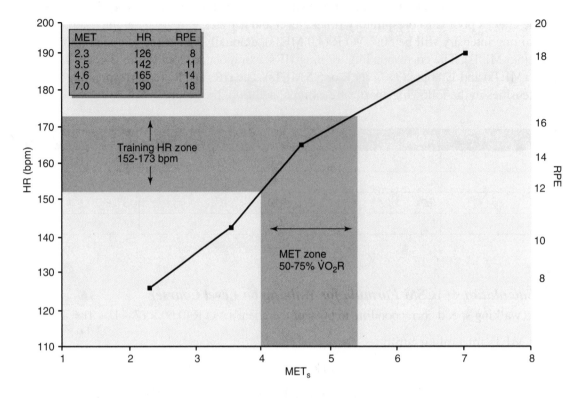

B.5 Plotting heart rate versus METs for graded exercise test.

Muscular Fitness Exercises and Norms

Appendix C.1 describes standardized testing protocols for 11 muscle groups using digital handheld dynamometry.

Appendix C.2 provides age-gender squat and bench press norms for untrained to elite lifters.

Appendix C.3 describes and illustrates some sample basic isometric exercises for a variety of muscle groups.

Appendix C.4 provides an extensive list of dynamic resistance training exercises. Exercises for the upper and lower extremities are organized by body region (e.g., chest, upper arm, thigh). For each exercise, equipment, body positions, joint actions, prime movers, and exercise variations are presented.

Appendix C.1 Standardized Testing Protocols for Digital Handheld Dynamometry

Muscle group	Position	Limb/joint position	Dynamometer placement
Elbow flexors	Supine	Shoulder 30° abducted, elbow 90° flexed, forearm supinated	Proximal to wrist on flexor surface of forearm
Elbow extensors	Supine	Same as for elbow flexors	Proximal to wrist on extensor surface of forearm
Shoulder extensors	Supine	Shoulder 90° anteflexed, elbow extended	Proximal to elbow on extensor surface of arm
Shoulder abductors	Supine	Shoulder 45° abducted, elbow extended	Proximal to lateral epicondyle of humerus
Wrist extensors	Sitting	Elbow 90° flexed, forearm supported and pronated, wrist in neutral position, fingers flexed	Proximal to 3rd metacarpal head
Hip flexors	Supine	Hip 90° flexed, knee relaxed, ankle supported by tester	Proximal to knee on anterior surface of thigh
Hip extensors	Supine	Hip 90° flexed, knee relaxed	Proximal to knee on posterior surface of thigh
Hip abductors	Supine	Hips 45° flexed, knees 90° flexed, contralateral knee supported by chest of tester	Lateral epicondyle of knee
Knee flexors	Sitting	Knee 90° flexed	Proximal to ankle on posterior surface of leg
Knee extensors	Sitting	Knee 90° flexed	Proximal to ankle on anterior surface of leg
Ankle dorsiflexors	Sitting	Knee 90° flexed, foot in neutral position	Proximal to metatarsophalangeal joints on dorsal surface of foot

Data from van den Beld et al. 2006.

Appendix C.2 1-RM Squat and Bench Press Norms for Adults

1-RM Squat Test Standards for Adult Men (Under 40 Years Old)

Body weight	Untrained	Novice	Intermediate	Advanced	Elite
114	77	143	176	237	320
123	83	154	193	259	347
132	88	171	204	281	369
148	99	187	231	314	408
165	110	204	248	342	446
181	121	220	270	369	480
198	127	231	287	391	507
220	132	243	298	408	529
242	138	254	309	424	551
275	143	259	320	435	568
319	149	270	325	446	579

Note: Measurements are in pounds.

In order for these standards to apply, squat must be performed with thighs traveling below parallel to floor.

Adapted with permission from http://www.kilgoreacademy.com/freebies.html. © Lon Kilgore PhD & Killustrated.

1-RM Squat Test Standards for Adult Women (Under 40 Years Old)

Body weight	Untrained	Novice	Intermediate	Advanced	Elite
97	44	83	99	132	165
106	50	88	105	143	176
115	53	99	116	149	193
123	55	105	121	160	198
132	61	110	132	171	209
148	66	121	138	187	231
165	72	127	149	198	254
181	77	138	165	215	270
198	83	149	176	231	292
212	88	160	187	243	303

Note: Measurements are in pounds.

In order for these standards to apply, squat must be performed with thighs traveling below parallel to floor.

Adapted with permission from http://www.kilgoreacademy.com/freebies.html. © Lon Kilgore PhD & Killustrated.

(continued)

1-RM Bench Press Standards for Adult Men (Under 40 Years Old)

Body weight	Untrained	Novice	Intermediate	Advanced	Elite
114	83	110	132	182	220
123	88	116	138	198	243
132	99	127	154	209	259
148	110	143	171	237	292
165	121	154	187	254	320
181	132	165	198	276	347
198	138	176	215	292	358
220	141	182	226	303	380
242	143	187	231	314	397
275	149	193	237	325	408
319	154	198	248	336	419

Note: Measurements are in pounds.

In order for these standards to apply, the bar must make contact with the chest above the bottom of the sternum with a momentary pause and be pressed to full elbow extension.

Adapted with permission from http://www.kilgoreacademy.com/freebies.html. © Lon Kilgore PhD & Killustrated.

1-RM Bench Press Standards for Adult Women (Under 40 Years Old)

Body weight	Untrained	Novice	Intermediate	Advanced	Elite
97	50	66	77	94	116
106	55	72	82	99	127
115	61	77	84	110	138
123	66	83	88	116	143
132	72	88	95	127	149
148	77	90	106	138	165
174	82	95	117	143	187
181	83	110	121	160	198
198	88	117	132	165	209
212	94	121	139	176	220

Note: Measurements are in pounds.

In order for these standards to apply, the bar must make contact with the chest above the bottom of the sternum with a momentary pause and be pressed to full elbow extension.

Adapted with permission from http://www.kilgoreacademy.com/freebies.html. © Lon Kilgore PhD & Killustrated.

Appendix C.3 Isometric Exercises

Video
C3.1

Exercise 1: Chest Push

Muscle groups: Shoulder and elbow flexors

Equipment: None

Description:

1. Lock hands together.
2. Keep forearms parallel to ground and hands close to chest.
3. Push hands together.

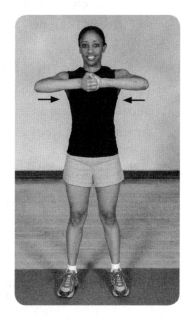

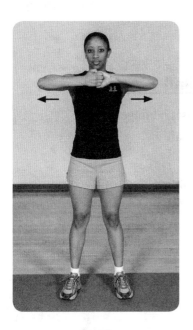

Exercise 2: Shoulder Pull

Muscle groups: Shoulder and elbow extensors

Equipment: None

Description:

1. Using same position as in chest push, attempt to pull hands apart.

Video
C3.2

Video
C3.3

Exercise 3: Triceps Extension

Muscle groups: Elbow extensors

Equipment: Towel or rope

Description:

1. Placing right hand over shoulder and left hand at small of back, grasp rope or towel behind back.
2. Attempt to pull towel or rope upward with right hand.
3. Change position of hands.

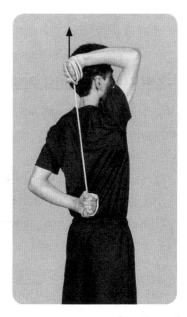

(continued)

Exercise 4: Arm Curls

Muscle groups: Elbow flexors

Equipment: Towel or rope

Description:

1. Stand with knees flexed about 45°.
2. Place rope or towel behind thighs, and grasp each end with hands shoulder-width apart.
3. Attempt to flex elbows.

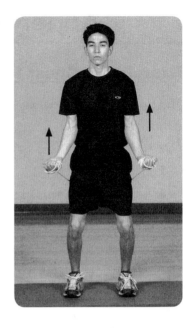

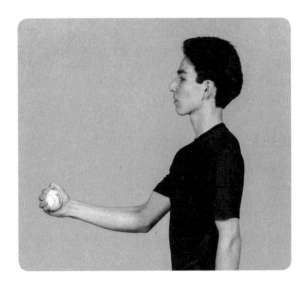

Exercise 5: Ball Squeeze

Muscle groups: Wrist and finger flexors

Equipment: Tennis ball

Description:

1. Hold tennis ball firmly in hand and squeeze maximally.

Exercise 6: Leg and Thigh Extensions

Muscle groups: Hip and knee extensors

Equipment: Rope

Description:

1. Stand on rope with knees flexed.
2. Grasp rope firmly with hands at sides, elbows fully extended.
3. Keeping trunk erect, attempt to extend legs by lifting upward.

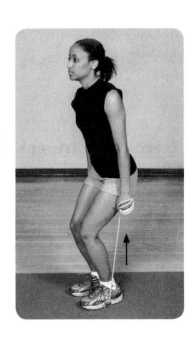

Exercise 7: Leg Press

Muscle groups: Hip and knee extensors

Equipment: Doorway

Description:

1. Sit in doorway facing side of door frame.
2. Grasp door frame behind feet.
3. Attempt to extend legs by pushing feet against door frame.

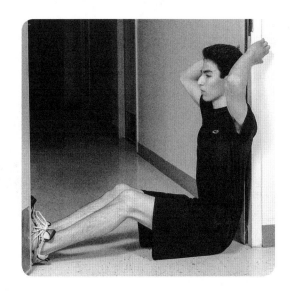

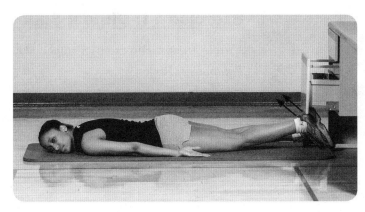

Exercise 8: Leg Curl

Muscle groups: Knee flexors

Equipment: Dresser or desk

Description:

1. Pull out lower dresser drawer slightly.
2. Lying prone, with knees flexed, hook heels under bottom of drawer.
3. Attempt to pull heels toward head.

Exercise 9: Knee Squeeze or Pull

Muscle groups: Hip adductors or abductors

Equipment: Chair

Description:

1. Sitting on chair with forearms crossed and hands on inside of knees, attempt to squeeze knees together (adductors).
2. Same position but place hands on outside of knees; attempt to pull knees apart (abductors).

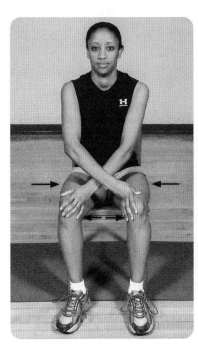
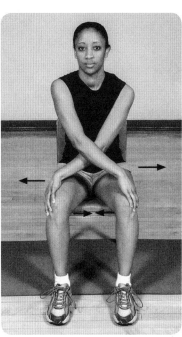

(continued)

Exercise 10: Pelvic Tilt

Muscle groups: Abdominals

Equipment: None

Description:

1. Lie supine with knees flexed and arms overhead.
2. Tighten abdominal muscles while pressing lower back into floor.

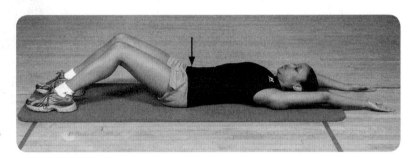

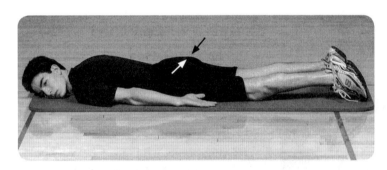

Exercise 11: Gluteal Squeeze

Muscle groups: Hip extensors and abductors

Equipment: None

Description:

1. Lie prone with legs together and fully extended.
2. Tighten and squeeze the buttocks together.

Appendix C.4: Dynamic Resistance Training Exercises

Exercise	Type[a]	Variations	Equipment[b]	Body position	Joint actions	Prime movers
Upper extremity						
Chest						
Bench press	M-J	Flat	B, D, M	Supine lying on flat bench	Shoulder horizontal adduction, elbow extension	Pectoralis major (midsternal), triceps brachii
		Incline	B, D, M	Sitting on incline bench	Shoulder flexion, elbow extension	Pectoralis major (clavicular), triceps brachii
		Decline	B, D	Supine lying on decline bench	Shoulder flexion, elbow extension	Pectoralis major (lower sternal), triceps brachii
Push-up	M-J	Hands wider than shoulders	None	Prone; BW supported by hands and feet	Shoulder horizontal adduction, elbow extension	Pectoralis major (midsternal), triceps brachii
		Hands narrower than shoulders	None	Same as above	Shoulder flexion, elbow extension	Pectoralis major (clavicular), ant deltoid, triceps brachii
Bar dip	M-J	Neutral grip	Parallel bars	Vertically supported by bars	Shoulder flexion, elbow extension	Pectoralis major (clavicular), ant deltoid, triceps brachii
		Pronated grip		Same as above	Shoulder adduction, elbow extension	Pectoralis major (midsternal), triceps brachii
Fly	S	Flat	D	Supine lying on flat bench	Shoulder adduction	Pectoralis major (midsternal)
Pullover (bent arm)	S	Flat	B, D	Supine lying on flat bench	Shoulder extension	Pectoralis major (lower sternal), post deltoid, latissimus dorsi

(continued)

From A.L. Gibson, D. R. Wagner, and V.H. Heyward, *Advanced Fitness Assessment and Exercise Prescription*, 8th ed. (Champaign, IL: Human Kinetics, 2019).

Appendix C.4: Dynamic Resistance Training Exercises   *(continued)*

Exercise	Type[a]	Variations	Equipment[b]	Body position	Joint actions	Prime movers
Upper extremity (cont.)						
Shoulders						
Overhead press	M-J	Military	B, D, M	Sitting or standing	Shoulder flexion, elbow extension	Pectoralis major (clavicular), ant deltoid, triceps brachii
		Behind the head	B	Sitting	Shoulder abduction, elbow extension	Ant/mid deltoid, supraspinatus
Upright row	M-J		B, D	Standing	Shoulder abduction, scapula upward rotation, elbow flexion	Mid deltoid, supraspinatus, trapezius (upper), brachialis
Front arm raise	S		B, C, D	Standing	Shoulder flexion	Pectoralis major (clavicular), ant deltoid
Lateral arm raise	S		C, D, M	Sitting or standing	Shoulder abduction	Mid deltoid, supraspinatus, pectoralis major (clavicular)
Reverse fly	S		C, D	Standing	Shoulder horizontal extension	Post deltoid, infraspinatus, teres minor
Upper arm						
Arm curl	S	Supinated grip	B, D, M	Standing or sitting on incline bench or preacher bench	Elbow flexion	Biceps brachii, brachialis
	S	Neutral grip	Same as above		Elbow flexion	Brachioradialis, brachialis, biceps brachii
	S	Pronated grip	Same as above		Elbow flexion	Brachialis
Triceps press-down	M-J		M	Seated	Shoulder flexion, elbow extension	Ant deltoid, pectoralis major (clavicular), triceps brachii

From A.L. Gibson, D. R. Wagner, and V.H. Heyward, *Advanced Fitness Assessment and Exercise Prescription*, 8th ed. (Champaign, IL: Human Kinetics, 2019).

Exercise	Type[a]	Variations	Equipment[b]	Body position	Joint actions	Prime movers
Upper extremity (cont.)						
Upper arm (cont.)						
Triceps extension	S		B	Supine lying on flat bench	Elbow extension	Triceps brachii
Triceps push-down	S	V-bar or strength bar	C	Standing	Elbow extension	Triceps brachii
French press	S		D	Standing or sitting	Elbow extension	Triceps brachii (medial head)
Overhead press	S		C, R	Standing with trunk flexed 45°	Elbow extension	Triceps brachii
Triceps kickback	S		D	Standing with one knee/hand on flat bench and trunk horizontal to floor	Elbow extension	Triceps brachii (long head)
Forearm						
Radioulnar rotation	S		D	Forearm/elbow supported on bench; hand free	Supination and pronation	Supinator, pronator teres, biceps brachii, brachioradialis
Wrist curl	S		D	Same as above	Wrist flexion	FCU, FCR
Reverse wrist curl	S		D	Same as above	Wrist extension	ECU, ECR (longus, brevis)
Radioulnar flexion	S		D	Standing with arm at side	Radial flexion, ulna flexion	FCR, ECR, FCU, ECU
Upper-mid back						
Lat pull-down	M-J	Pronated, wide grip	M	Sitting	Shoulder adduction, scapula adduction	Latissimus dorsi (upper), teres major, pectoralis major (upper), trapezius, rhomboids
	M-J	Narrow, neutral grip	M	Sitting	Shoulder extension, elbow flexion	Latissimus dorsi (lower), pectoralis major (lower sternal), biceps brachii

From A.L. Gibson, D. R. Wagner, and V.H. Heyward, *Advanced Fitness Assessment and Exercise Prescription*, 8th ed. (Champaign, IL: Human Kinetics, 2019).

(continued)

Appendix C.4: Dynamic Resistance Training Exercises (continued)

Exercise	Type[a]	Variations	Equipment[b]	Body position	Joint actions	Prime movers
Upper mid-back (cont.)						
Seated row	M-J	Neutral grip	M	Sitting	Shoulder extension, elbow flexion	Latissimus dorsi (lower), biceps brachii
	M-J	Pronated grip	M	Sitting with elbows horizontal to floor	Shoulder horizontal extension, elbow flexion	Post deltoid, latissimus dorsi (upper), infraspinatus, brachialis
Bent-over row	M-J	Neutral grip	D	Standing with trunk flexed 90°	Shoulder extension, elbow flexion	Latissimus dorsi, biceps brachii
	M-J	Pronated grip	D	Standing with trunk flexed 90° and elbows out	Shoulder horizontal extension, elbow flexion	Post deltoid, infraspinatus, latissimus dorsi, brachialis
Pull-up	M-J	Pronated grip	Pull-up bar	Vertically hanging from bar	Shoulder adduction, elbow flexion	Latissimus dorsi (upper), pectoralis major (sternal), brachialis
Chin-up	M-J	Supinated or neutral grip	Pull-up bar	Vertically hanging from bar	Shoulder extension, elbow flexion	Latissimus dorsi (lower), pectoralis major (sternal), biceps brachii
Shoulder shrug	S	Regular	B, D, M	Standing	Shoulder girdle (scapula and clavicle) elevation	Trapezius (upper), levator scapulae, rhomboids
	S	Elevation with shoulder roll		Standing	Shoulder girdle elevation, scapula adduction	Trapezius (mid), rhomboids
Lower back						
Trunk extension	M-J		M	Sitting with pelvis/thighs stabilized	Spinal extension	Erector spinae
Back raise	M-J		Glut-ham developer	Prone with pelvis supported; trunk flexed	Spinal extension	Erector spinae
Side bends	M-J		D	Standing	Spinal lateral flexion	Quadratus lumborum

From A.L. Gibson, D. R. Wagner, and V.H. Heyward, *Advanced Fitness Assessment and Exercise Prescription*, 8th ed. (Champaign, IL: Human Kinetics, 2019).

Exercise	Type[a]	Variations	Equipment[b]	Body position	Joint actions	Prime movers
Lower back (cont.)						
Isometric side support (side bridge)	M-J		None	Side-lying with BW supported by forearm and feet	None	Quadratus lumborum, abdominal obliques
Single-leg extension	M-J		None	Hands and knees	Spinal extension, hip extension	Erector spinae, gluteus maximus, hamstrings (upper)
Abdomen						
Curl-up	M-J	Bent knee	None	Supine lying with knees bent	Spinal flexion	Rectus abdominis
	M-J	With twist	None	Same as above	Spinal flexion	Abdominal obliques
Abdominal crunch	M-J		M	Sitting	Spinal flexion	Rectus abdominis
Reverse sit-up	M-J		None	Supine lying on floor on bench	Spinal flexion	Rectus abdominis (lower)
Lower extremity						
Hip						
Half squat	M-J		B, M	Standing	Hip extension, knee extension	Gluteus maximus, hamstrings (upper), quadriceps femoris
Leg press	M-J		M	Sitting	Hip extension, knee extension	Gluteus maximus, hamstrings (upper), quadriceps femoris
Lunge	M-J		B, D	Standing	Hip extension, knee extension	Gluteus maximus hamstrings (upper), quadriceps femoris
Glut-ham raise	M-J		Glut-ham developer	Prone with thighs supported and trunk flexed	Hip extension and knee flexion	Gluteus maximus, hamstrings

(continued)

From A.L. Gibson, D. R. Wagner, and V.H. Heyward, *Advanced Fitness Assessment and Exercise Prescription*, 8th ed. (Champaign, IL: Human Kinetics, 2019).

Appendix C.4: Dynamic Resistance Training Exercises (continued)

Exercise	Type[a]	Variations	Equipment[b]	Body position	Joint actions	Prime movers
Lower extremity (cont.)						
Hip (cont.)						
Hip flexion	S		C, M	Standing	Hip flexion	Iliopsoas, rectus femoris (upper)
Hip extension	S		C, M	Standing	Hip extension	Gluteus maximus, hamstrings (upper)
Hip adduction	S		M	Sitting or supine lying	Hip adduction	Adductor longus, brevis, and magnus; gracilis
Hip abduction	S		M	Sitting or supine lying	Hip abduction	Gluteus medius
Side leg raise	S		None	Lying on side	Hip abduction	Gluteus medius, hamstrings (upper)
Good morning exercise	S		B, D	Standing	Hip extension	Gluteus maximus, hamstrings (upper)
Thigh						
Leg extension	S		M	Seated	Knee extension	Quadriceps femoris
Leg curl	S	Straight	M	Prone lying, seated, or standing	Knee flexion	Hamstrings (lower)
	S	Knee externally rotated	M	Same as above	Knee flexion	Biceps femoris
	S	Knees internally rotated	M	Same as above	Knee flexion	Semitendinosus, semimembranosus
Lower leg						
Heel raise	S	Standing	D, M	Standing	Ankle plantar flexion	Gastrocnemius
	S	Seated	M	Sitting	Ankle plantar flexion	Soleus
Toe raise	S		Strength bar	Sitting	Ankle dorsiflexion	Tibialis anterior, peroneus tertius, extensor digitorum longus

Note: FCU = flexor carpi ulnaris; ECU = extensor carpi ulnaris; FCR = flexor carpi radialis; ECR = extensor carpi radialis.
[a]Type of exercise: M-J = multijoint exercise; S = single-joint exercise; [b]Equipment codes: B = barbell; C = cables; D = dumbbells; M = exercise machine; R = rope.

From A.L. Gibson, D. R. Wagner, and V.H. Heyward, *Advanced Fitness Assessment and Exercise Prescription*, 8th ed. (Champaign, IL: Human Kinetics, 2019).

Body Composition Assessments

Appendix D.1 presents prediction equations for estimating residual lung volume. Use these equations only when it is not possible to directly measure a client's residual lung volume.

Appendix D.2 describes and illustrates the standardized sites for skinfold measurements, and appendix D.3 describes the skinfold sites and measurement procedures for Jackson's generalized skinfold prediction equations for men and women.

Standardized sites for circumference (appendix D.4) and bony breadth (appendix D.5) measurements are also provided. Follow these procedures to identify and measure various sites.

Appendix D.6 contains the Ashwell Body Shape Chart. Use this chart to compare your clients' waist circumference to standing height.

Appendix D.1 Prediction Equations for Residual Volume

Population	Smoking history[a]	N	Equation[b]
MEN			
Boren, Kory, and Syner (1966)	Mixed	422	$RV = 0.0115 \text{ (age)} + 0.019 \text{ (HT)} - 2.24$ $r = .57$, *SEE* $= .53L$
Goldman and Becklake (1959)			$RV = 0.017 \text{ (age)} + 0.027 \text{ (HT)} - 3.477$
Berglund et al. (1963)			$RV = 0.022 \text{ (age)} + 0.0198 \text{ (HT)} - 0.015 \text{ (WT)} - 1.54$
WOMEN			
O'Brien and Drizd (1983)	Nonsmokers	926	$RV = 0.03 \text{ (age)} + 0.0387 \text{ (HT)} - 0.73 \text{ (BSA)} - 4.78$ $r = .66$, *SEE* $= .49$ L
Black, Offord, and Hyatt (1974)	Mixed	110	$RV = 0.021 \text{ (age)} + 0.023 \text{ (HT)} - 2.978$ $r = .70$, *SEE* $= .46L$
Goldman and Becklake (1959)			$RV = 0.009 \text{ (age)} + 0.032 \text{ (HT)} - 3.9$
Berglund et al. (1963)			$RV = 0.007 \text{ (age)} + 0.0268 \text{ (HT)} - 3.42$

[a]*Mixed* indicates that sample included both smokers and nonsmokers.

[b]Age (in yr); HT = height (in cm); BSA = body surface area (in m^2); WT = body mass (in kg).

Appendix D.2 Standardized Sites for Skinfold Measurements

Site	Direction of fold	Anatomical reference	Measurement
Chest	Diagonal	Axilla and nipple	Fold is taken between axilla and nipple as high as possible on anterior axillary fold, with measurement taken 1 cm below fingers.
Subscapular	Diagonal	Inferior angle of scapula	Fold is taken along natural cleavage line of skin just inferior to inferior angle of scapula, with caliper applied 1 cm below fingers.
Midaxillary	Horizontal	Xiphisternal junction (point were costal cartilage of ribs 5-6 articulates with sternum, slightly above inferior tip of xiphoid process)	Fold is taken on midaxillary line at level of xiphisternal junction.
Suprailiac	Oblique	Iliac crest	Fold is grasped posteriorly to midaxillary line and superiorly to iliac crest along natural cleavage of skin with caliper applied 1 cm below fingers.
Abdominal	Horizontal	Umbilicus	Fold is taken 3 cm lateral and 1 cm inferior to center of the umbilicus.
Triceps	Vertical (midline)	Acromion process of scapula and olecranon process of ulna	Using a tape measure, distance between lateral projection of acromion process and inferior margin of olecranon process is measured on lateral aspect of arm with elbow flexed 90°. Midpoint is marked on lateral side of arm. Fold is lifted 1 cm above marked line on posterior aspect of arm. Caliper is applied at marked level.
Biceps	Vertical (midline)	Biceps brachii	Fold is lifted over belly of the biceps brachii at the level marked from the triceps and on line with anterior border of the acromion process and the antecubital fossa. Caliper is applied 1 cm below fingers.
Thigh	Vertical (midline)	Inguinal crease and patella	Fold is lifted on anterior aspect of thigh midway between inguinal crease and proximal border of patella. Body weight is shifted to left foot, and caliper is applied 1 cm below fingers.
Calf	Vertical (medial aspect)	Maximal calf circumference	Fold is lifted at level of maximal calf circumference on medial aspect of calf with knees and hip flexed to 90°.

Adapted from Harrison et al. 1988.

(continued)

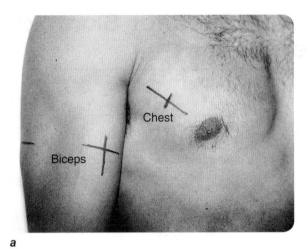
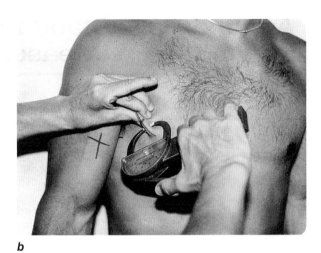

a **b**

FIGURE D.2.1 *(a)* Site and *(b)* measurement of the chest skinfold.

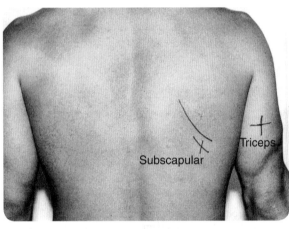
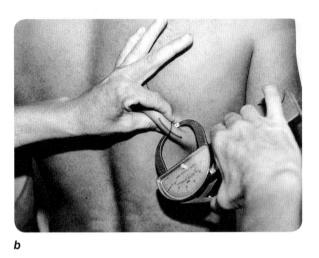

a **b**

FIGURE D.2.2 *(a)* Site and *(b)* measurement of the subscapular skinfold.

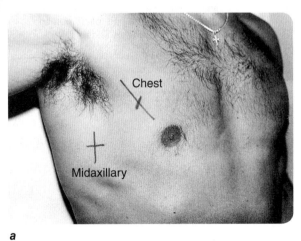
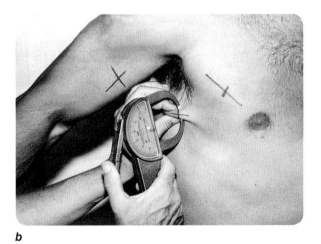

a **b**

FIGURE D.2.3 *(a)* Site and *(b)* measurement of the midaxillary skinfold.

Courtesy of Linda K. Gilkey. From A.L. Gibson, D. Wagner, and V.H. Heyward, *Advanced Fitness and Exercise Prescription,* 8th ed. (Champaign, IL: Human Kinetics, 2019).

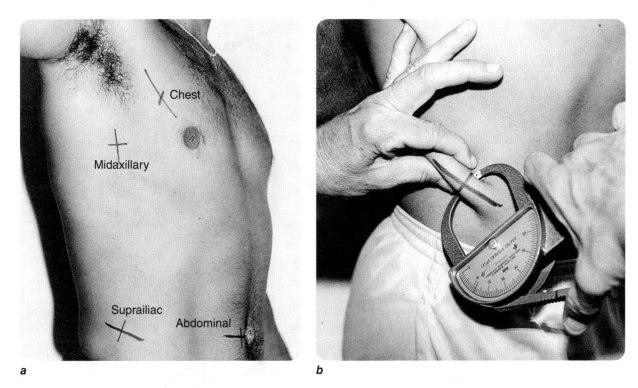

a

b

FIGURE D.2.4 *(a)* Site and *(b)* measurement of the suprailiac skinfold.

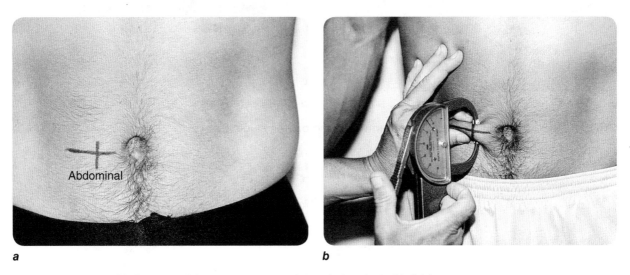

a

b

FIGURE D.2.5 *(a)* Site and *(b)* measurement of the abdominal skinfold.

Video
D2.3

Courtesy of Linda K. Gilkey. From A.L. Gibson, D. Wagner, and V.H. Heyward, *Advanced Fitness and Exercise Prescription,* 8th ed. (Champaign, IL: Human Kinetics, 2019).

(continued)

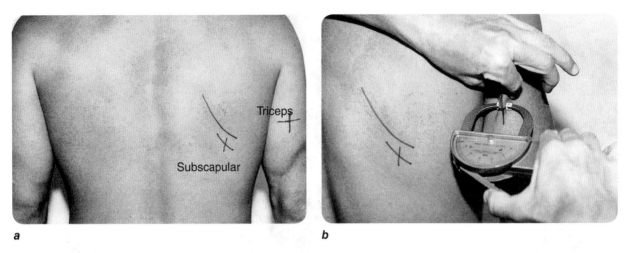

a   *b*

FIGURE D.2.6 *(a)* Site and *(b)* measurement of the triceps skinfold.

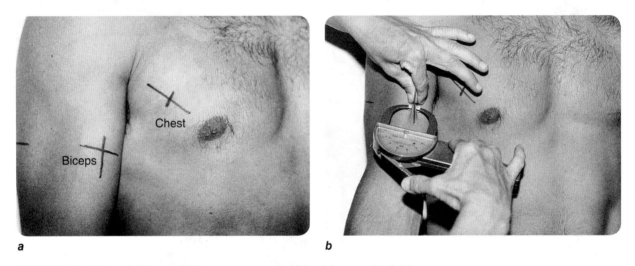

a   *b*

FIGURE D.2.7 *(a)* Site and *(b)* measurement of the biceps skinfold.

Courtesy of Linda K. Gilkey. From A.L. Gibson, D. Wagner, and V.H. Heyward, *Advanced Fitness and Exercise Prescription,* 8th ed. (Champaign, IL: Human Kinetics, 2019).

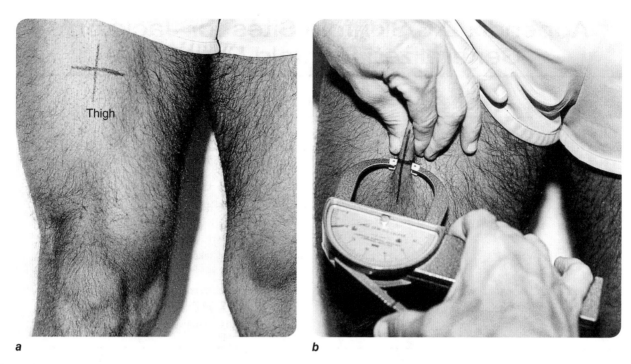

a

b

Video D2.4

FIGURE D.2.8 *(a)* Site and *(b)* measurement of the thigh skinfold.

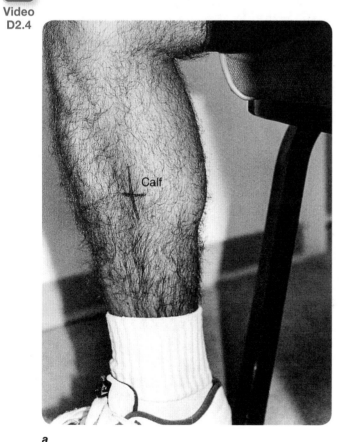

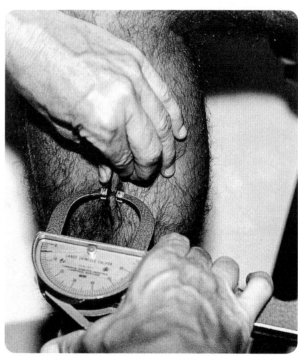

a

b

FIGURE D.2.9 *(a)* Site and *(b)* measurement of the calf skinfold.

Video D2.5

Appendix D.3 Skinfold Sites for Jackson's Generalized Skinfold Equations

Site	Direction of fold	Anatomical reference	Measurement
Chest	Diagonal	Axilla and nipple	Fold is taken 1/2 the distance between the anterior axillary line and nipple for men and 1/3 of this distance for women.
Subscapular	Oblique	Vertebral border and inferior angle of scapula	Fold is taken on diagonal line coming from the vertebral border, 1-2 cm below the inferior angle.
Midaxillary	Vertical	Xiphoid process of sternum	Fold is taken at level of xiphoid process along the midaxillary line.
Suprailiac	Diagonal	Iliac crest	Fold is taken diagonally above the iliac crest along the anterior axillary line.
Abdominal	Vertical	Umbilicus	Fold is taken vertically 2 cm lateral to the umbilicus.

Adapted from Jackson and Pollock 1978; Jackson, Pollock, and Ward 1980.

From A.L. Gibson, D. Wagner, and V.H. Heyward, *Advanced Fitness and Exercise Prescription,* 8th ed. (Champaign, IL: Human Kinetics, 2019).

Appendix D.4 Standardized Sites for Circumference Measurements

Site	Anatomical reference	Position	Measurement
Neck	Laryngeal prominence (Adam's apple)	Perpendicular to long axis of neck	Apply tape with minimal pressure just inferior to the Adam's apple.
Shoulder	Deltoid muscles and acromion processes of scapula	Horizontal	Apply tape snugly over maximum bulges of the deltoid muscles, inferior to acromion processes. Record measurement at end of normal expiration.
Chest	Fourth costosternal joints	Horizontal	Apply tape snugly around the torso at level of fourth costosternal joints. Record at end of normal expiration.
Waist	Narrowest part of torso, level of the natural waist between ribs and iliac crest	Horizontal	Apply tape snugly around the waist at level of narrowest part of torso. An assistant is needed to position tape behind the client. Take measurement at end of normal expiration.
Abdominal	Maximum anterior protuberance of abdomen, usually at umbilicus	Horizontal	Apply tape snugly around the abdomen at level of greatest anterior protuberance. An assistant is needed to position tape behind the client. Take measurement at end of normal expiration.
Hip (buttocks)	Maximum posterior extension of buttocks	Horizontal	Apply tape snugly around the buttocks. An assistant is needed to position tape on opposite side of body.
Thigh (proximal)	Gluteal fold	Horizontal	Apply tape snugly around thigh, just distal to the gluteal fold.
Thigh (mid)	Inguinal crease and proximal border of patella	Horizontal	With client's knee flexed 90° (right foot on bench), apply tape at level midway between inguinal crease and proximal border of patella.
Thigh (distal)	Femoral epicondyles	Horizontal	Apply tape just proximal to the femoral epicondyles.
Knee	Patella	Horizontal	Apply tape around the knee at midpatellar level with knee relaxed in slight flexion.
Calf	Maximum girth of calf muscle	Perpendicular to long axis of leg	With client sitting on end of table and legs hanging freely, apply tape horizontally around the maximum girth of calf.
Ankle	Malleoli of tibia and fibula	Perpendicular to long axis of leg	Apply tape snugly around the minimum circumference of leg, just proximal to the malleoli.
Arm (biceps)	Acromion process of scapula and olecranon process of ulna	Perpendicular to long axis of arm	With client's arms hanging freely at sides and palms facing thighs, apply tape snugly around the arm at level midway between the acromion process of scapula and olecranon process of ulna (as marked for triceps and biceps skinfolds)
Forearm	Maximum girth of forearm	Perpendicular to long axis of forearm	With client's arms hanging down and away from trunk and forearm supinated, apply tape snugly around the maximum girth of the proximal part of the forearm.
Wrist	Styloid processes of radius and ulna	Perpendicular to long axis of forearm	With client's elbow flexed and forearm supinated, apply tape snugly around wrist, just distal to the styloid processes of the radius and ulna.

Adapted from Callaway et al. 1988.

From A.L. Gibson, D.R. Wagner, and V.H. Heyward, *Advanced Fitness Assessment and Exercise Prescription,* 8th ed. (Champaign, IL: Human Kinetics, 2019).

Appendix D.5 Standardized Sites for Bony Breadth Measurements

Site	Anatomical reference	Position	Measurement
Biacromial (shoulder)	Lateral borders of acromion processes of scapula	Horizontal	With client standing, arms hanging vertically and shoulders relaxed, downward and slightly forward, apply blades of anthropometer to lateral borders of acromion processes. Measurement is taken from the rear.
Chest	Sixth rib on midaxillary line or fourth costosternal joints anteriorly	Horizontal	With client standing, arms slightly abducted, apply the large spreading caliper tips lightly on the sixth ribs on the midaxillary line. Take measurement at end of normal respiration.
Bi-iliac (bicristal)	Iliac crests	45° downward angle	With client standing, arms folded across the chest, apply anthropometer blades firmly at a 45° downward angle, at maximum breadth of iliac crest. Measurement is taken from rear.
Bitrochanteric	Greater trochanter of femur	Horizontal	With client standing, arms folded across the chest, apply anthropometer blade with considerable pressure to compress soft tissues. Measure maximum distance between the trochanters from the rear.
Knee	Femoral epicondyles	Diagonal or horizontal	With client sitting and knee flexed to 90°, apply caliper blades firmly on lateral and medial femoral epicondyles.
Ankle (bimalleolar)	Malleoli of tibia and fibula	Oblique	With client standing and weight evenly distributed, place the caliper blades on the most lateral part of lateral malleolus and most medial part of medial malleolus. Measurement is taken on an oblique plane from the rear.
Elbow	Epicondyles of humerus	Oblique	With client's elbow flexed 90°, arm raised to the horizontal, and forearm supinated, apply the caliper blades firmly to the medial and lateral humeral epicondyles at an angle that bisects the right angle at the elbow.
Wrist	Styloid process of radius and ulna, anatomical snuff box	Oblique	With client's elbow flexed 90°, upper arm vertical and close to torso, and forearm pronated, apply caliper tips firmly at an oblique angle to the styloid processes of the radius (at proximal part of anatomical snuff box) and ulna.

Video D5.1

Video D5.2

Adapted from Wilmore et al. 1988.

From A.L. Gibson, D.R. Wagner, and V.H. Heyward, *Advanced Fitness Assessment and Exercise Prescription,* 8th ed. (Champaign, IL: Human Kinetics, 2019).

Appendix D.6 Ashwell Body Shape Chart

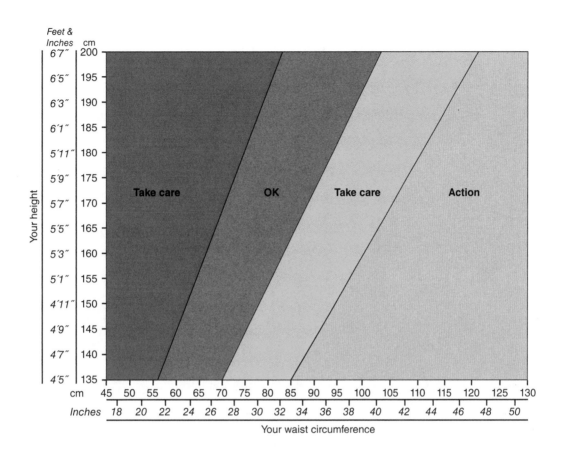

Energy Intake and Expenditure

You can use the Food Record and RDA Profile (appendix E.1) to obtain information about your clients' energy intake and daily energy needs.

Your clients may use the Physical Activity Log (appendix E.2) to record the type and duration of physical activities they engage in daily. This provides an estimate of their daily caloric expenditure due to activity. Appendix E.3 presents MET estimates of gross expenditure for conditioning exercises, sports, and recreational activities. You can use these estimates to calculate your clients' energy expenditure ($kcal \cdot min^{-1}$) for a variety of activities.

Appendix E.1 Food Record and RDA Profile

Food code	Amount	Description

From ESHA Research, Salem, OR.

Food code: This is generally for office use. If you have the food code list, however, use this space to more precisely describe your food item.

Amount: You can use common measures (cup, slice, etc.) or weight for your foods.

Food description: Be specific. For example, bread choices include soft and firm textures; vegetables may be raw or cooked fresh, frozen, or canned; meats should be lean only or lean with some fat; fruit juices are fresh, frozen, or canned; and cheese might be cream or skim, soft, hard, or cottage.

From ESHA Research, Salem, OR. From A.L. Gibson, D.R. Wagner, and V.H. Heyward, *Advanced Fitness Assessment and Exercise Prescription*, 8th ed. (Champaign, IL: Human Kinetics, 2019).

RDA Profile Information

Name: _____

Age: _____   Height: _____

Sex: Male_____   Weight: _____

      Female_____   Activity level: _____

                                                          (enter number from choices below)

      Pregnant _____

      Nursing _____

Most people engage in a variety of activities in a 24 hr period, and each activity can use a different amount of energy. Thus, any table of activity levels must depend on averages. Choose the level that represents your *normal daily average*.

1. Sedentary: Inactive, sometimes under someone else's care. Energy level is for basal metabolism plus about 15% for minimal activities.

2. Lightly active: Most professionals (lawyers, doctors, accountants, architects, etc.), office workers, shop workers, teachers, homemakers with mechanical appliances, unemployed persons.

3. Moderately active: Most persons in light industry, building workers (excluding heavy laborers), many farm workers, active students, department store workers, soldiers not in active service, people engaged in commercial fishing, homemakers without mechanical household appliances.

4. Very active: Full-time athletes, dancers, unskilled laborers, some agricultural workers (especially in peasant farming), forestry workers, army recruits, soldiers in active service, mine workers, steel workers.

5. Exceptionally active: Lumberjacks, blacksmiths, female construction workers, rickshaw pullers.

From ESHA Research, Salem, OR. From A.L. Gibson, D.R. Wagner, and V.H. Heyward, *Advanced Fitness Assessment and Exercise Prescription*, 8th ed. (Champaign, IL: Human Kinetics, 2019).

Appendix E.2 Physical Activity Log

Name: _____   Date: _____

Day and date	Activity	Duration (min)	x	kcal·min^{-1}	= Total (kcal)

From A.L. Gibson, D.R. Wagner, and V.H. Heyward, *Advanced Fitness Assessment and Exercise Prescription,* 8th ed. (Champaign, IL: Human Kinetics, 2019).

Appendix E.3 Gross Energy Expenditure for Conditioning Exercises, Sports, and Recreational Activities

METs	Description	METs	Description
CONDITIONING EXERCISES			

METs	Description	METs	Description
CONDITIONING EXERCISES			
5.0	Aerobic dancing, low impact	12.5	In-line skating, vigorous effort
8.5	Aerobics, step, with 6-8 in. step	8.0	Rope skipping, slow
10.0	Aerobics, step, with 10-12 in. step	10.0	Rope skipping, moderate
3.0	Bicycling, stationary, 50 W, very light effort	12.0	Rope skipping, fast
5.5	Bicycling, stationary, 100 W, light effort	9.5	Skiing, Nordic (machine)
7.0	Bicycling, stationary, 150 W, moderate effort	6.0	Slimnastics, Jazzercize
10.5	Bicycling, stationary, 200 W, vigorous effort	9.0	Stair-climbing (machine), step ergometer
12.5	Bicycling, stationary, 250 W, very vigorous effort	2.5	Stretching, hatha yoga
8.0	Calisthenics (e.g., push-ups, pull-ups, jumping jacks, sit-ups), vigorous	10.0	Swimming, laps, freestyle, fast, vigorous effort
3.5	Calisthenics, light or moderate effort	7.0	Swimming, laps, freestyle, slow, moderate or light effort
8.0	Circuit resistance training, including some aerobic activity and minimal rest (e.g., super circuit resistance training)	7.0	Swimming, backstroke
8.0	Elliptical training, machine, 125 strides·min⁻¹ with resistance	10.0	Swimming, breaststroke
3.5	Rowing (machine), 50 W, light effort	11.0	Swimming, butterfly
7.0	Rowing (machine), 100 W, moderate effort	11.0	Swimming, crawl, fast, vigorous effort
8.5	Rowing (machine), 150 W, vigorous effort	8.0	Swimming, crawl, slow, moderate or light effort
12.0	Rowing (machine), 200 W, very vigorous effort	8.0	Swimming, sidestroke
8.0	Running, 5 mph (12 min·mile⁻¹)	4.0	Swimming, treading water, moderate effort
9.0	Running, 5.2 mph (11.5 min·mile⁻¹)	4.0	Tai chi
10.0	Running, 6.0 mph (10 min·mile⁻¹)	5.0	Treading, walking, variable speed 2.5-4.0 mph and grade 0%-10%
11.0	Running, 6.7 mph (9 min·mile⁻¹)	11.0	Treading, running, variable speed 5.8-7.5 mph and grade 0%-10%
11.5	Running, 7.0 mph (8.5 min·mile⁻¹)	2.5	Walking, 2.0 mph
12.5	Running, 7.5 mph (8 min·mile⁻¹)	3.0	Walking, 2.5 mph
13.5	Running, 8 mph (7.5 min·mile⁻¹)	3.3	Walking, 3.0 mph
14.0	Running, 8.6 mph (7 min·mile⁻¹)	3.8	Walking, 3.5 mph
15.0	Running, 9 mph (6.5 min·mile⁻¹)	5.0	Walking, 4.0 mph
16.0	Running, 10 mph (6 min·mile⁻¹)	6.3	Walking, 4.5 mph
18.0	Running, 10.9 mph (5.5 min·mile⁻¹)	4.0	Water aerobics, water calisthenics

(continued)

From A.L. Gibson, D.R. Wagner, and V.H. Heyward, *Advanced Fitness Assessment and Exercise Prescription,* 8th ed. (Champaign, IL: Human Kinetics, 2019).

METs	Description	METs	Description
CONDITIONING EXERCISES			
9.0	Running, cross country	8.0	Water jogging
7.0	Jogging, general	3.0	Weightlifting (free weights/machines), light to moderate effort
6.0	Jogging/walking combination (jogging component less than 10 min)	6.0	Weightlifting (free weights/machines), powerlifting, bodybuilding, vigorous effort
4.5	Jogging on a mini-trampoline		
SPORTS AND RECREATIONAL ACTIVITIES			
3.5	Archery (nonhunting)	4.0	Curling
7.0	Badminton, competitive	4.8	Dancing, ballet or modern, twist, jazz, tap, jitterbug
4.5	Badminton, social singles or doubles	4.5	Dancing, Greek, Middle Eastern, belly, hula, flamenco, swing
5.0	Baseball, general	4.5	Dancing, ballroom, fast, disco, folk, square, line dancing, Irish step dancing, polka, contra, country
8.0	Basketball, game	3.0	Dancing, slow, waltz, foxtrot, samba, tango, mambo, cha-cha
4.5	Basketball, shooting baskets	5.5	Dancing, traditional American Indian dancing
6.5	Basketball, wheelchair	2.5	Darts, wall or lawn
8.5	Bicycling, BMX or mountain	3.0	Diving, springboard or platform
4.0	Bicycling, <10 mph, leisure, pleasure	6.0	Fencing
6.0	Bicycling, 10-11.9 mph	4.0	Fishing and hunting from riverbank and walking
8.0	Bicycling, 12-13.9 mph	2.5	Fishing and hunting from boat, sitting
10.0	Bicycling, 14-15.9 mph	6.0	Fishing in stream, in waders
12.0	Bicycling, 16-19 mph	2.0	Fishing, ice, sitting
16.0	Bicycling, ≥20 mph	2.5	Fishing and hunting, bow and arrow, crossbow
5.0	Bicycling, unicycle	2.5	Fishing and hunting, pistol shooting, trap shooting, standing
2.5	Billiards, pool	9.0	Football, competitive
2.5	Bird watching	2.5	Football or baseball, playing catch
3.0	Bowling	8.0	Football, touch, flag
3.0	Bowling, lawn	3.0	Frisbee, playing, general
12.0	Boxing, in ring	8.0	Frisbee, ultimate
6.0	Boxing, punching bag	3.0	Gardening, lawn work, general
9.0	Boxing, sparring	4.5	Golfing, walking and carrying clubs
7.0	Broomball	3.0	Golfing, miniature, driving range
3.0	Canoeing, 2.0-3.9 mph, light effort	4.3	Golfing, walking and pulling clubs
7.0	Canoeing, 4.0-5.9 mph, moderate effort	3.5	Golfing, power cart
12.0	Canoeing ≥6.0 mph, vigorous effort	4.0	Gymnastics, general
5.0	Children's games, hopscotch, dodgeball, tee ball, tetherball, playground	4.0	Hacky sack
5.0	Cricket (batting and bowling)	12.0	Handball, general
2.5	Croquet	8.0	Handball, team

From A.L. Gibson, D.R. Wagner, and V.H. Heyward, *Advanced Fitness Assessment and Exercise Prescription,* 8th ed. (Champaign, IL: Human Kinetics, 2019).

METs	Description	METs	Description
	SPORTS AND RECREATIONAL ACTIVITIES		
3.5	Hang gliding	14.0	Skiing, cross-country, >8.0 mph, racing
6.0	Hiking, cross country	5.0	Skiing, downhill, light effort
8.0	Hockey, field	6.0	Skiing, downhill, moderate effort
8.0	Hockey, ice	8.0	Skiing, downhill, vigorous effort, racing
4.0	Horseback riding, general	6.0	Skiing, water
3.0	Horseshoe pitching, quoits	7.0	Skimobiling
12.0	Jai alai	3.5	Skydiving
10.0	Judo, jujitsu, kick boxing, tae kwon do	7.0	Sledding, tobogganing, bobsledding, luge
4.0	Juggling	5.0	Snorkeling
5.0	Kayaking and whitewater rafting	8.0	Snowshoeing
7.0	Kickball	10.0	Soccer, competitive
8.0	Lacrosse	7.0	Soccer, casual, general
4.0	Motocross	5.0	Softball, fast or slow pitch
9.0	Orienteering	6.0	Softball, pitching
10.0	Paddleball, competitive	12.0	Squash
6.0	Paddleball, casual, general	3.0	Surfing, body or board
4.0	Paddle boating	6.0	Swimming, leisurely, not laps
8.0	Polo	8.0	Swimming, synchronized
6.5	Race walking	4.0	Table tennis, Ping-Pong
10.0	Racquetball, competitive	7.0	Tennis, general
7.0	Racquetball, casual, general	5.0	Tennis, doubles
11.0	Rock climbing, ascending	8.0	Tennis, singles
8.0	Rock climbing, rappelling	4.0	Track and field, shot, discus, hammer throw
12.5	Inline skating	6.0	Track and field, high jump, long jump, triple jump, javelin, pole vault
3.0	Sailing, boat and board sailing, wind surfing, ice surfing	10.0	Track and field, steeplechase, hurdles
7.0	Scuba diving, skin diving	3.5	Trampoline
3.0	Shuffleboard	8.0	Volleyball, competitive
5.0	Skateboarding	8.0	Volleyball, beach
7.0	Skating, roller or ice	3.0	Volleyball, noncompetitive
15.0	Skating, speed skating	10.0	Water polo
7.0	Skiing, cross-country, 2.5 mph, light effort	3.0	Water volleyball
8.0	Skiing, cross-country, 4.0-4.9 mph, moderate effort	7.0	Wallyball
9.0	Skiing, cross-country, 5.0-7.9 mph, vigorous effort	6.0	Wrestling

From A.L. Gibson, D.R. Wagner, and V.H. Heyward, *Advanced Fitness Assessment and Exercise Prescription,* 8th ed. (Champaign, IL: Human Kinetics, 2019).

Flexibility and Low Back Care Exercises

Appendix F.1 describes and illustrates selected static stretching exercises for flexibility. This information is organized by body region and muscle groups. Appendix F.2 summarizes Exercise Dos and Don'ts. For each contraindicated exercise, a safe alternative exercise is presented.

Recommended exercises for low back care programs are illustrated in appendix F.3. This appendix provides a description and identifies muscle groups involved for each exercise.

Appendix F.1 Selected Flexibility Exercises

ANTERIOR THIGH REGION

Muscle Groups: Quadriceps and Hip Flexors

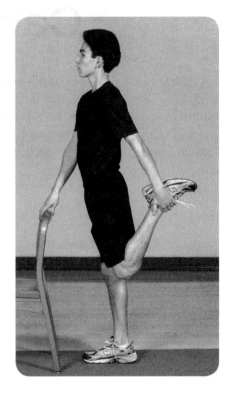

Exercise 1

Description: From a standing position, raise one foot toward hips and grasp ankle. Pull leg upward toward buttocks.

Exercise 2

Description: Lying on your side, flex the knee and grasp the ankle. Press the foot into the hand and squeeze pelvis forward. Do not pull the foot.

Exercise 3

Description: In a prone position, flex the knee and grasp ankle or foot with both hands. Do not pull on the foot. Keep knees on the floor and do not arch the back.

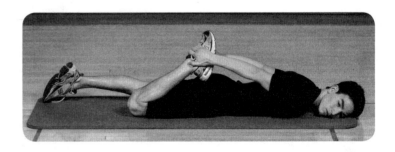

From A.L. Gibson, D.R. Wagner, and V.H. Heyward, *Advanced Fitness Assessment and Exercise Prescription*, 8th ed. (Champaign, IL: Human Kinetics, 2019).

Muscle Groups: Hamstrings and Hip Extensors

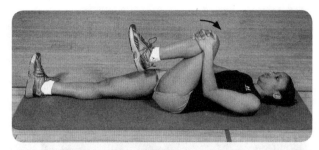

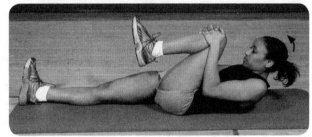

Video
F1.1

Exercise 1

Description: In a supine position, grasp knee and pull knee toward chest, then flex head to knee.

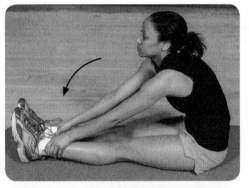

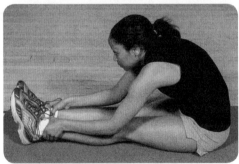

Exercise 2

Description: From a long-sitting position, grasp ankles and flex trunk to legs.

Exercise 3

Description: From a standing position, place your foot on a low step, keep the knee flexed slightly, and bend from the hips until you feel the stretch.

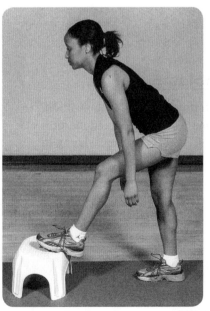

(continued)

From A.L. Gibson, D.R. Wagner, and V.H. Heyward, *Advanced Fitness Assessment and Exercise Prescription,* 8th ed. (Champaign, IL: Human Kinetics, 2019).

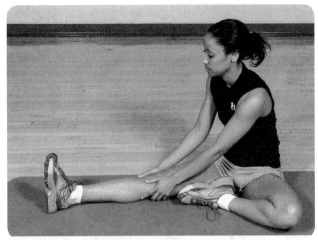

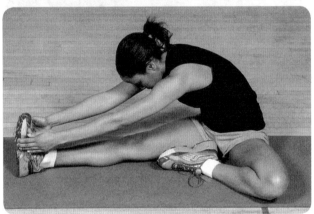

Exercise 4

Description: From a sitting position, with one knee flexed, flex the trunk keeping the spine extended until you feel tension.

Exercise 5

Description: From a lying position, with one leg extended and the other leg flexed, grasp leg with both hands and flex thigh to trunk.

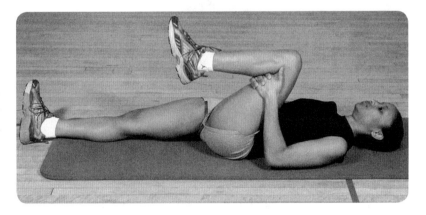

From A.L. Gibson, D.R. Wagner, and V.H. Heyward, *Advanced Fitness Assessment and Exercise Prescription,* 8th ed. (Champaign, IL: Human Kinetics, 2019).

Muscle Group: Hip Adductors

Exercise 1

Description: From a tailor-sitting position, with soles of feet together, place hands on inside of knees and push downward slightly.

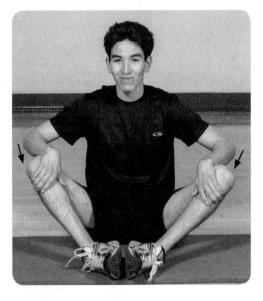

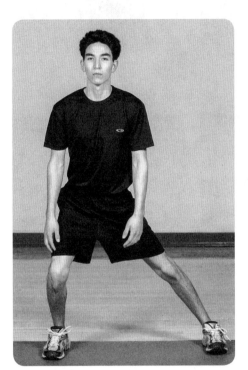

Exercise 2

Description: From a straddle-standing position, flex one knee and hip, lowering body closer to floor.

Exercise 3

Description: Standing on one leg while supporting yourself against wall or chair abduct hip, keeping leg straight. Have partner, if available, grasp ankle and passively stretch the muscle further.

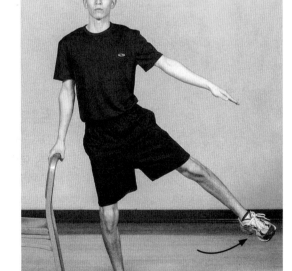

From A.L. Gibson, D.R. Wagner, and V.H. Heyward, *Advanced Fitness Assessment and Exercise Prescription,* 8th ed. (Champaign, IL: Human Kinetics, 2019).

LATERAL THIGH-TRUNK REGION

Muscle Groups: Hip Abductors and Trunk Lateral Flexors

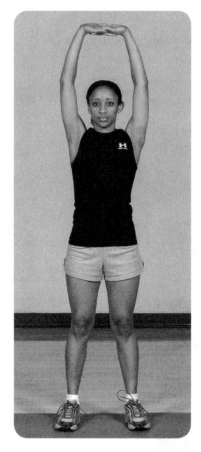 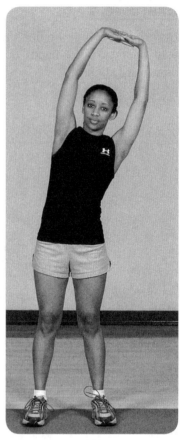

Exercise 1

Description: From standing position, with arms overhead, clasp hands together and laterally flex trunk to side no more than 20°.

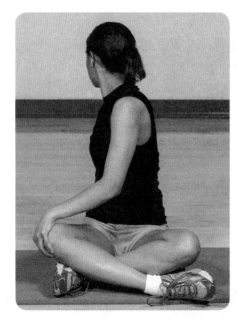

Exercise 2

Description: From a crossed-leg sitting position, rotate trunk to the right. Place hands on right side of upper leg and pull. Repeat to opposite side.

From A.L. Gibson, D.R. Wagner, and V.H. Heyward, *Advanced Fitness Assessment and Exercise Prescription,* 8th ed. (Champaign, IL: Human Kinetics, 2019).

Muscle Group: Plantar Flexors

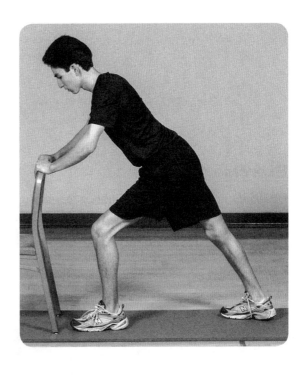

Exercise 1

Description: Assume front-leaning position against wall or chair with one foot ahead of the other. Flex hip, knee, and ankle to lower your body closer to the ground, keeping feet flat on floor.

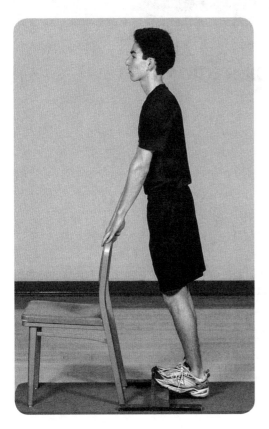

Exercise 2

Description: Standing with balls of feet on stairs, curb, or wood block, lower heels to floor.

From A.L. Gibson, D.R. Wagner, and V.H. Heyward, *Advanced Fitness Assessment and Exercise Prescription,* 8th ed. (Champaign, IL: Human Kinetics, 2019).

ANTERIOR LEG REGION

Muscle Group: Dorsiflexors

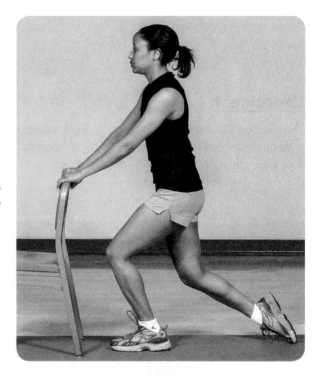

Exercise 1

Description: Standing with ankle of the nonsupporting leg fully extended, stretch the dorsiflexors by slowly flexing the knee of the supporting leg.

UPPER AND LOWER BACK REGIONS

Muscle Group: Trunk Extensors

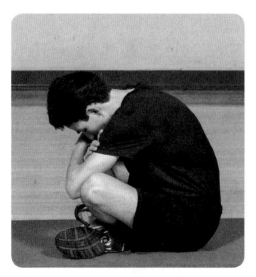

Exercise 1

Description: Sit with legs crossed and arms relaxed. Tuck chin and curl forward, attempting to touch forehead to knees.

From A.L. Gibson, D.R. Wagner, and V.H. Heyward, *Advanced Fitness Assessment and Exercise Prescription,* 8th ed. (Champaign, IL: Human Kinetics, 2019).

Exercise 2

Description: In a supine position, with knees flexed, grasp thighs below the knee caps and bring knees to chest. Flatten lower back to floor.

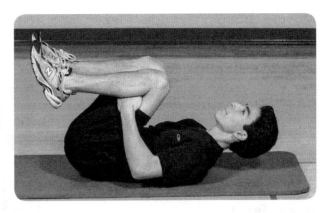

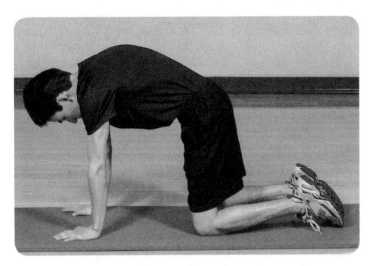

Exercise 3

Description: From a kneeling position, bring chin to chest. Contract abdomen and buttocks muscles while rounding lower back.

ANTERIOR CHEST, SHOULDER, AND ABDOMINAL REGIONS

Muscle Groups: Shoulder Flexors and Adductors, Trunk Flexors

Exercise 1

Description: In a prone position, push up until elbows are extended. Keep pelvis and hips on floor.

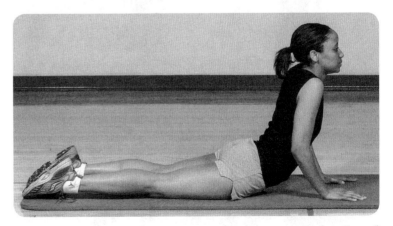

(continued)

From A.L. Gibson, D.R. Wagner, and V.H. Heyward, *Advanced Fitness Assessment and Exercise Prescription,* 8th ed. (Champaign, IL: Human Kinetics, 2019).

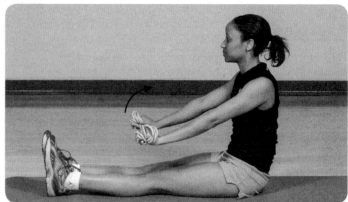

Exercise 2

Description: Grasp towel or rope with both hands. Rotate arms overhead behind trunk.

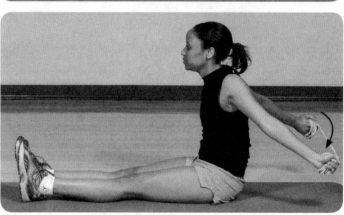

Video
F1.2

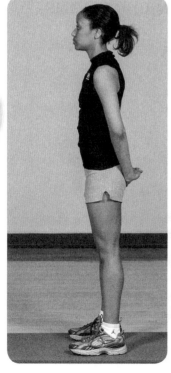

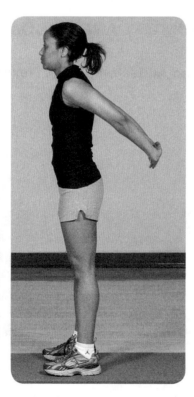

Exercise 3

Description: Clasp hands together behind trunk with elbows extended. Slowly raise arms upward.

From A.L. Gibson, D.R. Wagner, and V.H. Heyward, *Advanced Fitness Assessment and Exercise Prescription,* 8th ed. (Champaign, IL: Human Kinetics, 2019).

Appendix F.2 Exercise Dos and Don'ts

DON'T: Neck Hyperextension

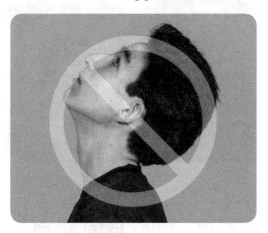

DO: Neck Lateral Flexion

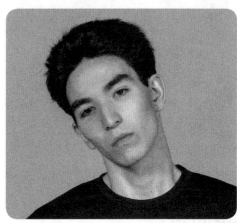

DON'T: Head Throws in a Crunch

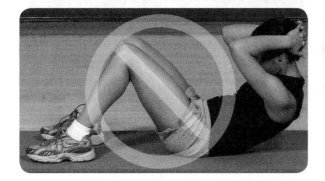

DO: Partial Sit-Ups

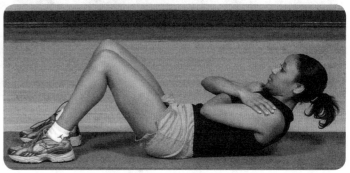

DON'T: Unsupported Hip/Trunk Flexion

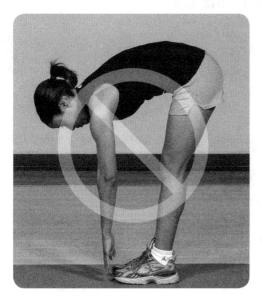

DO: Seated Hip/Trunk Flexion

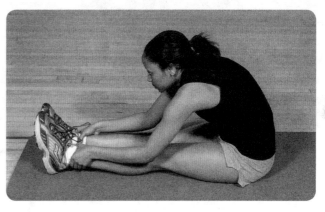

From A.L. Gibson, D.R. Wagner, and V.H. Heyward, *Advanced Fitness Assessment and Exercise Prescription,* 8th ed. (Champaign, IL: Human Kinetics, 2019).

(continued)

DON'T: The Plow

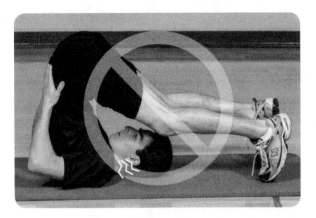

DO: Camel

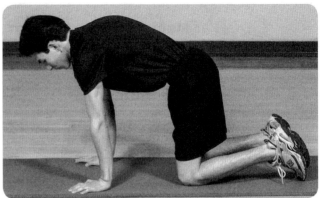

DON'T: Swan Lifts

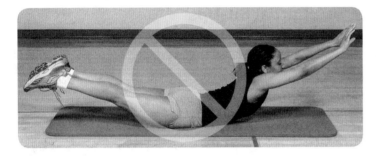

DO: Trunk Extensions

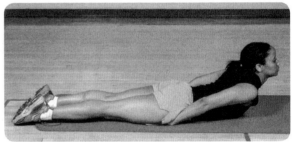

DON'T: V-Sits

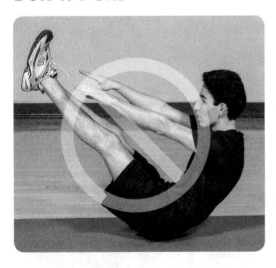

DO: Partial Sit-Ups

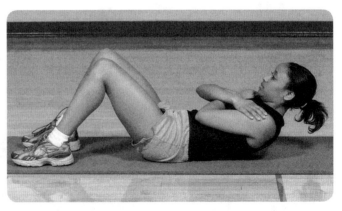

From A.L. Gibson, D.R. Wagner, and V.H. Heyward, *Advanced Fitness Assessment and Exercise Prescription,* 8th ed. (Champaign, IL: Human Kinetics, 2019).

DON'T: Leg Lifts With Trunk Hyperextended

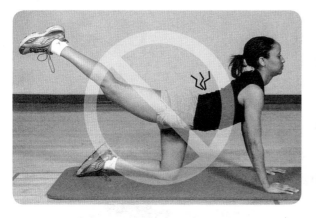

DO: Leg Lifts With Trunk and Leg in Straight Line

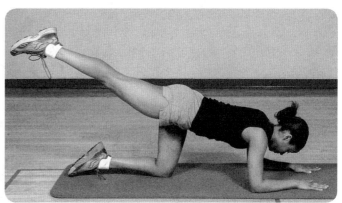

DON'T: Hamstring Stretch—Leg on Bar

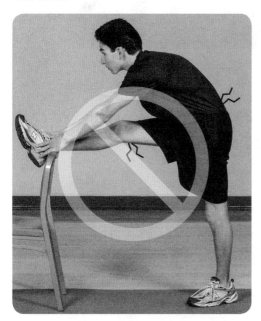

DO: Hamstring Stretch—Knee to Chest

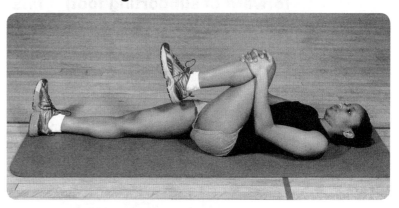

DON'T: Hurdler's Stretch

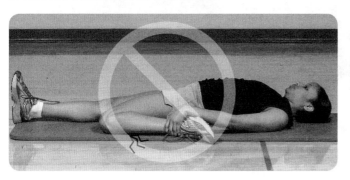

DO: Quad Stretch

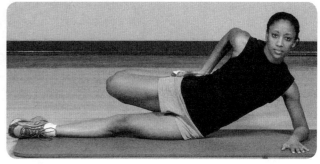

(continued)

From A.L. Gibson, D.R. Wagner, and V.H. Heyward, *Advanced Fitness Assessment and Exercise Prescription,* 8th ed. (Champaign, IL: Human Kinetics, 2019).

DON'T: Squats and Deep Knee Bends

DO: Half-Squats

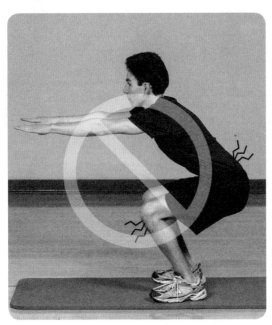

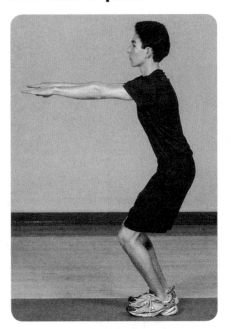

DON'T: Lunges (with knee forward of supporting foot)

DO: Lunges (with knee in line with supporting heel)

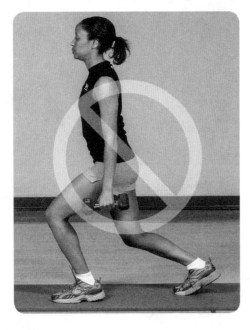

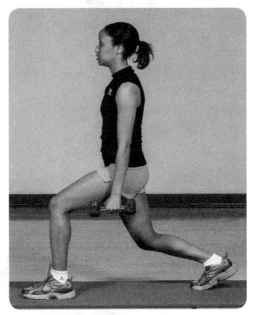

From A.L. Gibson, D.R. Wagner, and V.H. Heyward, *Advanced Fitness Assessment and Exercise Prescription,* 8th ed. (Champaign, IL: Human Kinetics, 2019).

DON'T: Fast Twists and Jump Twists

DO: Jump Without Twist

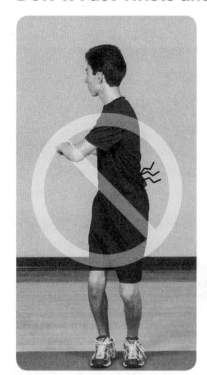 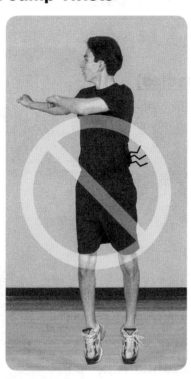 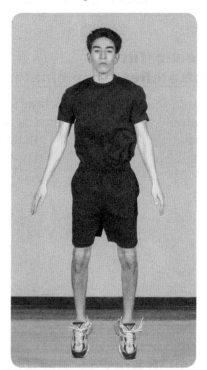

Appendix F.3 Exercises for Low Back Care

Pelvic Tilt (stretches abdominal muscles)

Lie on your back with knees bent, feet flat on the floor, and arms at your sides. Flatten the small of your back against the floor. (Your hips will tilt upward.) Hold.

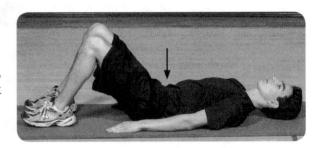

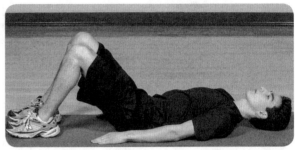

Double Knee to Chest (stretches hip, buttock, and lower back muscles)

Lie on your back with knees bent, feet flat on the floor, and arms at your sides. Raise both knees, one at a time, to your chest and hold both with your hands. Lower your legs, one at a time, to the floor and rest briefly.

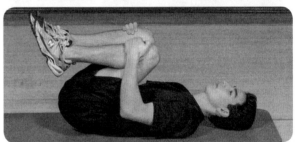

Trunk Flex (stretches back, abdominal, and leg muscles)

On your hands and knees, tuck in your chin and arch your back. Slowly sit back on your heels, letting your shoulders drop toward the floor. Hold.

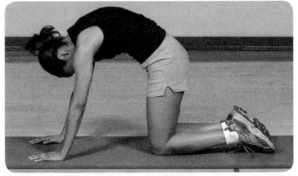

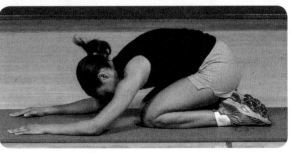

From A.L. Gibson, D.R. Wagner, and V.H. Heyward, *Advanced Fitness Assessment and Exercise Prescription,* 8th ed. (Champaign, IL: Human Kinetics, 2019).

Cat and Camel (strengthens back and abdominal muscles)

On your hands and knees with your head parallel to the floor, arch your back and then let it slowly sag toward the floor. Try to keep your arms straight.

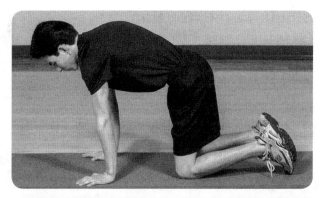

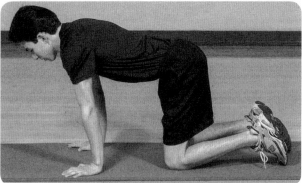

Partial Sit-Up (strengthens abdominal muscles)

Lie on your back with knees bent, feet flat on the floor, and arms crossed over your chest. Keeping your middle and lower back flat on the floor, raise your head and shoulders off the floor, and hold. Gradually increase your holding time.

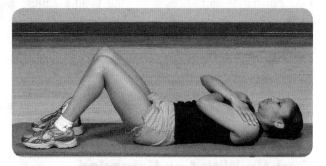

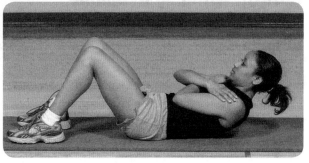

(continued)

Single-Leg Extension (strengthens hip and buttock muscles; stretches abdominal and leg muscles)

Lie on your abdomen with your arms folded under your chin. Slowly lift one leg—not too high—without bending it, while keeping your pelvis flat on the floor. Slowly lower your leg and repeat with the other leg.

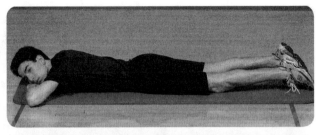

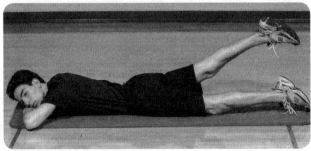

Single-Leg Extension Hold (strengthens trunk extensors)

On your hands and knees with your head parallel to the floor, extend your thigh and leg and hold this position. Raising the contralateral arm simultaneously is more difficult and increases the extensor muscle activity and spinal compression.

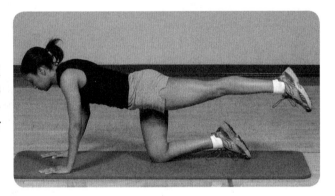

Curl-Up With Leg Extended (strengthens abdominal muscles)

Lie on your back with one knee flexed (foot flat on floor) and the other knee extended. Place your hands under the lumbar spine to preserve the neutral spine position. Slowly raise your head and shoulders off the floor.

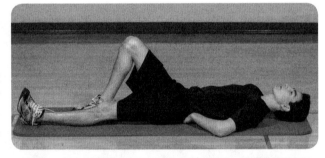

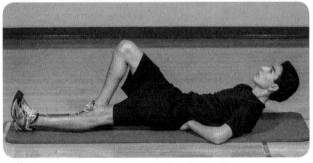

From A.L. Gibson, D.R. Wagner, and V.H. Heyward, *Advanced Fitness Assessment and Exercise Prescription,* 8th ed. (Champaign, IL: Human Kinetics, 2019).

Isometric Side Support or Side Bridge (strengthens lateral muscles of trunk and abdomen)

Assume a side support position with body supported by the knee, thigh, and forearm (flexed to 90°), and hold this position. Supporting the body with the feet, instead of the knee and thigh, increases the muscle activity and spinal load.

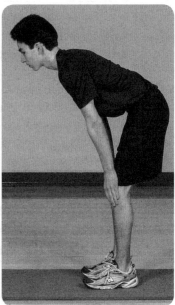

Standing Cat and Camel (strengthens back and abdominal muscles)

Stand with feet shoulder-width apart and with hands on knees. Straighten back and hold this position. Perform 10 to 20 repetitions.

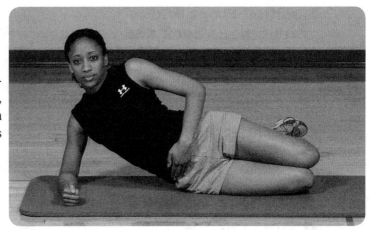

Bent-Knee Curl-Up (strengthens abdominal muscles)

Lie on your back with one knee bent and with foot flat on the floor. Place arms across chest. Lift shoulders off ground and hold this position momentarily. Perform 10 to 20 repetitions.

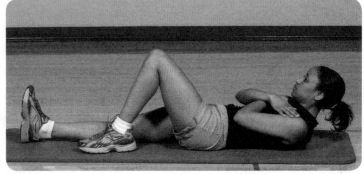

(continued)

From A.L. Gibson, D.R. Wagner, and V.H. Heyward, *Advanced Fitness Assessment and Exercise Prescription,* 8th ed. (Champaign, IL: Human Kinetics, 2019).

Modified Front Bridge (strengthens back and abdominal muscles)

Assume a front support position with the body supported by the forearms (elbows flexed to 90°), knees, and toes. Hold this position for 10 to 20 counts.

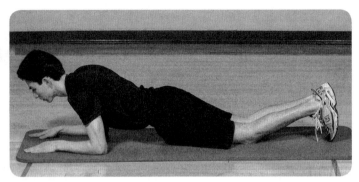

Modified Bird Dog (strengthens hip extensors)

Assume a front support position with the body supported by both hands (shoulder-width apart and elbows extended), one knee, and one foot. Extend unsupported leg so that thigh is parallel with the trunk. Hold this position momentarily. Perform 10 repetitions for each leg. Support the body with one arm to increase the difficulty of this exercise.

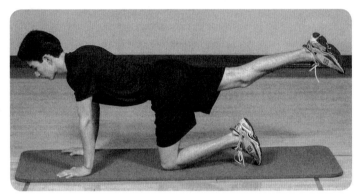

Standing McKenzie Exercise (stretches abdominal muscles; strengthens back extensors)

Assume a standing position with feet shoulder-width apart and with hands placed on hips. Extend the trunk and hold this position momentarily. Perform 10 repetitions.

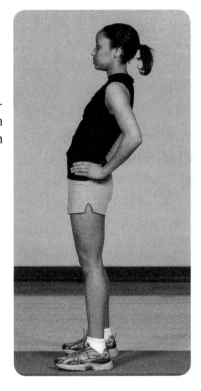

From A.L. Gibson, D.R. Wagner, and V.H. Heyward, *Advanced Fitness Assessment and Exercise Prescription,* 8th ed. (Champaign, IL: Human Kinetics, 2019).

List of Abbreviations

Terms

%BF	Percent body fat
A-mode	Amplitude modulation
ACSM	American College of Sports Medicine
ADL	Activities of daily living
ADP	Air displacement plethysmography
AIT	Aerobic interval training
APHRmax	Age-predicted maximal heart rate
ATP	Adenosine triphosphate
AV	Atrioventricular
AVG	Active video game
B-mode	Brightness modulation
BBS	Berg Balance Scale
BESS	Behavioral Error Scoring System
BIA	Bioelectrical impedance analysis
BIS	Bioimpedance spectroscopy
BM	Body mass
BMI	Body mass index
BMR	Basal metabolic rate
BP	Blood pressure
BSA	Body surface area
BV	Body volume
BW	Body weight
C	Circumference
CAAHEP	Commission on Accreditation of Allied Health Education Programs
CDC	Centers for Disease Control and Prevention
CE	Constant error
CHD	Coronary heart disease
CMJ	Countermovement jump
CR	Contract-relax
CRAC	Contract-relax with agonist contraction
CREP	Coalition for the Registration of Exercise Professionals
CRF	Cardiorespiratory fitness
CrP	Creatine phosphate
CSA	Cross-sectional area
CSEP	Canadian Society for Exercise Physiology
CTT	Counting talk test
CV	Cardiovascular
CVD	Cardiovascular disease
D	Skeletal diameter
Db	Body density
DBP	Diastolic blood pressure
DDR	Dance Dance Revolution
DOMS	Delayed-onset muscle soreness
DXA	Dual-energy X-ray absorptiometry
EAT	Exercise activity thermogenesis
ECG	Electrocardiogram
EDD	Exercise deficit disorder
EIM	Exercise is Medicine®
EIMD	Exercise-induced muscle damage
EMG	Electromyography
ePARmed-X+	electronic Physical Activity Readiness Medical Examination
ESH-IP	European Society of Hypertension International Protocol
FFB	Fat-free body
FFM	Fat-free mass
FITT-VP	Frequency, intensity, time, type of exercise, volume, and progression
FM	Fat mass
FRC	Functional residual lung capacity
FSR	Final stepping rate
GH	Growth hormone
GI	Glycemic index
GIS	Geographical information system
GPS	Global positioning system
GV	Volume of air in gastrointestinal tract
GWAS	Genome-wide associated study
GXT	Graded exercise test
HDL	High-density lipoprotein
HDL-C	High-density lipoprotein cholesterol
HIT	High-intensity interval training
HMB	β-hydroxy-β-methylbutyrate
HR	Heart rate
HRmax	Maximal heart rate
HRrest	Resting heart rate
HRR	Heart rate reserve
HT	Standing height
HT^2/R	Resistance index

HW	Hydrostatic weighing	REE	Resting energy expenditure
IDF	International Diabetes Federation	REP	Repetition
IHD	Ischemic heart disease	RER	Respiratory exchange ratio
IOM	Institute of Medicine	RLP	Reverse linear periodization
LDL	Low-density lipoprotein	RM	Repetition maximum
LDL-C	Low-density lipoprotein cholesterol	Rmc	Multiple correlation coefficient
LP	Linear periodization	RMR	Resting metabolic rate
LTPA	Leisure-time physical activity	ROM	Range of motion
MET	Metabolic equivalent of task	RPE	Rating of perceived exertion
MET·min	MET minutes	RV	Residual (lung) volume
MetS	Metabolic syndrome	SAD	Sagittal abdominal diameter
MIPA	Moderate-intensity physical activity	SAT	Subcutaneous adipose tissue
MRI	Magnetic resonance imaging	SBP	Systolic blood pressure
MVC	Maximal voluntary contraction	SCENIHR	Scientific Committee on Emerging and Newly Identified Health
MVPA	Moderate- to vigorous-physical activity		
N	Sample size	SEE	Standard error of estimate
NBFE	National Boards of Fitness Examiners	SHAPE	Society of Health and Physical Educators; commonly referred to as SHAPE America; formerly AAHPERD (American Alliance for Health, Physical Education, Recreation, and Dance)
NCCA	National Commission for Certifying Agencies		
NCD	Noncommunicable disease		
NCEP	National Cholesterol Education Program	SIT	Sprint interval training
NCEP-ATPIII	National Cholesterol Education Program – Adult Treatment Panel III	SKF	Skinfold
		ΣSKF	Sum of skinfolds
NEAT	non-exercise activity thermogenesis	SRP	Steep ramp cycling protocol
NHANES	National Health and Nutrition Examination Survey	SV	Stroke volume
		TBW	Total body water
NIDDM	Non-insulin-dependent diabetes mellitus	TC	Total cholesterol
NIH	National Institutes of Health	TC/HDL-C	Ratio of total cholesterol to HDL-cholesterol
NIR	Near-infrared interactance		
P	Power output	TE	Total error
PAL	Physical activity level	TEE	Total energy expenditure
PAR-Q	Physical Activity Readiness Questionnaire	TGV	Thoracic gas volume
PARmed-X	Physical Activity Readiness Medical Examination Questionnaire	TLC	Total lung capacity
		TLCNS	Total lung capacity, head not submerged
PEI	Physical efficiency index	TMS	Transcranial magnetic stimulation
PFA	Perceived functional ability	UWW	Underwater weight
PNF	Proprioceptive neuromuscular facilitation	UP	Undulating periodization
POMA	Performance-Oriented Mobility Assessment	VAT	Visceral adipose tissue
		VIPA	Vigorous-intensity physical activity
PRET	Perceptually regulated exercise tests	VLDL	Very low-density lipoprotein
$\dot{Q}$	Cardiac output	$\dot{V}O_2$	Volume of oxygen consumed per minute
ρ	Specific resistivity	$\dot{V}O_2max$	Maximal oxygen uptake
R	Resistance for bioimpedance analysis	$\dot{V}O_2R$	Oxygen uptake reserve
r	Pearson product–moment correlation	VT	Ventilatory threshold
RDA	Recommended dietary allowance	WBAN	Wireless body area network

WBV	Whole-body vibration		**kHz**	kilohertz
WHR	Waist-to-hip ratio		**km**	kilometer
WHO	World Health Organization		**L**	liter
WHTR	Waist-to-height ratio		**lb**	pound
Xc	Reactance		**m**	meter
YMCA	Young Men's Christian Association		**meq**	milli-equivalent
YYIR1C	Modified Yo-Yo Intermittent Recovery Level 1 test for children		**mg**	milligram
			mi	mile
Z	Impedance		**min**	minute

Units of Measure

			ml	milliliter
bpm	beats per minute		**mm**	millimeter
C	Celsius		**mmHg**	millimeters of mercury
cc	cubic centimeter		**mo**	month
cm	centimeter		**mph**	miles per hour
dl	deciliter		**N**	newton
F	Fahrenheit		**Nm**	newton-meter
ft-lb	foot-pound		**rpm**	revolutions per minute
g	gram		**sec**	second
hr	hour		**W**	watt
Hz	hertz		**wk**	week
in.	inch		**yr**	year
kcal	kilocalorie		**μg**	microgram
kg	kilogram		**μg RE**	retinol equivalent
kgm	kilogram-meter		**Ω**	ohm

Glossary

absolute $\dot{V}O_2$—Measure of rate of oxygen consumption and energy cost of non-weight-bearing activities; measured in $L \cdot min^{-1}$ or $ml \cdot min^{-1}$.

accelerometer—Device used to record body acceleration from minute to minute, providing detailed information about frequency, duration, intensity, and patterns of movement.

accommodating-resistance exercise—Type of exercise in which fluctuations in muscle force throughout the range of motion are matched by an equal counterforce as the speed of limb movement is kept at a constant velocity; isokinetic exercise.

acquired immune deficiency syndrome (AIDS)—Disease characterized as a deficiency in the body's immune system, caused by human immunodeficiency virus (HIV).

active-assisted stretching—Stretching technique that involves voluntarily moving a body part to the end of its active range of motion, followed by assistance in moving the body part beyond its active range of motion.

active stretching—Stretching technique that involves moving a body part without external assistance; voluntary muscle contraction.

activities of daily living (ADLs)—Normal everyday activities such as getting out of a chair or car, climbing stairs, shopping, dressing, and bathing.

acute-onset muscle soreness—Soreness or pain occurring during or immediately after exercise; caused by ischemia and accumulation of metabolic waste products in the muscle.

aerobic interval training (AIT)—Subclass of high-intensity interval training; consists of repeated combinations of near maximal (80%-95% $\dot{V}O_2R$) 4 min bouts of exercise and rest or recovery periods of similar duration.

air displacement plethysmography (ADP)—Densitometric method to estimate body volume using air displacement and pressure-volume relationships.

allele—One member of a pair or series of genes that occupy a specific position on a specific chromosome.

android obesity—Type of obesity in which excess body fat is localized in the upper body; upper body obesity; apple-shaped body.

aneurysm—Dilation of a blood vessel wall causing a weakness in the vessel's wall; usually caused by atherosclerosis and hypertension.

angina pectoris—Chest pain.

ankylosis—Limited range of motion at a joint.

anorexia nervosa—Eating disorder characterized by excessive weight loss.

anthropometry—Measurement of body size and proportions including skinfold thicknesses, circumferences, bony widths and lengths, stature, and body weight.

aortic stenosis—Narrowing of the aortic valve, obstructing blood flow from the left ventricle into the aorta.

Archimedes' principle—Principle stating that weight loss underwater is directly proportional to the volume of water displaced by the body's volume.

arrhythmia—Abnormal heart rhythm.

arteriosclerosis—Hardening of the arteries, or thickening and loss of elasticity in the artery walls that obstruct blood flow; caused by deposits of fat, cholesterol, and other substances.

asthma—Respiratory disorder characterized by difficulty in breathing and wheezing due to constricted bronchi.

ataxia—Impaired ability to coordinate movement characterized by staggering gait or postural imbalance.

atherosclerosis—Buildup and deposition of fat and fibrous plaque in the inner walls of the coronary arteries.

atrial fibrillation—Cardiac dysrhythmia in which the atria quiver instead of pumping in an organized fashion.

atrial flutter—Type of atrial tachycardia in which the atria contract at rates of 230 to 380 bpm.

atrophy—A wasting or decrease in size of a body part.

attenuation—Weakening of X-ray energy as it passes through fat, lean tissue, and bone.

augmented unipolar leads—Three ECG leads (aVF, aVL, aVR) that compare voltage across each limb lead to the average voltage across the two opposite electrodes.

auscultation—Method used to measure heart rate or blood pressure by listening to heart and blood sounds.

autogenic inhibition—A theory to explain the effectiveness of PNF stretching by claiming a decrease in the excitability of the targeted muscle due to inhibitory signals from the Golgi tendon organ during the static contraction portion of PNF.

autophagy—A cell-level recycling program that sequesters damaged organelles and misfolded proteins, breaks them down into smaller pieces, and reuses those smaller components to support cellular viability.

auxotonic muscle action—Type of dynamic muscle action in which there is variable muscle tension as a result of changing velocities and joint angles.

balance—Complex construct involving multiple biomechanical, neurological, and environmental systems.

ballistic stretching—Type of stretching exercise that uses a fast bouncing motion to produce stretch and increase range of motion.

basal metabolic rate (BMR)—Measure of minimal amount of energy needed to maintain basic and essential physiological functions.

behavior modification model—Psychological theory of change; clients become actively involved with the change process by setting short- and long-term goals.

β-hydroxy-β-methylbutyrate (HMB)—Dietary supplement known to increase lean body mass and strength of individuals engaging in resistance training.

bias—In regression analysis, a systematic over- or underestimation of actual scores caused by technical error or biological variability between validation and cross-validation samples; constant error.

biaxial joint—Joint allowing movement in two planes; condyloid and saddle joints.

bioelectrical impedance analysis (BIA)—Field method for estimating the total body water or fat-free mass using measures of impedance to current flowing through the body.

bioimpedance spectroscopy (BIS)—Type of bioimpedance analysis that combines upper body, lower body, and whole-body bioimpedance to estimate FFM and %BF; utilizes a range of electrical frequencies and allows for determination of extracellular water (low-level frequencies) and intracellular water (high-level frequencies).

Bland and Altman method—Statistical approach used to assess the degree of agreement between methods by calculating the 95% limits of agreement and confidence intervals; used to judge the accuracy of a prediction equation or method for estimating measured values of individuals in a group.

body composition—A component of physical fitness; absolute and relative amounts of muscle, bone, and fat tissues composing body mass.

body density (Db)—Overall density of fat, water, mineral, and protein components of the human body; total body mass expressed relative to total body volume.

body mass (BM)—Measure of the size of the body; body weight.

body mass index (BMI)—Crude index of obesity; body mass (kg) divided by height squared (m^2).

body surface area—Amount of surface area of the body estimated from the client's height and body weight.

body volume (BV)—Measure of body size estimated by water or air displacement.

body weight (BW)—Mass or size of the body; body mass.

bone strength—Function of mineral content and density of bone tissue; related to risk of bone fracture.

Boyle's law—Isothermal gas law stating that volume and pressure are inversely related.

bradycardia—Resting heart rate <60 bpm.

bronchitis—Acute or chronic inflammation of the bronchi of the lungs.

caloric threshold—Method to estimate duration of exercise based on the caloric cost of the exercise and to estimate the total amount of exercise needed per week for health benefits.

cardiac arrest—Sudden loss of heart function usually caused by ventricular fibrillation.

cardiomyopathy—Any disease that affects the structure and function of the heart.

cardiorespiratory endurance—Ability of heart, lungs, and circulatory system to efficiently supply oxygen to working muscles.

cardiovascular disease (CVD)—Disease of the heart, blood vessels, or both; types of cardiovascular disease include atherosclerosis, hypertension, coronary heart disease, congestive heart failure, and stroke.

center of pressure—Vertical force applied to the supporting base or a force platform during sitting or standing.

chest leads—Six ECG leads (V_1 to V_6) used to measure voltage across specific areas of the chest.

cholesterol—Waxy, fatlike substance found in all animal products (e.g., meats, dairy products, and eggs).

chylomicron—Type of lipoprotein derived from intestinal absorption of triglycerides.

circumference (C)—Measure of the girth of body segments.

cirrhosis—Chronic degenerative disease of the liver in which the lobes are covered with fibrous tissue; associated with chronic alcohol abuse.

claudication—Cramp-like pain in the calves due to poor circulation in leg muscle.

compound sets—Advanced resistance training system in which two sets of exercises for the same muscle group are performed consecutively, with little or no rest between sets.

computerized dynamic posturography—Computer system designed to assess the individual and composite functioning of sensory, motor, and biomechanical components of balance.

concentric muscle action—Type of dynamic muscle contraction in which muscle shortens as it exerts tension.

congestive heart failure—Impaired cardiac pumping caused by myocardial infarction, ischemic heart disease, or cardiomyopathy.

constant error (CE)—Average difference between measured and predicted values for cross-validation group; bias.

constant-resistance exercise—Type of exercise in which the external resistance remains the same throughout the range of motion (e.g., lifting free weights or dumbbells).

continuous exercise test—Type of graded exercise test that is performed with no rest between workload increments.

continuous training—One continuous aerobic exercise bout performed at low to moderate intensity.

contract-relax agonist contract (CRAC) technique—Type of proprioceptive neuromuscular facilitation technique in which the target muscle is isometrically contracted and then stretched; stretching is assisted by a submaximal contraction of the agonistic muscle group.

contract-relax (CR) technique—Type of proprioceptive neuromuscular facilitation technique in which the target muscle is isometrically contracted and then stretched.

contracture—Shortening of resting muscle length caused by disuse or immobilization.

core stability—Ability to maintain ideal alignment of neck, spine, scapulae, and pelvis while exercising.

core strengthening—Strengthening core muscle groups (erector spinae and abdominal movers and stabilizers) used for core stability.

coronary heart disease (CHD)—Disease of the heart caused by a lack of blood flow to heart muscle, resulting from atherosclerosis.

countermovement jump (CMJ)—Commonly employed jumping technique that includes a quick eccentric movement (flexion of hips and knees and backward swing of arms) followed immediately by an explosive concentric movement to propel the individual upward or forward.

counting talk test (CTT)—Method to monitor exercise intensity; measure of the client's ability to comfortably count out loud while exercising; based on the relationship between exercise intensity and pulmonary ventilation.

criterion method—Gold standard, or reference method; typically a direct measure of a component used to validate other tests.

cross-training—Type of training in which the client participates in a variety of exercise modes to develop one or more components of physical fitness.

cuff hypertension—Overestimation of blood pressure caused by use of a bladder that is too small for the arm circumference.

cyanosis—Bluish discoloration of skin caused by lack of oxygenated hemoglobin in the blood.

damping technique—Technique used to reduce the motion of the underwater weighing scale arm during the total body submersion process.

decision-making theory—Theory stating that individuals decide whether or not to engage in a behavior by weighing the perceived benefits and costs of that behavior.

delayed-onset muscle soreness (DOMS)—Soreness in the muscle occurring 24 to 48 hr after exercise.

densitometry—Measurement of body volume leading to calculation of total body density; hydrodensitometry and air displacement plethysmography are densitometric methods.

diabetes—Complex disorder of carbohydrate, fat, and protein metabolism resulting from a lack of insulin secretion (type 1) or defective insulin receptors (type 2).

diastolic blood pressure (DBP)—Lowest pressure in the artery during the cardiac cycle.

dietary thermogenesis—Energy needed for digesting, absorbing, transporting, and metabolizing foods.

diminishing returns principle—Training principle; as genetic ceiling is approached, rate of improvement slows or evens off.

discontinuous exercise test—Type of graded exercise test that is performed with 5 to 10 min of rest between increments in workload.

discontinuous training—Several intermittent, low- to high-intensity aerobic exercise bouts interspersed with rest or relief intervals.

dose-response relationship—The volume of physical activity is directly related to health benefits from that activity.

dual-energy X-ray absorptiometry (DXA)—Method used to measure total body bone mineral density and bone mineral content as well as to estimate fat and lean soft tissue mass.

dynamic balance—Ability to maintain an upright position while the center of gravity and base of support are moving.

dynamic flexibility—Measure of the rate of torque or resistance developed during stretching throughout the range of joint motion.

dynamic muscle action—Type of muscle contraction producing visible joint movement; concentric, eccentric, or isokinetic contraction.

dynamic stretching—Type of stretching exercise that uses slow, controlled movements that are repeated several times to produce stretch and increase range of motion.

dynapenia—Age-related loss in muscle strength.

dyslipidemia—Abnormal blood lipid profile.

dyspnea—Shortness of breath or difficulty breathing caused by certain heart conditions, anxiety, or strenuous exercise.

eccentric muscle action—Type of muscle contraction in which the muscle lengthens as it produces tension to resist gravity or decelerate a moving body segment.

eccentric training—Resistance training strategy that places an emphasis on eccentric muscle actions, often using specialized machines to administer an eccentric load.

edema—Accumulation of interstitial fluid in tissues such as the pericardial sac and joint capsules.

elastic deformation—Deformation of the muscle-tendon unit that is proportional to the load or force applied during stretching.

electrocardiogram (ECG)—A composite record of the electrical events in the heart during the cardiac cycle.

electrogoniometer—Flexible strain gauges that cross the joint to measure range of motion; capable of measuring range of motion in two planes simultaneously.

elevated blood pressure—Systolic blood pressure ranging from 120 to 129 mmHg and diastolic blood pressure lower than 80 mmHg.

embolism—Piece of tissue or thrombus that circulates in the blood until it lodges in a vessel.

emphysema—Pulmonary disease causing damage to alveoli and loss of lung elasticity.

exercise activity thermogenesis (EAT)—The portion of physical activity energy expenditure derived from exercise.

exercise deficit disorder (EDD)—Term associated with children who do not engage in at least 60 min/day of moderate- to vigorous-intensity physical activity.

exercise-induced hypertrophy—Increase in size of muscle as a result of resistance training.

exercise-induced muscle damage (EIMD)—Skeletal muscle damage induced through exercise.

exergaming—Interactive digital games in which the player physically moves to score points.

factorial method—Method used to assess energy needs; the sum of the resting metabolic rate and the additional calories expended during work, household chores, personal daily activities, and exercise.

false negative—An error in which individuals are incorrectly identified as having no risk factors when in fact they do have risk factors.

false positive—An error in which individuals are incorrectly identified as having risk factors when they do not have risk factors.

fat-free body (FFB)—All residual, lipid-free chemicals and tissues in the body, including muscle, water, bone, connective tissue, and internal organs.

fat-free mass (FFM)—*See* fat-free body; weight or mass of the fat-free body.

fat mass (FM)—All extractable lipids from adipose and other tissues in the body.

FITT-VP principle (FITT-VP)—Describes six components of an exercise prescription: frequency, intensity, time, type, volume, and progression of activity.

flexibility—Ability to move joints fluidly through complete range of motion without injury.

flexibility training—Systematic program of stretching exercises that progressively increases the range of motion of joints over time.

flexometer—Device for measuring range of joint motion using a weighted 360° dial and pointer.

free-motion machines—Resistance exercise machines that have adjustable seats, lever arms, and cable pulleys for exercising muscle groups in multiple planes.

functional balance—Ability to perform daily activities requiring balance (e.g., picking up an object from the floor).

functional fitness—Ability to perform everyday activities safely and independently without fatigue; requires aerobic endurance, flexibility, balance, agility, and muscular strength.

functional training—System of exercise progressions for specific muscle groups using a stepwise approach that increases the difficulty level (strength) and skill (balance and coordination) required for each exercise in the progression.

gait velocity—The speed of walking. Indirect measure of dynamic balance while walking used to detect mobility problems and risk of falling.

generalized prediction equations—Prediction equations that are applicable to a diverse, heterogeneous group of individuals.

genome-wide assessment studies (GWAS)—An investigation across the human genome that compares DNA variants of individuals presenting different phenotypes for a disease or trait; typically involves use of control group (disease or trait not present) and affected group with the disease or trait.

global positioning system (GPS)—System that uses 24 satellites and ground stations to calculate geographic locations and accurately track a specific activity.

glucose intolerance—Inability of the body to metabolize glucose.

goniometer—Protractor-like device used to measure joint angle at the extremes of the range of motion.

graded exercise test (GXT)—A multistage submaximal or maximal exercise test requiring the client to exercise at gradually increasing workloads; may be continuous or discontinuous; used to estimate $\dot{V}O_2$max.

Graves' disease—Disease associated with an overactive thyroid gland that secretes greater than normal amounts of thyroid hormones; also known as hyperthyroidism or thyrotoxicosis.

gross $\dot{V}O_2$—Total rate of oxygen consumption, reflecting the caloric cost of both rest and exercise.

gynoid obesity—Type of obesity in which excess fat is localized in the lower body; lower body obesity; pear-shaped body.

HbA1c—An indicator of the average blood glucose over the previous 2 to 3 mo; glycosylated hemoglobin.

HDL-cholesterol (HDL-C)—Cholesterol transported in the blood by high-density lipoproteins.

health belief model—Model suggesting that individuals will change a behavior because they perceive a threat of disease if they do not change.

healthy body weight—Body mass index from 18.5 to 25 kg/m^2.

heart block—Interference in the conduction of electrical impulses that control normal contraction of the heart muscle; may occur at sinoatrial node, atrioventricular node, bundle of His, or a combination of these sites.

heart rate monitor—Device used to assess heart rate and to monitor exercise intensity.

heart rate reserve (HRR)—Maximal heart rate minus the resting heart rate.

heart rate variability (HRV)—Differences in the time intervals between consecutive resting heart beats; reflects autonomic nervous system function.

hemiscan procedure—Used for clients who are too wide for the DXA scan table; client is positioned off center on the DXA scan table so that one side of the body is completely within the scan field.

hepatitis—Inflammation of the liver characterized by jaundice and gastrointestinal discomfort.

high blood pressure—Hypertension; chronic elevation of blood pressure.

high-density lipoprotein (HDL)—Type of lipoprotein involved in the reverse transport of cholesterol to the liver.

high-intensity interval training (HIT)—Style of cardiometabolic training based on repeated combinations of vigorous-intensity exertion followed by a rest or recovery period; commonly performed using an aerobic modality; combinations of exertion and rest can be manipulated so that training focuses on a specific metabolic pathway.

high intensity–low repetitions—Optimal training stimulus for strength development; 85% to 100% 1-RM or 1-RM to 6-RM.

hybrid sphygmomanometer—Device used to measure blood pressure that combines features of electronic and auscultatory devices.

hydrodensitometry—Method used to estimate body volume by measuring weight loss when the body is fully submerged; underwater weighing.

hydrostatic weighing (HW)—*See* hydrodensitometry.

hypercholesterolemia—Excess of total cholesterol, LDL-cholesterol, or both in blood.

hyperlipidemia—Excess lipids in blood.

hypermobility—Excessive range of motion at a joint.

hyperplasia—Increase in number of cells.

hypertension—High blood pressure; chronic elevation of blood pressure.

hyperthyroidism—Overactive thyroid gland that secretes greater than normal amounts of thyroid hormones; also known as thyrotoxicosis or Graves' disease.

hypertrophy—Increase in size of cells.

hypoglycemia—Low blood glucose level.

hypokalemia—Inadequate amount of potassium in the blood characterized by an abnormal ECG, weakness, and flaccid paralysis.

hypomagnesemia—Inadequate amount of magnesium in the blood resulting in nausea, vomiting, muscle weakness, and tremors.

hypothyroidism—Underactive thyroid gland that secretes lower than normal amounts of thyroid hormones; also known as myxedema.

hypoxia—Inadequate oxygen at the cellular level.

impedance (Z)—Measure of total amount of opposition to electrical current flowing through the body; function of resistance and reactance.

improvement stage—Stage of exercise program in which client improves most rapidly; frequency, intensity, duration are systematically increased; usually lasts 4 to 8 mo.

inclinometer—Gravity-dependent goniometer used to measure the angle between the long axis of the moving segment and the line of gravity.

initial conditioning stage—Stage of exercise program used as a primer to familiarize client with exercise training, usually lasting 4 wk.

initial values principle—Training principle; the lower the initial value of a component, the greater the relative gain and the faster the rate of improvement in that component; the higher the initial value, the slower the improvement rate.

insulin-dependent diabetes mellitus (IDDM)—Type 1 diabetes, caused by lack of insulin production by the pancreas.

interindividual variability principle—Training principle; individual responses to training stimulus are variable and depend on age, initial fitness level, and health status.

interval training—A repeated series of exercise work bouts interspersed with rest or relief periods.

ischemia—Decreased supply of oxygenated blood to a body part or organ; due to occlusion or restriction of blood flow.

ischemic heart disease—Pathologic condition of the myocardium caused by lack of oxygen to the heart muscle.

isokinetic muscle action—Maximal contraction of a muscle group at a constant velocity throughout entire range of motion.

isometric muscle action—Type of muscle contraction in which there is no visible joint movement; static contraction.

isotonic muscle action—Type of muscle contraction producing visible joint movement; dynamic contraction.

joint laxity—Looseness or instability of a joint, increasing risk of musculoskeletal injury.

Karvonen method—Method to prescribe exercise intensity as a percentage of the heart rate reserve added to the resting heart rate; percent heart rate reserve method.

kettlebell training—Type of resistance training that uses a cast-iron weight (resembling a cannonball with a handle) to perform ballistic exercises; improves strength, cardiorespiratory fitness, and flexibility.

kilocalorie (kcal)—Amount of heat needed to raise the temperature of 1 kg of water 1 °C; measure of energy need and expenditure.

lactate threshold—Exercise intensity at which blood lactate production exceeds blood lactate removal; denoted by an increase of 1 $mmol \cdot L^{-1}$ between two consecutive stages; an indication of when the primary metabolic pathway switches from mitochondrial oxidation to glycolysis.

LDL-cholesterol (LDL-C)—Cholesterol transported in the blood by low-density lipoproteins.

limb leads—Three ECG leads (I, II, III) measuring the voltage differential between left and right arms (I) and between the left leg and right (II) and left (III) arms.

limits of agreement—Statistical method used to assess the extent of agreement between methods; also known as the Bland and Altman method.

limits of stability—Measure of the maximum excursion of the center of gravity during maintenance of balance over a fixed supporting base.

linear periodization (LP)—Strength training method that progressively increases training intensity as training volume decreases between microcycles.

line of best fit—Regression line depicting relationship between reference measure and predictor variables in an equation.

line of gravity—Vertical projection of the center of gravity of the body to the supporting base.

line of identity—Straight line with a slope equal to 1 and an intercept equal to 0; used in a scatter plot to illustrate the differences in the measured and predicted scores of a cross-validation sample.

lipoprotein—Molecule used to transport and exchange lipids among the liver, intestine, and peripheral tissues.

low back pain—Pain produced by muscular weakness or imbalance resulting from lack of physical activity.

low-density lipoprotein (LDL)—Primary transporter of cholesterol in the blood; product of very low-density lipoprotein metabolism.

lower body obesity—Type of obesity in which excess body fat is localized in the lower body; gynoid obesity; pear-shaped body.

low intensity–high repetition—Optimal training stimulus for development of muscular endurance; ≤60% 1-RM or 15-RM to 20-RM.

lumbar stabilization—Maintaining a static position of the lumbar spine by isometrically cocontracting the abdominal wall and low back muscles during exercise.

macrocycle—Phase of periodized resistance training program usually lasting 9 to 12 mo; comprised of mesocycles.

maintenance stage—Stage of exercise program designed to maintain level of fitness achieved by end of improvement stage; should be continued on a regular, long-term basis.

masked hypertension—Condition in which individuals exhibit elevated BP readings outside the physician's office but have normal BP values in the office.

masked obesity—Condition in which individuals have a normal body mass index but carry an excessive amount of body fat.

maximal exercise test—Graded exercise test in which exercise intensity increases gradually until the $\dot{V}O_2$ plateaus or fails to rise with a further increase in workload.

maximum oxygen consumption—Maximum rate of oxygen utilization by muscles during exercise; $\dot{V}O_2$max.

maximum oxygen uptake ($\dot{V}O_2$max)—Maximum rate of oxygen utilization of muscles during aerobic exercise.

maximum voluntary contraction (MVC)—Measure of the maximum force exerted in a single contraction against an immovable resistance.

McArdle's syndrome—Inherited metabolic disease characterized by inability to metabolize muscle glycogen, resulting in excessive amounts of glycogen stored in skeletal muscles.

mesocycle—Phase of a periodized resistance training program usually lasting 3 to 4 mo; comprised of microcycles.

metabolic equivalents (METs)—The ratio of the person's working (exercising) metabolic rate to the resting metabolic rate.

metabolic syndrome (MetS)—A combination of cardiovascular disease risk factors associated with hypertension, dyslipidemia, insulin resistance, and abdominal obesity.

MET·min—Index of energy expenditure; product of exercise intensity (METs) and duration (min) of exercise.

microcycle—Phase of a periodized resistance training program usually lasting 1 to 4 wk.

miscuffing—Source of blood pressure measurement error caused by use of a blood pressure cuff that is not appropriately scaled for the client's arm circumference.

multicomponent model—Body composition model that takes into account interindividual variations in water, protein, and mineral content of the fat-free body.

multimodal exercise program—Type of exercise program that uses a variety of exercise modalities.

multiple correlation coefficient (R_{mc})—Correlation between reference measure and predictor variables in a prediction equation.

murmur—Low-pitched fluttering or humming sound.

muscle balance—Ratio of strength between opposing muscle groups, contralateral muscle groups, and upper and lower body muscle groups.

muscular endurance—Ability of muscle to maintain submaximal force levels for extended periods.

muscular power—Ability to exert force per unit of time; rate of performing work.

muscular strength—Maximal force or tension level produced by a muscle or muscle group.

musculoskeletal fitness—Ability of skeletal and muscular systems to perform work.

myocardial infarction—Heart attack.

myocardial ischemia—Lack of blood flow to the heart muscle.

myocarditis—Inflammation of the heart muscle caused by viral, bacterial, or fungal infection.

myxedema—Disease associated with an underactive thyroid gland that secretes lower than normal amounts of thyroid hormones; also known as hypothyroidism.

negative energy balance—Excess of energy expenditure in relation to energy intake.

net $\dot{V}O_2$—Rate of oxygen consumption in excess of the resting $\dot{V}O_2$; used to describe the caloric cost of exercise.

neuromotor training—Exercises to improve balance, agility, gait, coordination, and proprioception; especially beneficial as part of comprehensive exercise programs for older adults.

nonaxial joint—Type of joint allowing only gliding, sliding, or twisting rather than movement about an axis of rotation; gliding joint.

noncommunicable diseases (NCDs)— Diseases that cannot be transmitted from one person to another; cardiovascular diseases, diabetes, obesity, chronic respiratory disorders, and most cancers.

non-exercise activity thermogenesis (NEAT)—The portion of physical activity energy expenditure that is not from a defined exercise (e.g., fidgeting, activities of daily living).

non-insulin-dependent diabetes mellitus (NIDDM)—Type 2 diabetes; caused by decreased insulin receptor sensitivity.

normotensive—Referring to normal blood pressure, defined as values less than 120/80 mmHg.

obesity—Excessive amount of body fat relative to body mass; BMI of 30 kg/m^2 or more.

obesity paradox—The hypothesis that obesity can be both harmful (i.e., increasing risk of certain disorders) and protective (i.e., improving survival rates compared with those of nonobese individuals).

objectivity—Intertester reliability; ability of test to yield similar scores for a given individual when the same test is administered by different technicians.

objectivity coefficient—Correlation between pairs of test scores measured on the same individuals by two different technicians.

occlusion—Blockage or restriction of blood flow to a body part or organ.

one-repetition maximum (1-RM)—Maximal weight that can be lifted with good form for one complete repetition of a movement.

oscillometry—Method for measuring blood pressure that uses an automated electronic manometer to measure oscillations in pressure when the cuff is deflated.

osteoarthritis—Degenerative disease of the joints characterized by excessive amounts of bone and cartilage in the joint.

osteopenia—Low bone mineral mass; precursor to osteoporosis.

osteoporosis—Disorder characterized by low bone mineral and bone density; occurring most frequently in postmenopausal women and sedentary individuals.

overcuffing—Using a blood pressure cuff with a bladder too large for the arm circumference, leading to an underestimation of blood pressure.

overload principle—Training principle; physiological systems must be taxed beyond normal to stimulate improvement.

overweight—BMI between 25 and 29.9 kg/m^2 in adults; BMI greater than or equal to 95th percentile for age and sex in children.

pallor—Unnatural paleness or absence of skin color.

palpation—Method used to measure heart rate by feeling the pulse at specific anatomical sites.

palpitations—Racing or pounding of the heart.

passive stretching—Stretching technique that involves a body part being moved by an assistant as the client relaxes the target muscle group.

pedometer—A device used to count the number of steps taken throughout the day.

pelvic stabilization—Maintenance of a static position of the pelvis during performance of exercises for the low back extensor muscles.

percent body fat (%BF)—Fat mass expressed relative to body mass; relative body fat.

percent heart rate maximum (%HRmax)—Method used to prescribe exercise intensity as a percentage of the measured or age-predicted maximum heart rate.

percent heart rate reserve (%HRR) method—Method used to prescribe exercise intensity as a percentage of the heart rate reserve (HRR = HRmax − HRrest) added to the resting heart rate; Karvonen method.

percent $\dot{V}O_2$ reserve (%$\dot{V}O_2$R)—Method used to prescribe exercise intensity as a percentage of $\dot{V}O_2$ reserve ($\dot{V}O_2$R = $\dot{V}O_2$max − $\dot{V}O_2$rest) added to the resting $\dot{V}O_2$.

perceptually regulated exercise test (PRET)—Graded exercise test in which the 3 min workloads are incrementally progressed through intensities the client perceives as being equivalent to RPE values of 9, 11, 13, and 15 on the Borg 6 to 20 scale. Allows extrapolation to RPE values of 19 and 20 and, hence, $\dot{V}O_2$peak estimation via linear regression.

pericarditis—Inflammation of the pericardium caused by trauma, infection, uremia, or heart attack.

periodization—Advanced form of training that systematically varies the volume and intensity of the training exercises.

persuasive technology—A computer system, device, or application that is intentionally designed to change a person's attitude or behavior.

photoplethysmography (PPG)—A technology found in pulse oximeters and smart watches; uses light to determine heart rate by detecting changes in blood volume and blood flow in capillary beds.

physical activity level (PAL)—The ratio of total energy expenditure to basal metabolic rate; PAL = TEE / BMR.

physical fitness—Ability to perform occupational, recreational, and daily activities without undue fatigue.

Pilates—An exercise method introduced by Joseph Pilates that blends aspects of gymnastics, yoga, and martial arts to emphasize precision of body movement.

population-specific equations—Prediction equations intended only for use with individuals from a specific homogeneous group.

positive energy balance—Excess of energy intake in relation to energy expenditure.

prediabetes—Medical condition identified by fasting blood glucose or glycated hemoglobin levels above normal values yet below the threshold for diagnosis of diabetes.

PR interval—Part of ECG tracing that indicates delay in the impulse at the atrioventricular node.

progression principle—Training principle; training volume must be progressively increased to impose overload and stimulate further improvements.

proprioceptive neuromuscular facilitation (PNF)—Mode of stretching that increases range of joint motion through spinal reflex mechanisms such as reciprocal inhibition.

prosthesis—An artificial replacement of a missing body part, such as an artificial limb or joint.

pulmonary ventilation—Movement of air into and out of the lungs.

pulse pressure—Difference between the systolic and diastolic blood pressures.

P wave—Part of ECG tracing that reflects depolarization of the atria.

pyramiding—Advanced resistance training system in which a relatively light weight is lifted in the first set and progressively heavier weights are lifted in subsequent sets; light to heavy system.

QRS complex—Part of ECG tracing reflecting ventricular depolarization and contraction.

ramp protocols—Graded exercise tests that are individualized and that provide for continuous frequent increments (every 10-20 sec) in work rate so that $\dot{V}O_2$ increases linearly.

range of motion (ROM)—Degree of movement at a joint; measure of static flexibility.

rating of perceived exertion (RPE)—A scale used to measure a client's subjective rating of exercise intensity.

reactance (X_c)—Measure of opposition to electrical current flowing through the body due to the capacitance of cell membranes; a vector of impedance.

reactive balance—Ability to compensate and recover from perturbations while standing or walking.

reciprocal inhibition—Reflex that inhibits the contraction of antagonistic muscles when the prime mover is voluntarily contracted.

reference method—Gold standard, or criterion method; typically a direct measure of a component used to validate other tests.

regression line—Line of best fit depicting relationship between reference measure and predictor variables.

relative body fat (%BF)—Fat mass expressed as a percentage of total body mass; percent body fat.

relative strength—Muscular strength expressed relative to the body mass or lean body mass; 1-RM / BM.

relative $\dot{V}O_2$max—Rate of oxygen consumption expressed relative to the body mass (ml·kg^{-1}·min^{-1}) or lean body mass (ml·kg$_{FFM}$$^{-1}$·min^{-1}).

reliability—Ability of a test to yield consistent and stable scores across trials and over time.

reliability coefficient—Correlation depicting relationship between trial 1 and trial 2 scores or day 1 and day 2 scores of a test.

repetition maximum (RM)—Measure of intensity for resistance exercise expressed as maximum weight that can be lifted for a given number of repetitions.

repetitions—Number of times a specific exercise movement is performed in a set.

residual score—Difference between the actual and predicted scores (Y – Y').

residual volume (RV)—Volume of air remaining in the lungs following a maximal expiration.

resistance (R)—Measure of pure opposition to electrical current flowing through the body; a vector of impedance.

resistance index (ht^2/R)—Predictor variable in some BIA regression equations that is calculated by dividing standing height squared by resistance.

respiratory exchange ratio (RER)—Ratio of expired CO_2 to inspired O_2.

resting energy expenditure (REE)—Energy required to maintain essential physiological processes at rest; resting metabolic rate.

resting metabolic rate (RMR)—Energy required to maintain essential physiological processes in a relaxed, awake, and reclined state; resting energy expenditure.

reverse linear periodization (RLP)—Strength training method that progressively decreases training intensity as training volume increases between microcycles.

reversibility principle—Training principle; physiological gains from training are lost when an individual stops training (detraining).

rheumatic heart disease—Condition in which the heart valves are damaged by rheumatic fever, contracted from a streptococcal infection (strep throat).

rheumatoid arthritis—Chronic, destructive disease of the joints characterized by inflammation and thickening of the synovial membranes and swelling of the joints.

RPE-clamped protocol—Similar to PRET; client adjusts the workload to invoke a specific RPE value response per stage, with the final stage requiring a workload equivalent to the highest RPE possible on a given scale (e.g., 10 on the 0 to 10 scale or 20 on the Borg 6 to 20 scale).

sagittal abdominal diameter (SAD)—Measure of the anteroposterior thickness of the abdomen at the umbilical level.

sarcopenia—Age-related loss in muscle mass.

sedentarism—A lifestyle lacking in physical activity and dominated by excessive time spent sitting.

self-determination theory—Theory describing how the presence or absence of specific psychological needs affects behavior.

self-efficacy—Individuals' perception of their ability to perform a task and their confidence in making a specific behavioral change.

self-paced protocol—A free-form style of treadmill GXT in which the client adjusts (upward only) speed and incline periodically, with the stipulation that the client must reach the point of volitional exhaustion within 8 to 12 minutes.

sensitivity—Probability of a test correctly identifying individuals with risk factors for a specific disease.

set—Defines the number of times a specific number of repetitions of a given exercise is repeated; single or multiple sets.

skeletal diameter (D)—Measure of the width of bones.

skinfold (SKF)—Measure of the thickness of two layers of skin and the underlying subcutaneous fat.

social cognitive model—Psychological theory of behavior change; based on concepts of self-efficacy and outcome expectation.

specificity—Measure of a test's ability to correctly identify individuals with no risk factors for a specific disease.

specificity principle—Training principle; physiological and metabolic responses and adaptations to exercise training are specific to type of exercise and muscle groups involved.

sphygmomanometer—Device used to measure blood pressure manually, consisting of a blood pressure cuff and a manometer.

Spinning—Group-led exercise that involves stationary cycling at various cadences and resistances.

split routine—Advanced resistance training system in which different muscle groups are targeted on consecutive days to avoid overtraining.

sprint interval training (SIT)—Subclass of high-intensity interval training; based on repeated combinations of short (e.g., 30 sec) sprints and extended (e.g., 4 min) rest or recovery intervals.

stage 1 hypertension—Systolic blood pressure ranging from 130 to 139 mmHg or diastolic blood pressure ranging from 80 to 89 mmHg.

stage 2 hypertension—Systolic blood pressure ≥140 mmHg or diastolic blood pressure ≥90 mmHg.

stages of motivational readiness for change model—Psychological theory of behavior change; ability to make long-term behavioral change is based on the client's emotional and intellectual readiness; stages of readiness are precontemplation, contemplation, preparation, action, and maintenance.

standard error of estimate (SEE)—Measure of error for prediction equation; quantifies the average deviation of individual data points around the line of best fit.

static balance—Ability to maintain the center of gravity within the supporting base during standing or sitting.

static muscle action—Type of muscle contraction in which there is no visible joint movement; isometric contraction.

static flexibility—Measure of the total range of motion at a joint.

static stretching—Mode of exercise used to increase range of motion by placing the joint at the end of its range of motion and slowly applying torque to the muscle to stretch it further.

steep ramp cycling protocol (SRP)—Maximal exertion cycling protocol utilizing stage changes every 10 sec; magnitude of stage increments are determined by the rider's height.

stress relaxation—Decreased tension within musculotendinous unit when it is held at a fixed length during static stretching.

stretch tolerance—Measure of the amount of resistive force to stretch within target muscles that can be tolerated before experiencing pain.

stroke—Rupture or blockage of blood flow to the brain caused by an aneurysm, blood clot, or some other particle.

ST segment—Part of ECG tracing reflecting ventricular repolarization; used to detect coronary occlusion and myocardial infarct.

subcutaneous adipose tissue (SAT)—Fat located beneath the skin and above the muscle.

submaximal exercise test—Graded exercise test in which exercise is terminated at some predetermined submaximal heart rate or workload; used to estimate $\dot{V}O_2$max.

super circuit resistance training—Type of circuit resistance training that intersperses a short aerobic exercise bout between each resistance training exercise station.

supersetting—Advanced resistance training system in which exercises for agonist and antagonist muscle groups are done consecutively without rest.

syncope—Brief lapse in consciousness caused by lack of oxygen to the brain.

systolic blood pressure (SBP)—Highest pressure in the arteries during systole of the heart.

tachycardia—Resting heart rate >100 bpm.

talk test—Method to monitor exercise intensity; measure of the client's ability to converse comfortably while exercising; based on the relationship between exercise intensity and pulmonary ventilation.

tare weight—Weight of the chair or platform and its supporting equipment used in hydrostatic weighing.

telomeres—Repeated DNA sequences that determine structure and function of chromosomes.

terminal digit bias—Tendency of the technician to round BP values to the nearest 0 or 5 mmHg.

theory of planned behavior—An extension of the theory of reasoned action that takes into consideration the individual's perception of behavioral control.

theory of reasoned action—Theory that proposes a way to understand and predict an individual's behavior; intention is the most important determinant of behavior.

thoracic gas volume (TGV)—Volume of air in the lungs and thorax.

thrombus—Lump of cellular elements of the blood attached to the inner walls of an artery or vein, sometimes blocking blood flow through the vessel.

thyrotoxicosis—Overactive thyroid gland that secretes greater than normal amounts of thyroid hormones; also known as Graves' disease or hyperthyroidism.

tonic vibration reflex—Reflex that activates muscle spindles and alpha motor neurons of muscles stimulated by vibration loading.

total cholesterol (TC)—Absolute amount of cholesterol in the blood.

total energy expenditure (TEE)—Sum of energy expenditures for resting metabolic rate, dietary thermogenesis, and physical activity.

total energy expenditure (TEE) method—Method for determining energy expenditure measured by doubly labeled water or predicted from equations.

total error (TE)—Average deviation of individual scores of the cross-validation sample from the line of identity.

training volume—Total amount of training as determined by the number of sets and exercises for a muscle group, intensity, and frequency of training.

transcranial magnetic stimulation (TMS)—Method used to study adaptations in the central nervous system in response to strength training.

transcriptome signature of resistance exercise—The approximately 660 genes that are affected by resistance training.

transtheoretical model—Model describing the process a client goes through when adopting a change in health behavior.

treading—Type of group-led interval training that involves walking, jogging, and running at various speeds and grades on a treadmill with relief intervals interspersed.

triaxial joint—Type of joint allowing movement in three planes; ball-and-socket joint.

tri-sets—Advanced resistance training system in which three different exercises for the same muscle group are performed consecutively with little or no rest between the exercises.

T wave—Part of ECG tracing corresponding to ventricular repolarization.

two-component model—Body composition model that divides the body into fat and fat-free body components.

type A activity—Endurance activity requiring minimal skill or fitness (e.g., walking).

type B activity—Endurance activity requiring minimal skill but average fitness (e.g., jogging).

type C activity—Physical activity requiring both skill and physical fitness (e.g., swimming).

type D activity—Recreational sports that may improve physical fitness (e.g., basketball).

type 1 diabetes—Insulin-dependent diabetes, caused by lack of insulin production by the pancreas.

type 2 diabetes—Non-insulin-dependent diabetes, caused by decreased insulin receptor sensitivity.

ultrasound—A noninvasive alternative to SKFs for estimating subcutaneous body fat at specific sites; uses sound frequencies sent and received by a handheld probe (wand) to determine tissue interfaces and, hence, depth of various tissues at a specific site (e.g., from basal layer of the skin and start of subcutaneous adipose tissue layer to end of the subcutaneous adipose layer and start of underlying skeletal muscle); associated computer software displays and calculates the tissue thickness of interest.

undercuffing—Using a blood pressure cuff with a bladder too small for the arm circumference, leading to an overestimation of blood pressure.

underwater weight (UWW)—Method used to estimate body volume by measuring weight loss when the body is fully submerged; hydrostatic weighing.

underweight—BMI <18.5 kg/m^2.

undulating periodization (UP)—Strength training method that varies training intensity and volume weekly or even daily.

uniaxial joint—Type of joint allowing movement in one plane; hinge or pivot joint.

upper body obesity—Type of obesity in which excess fat is localized to the upper body; android obesity; apple-shaped body.

uremia—Excessive amounts of urea and other nitrogen waste products in the blood associated with kidney failure.

validity—Ability of a test to accurately measure, with minimal error, a specific component.

validity coefficient—Correlation between reference measure and predicted scores.

valvular heart disease—Congenital disorder of a heart valve characterized by obstructed blood flow, valvular degeneration, valvular stenosis, and regurgitation of blood.

variable-resistance exercise—Type of exercise in which resistance changes during the range of motion due to levers, pulleys, and cams.

ventilatory threshold—Point at which there is an exponential increase in pulmonary ventilation relative to exercise intensity and rate of oxygen consumption.

ventricular ectopy—Premature (out of sequence) contraction of the ventricles.

ventricular fibrillation—Cardiac dysrhythmia marked by rapid, uncoordinated, and unsynchronized contractions of the ventricles, so that no blood is pumped by the heart.

verification bout—Exercise against a constant load approximately 10% higher than the highest workload achieved during a maximal exertion ramped GXT; used to confirm $\dot{V}O_2$max was attained during a maximal exertion GXT effort that failed to meet the criterion of a plateau in oxygen consumption.

vertigo—Dizziness or inability to maintain normal balance in a standing or seated position.

very low-density lipoprotein (VLDL)—Lipoprotein made in the liver for transporting triglycerides.

visceral adipose tissue (VAT)—Fat located around the internal organs.

viscoelastic creep—A small increase in joint angle during constant-torque stretching, due to elongation of the muscle-tendon unit.

viscoelastic properties—Tension within the muscle-tendon unit caused by the elastic and viscous deformation of the unit when force is applied during stretching.

viscous deformation—Deformation of the muscle-tendon unit that is proportional to the speed at which tension is applied during stretching.

volume of exercise—Quantity of exercise determined by frequency, intensity, and time of exercise.

$\dot{V}O_2$max—Maximum rate of oxygen utilization of muscles during exercise.

$\dot{V}O_2$peak—Measure of highest rate of oxygen consumption during an exercise test regardless of whether or not a $\dot{V}O_2$ plateau is reached.

$\dot{V}O_2$reserve—The $\dot{V}O_2$max minus the $\dot{V}O_2$rest.

waist-to-height ratio (WHTR)—Waist circumference divided by standing height; used as a measure of abdominal obesity.

waist-to-hip ratio (WHR)—Waist circumference divided by hip circumference; used as a measure of upper body or abdominal obesity.

wearable technology—Data collection or data monitoring devices that may be worn during the day as well as during bouts of activity (e.g., heart rate monitors, pedometers, accelerometers); these devices do not restrict movement, thereby providing insights into physiological responses to activity and daily patterns of activity.

white coat effect—Acute elevation of blood pressure when measured in the doctor's office regardless of usual blood pressure readings outside of that environment or antihypertensive medication prescription status.

white coat hypertension—Condition in which individuals have normal blood pressure and are not taking any antihypertensive medications but become hypertensive when blood pressure is measured by a health professional.

whole-body vibration training (WBV)—Training method that uses whole-body mechanical vibration to increase strength, balance, and bone integrity.

References

Aagaard, P., Andersen, J.L., Bennekou, M., Larsson, B., Olesen, J.L., Crameri, R., Magnusson, S.P., and Kjaer, M. 2011. Effects of resistance training on endurance capacity and muscle fiber composition in young top-level cyclists. *Scandinavian Journal of Medicine and Science in Sports* 21(6): e298-e307.

Abercromby, A.F.J., Amonette, W.E., Layne, C.S., McFarlin, B.K., Hinman, M.R., and Paloski, W.H. 2007. Vibration exposure and biodynamic responses during whole-body vibration training. *Medicine & Science in Sports & Exercise* 39: 1794-1800.

Abraham, P., Noury-Desvaux, B., Gernigon, M., Mahe, G., Sauvaget, T., Leftheriotis, G., and LeFaucheur, A. 2012. The inter- and intra-unit variability of a low-cost GPS data logger/receiver to study human outdoor walking in view of health and clinical studies. *PLoS One* 7: e31338. doi:10.1371/journal.pone.0031338. Accessed November 10, 2012.

Abraham, W.M. 1977. Factors in delayed muscle soreness. *Medicine and Science in Sports* 9: 11-20.

Adams, J., Mottola, M., Bagnall, K.M., and McFadden, K.D. 1982. Total body fat content in a group of professional football players. *Canadian Journal of Applied Sport Sciences* 7: 36-44.

Ades, P.A., Savage, P.D., Marney, A.M., Harvey, J., and Evans, K.A. 2015. Remission of recently diagnosed type 2 diabetes mellitus with weight loss and exercise. *Journal of Cardiopulmonary Rehabilitation Prevention* 35: 193-197.

Ahlback, S.O., and Lindahl, O. 1964. Sagittal mobility of the hip-joint. *Acta Orthopaedica Scandinavica* 34: 310-313.

Ahluwalia, N., Dalmasso, P., Rasmussen, M., Lipsky, L., Currie, C., Haug, E., Kelly, C., Damsgaard, M.T., Due, P., Tabak, I., Ercan, O., Maes, L., Aasvee, K., and Cavallo, F. 2015. Trends in overweight prevalence among 11-, 13- and 15-year-olds in 25 countries in Europe, Canada and USA from 2002 to 2010. *European Journal of Public Health* 25(Suppl. 2): 28-32.

Ainsworth, B.E., Haskell, W.L., Whitt, M.C., Irwin, M.L., Swartz, A.M., Strath, S.J., O'Brien, W.L., Bassett, D.R. Jr., Schmitz, K.H., Emplaincourt, P.O., Jacobs, D.R., and Leon, A.S. 2000. Compendium of physical activities: An update of activity codes and MET intensities. *Medicine & Science in Sports & Exercise* 32(Suppl.): S498-S516.

Akuthota, V., Ferreiro, A., Moore, T., and Fredericson, M. 2008. Core stability exercise principles. *Current Sports Medicine Reports* 7: 39-44.

Albasini, A., Krause, M., and Rembitzki, I. 2010. *Using WBV therapy in physical therapy and sport.* London: Churchill Livingstone.

Alberti, K.G., Eckel, R.H., Grundy, S.M., Zimmet, P.Z., Cleeman, J.I., Donato, K.A., Fruchart, J-C., James, W.P., Loria, C.M., and Smith, S.C. Jr. 2009. Harmonizing the metabolic syndrome: A joint interim statement of the International Diabetes Federation Task Force on Epidemiology and Prevention; National Heart, Lung, and Blood Institute; American Heart Association; World Heart Federation; International Atherosclerosis Society; and International Association for the Study of Obesity. *Circulation* 120: 1640-1645.

Alcaraz, A.B., Perez-Gomez, J., Chavarrias, M., and Blazevich, A.J. 2011. Similarity in adaptations to high-resistance circuit vs. traditional strength training in resistance-trained men. *Journal of Strength and Conditioning Research* 25: 2519-2527.

Allen, L., Williams, J., Townsend, N., Mikkelsen, B., Roberts, N., Foster, C., and Wickramasinghe, K. 2017. Socioeconomic status and non-communicable disease behavioural risk factors in low-income and lower-middle-income countries: A systematic review. *Lancet Global Health 2017* 5: e277-e289.

Allison, M.K., Baglole, J.H., Martin, B.J., Macinnis, M.J., Gurd, B.J., and Gibala, M.J. 2017. Brief intense stair climbing improves cardiorespiratory fitness. *Medicine & Science in Sports & Exercise* 49: 298-307.

Allison, K.F., Keenan, K.A., Sell, T.C., Abt, J.P., Nagai, T., Deluzio, J., McGrail, M., and Lephart, S.M. 2015. Musculoskeletal, biomechanical, and physiological gender differences in the U.S. military. *U.S. Army Medical Department Journal* April-June: 22-32.

Al Kandari, J.R., Mohammad, S., Al-Hashem, R., Telahoun, G., and Barac-Nieto, M. 2016. Practical use of stairs to assess fitness, prescribe and perform physical activity training. *Health* 8: 1402-1410.

Almoallim, H., Alwafi, S., Albazli, K., Alotaibi, M., and Bazuhair, T. 2014. A simple approach of low back pain. *International Journal of Clinical Medicine* 5: 1087-1098.

Almuzaini, K.S., and Fleck, S.J. 2008. Modification of the standing long jump test enhances ability to predict anaerobic performance. *Journal of Strength and Conditioning Research* 22: 1265-1272.

Alter, M.J. 2004. *Science of flexibility*, 3rd ed. Champaign, IL: Human Kinetics.

Alves, A.R., Marta, C.C., Neiva, H.P., Izquierdo, M., and Marques, M.C. 2016. Does intrasession concurrent strength and aerobic training order influence training-induced explosive strength and $\dot{V}O_2$max in prepubescent children? *Journal of Strength and Conditioning Research* 30: 3267-3277.

Alway, S.E., Grumbt, W.H., Gonyea, W.J., and Stray-Gundersen, J. 1989. Contrasts in muscle and myofibers of elite male and female bodybuilders. *Journal of Applied Physiology* 67: 24-31.

Amaral, T.F., Restivo, M.T., Guerra, R.S., Marques, E., Chousal, M.F., and Mota, J. 2011. Accuracy of a digital skinfold system for measuring skinfold thickness and estimating body fat. *British Journal of Nutrition* 105: 478-484.

American Alliance for Health, Physical Education, Recreation and Dance. 1988. *The AAHPERD physical best program.* Reston, VA: Author.

American Cancer Society. 2017. ACS guidelines for nutrition and physical activity. www.cancer.org/healthy/eat-healthy-get-active/acs-guidelines-nutrition-physical-activity-cancer-prevention/guidelines.html. Accessed April 13, 2017.

American College of Sports Medicine. 2004. NCCA accreditation. *ACSM's Certified News* 14(3): 1.

American College of Sports Medicine. 2006. *ACSM's guidelines for exercise testing and prescription*, 7th ed. Philadelphia: Lippincott Williams & Wilkins.

American College of Sports Medicine. 2009. Appropriate physical activity intervention strategies for weight loss and prevention of weight regain for adults. *Medicine & Science in Sports & Exercise* 41: 459-471.

American College of Sports Medicine. 2014. *ACSM's guidelines for exercise testing and prescription*, 9th ed. Philadelphia: Lippincott Williams & Wilkins.

American College of Sports Medicine. 2018. *ACSM's guidelines for exercise testing and prescription*, 10th ed. Philadelphia: Lippincott Williams & Wilkins.

American Council on Exercise. 1997. Absolute certainty: Do abdominal trainers work any better than the average crunch? *ACE Fitness Matters* 3(2): 1-2.

American Diabetes Association. 2017. *Statistics about diabetes.* http://diabetes.org/diabetes-basics/statistics. Accessed April 9, 2017.

American Dietetic Association. 2000. Position of the American Dietetic Association, Dietitians of Canada, and the American College of Sports Medicine: Nutrition and athletic performance. *Journal of American Dietetic Association* 100: 1543-1556.

American Dietetic Association. 2003. *Let the evidence speak: Indirect calorimetry and weight management guides.* Chicago: Author.

American Fitness Professionals and Associates. 2004. AFPA news flash: What is the National Board of Fitness Examiners (NBFE) and how does it work? www.afpafitness.com.

American Heart Association. 2001. *International cardiovascular disease statistics.* Dallas: Author.

American Heart Association. 2004. *Heart disease and stroke statistics—2004 update.* Dallas: Author.

American Heart Association. 2012. Heart disease and stroke statistics 2012 update: A report from the American Heart Association Statistics Committee and Stroke Statistics Subcommittee. *Circulation* 125: e2-e220.

American Heart Association. 2017. Heart disease and stroke statistics 2017 update. *Circulation* 135. doi:10.1161/CIR.0000000000000485.

American Medical Association. 1988. *Guides to the evaluation of permanent impairment*, 3rd ed. Chicago, IL: Author.

American Society of Exercise Physiologists. 2018. Standards of practice. https://www.asep.org/organization/practice/.

American Society of Hand Therapists. 1992. *Clinical assessment recommendations*, 2nd ed. Chicago, IL: Author.

Aminian-Far, A., Hadian, M.R., Olyaei, G., Talebian, S., and Bakhtiary, A.H. 2011. Whole-body vibration and the prevention and treatment of delayed-onset muscle soreness. *Journal of Athletic Training* 46: 43-49.

Andersen, J.L., and Aagaard, P. 2000. Myosin heavy chain IIX overshooting in human skeletal muscle. *Muscle and Nerve* 23: 1095-1104.

Andersen, J.L., and Aagaard, P. 2010. Effects of strength training on muscle fiber types and size: Consequences for athletes training for high-intensity sport. *Scandinavian Journal of Medicine and Science in Sports* 20(Suppl. 2): S32-S38.

Anderson, G.S. 1992. The 1600 m and multistage 20 m shuttle run as predictive tests of aerobic capacity in children. *Pediatric Exercise Science* 4: 312-318.

Anderson, L.J., Erceg, D.N., and Schroeder, E.T. 2012. Utility of multifrequency bioelectrical impedance compared with dual-energy X-ray absorptiometry for assessment of total and regional body composition varies between men and women. *Nutrition Research* 32: 479-485.

Andres, S., Ziegenhagen, R., Trefflich, I., Pevny, S., Schultrich, K., Braun, H., Schänzer, W., Hirsch-Ernst, K.I., Schäfer, B., and Lampen, A. 2017. Creatine and creatine forms intended for sports nutrition. *Molecular Nutrition and Food Research* 61(6): article 1600772.

Andrews, A.W., Thomas, M.W., and Bohannon, R.W. 1996. Normative values for isometric muscle force measurements obtained with hand-held dynamometers. *Physical Therapy* 76: 248-259.

Androutsos, O., Gerasimidis, K., Karanikolou, A., Reilly, J.J., and Edwards, C.A. 2015. Impact of eating and drinking on body composition measurements by bioelectrical impedance. *Journal of Human Nutrition and Dietetics* 28: 165-171.

Ansai, J.H., Aurichio, T.R., Goncalves, R., and Rebelatto, J.R. 2016. Effects of two physical exercise protocols on physical performance related to falls in the oldest old: A randomized controlled trial. *Geriatrics and Gerontology International* 16: 492-499.

Antoine-Jonville, S., Sinnapah, S., and Hue, O. 2012. Relationship between body mass index and body composition in adolescents of Asian Indian origin and their peers. *European Journal of Public Health* 22: 887-889.

Antonio, J., and Gonyea, W.J. 1993. Skeletal muscle fiber hyperplasia. *Medicine & Science in Sports & Exercise* 25: 1333-1345.

Aragon, A.A., Schoenfeld, B.J., Wildman, R., Kleiner, S., VanDusseldorp, T., Taylor, L., Earnest, C.P., Arciero, P.J., Wilborn, C., Kalman, D.S., Stout, J.R., Willoughby, D.S., Campbell, B., Arent, S.M., Bannock, L., Smith-Ryan, A.E., and Antonio, J. 2017. International society of sports nutrition position stand: Diets and body composition. *Journal of the International Society of Sports Nutrition* 14: 16.

Ardern, C.I., Katzmarzyk, P.T., and Ross, R. 2003. Discrimination of health risk by combined body mass index and waist circumference. *Obesity Research* 11: 135-142.

Arem, H., Moore, S.C., Patel, A., Hartge, P., Berrington de Gonzalez, A., Visvanathan, K., Campbell, P.T., Freeman, M., Weiderpass, E., Adami, H.O., Linet, M.S., Lee, I-M., and Matthews, C.E. 2015. Leisure time physical activity and mortality: A detailed pooled analysis of the dose-response relationship. *JAMA Internal Medicine* 175: 959-967.

Arena, S.K., Simon, L., and Peterson, E.L. 2016. Aneroid blood pressure manometer calibration rates in physical therapy curricula: A descriptive study. *Cardiopulmonary Physical Therapy Journal* 27: 56-61.

Armstrong, R.B. 1984. Mechanisms of exercise-induced delayed onset muscular soreness: A brief review. *Medicine & Science in Sports & Exercise* 16: 529-538.

Artero, E.G., Espada-Fuentes, J.C., Arguelles-Cienfuegos, J., Roman, A., Gomez-Lopez, P.J., and Gutierrez, A. 2012. Effects of whole-body vibration and resistance training on knee extensors muscular performance. *European Journal of Applied Physiology* 112: 1371-1378.

Artero, E.G., España-Romero, V., Castro-Piñero, J., Ruiz, J.R., Jiménez-Pavón, D., Aparicio, V., Gatto-Cardia, M., Baena, P., Vicente-Rodríguez, G., Castillo, M.J., and Ortega, F.B. 2012. Criterion-related validity of field-based muscular fitness tests in youth. *Journal of Sports Medicine and Physical Fitness* 52(3): 263-272.

Asayama, K., Ohkubo, T., Hoshide, S., Kario, K., Ohya, Y., Rakugi, H., and Umemura, S., on behalf of the Japanese Society of Hypertension Working Group on Mercury Sphygmomanometer and Minamata Convention on Mercury. 2016. From mercury sphygmomanometer to electric device on blood pressure measurement: Correspondence of Minamata Convention on Mercury. *Hypertension Research* 39: 179-182.

Ashford, S., Edmunds, J., and French, D.P. 2010. What is the best way to change self-efficacy to promote lifestyle and recreational physical activity? A systematic review with meta-analysis. *British Journal of Health Psychology* 15: 265-280.

Ashwell, M., Gunn, P., and Gibson, S. 2011. Waist-to-height ratio is a better screening tool than waist circumference and BMI for adult cardiometabolic risk factors: Systematic review and meta-analysis. *Obesity Reviews.* doi:10.1111/j.1467-789X.2011.00952.x.

Ashwell, M., and Hsieh, S.D. 2005. Six reasons why the waist-to-height ratio is a rapid and effective global indicator for health risks of obesity and how its use could simplify the international public health message on obesity. *International Journal of Food Sciences and Nutrition* 56: 303-307.

Ashwell, M., Mayhew, L., Richardson, J., and Rickayzen, B. 2014. Waist-to-height ratio is more predictive of years of life lost than body mass index. *PLoS One* 9(9): e103483. doi:10.1371/journal.pone.0103483. Accessed August 14, 2017.

Ashwell, M., McCall, S.A., Cole, T.J., and Dixon, A.K. 1985. Fat distribution and its metabolic complications: Interpretations. In *Human body composition and fat distribution,* ed. N.G. Norgan, 227-242. Wageningen, Netherlands: Euronut.

Åstrand, I. 1960. Aerobic capacity in men and women with special reference to age. *Acta Physiologica Scandinavica* 49(Suppl. 169): S1-S92.

Åstrand, P.O. 1956. Human physical fitness with special reference to age and sex. *Physiological Reviews* 36: 307-335.

Åstrand, P.O. 1965. *Work tests with the bicycle ergometer.* Varberg, Sweden: AB Cykelfabriken Monark.

Åstrand, P.O., and Rodahl, K. 1977. *Textbook of work physiology.* New York: McGraw-Hill.

Åstrand, P.O., and Ryhming, I. 1954. A nomogram for calculation of aerobic capacity (physical fitness) from pulse rate during submaximal work. *Journal of Applied Physiology* 7: 218-221.

Atterhog, J.H., Jonsson, B., and Samuelsson, R. 1979. Exercise testing: A prospective study of complication rates. *American Heart Journal* 98: 572-580.

Aune, K.T., and Powers, J.M. 2017. Injuries in an extreme conditioning program. *Sports Health* 9: 52-58.

Avila, J.J., Gutierres, J.A., Sheehy, M.E., Lofgren, I.E., and Delmonico, M.J. 2010. Effect of moderate intensity resistance training during weight loss on body composition and physical performance in overweight older adults. *European Journal of Applied Physiology* 109: 517-525.

Axler, C.T., and McGill, S.M. 1997. Low back loads over a variety of abdominal exercises: Searching for the safest abdominal challenge. *Medicine & Science in Sports & Exercise* 29: 804-810.

Azevedo, L.F., Perlingeiro, P.S., Brum, P.C., Braga, A.M.W., Negrao, C.E., and de Matos, L.D.N.J. 2011. Exercise intensity optimization for men with high cardiorespiratory fitness. *Journal of Sports Sciences* 29: 555-561.

Bacon, A.P., Carter, R.E., Ogle, E.A., and Joyner, M.J. 2013. $\dot{V}O_2$max trainability and high intensity interval training in humans: A meta-analysis. *PLoS One* 8(9): e73182. doi:10.1371/journal.pone.00731825.

Baechle, T.R., Earle, R.W., and Wathen, D. 2000. Resistance training. In *Essentials of strength training and conditioning,* ed. T.R. Baechle and R.W. Earle. Champaign, IL: Human Kinetics.

Bahk, J., and Khang, Y-H. 2016. Trends in measures of childhood obesity in Korea from 1998 to 2012. *Journal of Epidemiology* 26: 199-207.

Bahr, R., Ingnes, I., Vaage, O., Sjersted, O.M., and Newsholme, E.A. 1987. Effect of duration of exercise on excess post-exercise O_2 consumption. *Journal of Applied Physiology* 62: 485-490.

Bai, Y., Welk, G.J., Nam, Y.H., Lee, J.A., Lee, J-M., Kin, Y., Meier, N.F., and Dixon, P.M. 2016. Comparison of consumer and research monitors under semistructured settings. *Medicine & Science in Sports & Exercise* 48(1): 151-158.

Bailey, B.W., and McInnis, K. 2011. Energy cost of exergaming: A comparison of the energy cost of 6 forms of exergaming. *Archives of Pediatric and Adolescent Medicine* 165: 597-602.

Baker, D., Wilson, G., and Carlyon, R. 1994. Periodization: The effect on strength of manipulating volume and intensity. *Journal of Strength and Conditioning Research* 8: 235-242.

Balachandran, A., Martins, M.M., De Faveri, F.G., Alan, O., Cetinkaya, F., and Signorile, J.F. 2016. Functional strength training: Seated machine vs standing cable training to improve physical function in elderly. *Experimental Gerontology* 82: 131-138.

Balady, G.J., Arena, R., Sietsema, K., Myers, J., Coke, L., Fletcher, G.F., Forman, D., Franklin, B., Guazzi, M., Gulati, M., Keteyian, S.J., Lavie, C.J., Macko, R., Mancini, D., and Milani, R.V. 2010. Clinician's guide to cardiopulmonary exercise testing in adults: A scientific statement from the American Heart Association. *Circulation* 122: 191-225.

Balke, B. 1963. A simple field test for the assessment of physical fitness. *Civil Aeromedical Research Institute Report,* 63-18. Oklahoma City: Federal Aviation Agency.

Balke, B., and Ware, R. 1959. An experimental study of physical fitness of Air Force personnel. *US Armed Forces Medical Journal* 10: 675-688.

Ball, T.E., and Rose, K.S. 1991. A field test for predicting maximum bench press lift of college women. *Journal of Applied Sport Science Research* 5: 169-170.

Ballor, D.L., and Keesey, R.E. 1991. A meta-analysis of the factors affecting exercise-induced changes in body mass, fat mass, and fat-free mass in males and females. *International Journal of Obesity* 15: 717-726.

Balsamo, S., Tibana, R.A., Nascimento, D., de Farias, G.L., Petruccelli, Z., de Santana, F., Martins, O.V., de Aguiar, F., Pereira, G.B., de Souza, J.C., and Prestes, J. 2012. Exercise order affects the total training volume and the ratings of perceived exertion in response to a super-set resistance training session. *International Journal of General Medicine* 5: 123-127.

Bandura, A. 1982. Self-efficacy mechanism in human agency. *American Psychologist* 37: 122-147.

Bankoski, A., Chen, K.Y., Harris, T.B., Berrigan, D., McClain, J.J., Troiano, R.P., Brychta, R.J., Koster, A., and Caserotti, P. 2011. Sedentary activity associated with metabolic syndrome independent of physical activity. *Diabetes Care* 34: 497-503.

Baranauskas, M.N., Johnson, K.E., Juvancic-Heltzel, J.A., Kappler, R.M., Richardson, L., Jamieson, S., and Otterstetter, R. 2017. Seven-site versus three-site method of body composition using BodyMetrix ultrasound compared to dual-energy X-ray absorptiometry. *Clinical Physiology and Functional Imaging* 37: 317-321.

Barbieri, E., Agostini, D., Polidori, E., Potenza, L., Guescini, M., Lucertini, F., Annibalini, G., Stocchi, L., DeSanti, M., and Stocchi, B. 2015. The pleiotropic effect of physical exercise on mitochondrial dynamics in aging skeletal muscle. *Oxidative Medicine and Cellular Longevity* doi:10.1155/2015/917085. Accessed May 6, 2017.

Barbosa, T.M., Marinho, D.A., Reis, V.M., Silva, A.J., and Bragada, J.A. 2009. Physiological assessment of heat-out aquatic exercises in healthy subjects: A qualitative review. *Journal of Sports Science and Medicine* 8: 179-189.

Bergamin, M., Zanuso, S., Alvar, B.A., Ermolao, A., and Zaccaria, M. 2012. Is water-based exercise training sufficient to improve physical fitness in the elderly? *European Review of Aging and Physical Activity* 9: 129-141.

Barker, A.R., Williams, C.A., Jones, A.M., and Armstrong, N. 2011. Establishing maximal oxygen uptake in young people during a ramp cycle test to exhaustion. *British Journal of Sports Medicine* 45: 498-503.

Barnes, J.N. 2015. Exercise, cognitive function, and aging. *Advances in Physiology Education* 39: 55-62.

Barry, G., van Schaik, P., MacSween, A., Dixon, J., and Martin, D. 2016. Exergaming (XBOX Kinect™) versus traditional gym-based exercise for postural control, flow and technology acceptance in healthy adults: A randomised controlled trial. *BMC Sports Science, Medicine and Rehabilitation* 8: 25. doi:10.1186/s13102-016-0050-0. Accessed November 15, 2016.

Bartlett, J.D., Close, G.L., Maclaren, D.P.M., Gregson, W., Drust, B., and Morton, J.P. 2011. High-intensity interval running is perceived to be more enjoyable than moderate-intensity continuous exercise: Implications for exercise adherence. *Journal of Sports Sciences* 29: 547-553.

Barquera, S., Pedroza-Tobias, A., Medina, C., Hernandez-Barrera, L., Bibbins-Domingo, K., Lozano, R., and Moran, A.E. 2015. Global overview of the epidemiology of atherosclerotic cardiovascular disease. *Archives of Medical Research* 46: 328-338.

Baumert, P., Lake, M.J., Stewart, C.E., Drust, B., and Erskine, R.M. 2016. Genetic variation and exercise-induced muscle damage: Implications for athletic performance, injury and ageing. *European Journal of Applied Physiology* 116: 1595-1625.

Baumgartner, R.N., Heymsfield, S.B., and Roche, A.F. 1995. Human body composition and the epidemiology of chronic disease. *Obesity Research* 3: 73-95.

Baumgartner, R.N., Heymsfield, S.B., Lichtman, S., Wang, J., and Pierson, R.N. 1991. Body composition in elderly people: Effect of criterion estimates on predictive equations. *American Journal of Clinical Nutrition* 53: 1-9.

Baumgartner, T.A. 1978. Modified pull-up test. *Research Quarterly* 49: 80-84.

Baumgartner, T.A., and Jackson, A.S. 1975. *Measurement for evaluation in physical education.* Boston: Houghton Mifflin.

Baumgartner, T.A., East, W.B., Frye, P.A., Hensley, L.D., Knox, D.F., and Norton, C.J. 1984. Equipment improvements and additional norms for the modified pull-up test. *Research Quarterly for Exercise and Sport* 55: 64-68.

Baun, W.B., Baun, M.R., and Raven, P.B. 1981. A nomogram for the estimate of percent body fat from generalized equations. *Research Quarterly for Exercise and Sport* 52: 380-384.

Baxter, C., McNaughton, L.R., Sparks, A., Norton, L., and Bentley, D. 2017. Impact of stretching on the performance and injury risk of long-distance runners. *Research in Sports Medicine* 25: 78-90.

Bazzocchi, A., Filonzi, G., Ponti, F., Albisinni, U., Guglielmi, F., and Battista, G. 2016. Ultrasound: Which role in body composition? *European Journal of Radiology* 85: 1469-1480.

Bazzocchi, A., Ponti, F., Albisinni, U., Battista, G., and Guglielmi, G. 2016. DXA: Technical aspects and application. *European Journal of Radiology* 85: 1481-1492.

Beardsley, C., and Contreras, B. 2014. The role of kettlebells in strength and conditioning: A review of the literature. *Strength and Conditioning Journal* 36(3): 64-70.

Beaulieu, J.E. 1980. *Stretching for all sports.* Pasadena, CA: Athletic Press.

Beenakker, E.A.C., van der Hoeven, J.H., Fock, J.M., and Maurits, N.M. 2001. Reference values of maximum isometric muscle force obtained in 270 children aged 4-16 years by hand-held dynamometry. *Neuromuscular Disorders* 11: 441-446.

Behm, D.G., Bambury, A., Farrell, C., and Power, K. 2004. Effect of acute static stretching on force, balance, reaction time and movement time. *Medicine & Science in Sports & Exercise* 36: 1397-1402.

Behm, D.G., Blazevich, A.J., Kay, A.D., and McHugh, M. 2016. Acute effects of muscle stretching on physical performance, range of motion, and injury incidence in healthy active individuals: A systematic review. *Applied Physiology, Nutrition, and Metabolism* 41: 1-11.

Behm, D.G., Drinkwater, E.J., Willardson, J.M., and Cowley, P.M. 2010a. The use of instability to train the core musculature. *Applied Physiology, Nutrition and Metabolism* 35: 91-108.

Behm, D.G., Drinkwater, E.J., Willardson, J.M., and Cowley, P.M. 2010b. Canadian Society for Exercise Physiology position stand: The use of instability to train the core in athletic and nonathletic conditioning. *Applied Physiology, Nutrition and Metabolism* 35: 109-112.

Behm, D.G., Faigenbaum, A.D., Falk, B., and Klentrou, P. 2008. Canadian Society for Exercise Physiology position paper: Resistance training in children and adolescents. *Applied Physiology, Nutrition, and Metabolism* 33: 547-561.

Behm, D.G., Young, J.D., Whitten, J.H.D., Reid, J.C., Quigley, P.J., Low, J., Li, Y., Lima, C.D., Hodgson, D.D., Chaouachi, A., Prieske, O., and Granacher, U. 2017. Effectiveness of traditional strength vs. power training on muscle strength, power and speed with youth: A systematic review and meta-analysis. *Frontiers in Physiology* 8: 423.

Behnke, A.R. 1961. Quantitative assessment of body build. *Journal of Applied Physiology* 16: 960-968.

Behnke, A.R., and Wilmore, J.H. 1974. *Evaluation and regulation of body build and composition.* Englewood Cliffs, NJ: Prentice Hall.

Beime, B., Deutsch, C., Gomez, T., Zwingers, T., Mengden, T., and Bramlage, P. 2016. Validation protocols for blood pressure-measuring devices: Status quo and development needs. *Blood Pressure Monitoring* 21: 1-8.

Bell, D.R., Guskiewicz, K.M., Clark, M.A., and Padua, D.A. 2011. Systematic review of the balance error scoring system. *Sports Health* 3: 287-295.

Beltz, N.M., Gibson, A.L., Janot, J.M., Kravitz, L., Mermier, C.M., and Dalleck, L.C. 2016. Graded exercise testing protocols for the determination of $\dot{V}O_2$max: Historical perspectives, progress, and future considerations. Journal of Sports Medicine 2016: article 3968393. doi:10.1155/2016/3968393. Accessed June 15, 2017.

Beltz, N., Erbes, D., Porcari, J.P., Martinez, R., Doberstein, S., and Foster, C. 2013. Effects of kettlebell training on aerobic capacity, muscular strength, balance, flexibility, and body composition. *Journal of Fitness Research* 2: 4-13.

Bemben, D.A., Palmer, I.J., Bemben, M.G., and Knehans, A.W. 2010. Effects of combined whole-body vibration and resistance training on muscular strength and bone metabolism in postmenopausal women. *Bone* 47: 650-656.

Bendiksen, M., Ahler, R., Clausen, H., Wedderkopp, N., and Krustrup, P. 2012. The use of Yo-Yo IR1 and Andersen testing for fitness and maximal heart rate assessments of 6-10 yr old school children. *Journal of Strength and Conditioning Research* [Epub ahead of print]. doi:10.1519/JSC.0b013e318270fd0b.

Benatti, F.B., and Ried-Larsen, M. 2015. The effects of breaking up prolonged sitting time: A review of experimental studies. *Medicine & Science in Sports & Exercise* 47: 2053-2061.

Benson, A.C., Bruce, L., and Gordon, B.A. 2015. Reliability and validity of a GPS-enabled iPhone™ "app" to measure physical activity. *Journal of Sports Sciences* 22: 1421-1428.

Bentzur, K.M., Kravitz, L., and Lockner, D.W. 2008. Evaluation of the Bod Pod for estimating percent body fat in collegiate track and field female athletes: A comparison of four methods. *Journal of Strength and Conditioning Research* 22: 1985-1991.

Berg, K.O., Wood-Dauphinee, S.L., Williams, J.I., and Maki, B. 1992. Measuring balance in the elderly: Validation of an instrument. *Canadian Journal of Public Health* 83(2): S7-S11.

Bergamin, M., Zanuso, S., Alvar, B.A., Ermolao, A., and Zaccaria, M. 2012. Is water-based exercise training sufficient to improve fitness in the elderly? *European Review of Aging and Physical Activity* 9: 129-141.

Bergen, G., Stevens, M.R., and Burns, E.R. 2016. Falls and fall injuries among adults aged ≥65 years—United States, 2014. *Morbidity and Mortality Weekly Report* 65: 993-998.

Bergeron, M.F., Nindl, B.C., Deuster, P.A., Baumgartner, N., Kane, S.F., Kraemer, W.J., Sexauer, L.R., Thompson, W.R., and O'Connor, F.G. 2011. Consortium for health and military performance and American College of Sports Medicine consensus paper on extreme conditioning programs in military personnel. *Current Sports Medicine Reports* 10(6): 383-389.

Berglund, E., Birath, G., Bjure, J., Grimby, G., Kjellmar, I., Sandvist, L., and Soderholm, B. 1963. Spirometric studies in normal subjects. I. Forced expirograms in subjects between 7 and 70 years of age. *Acta Medica Scandinavica* 173: 185-192.

Bergouignan, A., Legget, K.T., DeJong, N., Kealey, E., Nikolovski, J., Groppel, J.L., Jordan, C., O'Day, R., Hill, J.O., and Bessesen, D.H. 2016. Effect of frequent interruptions of prolonged sitting on self-perceived levels of energy, mood, food cravings and cognitive function. *International Journal of Behavioral Nutrition and Physical Activity* 13: 113. doi:10.1186/s12966-016-0437-z. Accessed April 6, 2017.

Bergsma-Kadijk, J.A., Baumeister, B., and Deurenberg, P. 1996. Measurement of body fat in young and elderly women: Comparison between a four-compartment model and widely used reference methods. *British Journal of Nutrition* 75: 649-657.

Berry, M.J., Cline, C.C., Berry, C.B., and Davis, M. 1992. A comparison between two forms of aerobic dance and treadmill running. *Medicine & Science in Sports & Exercise* 24: 946-951.

Best, J.R. 2011. Exergaming immediately enhances children's executive function. *Developmental Psychology* 48: 1501-1510.

Bielinski, R., Schultz, Y., and Jequier, E. 1985. Energy metabolism during the postexercise recovery in man. *American Journal of Clinical Nutrition* 42: 69-82.

Biering-Sorensen, F. 1984. Physical measurements as risk indicators for low-back trouble over a one-year period. *Spine* 9: 106-119.

Billinger, S.A., Loudon, J.K., and Gajewski, B.J. 2008. Validity of a total body recumbent stepper exercise test to assess cardiorespiratory fitness. *Journal of Strength and Conditioning Research* 22: 1556-1562.

Billinger, S.A., van Swearingen, E., McClain, M., Lentz, A.A., and Good, M.B. 2012. Recumbent stepper submaximal exercise test to predict peak oxygen uptake. *Medicine & Science in Sports & Exercise* 44: 1539-1544.

Biswas, A., Oh, P.I., Faulkner, G.E., Bajaj, R.R., Silver, M.A., Mitchell, M.S., and Alter, D.A. 2015. Sedentary time and its association with risk for disease incidence, mortality, and hospitalization in adults: A systematic review and meta-analysis. *Annals of Internal Medicine* 162: 123-132.

Bjorntorp, P. 1988. Abdominal obesity and the development of non-insulin diabetes mellitus. *Diabetes and Metabolism Reviews* 4: 615-622.

Black, D.M., and Rosen, C.J. 2016. Postmenopausal osteoporosis. *New England Journal of Medicine* 374: 254-262.

Black, L.F., Offord, K., and Hyatt, R.E. 1974. Variability in the maximum expiratory flow volume curve in asymptomatic smokers and nonsmokers. *American Review of Respiratory Diseases* 110: 282-292.

Blair, D., Habricht, J.P., Sims, E.A., Sylwester, D., and Abraham, S. 1984. Evidence of an increased risk for hypertension with centrally located body fat, and the effect of race and sex on this risk. *American Journal of Epidemiology* 119: 526-540.

Blair, S.N. 2009. Physical inactivity: The biggest public health problem of the 21st century. *British Journal of Sports Medicine* 43: 1-2.

Bland, J.M., and Altman, D.G. 1986. Statistical methods for assessing agreement between two methods of clinical measurement. *Lancet* 12: 307-310.

Bleakley, C., McDonough, S., Gardner, E., Baxter, G.D., Hopkins, J.T., and Davison, G.W. 2012. Cold-water immersion (cryotherapy) for preventing and treating muscle soreness after exercise. *Cochrane Database of Systematic Reviews* [online] 2: CD008262.

Bleakley, C.M., Charles, D., Porter-Armstrong, A., McNeill, M.D.J., McDonnough, S.M., and McCormack, B. 2015. Gaming for health: A systematic review of the physical and cognitive effects of interactive computer games in older adults. *Journal of Applied Gerontology* 34: NP166-NP189.

Blum, V., Carriere, E.G.J., Kolsters, W., Mosterd, W.L., Schiereck, P., and Wesseling, K.H. 1997. Aortic and peripheral blood pressure during isometric and dynamic exercise. *International Journal of Sports Medicine* 18: 30-34.

Bogaerts, A., Ameye, L., Bijlholt, M., Amuli, K., Heynickx, D., and Devlieger, R. 2017. INTER-ACT: Prevention of pregnancy complications through an e-health driven interpregnancy lifestyle intervention—study protocol of a multicentre randomized controlled trial. *BMC Pregnancy and Childbirth* 17: article 154.

Bogaerts, A.C.G., Delecluse, C., Claessens, A.L., Troosters, T., Boonen, S., Verschueren, S.M.P. 2009. Effects of whole body vibration training on cardiorespiratory fitness and muscle strength in older individuals (A 1-year randomized controlled trial). 2009. *Age and Ageing* 38: 448-454.

Bohannon, R.W. 1997. Reference values for extremity muscle strength obtained by hand-held dynamometry from adults aged 20 to 79 years. *Archives of Physical Medicine and Rehabilitation* 78: 26-32.

Bohannon, R.W. 2006a. Reference values for the timed up and go test: A descriptive meta-analysis. *Journal of Geriatric Physical Therapy* 29(2): 64-68.

Bohannon, R.W. 2006b. Single leg stance times. A descriptive meta-analysis of data from individuals at least 60 years of age. *Topics in Geriatric Rehabilitation* 22: 70-77.

Bohannon, R.W., Peolsson, A., Massy-Westropp, N., Desrosiers, J., and Bear-Lehman, J. 2006. Reference values for adult grip strength measured with a Jamar dynamometer: A descriptive meta-analysis. *Physiotherapy* 92: 11-15.

Bolam, K.A., Van Uffelen, J.G.Z., and Taaffe, D.R. 2013. The effect of physical exercise on bone density in middle-aged and older men: A systematic review. *Osteoporosis International* 24: 2749-2762.

Bompa, T.O., DiPasquale, M.D., and Cornacchia, L.J. 2003. *Serious strength training*, 2nd ed. Champaign, IL: Human Kinetics.

Bonge, D., and Donnelly, J.E. 1989. Trials to criteria for hydrostatic weighing at residual volume. *Research Quarterly for Exercise and Sport* 60: 176-179.

Bongers, B.C., de Vries, S.I., Helders, P.J.M., and Takken, T. 2013. The Steep Ramp Test in healthy children and adolescents: Reliability and validity. *Medicine & Science in Sports & Exercise* 45: 366-371.

Borde, R., Hortobagyi, T., and Granacher, U. 2015. Dose-response relationships of resistance training in healthy old adults: A systematic review and meta-analysis. *Sports Medicine* 45: 1693-1720.

Boren, H.G., Kory, R.C., and Syner, J.C. 1966. The Veteran's Administration-Army cooperative study of pulmonary function: II. The lung volume and its subdivisions in normal men. *American Journal of Medicine* 41: 96-114.

Borg, G. 1998. *Borg's perceived exertion and pain scales.* Champaign, IL: Human Kinetics.

Bouaziz, W., Lang, P.O., Schmitt, E., Kaltenbach, G., Geny, B., and Vogel, T. 2016. Health benefits of multicomponent training programmes in seniors: A systematic review. *International Journal of Clinical Practice* 70: 520-536.

Bouchard, C. 2008. Gene-environment interactions in the etiology of obesity: Defining the fundamentals. *Obesity* 16(Suppl.): S5-S10.

Bouchard, C., Blair, S.N., and Katzmarzyk, P.T. 2015. Less sitting, more physical activity, or more fitness? *Mayo Clinic Proceedings* 90: 1533-1540.

Bouchard, C., Perusse, L., Leblanc, C., Tremblay, A., and Theriault, G. 1988. Inheritance of the amount and distribution of human body fat. *International Journal of Obesity* 12: 205-215.

Bouchard, C., Tremblay, A., Despres, J.P., Nadeau, A., Lupien, P.J., Theriault, G., Dussault, J., Moorjani, S., Pinault, S., and Fournier, G. 1990. The response of long-term overfeeding in identical twins. *New England Journal of Medicine* 322: 1477-1482.

Bracko, M.R. 2004. Can we prevent back injuries? *ACSM's Health & Fitness Journal* 8(4): 5-11.

Brahler, C.J., and Blank, S.E. 1995. VersaClimbing elicits higher $\dot{V}O_2$max than does treadmill running or rowing ergometry. *Medicine & Science in Sports & Exercise* 27: 249-254.

Braith, R.W., Graves, J.E., Leggett, S.H., and Pollock, M.L. 1993. Effect of training on the relationship between maximal and submaximal strength. *Medicine & Science in Sports & Exercise* 25: 132-138.

Branch, J.D. 2003. Effect of creatine supplementation on body composition and performance: A meta-analysis. *International Journal of Sport Nutrition and Exercise Metabolism* 13: 198-226.

Bray, G.A. 1978. Definitions, measurements and classifications of the syndromes of obesity. *International Journal of Obesity* 2: 99-113.

Bray, G.A. 2004. The epidemic of obesity and changes in food intake: The fluoride hypothesis. *Physiological Behavior* 82: 115-121.

Bray, G.A., Frühbeck, G., Ryan, D.H., and Wilding, J.P.H. 2016. Management of obesity. *Lancet* 387: 1947-1956.

Bray, G.A., and Gray, D.S. 1988a. Anthropometric measurements in the obese. In *Anthropometric standardization reference manual*, ed. T.G. Lohman, A.F. Roche, and R. Martorell, 131-136. Champaign, IL: Human Kinetics.

Bray, G.A., and Gray, D.S. 1988b. Obesity. Part I—Pathogenesis. *Western Journal of Medicine* 149: 429-441.

Brehm, B.A. 1988. Elevation of metabolic rate following exercise—implications for weight loss. *Sports Medicine* 6: 72-78.

British Heart Foundation. 2006. Diet, physical activity, and obesity statistics, 2006 edition. www.bhf.org.

British Heart Foundation. 2015a. *Physical activity statistics 2015*. www.bhf.org.uk/publications/statistics/physical-activity-statistics-2015. Accessed March 19, 2017.

British Heart Foundation. 2015b. Cardiovascular disease statistics, 2015. bhf-cvd-satistics-2015-final.pdf. Accessed April 2, 2017.

Broadbent, S., Rousseau, J.J., Thorp, R.M., Choate, S.L., Jackson, F.S., and Rowlands, D.S. 2010. Vibration therapy reduces plasma IL6 and muscle soreness after downhill running. *British Journal of Sports Medicine* 44: 888-894.

Brogan, M., Ledesma, R., Coffino, A., and Chander, P. 2017. Freebie rhabdomyolysis: A public health concern. Spin class–induced rhabdomyolysis. *American Journal of Medicine* 130: 484-487.

Bronner, S., Agraharasamakulam, S., and Ojofeitimi, S. 2010. Reliability and validity of electrogoniometry measurement of lower extremity movement. *Journal of Medical Engineering & Technology* 34: 232-242.

Bronner, S., Pinsker, R., and Noah, J.A. 2015. Physiological and psychophysiological responses in experienced players while playing different dance exer-games. *Computers in Human Behavior* 51: 34-41.

Brooks, G.A., Butte, N.F., Rand, W.M., Flatt, J.P., and Caballero, B. 2004. Chronicle of the Institute of Medicine physical activity recommendation: How a physical activity recommendation came to be among dietary recommendations. *American Journal of Clinical Nutrition* 79(Suppl.): 921S-930S.

Brose, A., Parise, G., and Tarnopolsky, M.A. 2003. Creatine supplementation enhances isometric strength and body composition improvements following strength exercise training in older adults. *Journals of Gerontology, Series A: Biological Sciences and Medical Sciences* 58: 11-19.

Brouha, L. 1943. The step test: A simple method of measuring physical fitness for muscular work in young men. *Research Quarterly* 14: 31-36.

Brown, D.A., and Miller, W.C. 1998. Normative data for strength and flexibility of women throughout life. *European Journal of Applied Physiology* 78: 77-82.

Brown, G.A., Cook, C.M., Krueger, R.D., and Heelan, K.A. 2010. Comparison of energy expenditure on a treadmill vs. an elliptical device at a self-selected exercise intensity. *Journal of Strength and Conditioning Research* 24: 1643-1649.

Brozek, J., Grande, F., Anderson, J.T., and Keys, A. 1963. Densiometric analysis of body composition: Revision of some quantitative assumptions. *Annals of the New York Academy of Sciences* 110: 113-140.

Bruce, R.A., Kusumi, F., and Hosmer, D. 1973. Maximal oxygen intake and nomographic assessment of functional aerobic impairment in cardiovascular disease. *American Heart Journal* 85: 546-562.

Brzycki, M. 1993. Strength testing—predicting a one-rep max from reps-to-fatigue. *Journal of Physical Education, Recreation and Dance* 64 (1): 88-90.

Brzycki, M. 2000. Assessing strength. *Fitness Management* 16(7): 34-37.

Buch, A., Kis, O., Carmeli, E., Keinan-Boker, L., Berner, Y., Barer, Y., Shefer, G., Marcus, Y., and Stern, N. 2017. Circuit resistance training is an effective means to enhance muscle strength in older and middle aged adults: A systematic review and meta-analysis. *Ageing Research Reviews* 37: 16-27.

Buckthorpe, M., Morris, J., and Folland, J.P. 2012. Validity of vertical jump measurement devices. *Journal of Sports Sciences* 30: 63-69.

Bunt, J.C., Lohman, T.G., and Boileau, R.A. 1989. Impact of total body water fluctuations on estimation of body fat from body density. *Medicine & Science in Sports & Exercise* 21: 96-100.

Buresh, R., and Berg, K. 2002. Scaling oxygen uptake to body size and several practical applications. *Journal of Strength and Conditioning Research* 16: 461-465.

Burns, R.D., Hannon, J.C., Brusseau, T.A., Eisenman, P.A., Shultz, B.B., Saint-Maurice, P.F., Welk, G.J., and Mahar, M.T. 2016. Development of an aerobic capacity prediction model from one-mile run/walk performance in adolescents aged 13-15 years. *Journal of Sports Sciences* 34: 18-26.

Bushman, B., ed. 2011. *Complete guide to fitness & health*. Champaign, IL: Human Kinetics.

Bushman, B. 2012. Neuromotor exercise training. *ACSM's Health & Fitness Journal* 16(6): 4-7.

Byrne, J.M., Bishop, N.S., Caines, A.M., Crane, K.A., Feaver, A.M., and Pearcey, G.E.P. 2014. Effect of using a suspension training system on muscle activation during the performance of a front plank. *Journal of Strength and Conditioning Research* 28: 3049-3055.

Byrnes, W.C., Clarkson, P.M., and Katch, F.I. 1985. Muscle soreness following resistive exercise with and without eccentric contraction. *Research Quarterly for Exercise and Sport* 56: 283-285.

Cable, A., Nieman, D.C., Austin, M., Hogen, E., and Utter, A.C. 2001. Validity of leg-to-leg bioelectrical impedance measurement in males. *Journal of Sports Medicine and Physical Fitness* 41: 411-414.

Cadore, E.L., González-Izal, M., Pallarés, J.G., Rodriguez-Falces, J., Häkkinen, K., Kraemer, W.J., Pinto, R.S., and Izquierdo, M. 2014. Muscle conduction velocity, strength, neural activity, and morphological changes after eccentric and concentric training. *Scandinavian Journal of Medicine and Science in Sports* 24(5): e343-e352.

Cadore, E.L., Rodriguez-Manas, L., Sinclair, A., and Izquierdo, M. 2013. Effects of different exercise interventions on risk of falls, gait ability, and balance in physically frail older adults: A systematic review. *Rejuvenation Research* 16: 105-114.

Callaway, C.W., Chumlea, W.C., Bouchard, C., Himes, J.H., Lohman, T.G., Martin, A.D., Mitchell, C.D., Mueller, W.H., Roche, A.F., and Seefeldt, V.D. 1988. Circumferences. In *Anthropometric standardization reference manual*, ed. T.G. Lohman, A.F. Roche, and R. Martorell, 39-54. Champaign, IL: Human Kinetics.

Camhi, S.M., Bray, G.A., Bouchard, C., Greenway, F.L., Johnson, W.D., Newton, R.I., Ravussin, E., Ryan, D.H., Smith, S.R., and Katzmarzyk, P.T. 2011. The relationship of waist circumference and BMI to visceral, subcutaneous, and total body fat: Sex and race differences. *Obesity* 19: 402-408.

Campbell, N.R.C., Gelfer, M., Stergiou, G.S., Alpert, B.S., Myers, M.G., Rakotz, M.K., Padwal, R., Schutte, A.E., O'Brien, E., Lackland, D.T., Niebylski, M.L., Nilsoson, P.M., Redburn, K.A., Zhang, X-H., Prabhakaran, D., Ramirez, A.J., Schiffrin, E.L., Touyz, R.M., Wang, J-G., and Weber, M.A. 2016. A call to regulate manufacture and marketing of blood pressure devices and cuffs: A position statement from the World Hypertension League, International Society of Hypertension and supporting hypertension organizations. *Journal of Clinical Hypertension* 18: 378-379.

Canadian Society for Exercise Physiology. 2013. *Physical activity training for health (CSEP-PATH) resource manual.* Ottawa, ON: Author.

Candow, D.G., Chilibeck, P.D., Abeysekara, S., and Zello, G.A. 2011. Short-term heavy resistance training eliminates age-related deficits in muscle mass and strength in healthy older males. *Journal of Strength and Conditioning Research* 25: 326-333.

Cao, C., Liu, Y., Zhu, W., and Ma, J. 2016. Effect of active workstation on energy expenditure and job performance: A systematic review and meta-analysis. *Journal of Physical Activity and Health* 13: 562-571.

Cardinal, B.J., Park, E.A., Kim, M.S., and Cardinal, M.K. 2015. If exercise is medicine, where is exercise in medicine? Review of U.S. medical education curricula for physical-activity-related content. *Journal of Physical Activity and Health* 12: 1336-1342.

Carey, M.A., Laird, D.E., Murray, K.A., and Stevenson, J.R. 2010. Reliability, validity, and clinical usability of a digital goniometer. *Work* 36: 55-66.

Carneiro, N.H., Ribeiro, A.S., Nascimento, M.A., Gobbo, L.A., Schoenfeld, B.J., Achour Júnior, A., Gobbi, S., Oliveira, A.R., and Cyrino, E. 2015. Effects of different resistance training frequencies on flexibility in older women. *Clinical Interventions in Aging* 10: 531-538.

Carns, M.L., Schade, M.L., Liba, M.R., Hellebrandt, F.A., and Harris, C.W. 1960. Segmental volume reduction by localized and generalized exercise. *Human Biology* 32: 370-376.

Carpenter, D.M., and Nelson, B.W. 1999. Low back strengthening for the prevention and treatment of low back pain. *Medicine & Science in Sports & Exercise* 31: 18-24.

Carrick-Ranson, G., Hastings, J.L., Bhella, P.S., Shibata, S., Fujimoto, N., Palmer, D., Boyd, K., and Levine, B.D. 2012. The effect of age-related differences in body size and composition on cardiovascular determinants of $\dot{V}O_2$ max. *Journal of Gerontology.* doi:10.1093/gerona/gls220. Accessed December 18, 2012.

Carroll, T.J., Barton, J., Hsu, M., and Lee, M. 2009. The effect of strength training on the force of twitches evoked by corticospinal stimulation in humans. *Acta Physiologica* 197: 161-173.

Carter, B.D., Abnet, C.C., Feskanich, D., Freedman, N.D., Hartge, P., Lewis, C.E., Ockene, J.K., Prentice, R.L., Speizer, F.E. Thun, M.J., and Jacobs, E.J. 2015. Smoking and mortality: Beyond established causes. *New England Journal of Medicine* 372: 631-640.

Carter, N.D., Kannus, P., and Khan, K.M. 2001. Exercise in the prevention of falls in older people. A systematic literature review examining the rationale and the evidence. *Sports Medicine* 31: 427-438.

Carter, S., Hartman, Y., Holder, S., Thijssen, D.H., and Hopkins, N.D. 2017. Sedentary behavior and cardiovascular disease risk: Mediating mechanisms. *Exercise and Sports Sciences Reviews* 45: 80-86.

Casanova, C., Ceili, B.R., Barria, P., Casas, A., Cote, C., de Torres, J.P., Jardim, J., Lopez, M.V., Marin, J.M., Montes de Oca, M., Pinto-Plata, V., and Aguirre-Jaime, A. 2011. The 6 min walk distance in healthy subjects: Reference standards from seven countries. *European Respiratory Journal* 37: 150-156.

Casartelli, N., Muller, R., and Maffiuletti, N.A. 2010. Validity and reliability of the Myotest accelerometric system for the assessment of vertical jump height. *Journal of Strength and Conditioning Research* 24: 3186-3193.

Casiglia, E., Tikhonoff, V., Albertini, F., and Palatini, P. 2016. Poor reliability of wrist blood pressure self-measurement at home: A population-based study. *Hypertension.* doi:10.1161/HYPERTENSION AHA.116.07961. Accessed May 2, 2017.

Cataldo, D., and Heyward, V. 2000. Pinch an inch: A comparison of several high-quality and plastic skinfold calipers. *ACSM's Health & Fitness Journal* 4(3): 12-16.

Catenacci, V.A., Grunwald, G.K., Ingebrigtsen, J.P., Jakicic, J.M., McDermott, M.D., Phelan, S., Wing, R.R., Hill, J.O., and Wyatt, H.R. 2011. Physical activity patterns using accelerometry in the National Weight Control Registry. *Obesity* 19(6): 1163-1170.

Catley, M.J., and Tomkinson, G.R. 2013. Normative health-related fitness values for children: Analysis of 85347 test results on 9-17-year-old Australians since 1985. *British Journal of Sports Medicine* 47: 98-108.

Caton, J.R., Mole, P.A., Adams, W.C., and Heustis, D.S. 1988. Body composition analysis by bioelectrical impedance: Effect of skin temperature. *Medicine & Science in Sports & Exercise* 20: 489-491.

Cavallo, D.N., Tate, D.F., Ries, A.V., Brown, J.D., DeVellis, R.F., and Ammerman, A.S. 2012. A social media-based physical activity intervention: A randomized controlled trial. *American Journal of Preventive Medicine* 43: 527-532.

Cayir, Y., Menekse, S., and Akturk, Z. 2015. The effect of pedometer use on physical activity and body weight in obese women. *European Journal of Sport Science* 15: 351-356.

Centers for Disease Control and Prevention. 2013. National Health and Nutrition Examination Survey (NHANES): Body composition procedures manual. www.cdc.gov/nchs/data/nhanes/nhanes_13_14/2013_Body_Composition_DXA.pdf. Accessed August 6, 2017.

Centers for Disease Control and Prevention. 2014. National diabetes statistics report, 2014. www.cdc.gov/diabetes/pdfs/data/2014-report-estimates-of-diabetes-and-its-burden-in-the-united-states.pdf. Accessed April 9, 2017.

Centers for Disease Control and Prevention. 2015a. Heart disease facts. www.cdc.gov/heartdisease/facts.htm. Accessed April 2, 2017.

Centers for Disease Control and Prevention. 2015b. *Health, United States, 2015.* www.cdc.gov/nchs/hus/contents2015.htm#057. Accessed August 9, 2016.

Centers for Disease Control and Prevention. 2016. High Blood Pressure Facts. www.cdc.gov/bloodpressure/facts.htm. Accessed April 2, 2017.

Chalmers, G. 2004. Re-examination of the possible role of Golgi tendon organ and muscle spindle reflexes in proprioceptive neuromuscular facilitation muscle stretching. *Sports Biomechanics* 3: 159-183.

Chamberlin, B., and Gallagher, R. 2008. Exergames: Using video games to promote physical activity. Paper presented at Children, Youth and Families at Risk (CYFAR) Conference, San Antonio, TX.

Chandler, J.M., Duncan, P.W., and Studenski, S.A. 1990. Balance performance on the postural stress test: Comparison of young adults, healthy elderly, and fallers. *Physical Therapy* 70: 410-415.

Chapman, E.A., deVries, H.A., and Swezey, R. 1972. Joint stiffness: Effects of exercise on young and old men. *Journal of Gerontology* 27: 218-221.

Charlton, P.C., Mentiplay, B.F., Pua, Y-H., Clark, R.A. 2015. Reliability and concurrent validity of a smartphone, bubble inclinometer and motion analysis system for measurement of hip joint range of motion. *Journal of Science and Medicine in Sport* 18: 262-267.

Charro, M.A., Aoki, M.S., Coutts, A.J., Araujo, R.C., and Bacurau, R.F. 2010. Hormonal, metabolic and perceptual responses to different resistance training systems. *Journal of Sports Medicine and Physical Fitness* 50: 229-234.

Chen, C-H., Chen, T.C., Jan, M-H., and Lin, J-J. 2015. Acute effects of static active or dynamic active stretching on eccentric-exercise-induced hamstring muscle damage. *International Journal of Sports Physiology and Performance* 10: 346-352.

Chen, C., Nosaka, K., Chen, H., Lin, M., Tseng, K., and Chen, T.C. 2011. Effects of flexibility training on eccentric exercise-induced muscle damage. *Medicine & Science in Sports & Exercise* 43: 491-500.

Chen, G., Doumatey, A.P., Zhou, J., Lei, L., Bentley, A.B. Tekola-Ayele, F., Adebamowo, S.N., Baker, J.L., Fasanmade, O., Okafor, G., Eghan, B. Jr., Agyenum-Boateng, K., Amoult, A., Adebamowo, C., Acheampong, J., Johnson, T., Oli, J., Shriner, D., Adeyemo, A.A., and Rotimi, C.N. 2017. Genome-wide analysis identifies an African-specific variant in SEMA4D associated with body mass index. *Obesity* 25: 794-800.

Chen, Y-L., Chiou, W-K, Tzeng, Y-T., Lu, C-Y., and Chen, S-C. 2017. A rating of perceived exertion scale using facial expressions for conveying exercise intensity for children and young adults. *Journal of Science and Medicine in Sport* 20: 66-69.

Cherkas, L.F., Hunkin, J.L., Kato, B.S., Richards, J.B., Gardner, J.P., Surdulescu, G.L., Kimura, M., Lu, X., Spector, T.D., and Aviv, A. 2008. The association between physical activity in leisure time and leukocyte telomere length. *Archives of Internal Medicine* 168(2): 154-158.

Cheung, A.M., and Giangregorio, L. 2012. Mechanical stimuli and bone health: What is the evidence? *Current Opinions in Rheumatology* 24: 561-566.

Cheung, A.S., de Rooy, C., Hoermann, R., Gianatti, E.J., Hamilton, E.J., Roff, G., Zajac, J.D., and Grossmann, M. 2016. Correlation of visceral adipose tissue measured by Lunar Prodigy dual X-ray absorptiometry with MRI and CT in older men. *International Journal of Obesity* 40(8): 1325-1328.

Chidnok, W., DiMenna, F.J., Bailey, S.J., Burnley, M., Wilderson, D.P., and Vanhatalo, A. 2013. V̇O₂max is not altered by self-pacing during incremental exercise. *European Journal of Applied Physiology* 113: 529-539.

Chillon, P., Castro-Pinero, J., Ruiz, J.R., Soto, V.M., Carbonell-Baeza, A., Dafos, J., Vincente-Rodriguez, G., Castillo, M.J., and Ortega, F.B. 2010. Hip flexibility is the main determinant of the back-saver sit-and-reach test in adolescents. *Journal of Sport Sciences* 28: 641-648.

Cho, G-H., Rodriguez, D.A., and Evenson, K.R. 2011. Identifying walking trips using GPS data. *Medicine & Science in Sports & Exercise* 43: 365-372.

Cho, K., Tian, M., Lan, Y., Zhao, X., and Yan, L.L. 2013. Validation of the Omron HEM-7201 upper arm blood pressure monitor, for self-measurement in a high-altitude environment, according to the European Society of Hypertension International Protocol revision 2010. *Journal of Human Hypertension* 27: 487-491.

Chodzko-Zajko, W.J., Proctor, D.N., Fiatarone, S., Maria, A., Minson, C.T., Nigg, C.R., Claudio, R., Salem, G.J., and Skinner, J.S. 2009. Exercise and physical activity for older adults. ACSM position stand. *Medicine & Science in Sports & Exercise* 41: 1510-1530.

Christie, A., and Kamen, G. 2014. Cortical inhibition is reduced following short-term training in young and older adults. *Age* 36(2): 749-758.

Churchward-Venne, T.A., Murphy, C.H., Longland, T.M., and Phillips, S.M. 2013. Role of protein and amino acids in promoting lean mass accretion with resistance exercise and attenuating lean mass loss during energy deficit in humans. *Amino Acids* 45: 231-240.

Cipriani, D., Abel, B., and Pirrwitz, D. 2003. A comparison of two stretching protocols on hip range of motion: Implications for total daily stretch duration. *Journal of Strength and Conditioning Research* 17: 274-278.

Clark, B.C., and Manini, T.M. 2008. Sarcopenia ≠ dynapenia. *Journal of Gerontology* 63A: 829-834.

Clark, R.A., Bryant, A.L., Pua, Y., McCrory, P., Bennell, K., and Hunt, M. 2010. Validity and reliability of the Nintendo Wii balance board for assessment of standing balance. *Gait & Posture* 31: 307-310.

Clark, S., Iltis, P.W., Anthony, C.J., and Toews, A. 2005. Comparison of older adult performance during the functional-reach and limits-of-stability tests. *Journal of Aging and Physical Activity* 13: 266-275.

Clark, S., Rose, D.J., and Fujimoto, K. 1997. Generalizability of the limits of stability test in the evaluation of dynamic balance among older adults. *Archives of Physical Medicine and Rehabilitation* 78: 1078-1084.

Clarkson, P.M., Byrnes, W.C., McCormick, K.M., Turcotte, L.P., and White, J.S. 1986. Muscle soreness and serum creatine kinase activity following isometric, eccentric and concentric exercise. *International Journal of Sports Medicine* 7: 152-155.

Clarys, J.P., Martin, A.D., Drinkwater, D.T., and Marfell-Jones, M.J. 1987. The skinfold: Myth and reality. *Journal of Sports Sciences* 5: 3-33.

Cleary, M.A., Hetzler, R.K., Wages, J.J., Lentz, M.A., Stickley, C.D., and Kimura, I.F. 2011. Comparisons of age-predicted maximum heart rate equations in college-aged subjects. *Journal of Strength and Conditioning Research* 25: 2591-2597.

Clemons, J.M., Duncan, C.A., Blanchard, O.E., Gatch, W.H., Hollander, D.B., and Doucer, J.L. 2004. Relationships between the flexed-arm hang and select measures of muscular fitness. *Journal of Strength and Conditioning Research* 18: 630-636.

Clinical Exercise Physiology Association. 2013. State Updates. https://www.acsm-cepa.org/i4a/pages/index.cfm?pageid=3339. Accessed May 5, 2017.

Cloutier, L., Daskalopoulou, S.S., Padwal, R.S., Lamarre-Cliché, M., Bolli, P., McLean, D., Milot, A., Tobe, S.W., Tremblay, G., McKay, D.W., Townsend, R., Campbell, N., and Gelfer, M. 2015. A new algorithm for the diagnosis of hypertension in Canada. *Canadian Journal Cardiology* 31: 620-630.

Cobb, N.K., and Graham, A.L. 2012. Health behavior interventions in the age of Facebook. *American Journal of Preventive Medicine* 43: 571-572.

Cochrane, D. 2013. The sports performance application of vibration exercise for warm-up, flexibility and sprint speed. *European Journal of Sport Science* 13: 256-271.

Cohen, A. 2004. It's getting personal. *Athletic Business* July: 52-54, 56, 58, 60.

Cohen, A., Baker, J., and Ardern, C.I. 2016. Association between body mass index, physical activity, and health-related quality of life in Canadian adults. *Journal of Aging and Physical Activity.* 24: 32-38.

Colberg, S.R., Rubin, R.R., Sigal, R.J., Chasa-Taber, L., Fernall, B., Albright, A.L., Regensteiner, J.G., Braun, B., and Blissmer, B.J. 2010. Exercise and type 2 diabetes. *Diabetes Care.* 33: 2692-2696.

Cole, T.J., Bellizzi, M.C., Flegal, K.M., and Dietz, W.H. 2000. Establishing a standard definition for child overweight and obesity worldwide: International survey. *British Medical Journal* 320: 1240-1245.

Collins, M., Millard-Stafford, M., Sparling, P., Snow, T., Rosskopf, L., Webb, S., and Omer, J. 1999. Evaluation of the Bod Pod for assessing body fat in collegiate football players. *Medicine & Science in Sports & Exercise* 31: 1350-1356.

Collora, C. 2017. Exercise physiologist: Career overview. www.exercise-science-guide.com/careers/exercise-physiologist. Accessed May 5, 2017.

Comstock, B.A., Solomon-Hill, G., Flanagan, S.D., Earp, J.E., Luk, H.Y., Dobbins, K.A., Dunn-Lewis, C., Fragala, M.S., Ho, J.Y., Hatfield, D.L., Vingren, J.L., Denegar, C.R., Volek, J.S., Kupchak, B.R., Maresh, C.M., and Kraemer, W.J. 2011. Validity of the Myotest in measuring force and power production in the squat and bench press. *Journal of Strength and Conditioning Research* 25: 2293-2297.

Conley, D., Cureton, K., Dengel, D., and Weyand, P. 1991. Validation of the 12-min swim as a field test of peak aerobic power in young men. *Medicine & Science in Sports & Exercise* 23: 766-773.

Conley, D., Cureton, K., Hinson, B., Higbie, E., and Weyand, P. 1992. Validation of the 12-minute swim as a field test of peak aerobic power in young women. *Research Quarterly for Exercise and Sport* 63: 153-161.

Conlon, J.A., Newton, R.U., Tufano, J.J., Banyard, H.G., Hopper, A.J., Ridge, A.J., and Haff, G.G. 2016. Periodization strategies in older adults: Impact on physical function and health. *Medicine & Science in Sports & Exercise* 48: 2426-2436.

Conroy, R.M., Pyörälä, K., Fitzgerald, A.P., Sans, S., Menotti, A., DeBacker, G., DeBacquer, D., Ducimetière, P., Jousilahti, P., Keil, U., Njølstad, I., Oganov, R.G., Thomsen, T., Turnstall-Pedoe, H., Tverdal, A., Wedel, H., Whincup, P., Wilhelmsen, L., and Graham, I.M., on behalf of the SCORE project group. 2003. Estimation of ten-year risk of fatal cardiovascular disease in Europe: The SCORE project. *European Heart Journal* 24: 987-1003.

Coombes, J.S., Law, J., Lancashire, B., and Fassett, R.G. 2015. "Exercise is medicine": Curbing the burden of chronic disease and physical inactivity. *Asia-Pacific Journal of Public Health* 27: NP600-NP605.

Cooper Institute for Aerobics Research. 1992. *The Prudential FitnessGram test administration manual.* Dallas: Author.

Cooper Institute for Aerobics Research. 1994. *FitnessGram user's manual.* Dallas: Author.

Cooper Institute for Aerobics Research. 2005. *The fitness specialist certification manual.* Dallas: Author.

Cooper, K.H. 1968. A means of assessing maximal oxygen intake. *Journal of the American Medical Association* 203: 201-204.

Cooper, K.H. 1977. *The aerobics way.* New York: Evans.

Cooper, R., Naclerio, F., Allgrove, J., and Jimenez, A. 2012. Creatine supplementation with specific view to exercise/sports performance: An update. *Journal of the International Society of Sports Nutrition* 9: article 33.

Coquart, J., Tabben, M., Farooq, A., Tourney, C., and Eston, R. 2016. Submaximal, perceptually regulated exercise testing predicts maximal oxygen uptake: A meta-analysis study. *Sports Medicine* 46: 885-897.

Corbin, C.B., Dowell, L.J., Lindsey, R., and Tolson, H. 1978. *Concepts in physical education.* Dubuque, IA: Brown.

Costa, P.B., Graves, B.S., Whitehurst, M., and Jacobs, P.L. 2009. The acute effects of different durations of static stretching on dynamic balance performance. *Journal of Strength and Conditioning Research* 23: 141-147.

Costill, D.L., Coyle, E.F., Fink, W.F., Lesmes, G.R., and Witzmann, F.A. 1979. Adaptations in skeletal muscle following strength training. *Journal of Applied Physiology* 46: 96-99.

Costill, D.L., and Fox, E.L. 1969. Energetics of marathon running. *Medicine and Science in Sports* 1: 81-86.

Costill, D.L., Thomason, H., and Roberts, E. 1973. Fractional utilization of the aerobic capacity during distance running. *Medicine and Science in Sports* 5: 248-252.

Cote, D.K., and Adams, W.C. 1993. Effect of bone density on body composition estimates in young adult black and white women. *Medicine & Science in Sports & Exercise* 25: 290-296.

Cotten, D.J. 1971. A modified step test for group cardiovascular testing. *Research Quarterly* 42: 91-95.

Cotten, D.J. 1972. A comparison of selected trunk flexibility tests. *American Corrective Therapy Journal* 26: 24.

Coughlan, G.F., Fullam, K., Delahunt, E., Gissane, C., and Caulfield, B.M. 2012. A comparison between performance on selected directions of the star excursion balance test and the Y balance test. *Journal of Athletic Training* 47: 366-371.

Cowell, J.F., Cronin, J., and Brughelli, M. 2012. Eccentric muscle actions and how the strength and conditioning specialist might use them for a variety of purposes. *Strength and Conditioning Journal* 34: 33-48.

Coyle, E.F. 1995. Fat metabolism during exercise. *Sports Science Exchange* 8(6).

Coyle, E.F., Feiring, D.C., Rotkis, T.C., Cote, R.W. III, Roby, F.B., Lee, W., and Wilmore, J.H. 1981. Specificity of power improvements through slow and fast isokinetic training. *Journal of Applied Physiology* 51: 1437-1442.

Crandall, C.J., Hovey, K.M., Cauley, J.A., Andrews, C.A., Curtis, J.R., Wactawski-Wende, J., Wright, N.C., Li, W., and LeBoff, M.S. 2015. Wrist fracture and risk of subsequent fracture: Findings from the Women's Health Initiative Study. *Journal of Bone and Mineral Research* 11: 2086-2095.

Crandall, K.J., Zagdsuren, B., Schafer, M.A., and Lyons, T.S. 2016. Static and active workstations for improving workplace physical activity and sitting time. *International Journal of Human Movement and Sports Sciences* 4: 20-25.

Crewther, B.T., Kilduff, L.P., Cunningham, D.J., Cook, C., Owen, N., and Yang, G.Z. 2011. Validating two systems for estimating force and power. *International Journal of Sports Medicine* 32: 254-258.

Cribb, P.J., Williams, A.D., and Hayes, A. 2007. A creatine-carbohydrate supplement enhances responses to resistance training. *Medicine & Science in Sports & Exercise* 39: 1960-1968.

Cribb, P.J., Williams, A.D., Hayes, A., and Carey, M.F. 2006. The effect of whey isolate on strength, body composition, and plasma glutamine. *International Journal of Sports Nutrition and Exercise Metabolism* 16: 494-509.

Cribb, P.J., Williams, A.D., Stathis, C.G., Carey, M.F., and Hayes, A. 2007. Effect of whey isolate, creatine, and resistance training on muscle hypertrophy. *Medicine & Science in Sports & Exercise* 39: 298-307.

Critoph, C.H., Patel, V., Mist, B., Thomas, M.D., and Elliott, P.M. 2013. Non-invasive assessment of cardiac output at rest and during exercise by finger plethysmography. *Clinical Physiology and Functional Imaging* 33: 338-343.

Crommett, A., Kravitz, L., Wongsathikun, J., and Kemerly, T. 1999. Comparison of metabolic and subjective response of three modalities in college-age subjects. *Medicine & Science in Sports & Exercise* 31(Suppl.): S158 [abstract].

Crook, T.A., Armbya, N., Cleves, M.A., Badger, T.M., and Andres, A. 2012. Air displacement plethysmography, dual-energy X-ray absorptiometry, and total body water to evaluate body composition in preschool-age children. *Journal of the Academy of Nutrition and Dietetics* 112: 1993-1998.

Cug, M. 2017. Stance foot alignment and hand positioning alter star excursion balance test scores in those with chronic ankle instability: What are we really assessing? *Physiotherapy Theory and Practice* 33: 316-322.

Cullinen, K., and Caldwell, M. 1998. Weight training increases fat-free mass and strength in untrained young women. *Journal of the American Dietetic Association* 98(4): 414-418.

Curb, J.D., Ceria-Ulep, C.D., Rodriquez, B.L., Grove, J., Guralnik, J., Willcox, B.J., Donlon, T.A., Masaki, K.H., and Chen, R. 2006. Performance-based measures of physical function for high-function populations. *Journal of the American Geriatrics Society* 54: 737-742.

Cureton, K.J., Collins, M.A., Hill, D.W., and McElhannon, F.M. Jr. 1988. Muscle hypertrophy in men and women. *Medicine & Science in Sports & Exercise* 20: 338-344.

Cureton, K.J., Sloniger, M., O'Bannon, J., Black, D., and McCormack, W. 1995. A generalized equation for prediction of $\dot{V}O_2$peak from 1-mile run/walk performance. *Medicine & Science in Sports & Exercise* 27: 445-451.

Cureton, K.J., Sparling, P.B., Evans, B.W., Johnson, S.M., Kong, U.D., and Purvis, J.W. 1978. Effect of experimental alterations in excess weight on aerobic capacity and distance running performance. *Medicine and Science in Sports* 10: 194-199.

Cureton, T.K., and Sterling, L.F. 1964. Interpretation of the cardiovascular component resulting from the factor analysis of 104 test variables measured in 100 normal young men. *Journal of Sports Medicine and Physical Fitness* 4: 1-24.

Cuthbertson, D.J., Steele, T., Wilding, J.P., Halford, J.C., Harrold, J.A., Hamer, M., and Karpe, F. 2017. What have human experimental overfeeding studies taught us about adipose tissue expansion and susceptibility to obesity and metabolic complications? *International Journal of Obesity* 41: 853-865.

Cyrino, E.S., Okano, A.H., Glaner, M.F., Ramanzini, M., Gobbo, A., Makoski, A., Bruna, N., Cordeiro de Melo, J., and Tassi, G.N. 2003. Impact of the use of different skinfold calipers for the analysis of the body composition. *Revista Brasileira de Medicina do Esporte* 9: 150-153.

dabl® Educational Trust. 2017. Classification of sphygmomanometers. www.dableducational.org/sphygmomanometers.html. Accessed April 29, 2017.

da Silva, D.F., Bianchini, J.A.A., Lopera, C.A., Capelato, D.A., Hintze, L.J., Narido, C.C.S., Ferraro, Z.M., and Junior, N.N. 2015. Impact of readiness to change behavior on the effects of a multidisciplinary intervention in obese Brazilian children and adolescents. *Appetite* 87: 229-235.

Dalleck, L.C., Kravitz, L., and Roberts, R.A. 2006. Development of a submaximal test to predict elliptical cross-trainer $\dot{V}O_2$max. *Journal of Strength and Conditioning Research* 20: 278-283.

Dalleck, L.C., Roos, K.A., Byrd, B.R., and Weatherwax, R.M. 2015. Zumba Gold®: Are the physiological responses sufficient to improve fitness in middle-age to older adults? *Journal of Sports Science and Medicine* 14: 689-690.

Daly, R.M. 2017. Exercise and nutritional approaches to prevent frail bones, falls and fractures: An update. *Climacteric* 20: 119-124.

Danaei, G., Finucane, M.M., Lu, Y., Singh, G.M., Cowan, M.J., Paciorek, C.J., Lin, J.K, Farzadfar, F., Khang, Y-H., Stevens, G.A., Rao, M., Ali, M.K., Riley, L.M., Robinson, C.A., and Ezzati, M. 2011. National, regional, and global trends in fasting plasma glucose and diabetes prevalence since 1980: Systematic analysis of health examination surveys and epidemiological studies with 370 country-years and 2.7 million participants. *Lancet* 378: 31-40.

Davin, J., and Callaghan, M. 2016. BET2: Core stability versus conventional exercise for treating non-specific low back pain. *Emergency Medicine Journal* 33: 162-163.

Davis, D.S., Quinn, R.O., Whiteman, C.T., Williams, J.D., and Young, C.R. 2008. Concurrent validity of four clinical tests to measure hamstring flexibility. *Journal of Strength and Conditioning Research* 22: 583-588.

Davis, J.A., Dorado, S., Keays, K.A., Reigel, R.A., Valencia, K.S., and Pham, P.H. 2007. Reliability and validity of the lung volume measurement made by the Bod Pod body composition system. *Clinical Physiology and Functional Imaging* 27: 42-46.

Dawes, J. 2017. *Complete guide to TRX suspension training.* Champaign, IL: Human Kinetics.

Day, J.R., Rossiter, H.B., Coats, E.M., Skasick, A., and Whipp, B.J. 2003. The maximally attainable $\dot{V}O_2$ during exercise in humans: The peak vs. maximum issue. *Journal of Applied Physiology* 95: 1901-1907.

de Bruin, E.D., Swanenburg, J., Betschon, E., and Murer, K. 2009. A randomized controlled trial investigating motor skill training as a function of attentional focus in old age. *BMC Geriatrics* 9: 15-24.

Deci, E.L., and Ryan, R.M. 2000. The "what" and "why" of goal pursuits: Human needs and the self-determination of behavior. *Psychological Inquiry* 11(4): 227-268.

deJong, A. 2010. Active video gaming: An opportunity to increase energy expenditure throughout aging. *ACSM's Health & Fitness Journal* 14: 44-46.

del Consuelo Velazquez-Alva, M., Irogyen-Camacho, M.E., Huerta-Huerta, R., and Delgadillo-Velazquez, J. 2014. A comparison of dual energy X-ray absorptiometry and two bioelectrical impedance analyzers to measure body fat percentage and fat-free mass index in a group of Mexican young women. *Nutrición Hospitalaria* 29: 1038-1046.

Delecluse, C., Roelants, M., and Verschueren, S. 2003. Strength increase after whole-body vibration compared with resistance training. *Medicine & Science in Sports & Exercise* 35: 1033-1041.

Demerath, E.W., Guo, S.S., Chumlea, W.C., Towne, B., Roche, A.F., and Siervogel, R.M. 2002. Comparison of percent body fat estimates using air displacement plethysmography and hydrodensitometry in adults and children. *International Journal of Obesity and Related Metabolic Disorders* 26: 389-397.

de Melo dos Santos, R., Costa e Costa, F., Saraiva, T.S., Maniglia de Resende, M., Carvalho, N.C.S., Beda, A., and Callegari, B. 2015. Short-term adaptations in sedentary individuals during indoor cycling classes. *Archives of Sports Medicine* 32: 374-381.

Demont, R.G., Lephart, S.M., Giraldo, J.L., Giannantonio, F.P., Yuktanandana, P., and Fu, F.H. 1999. Comparison of two abdominal training devices with an abdominal crunch using strength and EMG measurements. *Journal of Sports Medicine and Physical Fitness* 39: 253-258.

Dempster, P., and Aitkens, S. 1995. A new air displacement method for the determination of human body composition. *Medicine & Science in Sports & Exercise* 27: 1692-1697.

Demura, S., Yamaji, S., Goshi, F., Kobayashi, H., Sato, S., and Nagasawa, Y. 2002. The validity and reliability of relative body fat estimates and the construction of new prediction equations for young Japanese adult males. *Journal of Sports Sciences* 20: 153-164.

Deschenes, M.R., and Kraemer, W.J. 2002. Performance and physiologic adaptations to resistance training. *American Journal of Physical Medicine and Rehabilitation* 8(Suppl.): S3-S16.

Desgorces, F.D., Berthelot, G., Dietrich, G., and Testa, M.S.A. 2010. Local muscular endurance and prediction of 1 repetition maximum for bench in 4 athletic populations. *Journal of Strength and Conditioning Research* 24: 394-400.

Despres, J.P., and Lamarche, B. 1994. Low-intensity endurance training, plasma lipoproteins, and the risk of coronary heart disease. *Journal of Internal Medicine* 236: 7-22.

Despres, J.P., Bouchard, C., Tremblay, A., Savard, R., and Marcotte, M. 1985. Effects of aerobic training on fat distribution in male subjects. *Medicine & Science in Sports & Exercise* 17: 113-118.

Deurenberg, P. 2001. Universal cut-off BMI points for obesity are not appropriate. *British Journal of Nutrition* 85: 135-136.

Deurenberg, P., and Deurenberg-Yap, M. 2001. Differences in body-composition assumptions across ethnic groups: Practical consequences. *Current Opinion in Clinical Nutrition and Metabolic Care* 4: 377-383.

Deurenberg, P., and Deurenberg-Yap, M. 2002. Validation of skinfold thickness and hand-held impedance measurements for estimation of body fat percentage among Singaporean Chinese, Malay and Indian subjects. *Asia Pacific Journal of Clinical Nutrition* 11: 1-7.

Deurenberg, P., van der Kooy, K., Evers, P., and Hulshof, T. 1990. Assessment of body composition by bioelectrical impedance in a population aged >60 y. *American Journal of Clinical Nutrition* 51: 3-6.

Deurenberg, P., van der Kooy, K., and Leenan, R. 1989. Differences in body impedance when measured with different instruments. *European Journal of Clinical Nutrition* 43: 885-886.

Deurenberg, P., Weststrate, J.A., Paymans, I., and van der Kooy, K. 1988. Factors affecting bioelectrical impedance measurements in humans. *European Journal of Clinical Nutrition* 42: 1017-1022.

Deurenberg, P., Yap, M., and van Staveren, W.A. 1998. Body mass index and percent body fat: A meta analysis among different ethnic groups. *International Journal of Obesity* 22: 1164-1171.

Deurenberg-Yap, M., Schmidt, G., van Staveren, W.A., Hautvast, J.G.A.J., and Deurenberg, P. 2001. Body fat measurement among Singaporean Chinese, Malays and Indians: A comparative study using a four-compartment model and different two-compartment models. *British Journal of Nutrition* 85: 491-498.

deVries, H.A. 1961. Prevention of muscular distress after exercise. *Research Quarterly* 32: 177-185.

deVries, H.A. 1962. Evaluation of static stretching procedures for improvement of flexibility. *Research Quarterly* 33: 222-229.

deVries, H.A., and Klafs, C.E. 1965. Prediction of maximal oxygen intake from submaximal tests. *Journal of Sports Medicine and Physical Fitness* 5: 207-214.

de Vries, R.A.J., Truong, K.P., Swint, S., Drossaert, C.H.C., and Evers, V. 2016. Crowd-designed motivation: Motivational messages for exercise adherence based on behavior change theory. *Persuasive Technology*. doi:10.1007/978-3-319-31510-2_4. Accessed May 3, 2017.

deWeijer, V.C., Gorniak, G.C., and Shamus, E. 2003. The effect of static stretch and warm-up exercise on hamstring length over the course of 24 hours. *Journal of Orthopaedic and Sports Physical Therapy* 33: 727-733.

Dewit, O., Fuller, N.J., Fewtrell, M.S., Elia, M., and Wells, J.C.K. 2000. Whole body air displacement plethysmography compared with hydrodensitometry for body composition analysis. *Archives of Disease in Childhood* 82: 159-164.

Dickin, D.C. 2010. Obtaining reliable performance measures on the sensory organization test: Altered testing sequence in young adults. *Clinical Journal of Sport Medicine* 20: 278-285.

Dickin, D.C., and Clark, S. 2007. Generalizability of the sensory organization test in college-aged males: Obtaining a reliable performance measure. *Clinical Journal of Sport Medicine* 17: 109-115.

Dickinson, R.V. 1968. The specificity of flexibility. *Research Quarterly* 39: 792-793.

Disch, J., Frankiewicz, R., and Jackson, A. 1975. Construct validation of distance run tests. *Research Quarterly* 46: 169-176.

Dishman, R.K. 1994. Prescribing exercise intensity for healthy adults using perceived exertion. *Medicine & Science in Sports & Exercise* 26: 1087-1094.

Dishman, R.K., Jackson, A.S., and Bray, M.S. 2014. Self-regulation of exercise behavior in the TIGER Study. *Annals of Behavioral Medicine* 48: 80-91.

Dishman, R.K., Sallis, J.F., and Orenstein, D.R. 1985. The determinants of physical activity and exercise. *Public Health Reports* 100: 158-171.

Dolezal, B.A., and Potteiger, J.A. 1998. Concurrent resistance and endurance training influence basal metabolic rate in nondieting individuals. *Journal of Applied Physiology* 85: 695-700.

Domene, P.A., Moir, J.J., Pummell, E., and Easton, C. 2016. Salsa dance and Zumba fitness: Acute responses during community-based classes. *Journal of Sport and Health Science* 5: 190-196.

Donahue, B., Turner, D., and Worrell, T. 1994. The use of functional reach as a measurement of balance in boys and girls without disabilities ages 5 to 15 years. *Pediatric Physical Therapy* 6: 189-193.

Donahue, C.P., Lin, D.H., Kirschenbaum, D.S., and Keesey, R.E. 1984. Metabolic consequence of dieting and exercise in the treatment of obesity. *Journal of Counseling and Clinical Psychology* 52: 827-836.

Donath, L., Rossler, R., and Faude, O. 2016. Effects of virtual reality training (exergaming) compared to alternative exercise training and passive control on standing balance and functional mobility in healthy community-dwelling seniors: A meta-analytical review. *Sports Medicine* 46: 1293-1309.

Donath, L., Roth, R., Hürlimann, C., Zahner, L., and Faude, O. 2016. Pilates vs. balance training in healthy community-dwelling seniors: A 3-arm, randomized controlled trial. *International Journal of Sports Medicine* 37: 202-210.

Donnelly, J.R., Brown, T.E., Israel, R.G., Smith-Sintek, S., O'Brien, K.F., and Caslavka, B. 1988. Hydrostatic weighing without head submersion: Description of a method. *Medicine & Science in Sports & Exercise* 20: 66-69.

Dourado, V.Z., and McBurnie, M.A. 2012. Allometric scaling of 6 min walking distance by body mass as a standardized measure of exercise capacity. *European Journal of Applied Physiology* 112: 2503-2510.

Downs, D.S. 2006. Understanding exercise intention in an ethnically diverse sample of postpartum women. *Journal of Sport and Exercise Psychology* 28: 159-180.

Drenowatz, C., Hand, G.A., Sagner, M., Shook, R.P., Burgess, S., and Blair, S.N. 2015. The prospective association between different types of exercise and body composition. *Medicine & Science in Sports & Exercise* 47: 2535-2541.

Drenowatz, C., Hill, J.O., Peters, J.C., Soriano-Maldonado, A., and Blair, S.N. 2017. The association of change in physical activity and body weight in the regulation of total energy expenditure. *European Journal of Clinical Nutrition* 71: 377-382.

Drystad, S.M., Edvardsen, E., Hansen, B.H., and Anderssen, S.A. 2017. Waist circumference thresholds and cardiorespiratory fitness. *Journal of Sport and Health Science* [Epub ahead of print]. doi:10.1016/j.jshs.2017.03.011. Accessed August 5, 2017.

Dubin, D. 2000. *Rapid interpretation of EKGs: An interactive course,* 6th ed. Tampa: Cover.

Dubow, J., and Fink, M.E. 2011. Impact of hypertension on stroke. *Current Atherosclerosis Reports* 13: 298-305.

Ducimetier, P., Richard, J., and Cambien, F. 1989. The pattern of subcutaneous fat distribution in middle-aged men and the risk of coronary heart disease: The Paris prospective study. *International Journal of Obesity* 10: 229-240.

Duncan, P.W., Studenski, S., Chandler, J., and Prescott, B. 1992. Functional reach: Predictive validity in a sample of elderly male veterans. *Journal of Gerontology* 47(3): M93-M98.

Duncan, P.W., Weiner, D.K., Chandler, J., and Studenski, S. 1990. Functional reach: A new clinical measure of balance. *Journal of Gerontology* 45: M192-M197.

Eather, N., Morgan, P.J., and Lubans, D.R. 2016. Improving health-related fitness in adolescents: The CrossFit Teens™ randomized controlled trial. *Journal of Sports Sciences* 34: 209-223.

Ebbeling, C., Ward, A., Puleo, E., Widrick, J., and Rippe, J. 1991. Development of a single-stage submaximal treadmill walking test. *Medicine & Science in Sports & Exercise* 23: 966-973.

Eckert, S., and Horstkotte, D. 2002. Comparison of Portapres non-invasive blood pressure measurement in the finger with intra-aortic pressure measurement during incremental bicycle exercise. *Blood Pressure Monitoring* 7: 179-183.

Edgerton, V.R. 1970. Morphology and histochemistry of the soleus muscle from normal and exercised rats. *American Journal of Anatomy* 127: 81-88.

Edgerton, V.R. 1973. Exercise and the growth and development of muscle tissue. In *Physical activity, human growth and development,* ed. G.L. Rarick, 1-31. New York: Academic Press.

Edinborough, L., Fisher, J.P., and Steele, J. 2016. A comparison of the effect of kettlebell swings and isolated lumbar extension training on acute torque production of the lumbar extensors. *Journal of Strength and Conditioning Research* 30: 1189-1195.

Edvardsen, E., Hem, E., and Anderssen, S.A. 2014. End criteria for reaching maximal oxygen uptake must be strict and adjusted to sex and age: A cross-sectional study. *PLOS One* 9: 1 e85276. doi:10.1371/journal.pone.0085276. Accessed June 15, 2017.

Edwards, D.A., Hammond, W.H., Healy, M.J., Tanner, J.M., and Whitehouse, R.H. 1955. Design and accuracy of calipers for measuring subcutaneous tissue thickness. *British Journal of Nutrition* 9: 133-143.

Edwards, H.L., Simpson, J.A.R., and Buchholz, A.C. 2011. Air displacement plethysmography for fat-mass measurement in healthy young women. *Canadian Journal for Dietetic Practice and Research* 72: 85-87.

Edwards, M.K., Addoh, O., and Loprinzi, P.D. 2016. Predictive validity of the ACC/AHA pooled cohort equations in predicting residual-specific mortality in a national prospective cohort study of adults in the United States. *Postgraduate Medicine* 128: 865-868.

Egaña, M., and Donne, B. 2004. Physiological changes following a 12 week gym based stair-climbing, elliptical trainer and treadmill running program in females. *Journal of Sports Medicine and Physical Fitness* 44: 141-146.

Egli, T., Bland, H.W., Melton, B.F., and Czech, D.R. 2011. Influence of age, sex, and race on college students' exercise motivation of physical activity. *Journal of American College Health* 59: 399-406.

Ehrampoush, E., Arasteh, P., Homayounfar, R., Cheraghpour, M., Alipour, M., Naghizadeh, M.M., Hadibarhaghtalab, M., Daboodi, S.H., Askari, A., and Razaz, J.M. 2016. New anthropometric indices or old ones: Which is the better predictor of body fat? *Diabetes & Metabolic Syndrome: Clinical Research Reviews* [Epub ahead of print]. doi:10.1016/j.dsx.2016.08.027. Accessed August 14, 2017.

Ehrler, F., Weber, C., and Lovis, C. 2016. Influence of pedometer position on pedometer accuracy at various walking speeds: A comparative study. *Journal of Medical Internet Research* 18: e268. doi:10.2196/jmir.5916. Accessed May 10, 2017.

Eickhoff-Shemek, J., and Herbert, D.L. 2007. Is licensure in your future? Issues to consider—part 1. *ACSM's Health & Fitness Journal* 11(5): 35-37.

Eickhoff-Shemek, J., and Herbert, D.L. 2008a. Is licensure in your future? Issues to consider—part 2. *ACSM's Health & Fitness Journal* 12 (1): 36-38.

Eickhoff-Shemek, J., and Herbert, D.L. 2008b. Is licensure in your future? Issues to consider—part 3. *ACSM's Health & Fitness Journal* 12 (3): 36-38.

Eijsvogels, T.M.H., and Thompson, P.D. 2015. Exercise is Medicine: At any dose? *Journal of the American Medical Association* 314: 1915-1916.

Ekelund, U., Steene-Johannessen, J., Brown, W.J., Fagerland, M.W., Owen, N., Powell, K.E., Bauman, A., and Lee, I-M. 2016. Does physical activity attenuate, or even eliminate, the detrimental association of sitting time with mortality? A harmonized meta-analysis of data from more than 1 million men and women. *Lancet* 388: 1302-1310.

El-Amrawy, F., Pharm, B., and Nounou, M.I. 2015. Are currently available wearable devices for activity tracking and heart rate monitoring accurate, precise, and medically beneficial? *Health Informatics Research* 21: 315-320.

Ellis, K.J., Bell, S.J., Chertow, G.M., Chumlea, W.C., Knox, T.A., Kotler, D.P., Lukaski, H.C., and Schoeller, D.A. 1999. Bioelectrical impedance methods in clinical research: A follow-up to the NIH technology assessment conference. *Nutrition* 15: 874-880.

Elsen, R., Siu, M.L., Pineda, O., and Solomons, N.W. 1987. Sources of variability in bioelectrical impedance determinations in adults. In *In vivo body composition studies,* ed. K.J. Ellis, S. Yasamura, and W.D. Morgan, 184-188. London: Institute of Physical Sciences in Medicine.

Emery, C.A. 2003. Is there a clinical standing balance measurement appropriate for use in sports medicine? A review of the literature. *Journal of Science and Medicine in Sport* 6: 492-504.

Emery, C.A., Cassidy, J.D., Klassen, T.P., Rosychuk, R.J., and Rowe, B.H. 2005. Development of a clinical static and dynamic standing balance measurement tool appropriate for use in adolescents. *Physical Therapy* 85(6): 502-514.

Emmanuel, J. 2013. Guidance on maintaining and calibrating non-mercury clinical thermometers and sphygmomanometers. UNDP GEF Global Healthcare Waste Project. https://noharm.org/sites/default/files/lib/downloads/mercury/Guidance_Hg_2013.pdf. Accessed April 29, 2017.

Englund, D.A., Sharp, R.L., Selsby, J.T., Ganesan, S.S., and Franke, W.D. 2017. Resistance training performed at distinct angular velocities elicits velocity-specific alterations in muscle strength and mobility status in older adults. *Experimental Gerontology* 91: 51-56.

Enwemeka, C.S. 1986. Radiographic verification of knee goniometry. *Scandinavian Journal of Rehabilitation Medicine* 18: 47-49.

Epstein, L.H., Beecher, M.D., Graf, J.L., and Roemmich, J.L. 2007. Choice of interactive dance and bicycle games in overweight and non-overweight youth. *Annals of Behavioral Medicine* 33: 124-131.

Esco, M.R., Olson, M.S., Williford, H.N., Lizana, S.N., and Russell, A.R. 2011. The accuracy of hand-to-hand bioelectrical impedance analysis in predicting body composition in college-age female athletes. *Journal of Strength and Conditioning Research* 25: 1040-1045.

Esco, M.R., Snarr, R.L., Leatherwood, M.D., Chamberlain, N.A., Redding, M.L., Flatt, A.A., Moon, J.R., and Williford, H.N. 2015. Comparison of total and segmental body composition using DXA and multifrequency bioimpedance in collegiate female athletes. *Journal of Strength and Conditioning Research* 29: 918-925.

Esmarck, B., Andersen, J.L., Olsen, S., Richter, E.A., Mizuno, M., and Kjaer, M. 2001. Timing of postexercise protein intake is important for muscle hypertrophy with resistance training in elderly humans. *Journal of Physiology* 535: 301-311.

Eston, R., Evans, H., Faulkner, J., Lambrick, D., Al-Rahamneh, H., and Parfitt, G. 2012. A perceptually regulated, graded exercise test predicts peak oxygen update during treadmill exercise in active and sedentary participants. *European Journal of Applied Physiology* 112: 3459-3468.

Evans, E.M., Rowe, D.A., Misic, M.M., Prior, B.M., and Arngrimsson, S.A. 2005. Skinfold prediction equation for athletes developed using a four-component model. *Medicine & Science in Sports & Exercise* 37: 2006-2011.

Evans, H., Parfitt, G., and Eston, R. 2014. Use of a perceptually-regulated test to measure maximal oxygen uptake is valid and feels better. *European Journal of Sport Science.* 14: 452-458.

Evans, H.J.L., Ferrar, K.E., Smith, A.E., Parfitt, F., and Eston, R.G. 2015. A systematic review of methods to predict maximal oxygen uptake from submaximal, open circuit spirometry in healthy adults. *Journal of Science and Medicine in Sport* 18: 183-188.

Evans, W., and Rosenberg, I. 1992. *Biomarkers.* New York: Simon & Schuster.

Fahey, T.D., Rolph, R., Moungmee, P., Nagel, J., and Mortara, S. 1976. Serum testosterone, body composition, and strength of young adults. *Medicine and Science in Sports* 8: 31-34.

Falatic, J.A., Plato, P.A., Holder, C., Fiinch, D., Han, K., and Cisar, C.J. 2015. Effects of kettlebell training on aerobic capacity. *Journal of Strength and Conditioning Research* 29: 1943-1947.

Faigenbaum, A.D., Kraemer, W.J., Blimkie, C.J.R., Jeffreys, I., Micheli, L.J., Nitka, M., and Rowland, T.W. 2009. Youth resistance training: Updated position statement paper from the National Strength and Conditioning Association. *Journal of Strength & Conditioning Research* 23: S60-S79.

Faigenbaum, A.D., Milliken, L.A., and Westcott, W.L. 2003. Maximal strength testing in healthy children. *Journal of Strength and Conditioning Research* 17: 162-166.

Faigenbaum, A.D., and Myer, G.D. 2011. Exercise deficit disorder: Play now or pay later. *Current Sports Medicine Reports* 11: 196-200.

Faigenbaum, A.D., Westcott, W.L., Loud, R.L., and Long, C. 1999. The effects of different resistance training protocols on muscular strength and endurance development in children. *Pediatrics* 104(1): e5.

Fairbarn, M.S., Blackie, S.P., McElvaney, N.G., Wiggs, B.R., Pare, P.D., and Purdy, R.L. 1994. Prediction of heart rate and oxygen uptake during incremental and maximal exercise in healthy adults. *Chest* 105: 1365-1369.

Farrar, R.E., Mayhew, J.L., and Koch, A.J. 2010. Oxygen cost of kettlebell swings. *Journal of Strength and Conditioning Research* 24: 1034-1036.

Farthing, J.P., and Chilibeck, P.D. 2003. The effects of eccentric and concentric training at different velocities on muscle hypertrophy. *European Journal of Applied Physiology* 89: 578-586.

Faulkner, S.H., Pugh, J.K., Hood, T.M., Menon, K., King, J.A., Nimmo, M.A. 2015. Group studio cycling: An effective intervention to improve cardiometabolic health in overweight physically inactive individuals. *Journal of Fitness Research* 4: 16-25.

Feigenbaum, M.S., and Pollock, M.L. 1999. Prescription of resistance training for health and disease. *Medicine & Science in Sports & Exercise* 31: 38-45.

Feland, J.B., and Marin, H.N. 2004. Effect of submaximal contraction intensity in contract-relax proprioceptive neuromuscular facilitation stretching. *British Journal of Sports Medicine* 38: e18.

Femina, H.A., Beevi, M.E., Miranda, J., Pedersen, C.F., and Wagner, S. 2016. An evaluation of commercial pedometers for monitoring slow walking speed populations. *Telemedicine and e-Health* 22: 441-449.

Fenstermaker, K., Plowman, S., and Looney, M. 1992. Validation of the Rockport walking test in females 65 years and older. *Research Quarterly for Exercise and Sport* 63: 322-327.

Ferber, R., Osternig, L., and Gravelle, D. 2002. Effect of PNF stretch techniques on knee flexor muscle EMG activity in older adults. *Journal of Electromyography and Kinesiology* 12: 391-397.

Ferguson, T., Rowlands, A.V., Olds, T., and Maher, C. 2015. The validity of consumer-level activity monitors in healthy adults worn in free-living conditions: A cross-sectional study. *International Journal of Behavioral Nutrition and Physical Activity* 12: 42. doi:10.1186/s12966-015-0201-9.

Ferland, M., Despres, J.P., Tremblay, A., Pinault, S., Nadeau, A., Moorjani, S., Lupien, P.J., Theriault, G., and Bouchard, C. 1989. Assessment of adipose distribution by computed axial tomography in obese women: Association with body density and anthropometric measurements. *British Journal of Nutrition* 61: 139-148.

Ferrar, K., Evans, H., Smith, A., Parfitt, G., and Eston, R. 2014. A systematic review and meta-analysis of submaximal exercise-based equations to predict maximal oxygen uptake in young people. *Pediatric Exercise Science* 26: 342-357.

Ferreira, H.R., Gill, P., Filho, J.F., and Fernandes, L.C. 2015. Effects of 12-weeks of supplementation with β-hydroxy-β-methylbutyrate-ca (HMB-Ca) on athletic performance. *Journal of Exercise Physiology Online* 18(2): 85-94.

Ferreira, H.R., Rodacki, A.L.F., Gill, P., Tanhoffer, R., Filho, J.F., and Fernandes, L.C. 2013. The effects of supplementation of β-hydroxy-β-melthylbutyrate on inflammatory markers in high performance athletes. *Journal of Exercise Physiology Online* 16(1): 53-63.

Fess, E.E. 1992. Grip Strength. In *Clinical assessment recommendations,* American Society of Hand Therapists, 41-45, Chicago, IL: American Society of Hand Therapists.

Fields, D.A., and Allison, D.B. 2012. Air-displacement plethysmography pediatric option in 2-6 year olds using the four-compartment model as a criterion method. *Obesity* 20: 1732-1737.

Fields, D.A., and Goran, M.I. 2000. Body composition techniques and the four-compartment model in children. *Journal of Applied Physiology* 89: 613-620.

Fields, D.A., Goran, M.I., and McCrory, M.A. 2002. Body-composition assessment via air-displacement plethysmography in adults and children: A review. *American Journal of Clinical Nutrition* 75: 453-467.

Fields, D.A., Hunter, G.R., and Goran, M.I. 2000. Validation of the Bod Pod with hydrostatic weighing: Influence of body clothing. *International Journal of Obesity* 24: 200-205.

Fields, D.A., Wilson, G.D., Gladden, L.B., Hunter, G.R., Pascoe, D.D., and Goran, M.I. 2001. Comparison of the Bod Pod with the four-compartment model in adult females. *Medicine & Science in Sports & Exercise* 33: 1605-1610.

Fisher, G., Brown, A.W., Brown, M.M.B., Alcorn, A., Noles, C., Winwood, L., Resuehr, H., George, B., Jeansonne, M.M., and Allison, D.B. 2015. High intensity interval- vs. moderate intensity-training for improving cardiometabolic health in overweight or obese males: A randomized controlled trial. *PLoS One* 10: e0138853. doi:10.1371/journal.pone.0138853. Accessed July 27, 2017.

Fitzmaurice, C., and the Global Burden of Disease Cancer Collaboration. 2017. Global, regional, and national cancer incidence, mortality, years of life lost, years lived with disability, and disability-adjusted life-years for 32 cancer groups, 1990 to 2015: A systematic analysis for the Global Burden of Disease study. *JAMA Oncology* 3: 524-548.

Fleck, S.J. 1999. Periodized strength training: A critical review. *Journal of Strength and Conditioning Research* 13(1): 82-89.

Fleck, S.J., and Falkel, J.E. 1986. Value of resistance training for the reduction of sports injuries. *Sports Medicine* 3: 61-68.

Fleck, S.J., and Kraemer, W.J. 2014. *Designing resistance training programs,* 4th ed. Champaign, IL: Human Kinetics.

Flegal, K.M., Carroll, M.D., Kit, B.K., and Ogden, C.L. 2012. Prevalence of obesity and trends in the distribution of body mass index among US adults, 1999-2010. *Journal of the American Medical Association* 307: 491-497.

Flegal, K.M., Kruszon-Moran, D., Carroll, M.D., Fryar, C.D., and Ogden, C.L. 2016. Prevalence of obesity and trends in the distribution of body mass index among US adults, 2005 to 2014. *Journal of the American Medical Association* 315: 2284-2291.

Flegal, K.M., Shepherd, J.A., Looker, A.C., Graubard, B.I., Borrud, L.G., Ogden, C.L., Harris, T.B., Everhart, J.E., and Schenker, N. 2009. Comparisons of percentage body fat, body mass index, waist circumference, and waist-stature ratio in adults. *American Journal of Clinical Nutrition* 89: 500-508.

Fletcher, G.F., Ades, P.A., Kligfield, P., Arena, R., Balacy, G.J., Bittner, V.A., Coke, L.A., Fleg, J.L., Forman, D.E., Gerber, T.C., Gulati, M., Madan, K., Rhodes, J., Thompson, P.D., Williams, M.A., on behalf of the American Heart Association Exercise, Cardiac Rehabilitation, and Prevention Committee of the Council on Clinical Cardiology, Council on Nutrition, Physical Activity and Metabolism, Council on Cardiovascular and Stroke Nursing, and Council on Epidemiology and Prevention. 2013. Exercise standards for testing and training: A scientific statement from the American Heart Association. *Circulation* 128: 873-934.

Fogelholm, G.M., Sievanan, H.T., Kukkonen-Harjula, K., Oja, P., and Vuori, I. 1993. Effects of a meal and its electrolytes on bioelectrical impedance. In *Human body composition: In vivo methods, models and assessment,* ed. K.J. Ellis and J.D. Eastman, 331-332. New York: Plenum Press.

Fogg, B.J. 2003. *Persuasive technology: Using computers to change what we think and do.* New York: Morgan Kaufmann.

Fogg, B.J., and Eckles, D., eds. 2007. *Mobile persuasion: 20 perspectives on the future of behavior change.* Palo Alto, CA: Stanford University.

Fohlin, L. 1977. Body composition, cardiovascular and renal function in adolescent patients with anorexia nervosa. *Acta Paediatrica Scandinavica* 268(Suppl.): S7-S20.

Forbes, G.B. 1976. Adult decline in the lean body mass. *Human Biology* 48: 151-173.

Forbes, S.C., Little, J.P., and Candow, D.G. 2012. Exercise and nutritional interventions for improving aging muscle health. *Endocrine* 42: 29-38.

Ford, G.S., Mazzone, M.A., and Taylor, K. 2005. The effect of 4 different durations of static hamstring stretching on passive knee-extension range of motion. *Journal of Sport Rehabilitation* 14: 95-107.

Fornetti, W.C., Pivarnik, J.M., Foley, J.M., and Fiechtner, J.J. 1999. Reliability and validity of body composition measures in female athletes. *Journal of Applied Physiology* 87: 1114-1122.

Fort, A., Romero, D., Bagur, C., and Guerra, M. 2012. Effects of whole-body vibration training on explosive strength and postural control in young female athletes. *Journal of Strength and Conditioning Research* 26: 926-936.

Foster, C., Jackson, A.S., Pollock, M.L., Taylor, M.M., Hare, J., Sennett, S.M., Rod, J.L., Sarwar, M., and Schmidt, D.H. 1984. Generalized equations for predicting functional capacity from treadmill performance. *American Heart Journal* 107: 1229-1234.

Foster, C., Pollock, M.L., Rod, J.L., Dymond, D.S., Wible, G., and Schmidt, D.H. 1983. Evaluation of functional capacity during exercise radionuclide angiography. *Cardiology* 70: 85-93.

Forouzanfar, M., Dajani, H.R., Groza, V.Z., Bolic, M., Rajan, S., and Batkin, I. 2015. Oscillometric blood pressure estimation: Past, present, and future. *IEEE Reviews in Biomedical Engineering* 8: 44-63.

Fox, E.L. 1973. A simple, accurate technique for predicting maximal aerobic power. *Journal of Applied Physiology* 35: 914-916.

Franchignoni, F., Tesio, L., Martino, M.T., and Ricupero, C. 1998. Reliability of four simple, quantitative tests of balance and mobility in healthy elderly females. *Aging* 10(1): 26-31.

Francis, P.R., Kolkhorst, F.W., Pennuci, M., Pozos, R.S., and Buono, M.J. 2001. An electromyographic approach to the evaluation of abdominal exercises. *ACSM's Health & Fitness Journal* 5(4): 8-14.

Franklin, S.S., Thijs, L., Asayama, K., Li, Y., Hansen, T.W., Boggia, J., Jacobs, L., Zhang, Z., Kikuya, M., Björklund-Bodegård, K., Ohkubo, T., Yang, W-Y., Jeppesen, J., Dolan, E., Kuznetsova, T., Stolarz-Skrzpek, K., Tikhonoff, V., Malyutina, S., Casiglia, E., Nikitin, Y., Lind, L., Sandoya, E., Kawecka-Jaszcz, K., Filipovsky, J., Imai, Y., Wang, J-G., O-Brien, E., and Staessen, J.A., on behalf of the IDACCO Investigators. 2016. The cardiovascular risk of white-coat hypertension. *Journal of the American College of Cardiology* 68: 2033-2043.

Frederick, A., and Frederick, C. 2017. *Stretch to win*, 2nd ed. Champaign, IL: Human Kinetics.

Freedman, D.S., Blanck, J.M., Dietz, W.H., DasMahapatra, P., Srinivasan, S.R., and Berenson, G.S. 2012. Is the body adiposity index (hip circumference/height$^{1.5}$) more related to skinfold thicknesses and risk factor levels than is BMI? The Bogalusa Heart Study. *British Journal of Nutrition.*

doi:10.1017/S0007114512000979.

Freedman, D.S., and Ford, E.S. 2015. Are the recent secular increases in the waist circumferences independent of changes in BMI? *American Journal of Clinical Nutrition* 101: 425-431.

Freitas, S.R., Vilarinho, D., Vaz, J.R., Bruno, P.M., Costa, P.B., and Mil-ho-mens, P. 2015. Responses to static stretching are dependent on stretch intensity and duration. *Clinical Physiology and Functional Imaging* 35: 478-484.

Friden, J. 2002. Delayed onset muscle soreness. *Scandinavian Journal of Medicine and Science in Sports* 12: 327-328.

Friden, J., Sjostrom, M., and Ekblom, B. 1983. Myofibrillar damage following intense eccentric exercise in man. *International Journal of Sports Medicine* 4: 170-176.

Friedl, K.E., DeLuca, J.P., Marchitelli, L.J., and Vogel, J.A. 1992. Reliability of body-fat estimations from a four-compartment model by using density, body water, and bone mineral measurements. *American Journal of Clinical Nutrition* 55: 764-770.

Frisancho, A.R. 1984. New standard of weight and body composition by frame size and height for assessment of nutritional status of adults and the elderly. *American Journal of Clinical Nutrition* 40: 808-819.

Frohlich, M., Emrich, E., and Schmidtbleicher, D. 2010. Outcome effects of single-set versus multiple-set training—An advanced replication study. *Research in Sports Medicine* 18: 157-175.

Fry, A.C. 2004. The role of resistance exercise intensity on muscle fibre adaptations. *Sports Medicine* 34: 663-679.

Fullam, K., Caulfield, B., Coughlan, G.F., and Delahunt, E. 2014. Kinematic analysis of selected reach directions of the star excursion balance test compared with the Y-balance test. *Journal of Sport Rehabilitation* 23: 27-35.

Gába, A., Kapuš, O., Cuberek, R., and Botek, M. 2015. Comparison of multi- and single-frequency bioelectrical impedance analysis with dual-energy X-ray absorptiometry for assessment of body composition in post-menopausal women: Effects of body mass index and accelerometer-determined physical activity. *Journal of Nutrition and Human Dietetics* 28: 390-400.

Gajdosik, R.L., Vander Linden, D.W., and Williams, A.K. 1999. Influence of age on length and passive elastic stiffness characteristics of the calf muscle-tendon unit of women. *Physical Therapy* 79: 827-838.

Gallagher, D., Visser, M., Sepulveda, D., Pierson, R.N., Harris, T., and Heymsfield, S.B. 1996. How useful is body mass index for comparison of body fatness across age, sex, and ethnic groups? *American Journal of Epidemiology* 143: 228-239.

Gallagher, M.R., Walker, K.Z., and O'Dea, K. 1998. The influence of a breakfast meal on the assessment of body composition using bioelectrical impedance. *European Journal of Clinical Nutrition* 52: 94-97.

Garatachea, N., Pareja-Galeano, H., Sanchis-Gomar, F., Santos-Lozano, A., Fiuza-Luces, C., Morán, M., Emanuele, E., Joyner, M.J., and Lucia, A. 2015. Exercise attenuates the major hallmarks of aging. *Rejuvenation Research* 18: 57-89.

Garber, C.E., Blissmer, B., Deschenes, M.R., Franklin, B.A.,

Lamonte, M.J., Lee, I., Nieman, D.C., and Swain, D.P. 2011. Quantity and quality of exercise for developing and maintaining cardiorespiratory, musculoskeletal, and neuromotor fitness in apparently healthy adults: Guidance for prescribing exercise. *Medicine & Science in Sports & Exercise* 43: 1334-1359.

Garcia, T.B. 2015. *12-lead ECG: The art of interpretation.* Burlington, MA: Jones and Bartlett Learning.

Garnacho-Castano, M.V., Lopez-Lastra, S., and Mate-Munoz, J.L. 2015. Reliability and validity assessment of a linear position transducer. *Journal of Sports Science and Medicine* 14: 128-136.

GBD 2015 Mortality and Causes of Death Collaborators. 2016. Global, regional, and national life expectancy, all-cause mortality, and cause-specific mortality for 249 causes of death, 1980-2015: A systematic analysis for the Global Burden of Disease Study 2015. *Lancet* 388: 1459-1544.

Gellish, R.L., Goslin, B.R., Olson, R.E., McDonald, A., Russi, G.D., and Moudgil, V.K. 2007. Longitudinal modeling of the relationship between age and maximal heart rate. *Medicine & Science in Sports & Exercise* 39: 822-829.

Gennuso, K.P., Gangnon, R.E., Thraen-Borowski, K.M., and Colbert, L.H. 2015. Dose-response relationships between sedentary behavior and the metabolic syndrome and its components. *Diabetologia* 58: 485-492.

Gentil, P., de Lira, C.A.B., Filho, S.G.C., La Scala Teixeira, C.V., Steele, J., Fisher, J., Carneiro, J.A., and Campos, M.H. 2017. High intensity interval training does not impair strength gains in response to resistance training in premenopausal women. *European Journal of Applied Physiology* 117: 1257-1265.

Genton, L., Hans, D., Kyle, U.G., and Pichard, C. 2002. Dual-energy X-ray absorptiometry and body composition: Differences between devices and comparison with reference methods. *Nutrition* 18: 66-70.

George, J.D., Stone, W.J., and Burkett, L.N. 1997. Non-exercise $\dot{V}O_2$max estimation for physically active students. *Medicine & Science in Sports & Exercise* 29: 415-423.

George, J., Vehrs, P., Allsen, P., Fellingham, G., and Fisher, G. 1993. $\dot{V}O_2$max estimation from a submaximal 1-mile track jog for fit college-age individuals. *Medicine & Science in Sports & Exercise* 25: 401-406.

Gesche, H., Grosskaurth, D., Kuchler, G., and Patzak, A. 2012. Continuous blood pressure measurement by using the pulse transit time: Comparison to a cuff-based method. *European Journal of Applied Physiology* 112: 309-315.

Gettman, L.R., Ayres, J.J., Pollock, M.L., and Jackson, A. 1978. The effect of circuit weight training on strength, cardiorespiratory function, and body composition of adult men. *Medicine and Science in Sports* 10: 171-176.

Gettman, L.R., and Pollock, M.L. 1981. Circuit weight training: A critical review of its physiological benefits. *The Physician and Sportsmedicine* 9: 44-60.

Gibbons, R.J., Balady, G.J., Bricker, J.T., Chaitman, B.R., Fletcher, G.F., Froelicher, V.F., Mark, D.B., McCallister, B.D., Mooss, A.N., O'Reilly, M.G., and Winters, W.L. Jr. 2002. *ACC/AHA* 2002 guideline update for exercise testing: A report of the American College of Cardiology/American Heart Association Task Force on Practice Guidelines (Committee on Exercise Testing). www.acc.org/clinical/guidelines/exercise/dirIndex.htm.

Gibby, J.T., Njeru, D.K., Cvetko, S.T., Heiny, E.L., Creer, A.R., and Gibby, W.A., 2017. Whole-body computed tomography-based body mass and body fat quantification: A comparison to hydrostatic weighing and air displacement plethysmography. *Journal of Computer Assisted Tomography* 41: 302-308.

Gibson, A., Heyward, V., and Mermier, C. 2000. Predictive accuracy of Omron Body Logic Analyzer in estimating relative body fat of adults. *International Journal of Sport Nutrition and Exercise Metabolism* 10: 216-227.

Gibson, A.L., Beam, J.R., Alencar, M.K., Zuhl, M.N., and Mermier, C.M. 2015. Time course of supine and standing shifts in total body, intracellular and extracellular water for a sample of healthy adults. *European Journal of Clinical Nutrition* 69: 14-19.

Gibson, A.L., Holmes, J.C., Desautels, R.L., Edmonds, L.B., and Nuudi, L. 2008. Ability of new octapolar bioimpedance spectroscopy analyzers to predict 4-component-model percentage body fat in Hispanic, black, and white adults. *American Journal of Clinical Nutrition* 87: 332-338.

Gibson, A.L., Roper, J.L., and Mermier, C.M. 2016. Intraindividual variability in test-retest air displacement plethysmography measurements of body density for men and women. *International Journal of Sport Nutrition and Exercise Metabolism* 26: 404-412.

Gillespie, B.D., McCormick, J.J., Mermier, C.M., and Gibson, A.L. 2015. Talk test as a practical method to estimate exercise intensity in highly trained competitive male cyclists. *Journal of Strength and Conditioning Research* 29: 894-898.

Gillen, J.G., Martin, B.J. MacInnis, M.J., Skelly, L.E., Tarnopolsky, M.A., and Gibala, M.J. 2016. Twelve weeks of sprint interval training improves indices of cardiometabolic health similar to traditional endurance training despite a five-fold lower exercise volume and time commitment. *PLoS One* 11: e0154075. doi:10.1371/journal.pone.0154075. Accessed July 30, 2017.

Gillman, M.W. 2008. The first months of life: A critical period for development of obesity. *American Journal of Clinical Nutrition* 87: 1587-1589.

Girouard, C.K., and Hurley, B.F. 1995. Does strength training inhibit gains in range of motion from flexibility training in older adults? *Medicine & Science in Sports & Exercise* 27: 1444-1449.

Gledhill, N., and Jamnik, R. 1995. Determining power outputs for cycle ergometers with different sized flywheels. *Medicine & Science in Sports & Exercise* 27: 134-135.

Gleichauf, C.N., and Rose, D.A. 1989. The menstrual cycle's effect on the reliability of bioimpedance measurements for assessing body composition. *American Journal of Clinical Nutrition* 50: 903-907.

Glowacki, S.P., Martin, S.E., Maurer, A., Baek, W., Green, J.S., and Crouse, S.F. 2004. Effects of resistance, endurance, and concurrent exercise on training outcomes in men. *Medicine & Science in Sports & Exercise* 36: 2119-2127.

Goble, D.J., Cone, B.L., and Fling, B.W. 2014. Using the Wii Fit as a tool for balance assessment and neurorehabilitation:

The first half decade of "Wii-search." *Journal of NeuroEngineering and Rehabilitation* 11: 12.

Gökbayrak, N.S., Paiva, A.L., Blissmer, B.J., and Prochaska, J.O. 2015. Predictors of relapse among smokers: Transtheoretical effort variables, demographics, and smoking severity. *Addictive Behaviors* 42: 176-179.

Goldberg, A., Etlinger, J., Goldspink, D., and Jablecki, C. 1975. Mechanism of work-induced hypertrophy of skeletal muscle. *Medicine and Science in Sports* 7: 185-198.

Goldenberg, L., and Twist, P. 2016. *Strength ball training, 3rd ed.* Champaign, IL: Human Kinetics.

Golding, L. 2000. *The Y's way to physical fitness.* Champaign, IL: Human Kinetics.

Goldman, H.I., and Becklake, M.R. 1959. Respiratory function tests: Normal values at medium altitudes and the prediction of normal results. *American Review of Tuberculosis and Respiratory Diseases* 79: 457-467.

Gonyea, W.J., Ericson, G.C., and Bonde-Petersen, F. 1977. Skeletal muscle fiber splitting induced by weight-lifting exercise in cats. *Acta Physiologica Scandinavica* 99: 105-109.

Goode, A.P., Hall, K.S., Batch, B.C., Huffman, K.M., Hastings, S.N., Allen, K.D., Shaw, R.J., Kanach, F.A., McDuffie, J.R., Kosinski, A.S., Williams, J.W. Jr., and Gierisch, J.M. 2017. The impact of interventions that integrate accelerometers on physical activity and weight loss: A systematic review. *Annals of Behavioral Medicine* 51(1): 79-93.

Goodman, J.M., Thomas, S.G., and Burr, J. 2011. Evidence-based risk assessment and recommendations for exercise testing and physical activity clearance in apparently healthy individuals. *Applied Physiology, Nutrition, and Metabolism* 36: S14-S32.

Goran, M.I., Allison, D.B., and Poehlman, E.T. 1995. Issues relating to normalization of body fat content in men and women. *International Journal of Obesity* 19: 638-643.

Goran, M.I., Toth, M.J., and Poehlman, E.T. 1998. Assessment of research-based body composition techniques in healthy elderly men and women using the 4-component model as a criterion method. *International Journal of Obesity* 22: 135-142.

Gordon, D.J., Probstfield, J.L., Garrison, R.J., Neaton, J.D., Castelli, W.P., Knoke, J.D., Jacobs, D.R., Bangdiwala, S., and Tyroler, H.A. 1989. High-density lipoprotein cholesterol and cardiovascular disease: Four prospective American studies. *Circulation* 79: 8-15.

Gordon-Larsen, P., Hou, N., Sidney, S., Sternfeld, B., Lewis, C., Jacobs, D. Jr., and Popkin, B. 2009. Fifteen-year longitudinal trends in walking patterns and their impact on weight change. *American Journal of Clinical Nutrition* 89: 19-26.

Gordon, C.M., Zemel, B.S., Wren, T.A.L., Leonard, M.B., Bachrach, L.K., Rauch, F., Gilsanz, V., Rosen, C.J, and Winer, K.K. 2017. The determinants of peak bone mass. *Journal of Pediatrics* 180: 261-269.

Gordon, R., and Bloxham, S. 2016. A systematic review of the effects of exercise and physical activity on non-specific chronic low back pain. *Healthcare* 4: 22. doi:10.3390/healthcare402002. Accessed April 15, 2017.

Gosselin, L.E., Kozlowski, K.F., de Vinney-Boymel, L., and Hambridge, C. 2012. Metabolic response of different high-intensity aerobic interval exercise protocols. *Journal of Strength and Conditioning Research* 26: 2866-2871.

Gothe, N.P., and McAuley, E. 2016. Yoga is as good as stretching-strengthening exercises in improving functional fitness outcomes: Results from a randomized controlled trial. *Journals of Gerontology, Series A: Biological Sciences and Medical Sciences* 71: 406-411.

Granacher, U. 2011. *Balance and strength performance in children, adolescents, and seniors.* Hamburg, Germany: Verlag Dr. Kovac.

Granacher, U., Gollhofer, A., Hortobagyi, T., Kressig, R.W., and Muehlbauer, T. 2013. The importance of trunk muscle strength for balance, functional performance, and fall prevention in seniors: A systematic review. *Sports Medicine* 43: 627-641.

Granacher, U., Gruber, M., and Gollhofer. 2010. Force production capacity and functional reflex activity in young and elderly men. *Aging Clinical and Experimental Research* 22: 374-382.

Granacher, U., Kressig, R.W., Borde, R., Lesinski, M., Bohm, S., Mersmann, F., and Arampatzis, A. 2017. Muscular strength and balance in old age: Effects and dose-response relationships following resistance and balance training. *Neurologie und Rehabilitation* 23: 61-76.

Granacher, U., Muehlbauer, T., Zahner, L., Gollhofer, A., and Kressig, R.W. 2011. Comparison of traditional and recent approaches in the promotion of balance and strength in older adults. *Sport Medicine* 41: 377-400.

Granacher, U., Muehlbauer, T., and Gruber, M. 2012. A qualitative review of balance and strength performance in healthy older adults: Impact for testing and training. *Journal of Aging Research* 2012: 708905. doi:10.1155/2012/708905. Accessed November 30, 2012.

Gras, L.Z., Ganley, K.J., Bosch, P.R., Mayer, J.E., and Pohl, P.S. 2017. Convergent validity of the sharpened Romberg. *Physical and Occupational Therapy in Geriatrics* [Epub ahead of print]. Epub: doi:10.1080/02703181.2017.1307897

Graversen, P., Abildstrøm, S.Z., Jespersen, L., Borglykke, A., and Prescott, E. 2016. Cardiovascular risk prediction: Can Systematic COronary Risk Evaluation (SCORE) be improved by adding simple risk markers? Results from the Copenhagen City Heart Study. *European Journal of Preventive Cardiology* 23: 1546-1556.

Graves, J.D., Webb, M., Pollock, M.L., Matkozich, J., Leggett, S.H., Carpenter, D.M., Foster, D.N., and Cirulli, J. 1994. Pelvic stabilization during resistance training: Its effect on the development of lumbar extension strength. *Archives of Physical Medicine and Rehabilitation* 75: 211-215.

Graves, J.E., Pollock, M.L., Colvin, A.B., Van Loan, M., and Lohman, T.G. 1989. Comparison of different bioelectrical impedance analyzers in the prediction of body composition. *American Journal of Human Biology* 1: 603-611.

Graves, L., Stratton, G., Ridgers, N.D., and Cable, N.T. 2007. Comparison of energy expenditure in adolescents when playing new generation and sedentary computer games: Cross-sectional study. *British Medical Journal* 335: 1282-1284.

Gray, D.S., Bray, G.A., Gemayel, N., and Kaplan, K. 1989. Effect of obesity on bioelectrical impedance. *American Journal of Clinical Nutrition* 50: 255-260.

Gray, M., and Paulson, S. 2014. Developing a measure of muscular power during a functional task for older adults. *BMC Geriatrics* 14: 145.

Green, J.M., Crews, T.R., Pritchett, R.C., Mathfield, C., and Hall, L. 2004. Heart rate and ratings of perceived exertion during treadmill and elliptical exercise training. *Perceptual and Motor Skills* 98: 340-348.

Greene, P.F., Durall, C.J., and Kernozek, T.W. 2012. Intersession reliability and concurrent validity of isometric endurance tests for the lateral trunk muscles. *Journal of Sport Rehabilitation* 21: 161-166.

Greene, W.B., and Heckman, J.D. 1994. *The clinical measurement of joint motion.* Rosemont, IL: American Academy of Orthopaedic Surgeons.

Grembowski, D., Patrick, D., Diehr, P., Durham, M., Beresford, S., Kay, E., and Hecht, J. 1993. Self-efficacy and health behavior among older adults. *Journal of Health and Social Behavior* 34(6): 89-104.

Grenier, S.G., Russell, C., and McGill, S.M. 2003. Relationships between lumbar flexibility, sit-and-reach test, and a previous history of low back discomfort in industrial workers. *Canadian Journal of Applied Physiology* 28: 165-177.

Gribble, P.A., and Hertel, J. 2003. Considerations for normalizing measures of the star excursion balance test. *Measurement in Physical Education and Exercise Science* 7: 89-100.

Grier, T., Canham-Chervak, M., McNulty, V., and Jones, B.H. 2013. Extreme conditioning programs and injury risk in a US Army Brigade Combat Team. *U.S. Army Medical Department Journal* (1 October): 36-47.

Griffin, S., Robergs, R., and Heyward, V. 1997. Assessment of exercise blood pressure: A review. *Medicine & Science in Sports & Exercise* 29: 149-159.

Grossman, J.C., and Deitrick, R.W. 2015. Air displacement plethysmography and resistance exercise. *Internet Journal of Allied Health Sciences and Practice.* http://nsuworks.nova.edu/ijahsp/vol13/iss2/4. Accessed August 5, 2017.

Gruber, J.J., Pollock, M.L., Graves, J.E., Colvin, A.B., and Braith, R.W. 1990. Comparison of Harpenden and Lange calipers in predicting body composition. *Research Quarterly for Exercise and Sport* 61: 184-190.

Guariglia, D.A., Pereira, L.M., Dias, J.M., Pereira, H.M., Menacho, M.O., Silva, D.A., Ayrino, E.S., and Cardoso, J.R. 2011. Time-of-day effect on hip flexibility associated with the modified sit-and-reach test in males. *International Journal of Sports Medicine* 32: 947-952.

Gudivaka, R., Schoeller, D., and Kushner, R.F. 1996. Effect of skin temperature on multifrequency bioelectrical impedance analysis. *Journal of Applied Physiology* 81: 838-845.

Guglani, R., Shenoy, S., and Singh, J. 2014. Effect of progressive pedometer based walking intervention on quality of life and general well being among patients with type 2 diabetes. *Journal of Diabetes & Metabolic Disorders* 13: 110-120.

Guidetti, L., Sgadari, A., Buzzachera, C.F., Broccatelli, M., Utter, A.C., Goss, F.L., and Baldari, C. 2011. Validation of the OMNI-cycle scale of perceived exertion in the elderly. *Journal of Aging and Physical Activity* 19: 214-224.

Guimaraes, R.M., and Isaacs, B. 1980. Characteristics of gait in old people who fall. *International Rehabilitation Medicine* 2: 177-180.

Guimarães-Ferreira, L., Cholewa, J.M., Naimo, M.A., Zhi, X.I., Magagnin, D., de Sá, R.B., Streck, E.L., Teixeira Tda, S., and Zanchi, N.E. 2014. Synergistic effects of resistance training and protein intake: Practical aspects. *Nutrition* 30(10): 1097-1103.

Guralnik, J.M., Seeman, T.E., Tinetti, M.E., Nevitt, M.C., and Berkman, L.F. 1994. Validation and use of performance measures of functioning in a non-disabled older population: MacArthur studies of successful aging. *Aging Clinical and Experimental Research* 6: 410-419.

Guskiewicz, K.M. 2011. Balance assessment in the management of sport-related concussion. *Clinics in Sports Medicine* 30: 89-102.

Guskiewicz, K.M., and Perrin, D.H. 1996. Research and clinical applications of assessing balance. *Journal of Sport Rehabilitation* 5: 45-63.

Gustavsen, P.H., Hoegholm, A., Bang, L.E., and Kristensen, K.S. 2003. White coat hypertension is a cardiovascular risk factor. A 10-year follow-up study. *Journal of Human Hypertension* 17: 811-817.

Guy, J.A., and Micheli, L.J. 2001. Strength training for children and adolescents. *Journal of the American Academy of Orthopaedic Surgeons* 9: 29-36.

Habash, D. 2002. Tactile and interpersonal techniques for fatfold anthropometry. School of Medicine. Ohio State University. Unpublished paper.

Habib, Z., and Westcott, S. 1998. Assessment of anthropometric factors on balance tests in children. *Pediatric Physical Therapy* 10: 101-109.

Haff, G.G. 2016. Periodization. In *Essentials of strength training and conditioning, 4th ed.,* ed. G.G. Haff and N.T. Triplett, 583-604. Champaign, IL: Human Kinetics.

Hagerman, F. 1993. *Concept II rowing ergometer nomogram for prediction of maximal oxygen consumption* [abstract]. Morrisville, VT: Concept II.

Hall, K.D., Sacks, G., Chandramohan, D., Chow, C.C., Wang, C., Gortmaker, S.L., and Swinburn, B.A. 2011. Quantification of the effect of energy imbalance on bodyweight. *Lancet* 378(9793): 826-837.

Halvarsson, A., Dohrn, I-M., and Stahle, A. 2015. Taking balance training for older adults one step further: The rationale for and description of a proven balance training programme. *Clinical Rehabilitation* 29: 417-425.

Han, L., and Yang, F. 2015. Strength or power, which is more important to prevent slip-related falls? *Human Movement Science* 44: 192-200.

Handelsman, Y., Bloomgarden, Z.T., Grungerger, G., Umpierrrez, G., Zimmerman, R.S., Bailey, T.S., Blonde, L., Bray, G.A., Cohen, A.J., Dagogo-Jack, S., Davidson, J.A., Einhorn, D., Ganda, O.P., Garber, A.J., Garvey, W.T., Henry, R.R., Hirsch, I.B., Horton, E.S., Hurley, D.L., Jellinger, P.S., Jovanovič, L., Lebovitz, H.E., LeRoith, D., Levy, P., McGill, J.G., Mechanick, J.I., Mestman, J.H., Moghissi, E.S., Orzeck, E.A., Pessah-Pollack, R., Rosenblit, P.D., Vinik, A.I., Wyne, K., and Zzangeneh, F. 2015. American Association of Clinical Endocrinologists and American College of Endocrinology:

Clinical practice guidelines for developing a diabetes mellitus comprehensive care plan—2015. *Endocrine Practice* 21(Suppl. 1): 1-87.

Hansen, D., Jacobs, N., Bex, S., D'Haene, G., Dendale, P. and Claes, N., 2011. Are fixed-rate step tests medically safe for assessing physical fitness? *European Journal of Applied Physiology* 111: 2593-2599.

Harmer, P., and Li, F. 2008. Tai chi and falls prevention in older people. *Medicine and Sport Science* 52: 124-134.

Harridge, S.D. 2007. Plasticity of human skeletal muscle: Gene expression to in vivo function. *Experimental Physiology* 92: 783-797.

Harries, S.K., Lubans, D.R., and Callister, R. 2015. Systematic review and meta-analysis of linear and undulating periodized resistance training programs on muscular strength. *Journal of Strength and Conditioning Research* 29: 1113-1125.

Harris, J.A., and Benedict, F.G. 1919. *A biometric study of basal metabolism in man* (publication no. 279). Washington, D.C.: Carnegie Institute.

Harris, M.L. 1969. A factor analytic study of flexibility. *Research Quarterly* 40: 62-70.

Harrison, G.G., Buskirk, E.R., Carter, L.J.E., Johnston, F.E., Lohman, T.G., Pollock, M.L., Roche, A.F., and Wilmore, J.H. 1988. Skinfold thicknesses and measurement technique. In *Anthropometric standardization reference manual,* ed. T.G. Lohman, A.F. Roche, and R. Martorell, 55-70. Champaign, IL: Human Kinetics.

Harrop, B.J., and Woodruff, S.J. 2015. Effects of acute and 2-hour postphysical activity on the estimation of body fat made by the Bod Pod. *Journal of Strength and Conditioning Research* 29: 1527-1533.

Hartley, L.H. 1975. Growth hormone and catecholamine response to exercise in relation to physical training. *Medicine and Science in Sports* 7: 34-36.

Hartley, L.H., Mason, J.W., Hogan, R.P., Jones, L.G., Kotchen, T.A., Mougey, E.H., Wherry, R., Pennington, L., and Ricketts, P. 1972. Multiple hormonal responses to graded exercise in relation to physical conditioning. *Journal of Applied Physiology* 33: 602-606.

Hartley-O'Brien, S.J. 1980. Six mobilization exercises for active range of hip flexion. *Research Quarterly for Exercise and Sport* 51: 625-635.

Hasanpour-Dehkordi, A., Dehghani, A., and Solati, K. 2017. A comparison of the effects of Pilates and McKenzie training on pain and general health in men with chronic low back pain: A randomized trial. *Indian Journal of Palliative Care* 23: 36-40.

Haskell, W.L., Lee, I.M., Pate, R.R., Powell, K.E., Blair, S.N., Franklin, B.A., Macera, C.A., Heath, G.W., Thompson, P.D., and Bauman, A. 2007. Physical activity and public health: Updated recommendation for adults from the American College of Sports Medicine and the American Heart Association. *Medicine & Science in Sports & Exercise* 39(8): 1423-1434.

Hass, C.J., Garzarella, L., De Hoyas, D., and Pollock, M. 2000. Single versus multiple sets in long-term recreational weightlifters. *Medicine & Science in Sports & Exercise* 32: 235-242.

Hastuti, J., Kagawa, M., Byrne, N.M., and Hills, A.P. 2016. Proposal of new body composition prediction equations from bioelectrical impedance for Indonesian men. *European Journal of Clinical Nutrition* 70: 1271-1277.

Hawk, C., Hyland, J.K., Rupert, R., Colonvega, M., and Hall, S. 2006. Assessment of balance and risk for falls in a sample of community-dwelling adults aged 65 and older. *Chiropractic & Osteology* 14: 3-10.

Hawkins, M.N., Raven, P.B., Snell, P.G., Stray-Gundersen, J., and Levine, B.D. 2007. Maximal oxygen uptake as a parametric measure of cardiorespiratory capacity. *Medicine & Science in Sports & Exercise* 39: 103-107.

Hayes, A., and Cribb, P.J. 2008. Effect of whey protein isolate on strength, body composition, and muscle hypertrophy during resistance training. *Current Opinion in Clinical Nutrition and Metabolic Care* 11: 40-44.

Hayes, P.A., Sowood, P.J., Belyavin, A., Cohen, J.B., and Smith, F.W. 1988. Sub-cutaneous fat thickness measured by magnetic resonance imaging, ultrasound, and calipers. *Medicine & Science in Sports & Exercise* 20: 303-309.

Health Canada. 2003. *Canada's physical activity guide to healthy active living.* Version 9. www.hc-sc.ca/english/lifestyles/index.html.

Hebden, L., Balestracci, K., McGeechan, K., Denney-Wilson, E., Harris, M., Bauman, A., and Allman-Farnelli, M. 2013. 'TXT2BFIT' a mobile phone-based healthy lifestyle program for preventing unhealthy weight gain in young adults: Study protocol for a randomized controlled trial. *Trials* 14: 75. www.trialsjournal.com/content/14/1/7.

Hegedus, E.J., McDonough, S.M., Bleakley, C., Baxter, D., and Cook, C.E. 2015. Clinician-friendly lower extremity physical performance tests in athletes: A systematic review of measurement properties and correlation with injury. Part 2—the tests for hip, thigh, foot and ankle including the star excursion balance test. *British Journal of Sports Medicine* 49: 649-656.

Heil, D.P. 1997. Body mass scaling of peak oxygen uptake in 20- to 79-year-old adults. *Medicine & Science in Sports & Exercise* 29: 1602-1608.

Heinrich, K.M., Patel, P.M., O'Neal, J.L., and Heinrich, B.S. 2014. High-intensity compared to moderate-intensity training for exercise initiation, enjoyment, adherence, and intentions: An intervention study. *BMC Public Health* 14: article 789.

Henschke, N., and Lin, C.C. 2011. Stretching before or after exercise does not reduce delayed-onset muscle soreness. *British Journal of Sport Medicine* 45: 1249-1250.

Henwood, T.R., and Taaffe, D.R. 2003. Beneficial effects of high-velocity resistance training in older adults. *Medicine & Science in Sports & Exercise* 35(Suppl.): S292 [abstract].

Herbert, D.L. 1995. First state licenses exercise physiologists. *Fitness Management* October: 26-27.

Herbert, D.L. 2004. New law to regulate personal trainers proposed in Oregon. *The Exercise Standards and Malpractice Reporter* 18(2): 17, 20-24.

Herbert, R.D., de Noronha, M., and Kamper, S.J. 2011. Stretching to prevent or reduce muscle soreness after exercise. *Cochrane Database of Systematic Reviews* [online] 7: CD004577.

Herda, T.J., Costa, P.B., Walter, A.A., Ryan, E.D., Hoge, K.M., Kerksick, C.M., Stout, J.R., and Cramer, J.T. 2011. Effects of two modes of static stretching on muscle strength and stiffness. *Medicine & Science in Sports & Exercise* 43: 1777-1784.

Herda, T.J., Herda, N.D., Costa, P.B., Walter-Herda, A.A., Valdez, A.M., and Cramer, J.T. 2013. The effects of dynamic stretching on the passive properties of the muscle-tendon unit. *Journal of Sports Sciences* 31: 479-487.

Herman, T., Giladi, N., and Hausdorff, J.M. 2011. Properties of the 'timed up and go' test: More than meets the eye. *Gerontology* 57: 203-210.

Hermansen, L., and Saltin, B. 1969. Oxygen uptake during maximal treadmill and bicycle exercise. *Journal of Applied Physiology* 26: 31-37.

Hertel, J., Braham, R.A., Hale, S.A., and Olmsted-Kramer, L.C. 2006. Simplifying the star excursion balance test: Analyses of subjects with and without chronic ankle instability. *Journal of Orthopaedic & Sports Physical Therapy* 36: 131-137.

Hertel, J., Miller, S.J., and Denegar, C.R. 2000. Intratester and intertester reliability during the star excursion balance tests. *Journal of Sport Rehabilitation* 9: 104-116.

Hess, J.A., and Woollacott, M. 2005. Effect of high-intensity strength-training on functional measures of balance ability in balance-impaired older adults. *Journal of Manipulative and Physiological Therapeutics* 28: 582-590.

Hettinger, T., and Muller, E.A. 1953. Muskelleistung und muskeltraining. *European Journal of Applied Physiology* 15: 111-126.

Heymsfield, S.B., Peterson, C.M., Thomas, D.M., Heo, M., and Schuna, J.M. Jr. 2016. Why are there race/ethnic differences in adult body mass index-adiposity relationships? A quantitative critical review. *Obesity Reviews* 17: 262-275.

Heymsfield, S.B., Wang, J., Lichtman, S., Kamen, Y., Kehayias, J., and Pierson, R.N. 1989. Body composition in elderly subjects: A critical appraisal of clinical methodology. *American Journal of Clinical Nutrition* 50: 1167-1175.

Heyward, V.H., and Wagner, D.R. 2004. *Applied body composition assessment,* 2nd ed. Champaign, IL: Human Kinetics.

Hickson, R.C., and Rosenkoetter, M.A. 1981. Reduced training frequencies and maintenance of increased aerobic power. *Medicine & Science in Sports & Exercise* 13: 13-16.

Higgins, P.B., Fields, D.A., Hunter, G.R., and Gower, B.A. 2001. Effect of scalp and facial hair on air displacement plethysmography estimates of percentage of body fat. *Obesity Research* 9: 326-330.

Hill, J.O., and Melanson, E.L. 1999. Overview of the determinants of overweight and obesity: Current evidence and research issues. *Medicine & Science in Sports & Exercise* 31(Suppl.): S515-S521.

Hillsdon, M., Coombes, E., Griew, P., and Jones, A. 2015. An assessment of the relevance of the home neighbourhood for understanding environmental influences on physical activity: How far from home do people roam? *International Journal of Behavioral Nutrition* 12: 100. doi:10.1186/s12966-015-0260-y. Accessed May 25, 2017.

Himes, J.H., and Frisancho, R.A. 1988. Estimating frame size. In *Anthropometric standardization reference manual,* ed. T.G. Lohman, A.F. Roche, and R. Martorell, 121-124. Champaign, IL: Human Kinetics.

Hindle, K.B., Whitcomb, T.J., Briggs, W.O., and Hong, J. 2012. Proprioceptive neuromuscular facilitation (PNF): Its mechanisms and effects on range of motion and muscular function. *Journal of Human Kinetics* 31: 105-113.

Hirsh, J. 1971. Adipose cellularity in relation to human obesity. *Advances in Internal Medicine* 17: 289-300.

Ho, M., Garnett, S.P., Baur, L.A., Burrows, T., Stewart, L., Neve, M., and Collins, C. 2013. Impact of dietary and exercise interventions on weight change and metabolic outcomes in obese children and adolescents: A systematic review and meta-analysis of randomized trials. *JAMA Pediatrics* 167: 759-768.

Ho, N-T-V.S., Olds, T., Schranz, N., and Maher, C. 2017. Secular trends in the prevalence of childhood overweight and obesity across Australian states: A meta-analysis. *Journal of Science and Medicine in Sport* 20: 480-488.

Hodgkins, J., and Skubic, V. 1963. Cardiovascular efficiency test scores for college women in the United States. *Research Quarterly* 34: 454-461.

Hoeger, W.W.K. 1989. *Lifetime physical fitness and wellness.* Englewood Cliffs, NJ: Morton.

Hoeger, W.W.K., and Hopkins, D.R. 1992. A comparison of the sit-and-reach and the modified sit-and-reach in the measurement of flexibility in women. *Research Quarterly for Exercise and Sport* 63: 191-195.

Hoeger, W.W.K., Hopkins, D.R., Button, S., and Palmer, T.A. 1990. Comparing the sit and reach with the modified sit and reach in measuring flexibility in adolescents. *Pediatric Exercise Science* 2: 156-162.

Hofsteenge, G.H., Chinapaw, M.J.M., Delemarre-van de Waal, H.A., and Weijs, P.J.M. 2010. Validation of predictive equations for resting energy expenditure in obese adolescents. *American Journal of Clinical Nutrition* 91: 1244-1254.

Hogrel, J-Y. 2015. Grip strength measured by high precision dynamometry in healthy subjects from 5 to 80 years. *BMC Musculoskeletal Disorders.* 16: 139.

Hoppeler, H. 2016. Moderate load eccentric exercise: A distinct novel training modality. *Frontiers in Physiology* 7: article 483.

Hoshang Bakhtiary, A., Aminian-Far, A., and Hedayati, R. 2013. Acute effects of static stretch on the static and dynamic balance indices in the young healthy non-athletic females. *Koomesh* 14: 431-438.

Houtkooper, L.B., Going, S.G., Lohman, T.G., Roche, A.F., and VanLoan, M. 1992. Bioelectrical impedance estimation of fat-free body mass in children and youth: A cross-validation study. *Journal of Applied Physiology* 72: 366-373.

Houtkooper, L.B., Going, S.B., Westfall, C.H., Lohman, T.G. 1989. Prediction of fat-free body corrected for bone mass from impedance and anthropometry in adult females. *Medicine & Science in Sports & Exercise* 21: 539 [abstract].

Howatson, G., and van Someren, K.A. 2008. The prevention and treatment of exercise-induced muscle damage. *Sports Medicine* 38: 483-503.

Howe, T.E., Rochester, L., Jackson, A., and Blair, V.A. 2007. Exercise for improving balance in older people (review). *Cochrane Database of Systematic Reviews* 4: CD004963.

Howe, T.E., Rochester, L., Neil, F., Skelton, D.A., and Ballinger, C. 2011. Exercise for improving balance in older people (review). *Cochrane Database of Systematic Reviews* 11: CD004963. doi:10.1002/14651858.CD004963.

Howley, E.T. 2007. V̇O₂max and the plateau—needed or not? *Medicine & Science in Sports & Exercise* 39: 101-102.

Howley, E. 2008. Physical activity guidelines for Americans. *President's Council on Physical Fitness and Sports Research Digest Series* 9(4): December.

Howley, E.T., Colacino, D.L., and Swensen, T.C. 1992. Factors affecting the oxygen cost of stepping on an electronic stepping ergometer. *Medicine & Science in Sports & Exercise* 24: 1055-1058.

Hoxie, R.E. Rubenstein, L.Z., Hoenig, H., and Gallagher, B.R. 1994. The older pedestrian. *Journal of the American Geriatrics Society* 42: 444-450.

Hsieh, S.D., Yoshinaga, H., and Muto, T. 2003. Waist-to-height ratio, a simple and practical index for assessing central fat distribution and metabolic risk in Japanese men and women. *International Journal of Obesity* 27: 610-616.

Huang, Y., Cai, X., Liu, C., Zhu, D., Hua, J., Hu, Y., Peng, J., and Xu, D. 2015. Prehypertension and the risk of coronary heart disease in Asian and Western populations: A meta-analysis. *Journal of the American Heart Association.* doi:10.1161/JAHA.114.001519. Accessed April 23, 2017.

Huang, Y., and Liu, X. 2015. Improvement of balance control ability and flexibility in the elderly tai chi chuan (TCC) practitioners: A systematic review and meta-analysis. *Archives of Gerontology and Geriatrics* 60: 233-238.

Hubley-Kozey, C.L. 1991. Testing flexibility. In *Physiological testing of the high-performance athlete,* ed. J.D. MacDougall, H.A. Wenger, and H.J. Green, 309-359. Champaign, IL: Human Kinetics.

Hübscher, M., Zech, A., Pfeifer, K., Hänsel, F., Vogt, L., and Banzer, W. 2010. Neuromuscular training for sports injury prevention: A systematic review. *Medicine & Science in Sports & Exercise* 42: 413-421.

Hudson, J., Hiripi, E., Pope, H., and Kessler, R. 2007. The prevalence and correlates of eating disorders in the National Comorbidity Survey Replication. *Biological Psychiatry* 61(3): 348-358.

Hui, S.C., and Yuen, P.Y. 2000. Validity of the modified back-saver sit-and-reach test: A comparison with other protocols. *Medicine & Science in Sports & Exercise* 32: 1655-1659.

Hui, S.C., Yuen, P.Y., Morrow, J.R., and Jackson, A.W. 1999. Comparison of the criterion-related validity of sit-and-reach tests with and without limb length adjustment in Asian adults. *Research Quarterly for Exercise and Sport* 70: 401-406.

Hui, S.S-C., Xie, Y.J., Woo, J., and Kwok, T.C-Y. 2015. Effects of tai chi and walking exercises on weight loss, metabolic syndrome parameters, and bone mineral density: A cluster randomized controlled trial. *Evidence-Based Complementary and Alternative Medicine.* doi:10.1155/2015/976123. Accessed April 16, 2017.

Hulsey, C.R., Soto, D.T., Koch, A.J., and Mayhew, J.L. 2012. Comparison of kettlebell swings and treadmill running at

equivalent rating of perceived values. *Journal of Strength and Conditioning Research* 26: 1203-1207.

Human Kinetics. 1995. *Practical body composition kit.* Champaign, IL: Author.

Hunt, T.N., Ferrara, M.S., Bornstein, R.A., and Baumgartner, T.A. 2009. The reliability of the modified balance error scoring system. *Clinical Journal of Sports Medicine* 19: 471-475.

Hunter, G.R., Brock, D.W., Byrne, N.M., Chandler-Laney, P.C., Del Corral, P., and Gower, B.A. 2010. Exercise training prevents regain of visceral fat for 1 year following weight loss. *Obesity* 18: 690-695.

Hunter, G.R., Wetzstein, C.J., McLafferty, C.L., Zuckerman, P.A., Landers, K.A., and Bamman, M.M. 2001. High-resistance versus variable-resistance training in older adults. *Medicine & Science in Sports & Exercise* 33: 1759-1764.

Hurkmans, H.L., Ribbers, G.M., Streur-Kranenburg, M.F., Stam, H.J., and van den Berg-Emons, R. 2011. Energy expenditure in chronic stroke patients playing Wii Sports: A pilot study. *Journal of NeuroEngineering and Rehabilitation* 8: 38-44.

Hurst, P.R., Walsh, D.C.I., Conlon, C.A., Ingram, M., Kruger, R., and Stonehouse, W. 2016. Validity and reliability of bioelectrical impedance analysis to estimate body fat percentage against air displacement plethysmography and dual-energy X-ray absorptiometry. *Nutrition and Dietetics* 73: 197-204.

Husu, P., and Suni, J. 2012. Predictive validity of health-related fitness tests on back pain and related disability: A 6-year follow-up study among high-functioning older adults. *Journal of Physical Activity and Health* 9: 249-258.

Hyldahl, R.D., and Hubal, M.J. 2014. Lengthening our perspective: Morphological, cellular, and molecular responses to eccentric exercise. *Muscle and Nerve* 49: 155-170.

Idema, R.N., van den Meiracker, A.H., and Imholz, B.P.M. 1989. Comparison of Finapres non-invasive beat-to-beat finger blood pressure with intrabrachial artery pressure during and after bicycle ergometry. *Journal of Hypertension* 7(Suppl. 6): S58-S59.

Ikai, M., and Fukunaga, T. 1968. Calculation of muscle strength per unit cross-sectional area of human muscle by means of ultrasonic measurement. *European Journal of Applied Physiology* 26: 26-32.

Imboden, M.T., Nelson, M.B., Kaminsky, L.A., and Montoye, A.H.K. 2017. Comparison of four Fitbit and Jawbone activity monitors with a research-grade ActiGraph accelerometer for estimating physical activity and energy expenditure. *British Journal of Sports Medicine* 0:1. doi:10.1136/bjsports-2016-096990. Accessed May 18, 2017.

Imtiyaz, S., Veqar, Z., and Shareef, M.Y. 2014. To compare the effect of vibration therapy and massage in prevention of delayed onset muscle soreness (DOMS). *Journal of Clinical and Diagnostic Research* 8: 133-136.

Instebo, A., Helgheim, V., and Greve, G. 2012. Repeatability of blood pressure measurements during treadmill exercise. *Blood Pressure Monitoring* 17: 69-72.

Institute of Medicine. 2002/2005. *Dietary reference intakes for energy, carbohydrates, fiber, fat, fatty acids, cholesterol, protein, and amino acids*. Washington, D.C.: National Academies Press.International Association for the Study of Obesity. 2012. Estimates of relative risk of disease per unit of BMI above 22 kg/m². www.iaso.org/policy/healthimpactobesity/estimatesrelativerisk. Accessed October 5, 2012.

International Atomic Energy Association. 2010. Dual energy X-ray absorptiometry for bone mineral density and body composition assessment. *IAEA Human Health Series* number 15, Vienna.

International Diabetes Foundation. 2006. IDF consensus worldwide definition of the metabolic syndrome. www.idf.org/e-library/consensus-statements.html. Accessed August 14, 2017.

International Osteoporosis Foundation. 2015. Epidemiology. www.iofbonehealth.org/health-professionals/about-osteoporosis/epidemiology.

Invergo, J.J., Ball, T.E., and Looney, M. 1991. Relationship of pushups and absolute muscular endurance to bench press strength. *Journal of Applied Sport Science Research* 5: 121-125.

Irving, B.A., Davis, C.K., Brock, D.W., Weltman, J.Y., Swift, D., Barrett, E.J., Gaesser, G.A., and Weltman, A. 2008. Effect of exercise training intensity on abdominal visceral fat and body composition. *Medicine & Science in Sports & Exercise* 40: 1863-1872.

Isacowitz, R. 2014. *Pilates, 2nd ed.* Champaign, IL: Human Kinetics.

Ishikawa, J., Ishikawa, Y., Edmondson, D., Pickering, T.G., and Schwartz, J.E. 2011. Age and the difference between awake ambulatory blood pressure and office blood pressure: A meta-analysis. *Blood Pressure Monitoring* 16: 159-167.

Ishikawa, S., Kim, Y., Kang, M., and Morgan, D.W. 2013. Effects of weight-bearing exercise on bone health in girls: A meta-analysis. *Sports Medicine* 43: 875-892.

Ismail, I., Keating, S.E., Baker, M.K., and Johnson, N.A. 2012. A systematic review and meta-analysis of the effect of aerobic vs. resistance exercise training on visceral fat. *Obesity Reviews* 13: 68-91.

Ito, T., Shirado, O., Suzuki, H., Takahaski, M., Kaneda, K., and Strax, T.E. 1996. Lumbar trunk muscle endurance testing: An expensive alternative to a machine for evaluation. *Archives of Physical Medicine and Rehabilitation* 77: 75-79.

Jackson, A. 1984. Research design and analysis of data procedures for predicting body density. *Medicine & Science in Sports & Exercise* 16: 616-620.

Jackson, A.S., Ellis, K.J., McFarlin, B.K., Sailors, M.H., and Bray, M.S. 2009. Cross-validation of generalized body composition equations with diverse young men and women: The Training Intervention and Genetics of Exercise Response (TIGER) Study. *British Journal of Nutrition* 101: 871-878.

Jackson, A.S., and Pollock, M.L. 1976. Factor analysis and multivariate scaling of anthropometric variables for the assessment of body composition. *Medicine & Science in Sports & Exercise* 8: 196-203.

Jackson, A.S., and Pollock, M.L. 1978. Generalized equations for predicting body density of men. *British Journal of Nutrition* 40: 497-504.

Jackson, A.S., and Pollock, M.L. 1985. Practical assessment of body composition. *The Physician and Sportsmedicine* 13: 76-90.

Jackson, A.S., Pollock, M.L., Graves, J.E., and Mahar, M.T. 1988. Reliability and validity of bioelectrical impedance in determining body composition. *Journal of Applied Physiology* 64: 529-534.

Jackson, A.S., Pollock, M.L., and Ward, A. 1980. Generalized equations for predicting body density of women. *Medicine & Science in Sports & Exercise* 12: 175-182.

Jackson, A.W., and Langford, N.J. 1989. The criterion-related validity of the sit-and-reach test: Replication and extension of previous findings. *Research Quarterly for Exercise and Sport* 60: 384-387.

Jackson, A.W., Morrow, J.R., Brill, P.A., Kohl, H.W., Gordon, N.F., and Blair, S.N. 1998. Relations of sit-up and sit-and-reach tests to low back pain in adults. *Journal of Orthopaedic and Sports Physical Therapy* 27: 22-26.

Jäger, R., Kerksick, C.M., Campbell, B.I., Cribb, P.J., Wells, S.D., Skwiat, T.M., Purpura, M., Ziegenfuss, T.N., Ferrando, A.A., Arent, S.M., Smith-Ryan, A.E., Stout, J.R., Arciero, P.J., Ormsbee, M.J., Taylor, L.W., Wilborn, C.D., Kalman, D.S., Kreider, R.B., Willoughby, D.S., Hoffman, J.R., Krzykowski, J.L., and Antonio, J. 2017. International society of sports nutrition position stand: Protein and exercise. *Journal of the International Society of Sports Nutrition* 14: 20.

Jahnke, R., Larkey, L., Rogers, C., Etnier, J., and Lin, F. 2010. A comprehensive review of health benefits of qigong and tai chi. *American Journal of Health Promotion* 24: e1-e25.

Jakicic, J.M., Davis, K.K., Rogers, R.J., King, W.C., Marcus, M.D., Helsel, D., Rickman, A.D., Wahed, A.S., and Belle, S.H. 2016. Effect of wearable technology combined with a lifestyle intervention on long-term weight loss: The IDEA randomized clinical trial. *Journal of the American Medical Association* 316(11): 1161-1171.

James, P.A., Oparil, S., Carter, B.L., Cushman, W.C., Dennison-Himmelfarb, C., Handler, J., Lackland, D.T., LeFevre, M.L., MacKenzie, T.D., Ogedegbe, O., Smith, S.C. Jr., Svetkey, L.P., Taler, S.J., Townsend, R.R., Wright, J.T. Jr., Narva, A.S., and Ortiz, E. 2014. 2014 Evidence-based guideline for the management of high blood pressure in adults: Report from the panel members appointed to the Eighth Joint National Committee (JNC8). *Journal of the American Medical Association* 311: 507-520.

Jankowska, M.M., Schipperijn, J., and Kerr, J. 2015. A framework for using GPS in physical activity and sedentary behavior studies. *Exercise and Sport Sciences Reviews* 43: 48-56.

Jankowski, M., Niedzielska, A., Brzezinski, M., and Drabik, J. 2015. Cardiorespiratory fitness in children: A simple screening test for population studies. *Pediatric Cardiology* 36(1): 27-32.

Janssen, P. 2001. *Lactate Threshold Training*. Champaign, IL: Human Kinetics.

Jay, K., Frisch, D., Hansen, K., Zebis, M.K., Andersen, C.H., Mortensen, O.S., and Andersen, L.L. 2011. Kettlebell training for musculoskeletal and cardiovascular health: A randomized controlled trial. *Scandinavian Journal of Work, Environment and Health* 37: 196-203.

Jdanov, D.A., Deev, A.D., Jasilionis, D., Shalnova, S.A., Shkolnikova, M.A., and Shkolnikov, V.M. 2014. Recalibration of the SCORE risk chart for the Russian population. *European Journal of Epidemiology* 29: 621-628.

Jeans, E.A., Foster, C., Porcari, J.P., Gibson, M., and Doberstein, S. 2011. Translation of exercise testing to exercise prescription using the Talk Test. *Journal of Strength and Conditioning Research* 25: 590-596.

Jenkins, W.L., Thackaberry, M., and Killian, C. 1984. Speed-specific isokinetic training. *Journal of Orthopaedic and Sports Physical Therapy* 6: 181-183.

Jeter, P.E., Nkodo, A-F., Moonaz, S.H., and Dagnelie, G. 2014. A systematic review of yoga for balance in a healthy population. *Journal of Alternative and Complementary Medicine* 20: 221-232.

Johansson, J., Nordström, A., and Nordström, P. 2015. Objectively measured physical activity is associated with parameters of bone in 70-year-old men and women. *Bone* 81: 72-79.

Johns, R.J., and Wright, V. 1962. Relative importance of various tissues in joint stiffness. *Journal of Applied Physiology* 17: 824-828.

Johnson, A.W., Mitchell, U.H., Meek, K., and Feland, J.B. 2014. Hamstring flexibility increases the same with 3 or 9 repetitions of stretching held for a total time of 90s. *Physical Therapy in Sport* 15: 101-105.

Johnson, B.L., and Nelson, J.K., eds. 1986. *Practical measurements for evaluation in physical education.* Minneapolis: Burgess.

Jones, B.H., and Knapik, J.J. 1999. Physical training and exercise-related injuries. *Sports Medicine* 27: 111-125.

Jones, C.J., Rikli, R.E., Max, J., and Noffal, G. 1998. The reliability and validity of a chair sit-and-reach test as a measure of hamstring flexibility in older adults. *Research Quarterly for Exercise and Sport* 69: 338-343.

Jones, D.W., Frohlich, E.D., Grim, C.M., Grim, C.E., and Taubert, K.A. 2001. Mercury sphygmomanometers should not be abandoned: An advisory statement from the Council for High Blood Pressure Research, American Heart Association. *Hypertension* 37: 185-186.

Jones, H.A., Putt, G.E., Rabinovitch, A.E., Hubbard, R., and Snipes, D. 2017. Parenting stress, readiness to change, and child externalizing behaviors in families of clinically referred children. *Journal of Child and Family Studies* 26: 225-233.

Jones, M.T., and Lorenzo, D.C. 2013. Assessment of power, speed, and agility in athletic, preadolescent youth. *Journal of Sports Medicine and Physical Fitness* 53: 693-700.

Jørstad, J.T., Boekholdt, S.M., Wareham, N.J., Khaw, K.T., and Peters, R.J.G. 2017. The Dutch SCORE-based risk charts seriously underestimate the risk of cardiovascular disease. *Netherlands Heart Journal* 25: 173-180.

Joshua, A.M., D'Souza, V., Unnikrishnan, B., Mithra, P., Kamath, A., Acharya, V., and Venugopal, A. 2014. Effectiveness of progressive resistance training versus traditional balance exercise in improving balance among the elderly—a randomized controlled trial. *Journal of Clinical and Diagnostic Research* 8: 98-102.

Jowko, E., Ostaszewski, P., and Jank, M. 2001. Creatine and β-hydroxy-β-methylbutyrate (HMB) additively increase lean body mass and muscle strength during weight-training program. *Nutrition* 17: 558-566.

Judex, S., and Rubin, C.T. 2010. Is bone formation induced by high-frequency mechanical signals modulated by muscle activity? 2010. *Journal of Musculoskeletal and Neuronal Interactions* 10: 3-11.

Juker, D., McGill, S., Kropf, P., and Steffen, T. 1998. Quantitative intramuscular myoelectric activity of lumbar portions of psoas and the abdominal wall during a wide variety of tasks. *Medicine & Science in Sports & Exercise* 30: 301-310.

Kahn, H.S., Gu, Q., Bullard, K.M., Freedman, D.S., Ahluwalia, N., and Ogden, C.L. 2014. Population distribution of the sagittal abdominal diameter (SAD) from a representative sample of US adults: Comparison of SAD, waist circumference and body mass index for identifying dysglycemia. *PLoS One* 9(10): e108707. doi:10.1371/journal.pone.0108707. Accessed August 14, 2017.

Kahraman, B.O., Sengul, Y.S., Kahraman, T., and Kalemci, O. 2016. Developing a reliable core stability assessment battery for patients with nonspecific low back pain. *Spine* 41: E844-E850.

Kallioinen, N., Hill, A., Horswill, M.S., Ward, H.E., and Watson, M.O., 2017. Sources of inaccuracy in the measurement of adult patients' resting blood pressure in clinical settings: A systematic review. *Journal of Hypertension* 35: 421-441.

Kalisch, T., Kattenstroth, J.C., Noth, S., Tegenthoff, M., and Dinse, H.R. 2011. Rapid assessment of age-related differences in standing balance. *Journal of Aging Research* 2011: 160490. doi:10.4061/2011/160490. Accessed November 2012.

Kametas, N.A., McAuliffe, F., Krampl, E., Nicolaides, K.H., and Shennan, A.H. 2006. Can aneroid sphygmomanometers be used at altitude? *Journal of Human Hypertension* 20: 517-522.

Kaminsky, L.A., and Whaley, M.H. 1998. Evaluation of a new standardized ramp protocol: The BSU/Bruce ramp protocol. *Journal of Cardiopulmonary Rehabilitation* 18: 438-444.

Kamioka, H., Tsutani, K., Katsumata, Y., Yoshizaki, T., Okuizumi, H., Okada, S., Park, S.J., Kitayuguchi, J., Abe, T., and Mutoh, Y. 2016. Effectiveness of Pilates exercise: A quality evaluation and summary of systematic reviews based on randomized controlled trials. *Complementary Therapies in Medicine* 25: 1-19.

Kanis, J.A., Borgstrom, F., De Laet, C., Johansson, H., Johnell, O., Jonsson, B., Oden, A., Zethraeus, N., Pfleger, B., and Khaltaev, N. 2005. Assessment of fracture risk. *Osteoporosis International* 16: 581-589.

Kanis, J.A., Oden, A., McCloskey, E.V., Johansson, H., Wahl, D.A., and Cooper, C. 2012. A systematic review of hip fracture incidence and probability of fracture.

Katanista, A., Król-Zieli⊠ska, M., Borowiec, J., Glapa, A., Lisowski, P., and Bronikowski, M. 2015. Physical activity of female children and adolescents based on step counts: Meeting the recommendation and relation to VMI. *Biomedical Human Kinetics* 7: 66-72.

Katch, F.I., Clarkson, P.M., Kroll, W., McBride, T., and Wilcox, A. 1984. Effects of sit-up exercise training on adipose cell size and adiposity. *Research Quarterly for Exercise and Sport* 55: 242-247.

Katch, F.I., McArdle, W.D., Czula, R., and Pechar, G.S. 1973. Maximal oxygen intake, endurance running performance, and body composition in college women. *Research Quarterly* 44: 301-312.

Kattus, A.A., Hanafee, W.N., Longmire, W.P., MacAlpin, R.N., and Rivin, A.U. 1968. Diagnosis, medical and surgical management of coronary insufficiency. *Annals of Internal Medicine* 69: 115-136.

Kaur, J. 2014. A comprehensive review on metabolic syndrome. *Cardiology Research and Practice.* doi:10.1155/2014/943162. Accessed April 13, 2017.

Kay, A.D., Dods, S., and Blazevich, A.J. 2016. Acute effects of contract-relax (CR) stretch versus a modified CR technique. *European Journal of Applied Physiology* 116: 611-621.

Keim, N.L., Blanton, C.A., and Kretsch, M.J. 2004. America's obesity epidemic: Measuring physical activity to promote an active lifestyle. *Journal of the American Dietetic Association* 104: 1398-1409.

Kell, A.B. 2011. The influence of periodized resistance training on strength changes in men and women. *Journal of Strength and Conditioning Research* 25: 735-744.

Kelley, G.A., and Kelley, K.S. 2006. Aerobic exercise and lipids and lipoproteins in men: A meta-analysis of randomized controlled trials. *Journal of Men's Health & Gender* 3(1): 61-70.

Kendall, K.L., Fukuda, D.H., Hyde, P.N., Smith-Ryan, A.E., Moon, J.R., and Stout, J.R. 2017. Estimating fat-free mass in elite-level male rowers: A four-compartment model validation of laboratory and field methods. *Journal of Sports Sciences* 35(7): 624-633.

Kendrick, D., Kumar, A., Carpenter, H., Zijlstra, G.A., Skelton, D.A., Cook, J.R., Stevens, Z., Belcher, C.M., Haworth, D., Gawler, S.J., Gage, H., Masud, T., Bowling, A., Pearl, M., Morris, R.W., Iliffe, S., and Delbaere, K. 2014. Exercise for reducing fear of falling in older people living in the community. *Cochrane Database of Systematic Reviews* 11: CD009848.

Kerr, A., Slater, G.J., Byrne, N., and Nana, A. 2016. Reliability of 2 different positioning protocols for dual-energy X-ray absorptiometry measurement of body composition in healthy adults. *Journal of Clinical Densitometry: Assessment & Management of Musculoskeletal Health* 19: 282-289.

Kesäniemi, A., Riddoch, C.J., Reeder, B., Blair, S.N., and Sorensen, T.I.A. 2010. Advancing the future of physical activity guidelines in Canada: An independent expert panel interpretation of the evidence. *International Journal of Behavioral Nutrition and Physical Activity* 7: 41. www.ijbnpa.org/content/7/1/41. Accessed August 25, 2012.

Kessler, H.S., Sisson, S.B., and Short, K.R. 2012. The potential for high-intensity interval training to reduce cardiometabolic disease risk. *Sports Medicine* 42: 489-509.

Keys, A., and Brozek, J. 1953. Body fat in adult man. *Physiological Reviews* 33: 245-325.

Khaled, M.A., McCutcheon, M.J., Reddy, S., Pearman, P.L., Hunter, G.R., and Weinsier, R.L. 1988. Electrical impedance in assessing human body composition: The BIA method. *American Journal of Clinical Nutrition* 47: 789-792.

Kibar, S., Yardimci, F.O., Evcik, D., Ay, S., Alhan, A., Manco, M., and Ergin, E.S. 2016. Can a Pilates exercise program be effective on balance, flexibility and muscle endurance? A randomized controlled trial. *Journal of Sports Medicine and Physical Fitness* 56: 1139-1146.

Kibler, W.B., Press, J., and Sciascia, A. 2006. The role of core stability in athletic function. *Sports Medicine* 36: 189-198.

Kidgell, D.J., and Pearce, A.J. 2011. What has transcranial magnetic stimulation taught us about neural adaptations to strength training? A brief review. *Journal of Strength and Conditioning Research* 25: 3208-3217.

Kidgell, D.J., Stokes, M.A., Castricum, T.J., and Pearce, A.J. 2010. Neurophysiological responses after short-term strength training of the biceps brachii muscle. *Journal of Strength and Conditioning Research* 24: 3123-3132.

Kim, H.I., Kim, J.T., Yu, S.H., Kwak, S.H., Jang, H.C., Park, K.S., Kim, S.Y., Lee, H.K., and Cho, Y.M. 2011. Gender differences in diagnostic values of visceral fat and waist circumference for predicting metabolic syndrome in Koreans. *Journal of Korean Medicine and Science* 26: 906-913.

Kim, J.C., Chon, J., Kim, H.S., Lee, J.H., Yoo, S.D., Kim, D.H., Lee, S.A., Han, Y.J., Lee, H.S., Lee, B.Y., Soh, Y.S., and Won, C.W. 2017. The association between fall history and physical performance tests in the community-dwelling elderly: A cross-sectional analysis. *Annals of Rehabilitation Medicine* 41(2): 239-247.

Kim, J.H., Ko, J.H., Lee, D., Lim, I., and Bang, H. 2012. Habitual physical exercise has beneficial effects on telomere length in postmenopausal women. *Menopause* 19. doi:10.1097/gme.0b013e3182503e97.

Kim, P.S., Mayhew, J.L., and Peterson, D.F. 2002. A modified bench press test as a predictor of 1 repetition maximum bench press strength. *Journal of Strength and Conditioning Research* 16: 440-445.

Kim, Y., and Welk, G.J. 2015. Criterion validity of competing accelerometry-based activity monitoring devices. *Medicine & Science in Sports & Exercise* 47: 2456-2463.

Kirby, R.L., Simms, F.C., Symington, V.J., and Garner, J.B. 1981. Flexibility and musculoskeletal symptomatology in female gymnasts and age-matched controls. *American Journal of Sports Medicine* 9: 160-164.

Klein, I.E., White, J.B., and Rana, S.R. 2016. Comparison of physiological variables between the elliptical bicycle and run training in experienced runners. *Journal of Strength and Conditioning Research* 30: 2998-3006.

Klein, P.J., Fiedler, R.C., and Rose, D.J. 2011. Rasch analysis of the Fullerton advanced balance (FAB) scale. *Physiotherapy Canada* 63: 115-125.

Klein, S., Allison, D.B., Heymsfield, S.B., Kelley, D.E., Leibel, R.L., Nonas, C., and Kahn, R. 2007. Waist circumference and cardiometabolic risk: A consensus statement from Shaping America's Health: Association for Weight Management and Obesity Prevention; NAASO, the Obesity Society; the American Society for Nutrition; and the American Diabetes Association. *American Journal of Clinical Nutrition* 85: 1197-1202.

Kline, G.M., Porcari, J.P., Hintermeister, R., Freedson, P.S., Ward, A., McCarron, R.F., Ross, J., and Rippe, J.M. 1987. Estimation of $\dot{V}O_2$max from a one-mile track walk, gender, age, and body weight. *Medicine & Science in Sports & Exercise* 19: 253-259.

Kloubec, J. 2011. Pilates: How does it work and who needs it? *Muscles, Ligaments and Tendons Journal* 1: 61-66.

Knapik, J.J. 2015. Extreme conditioning programs: Potential benefits and potential risks. *Journal of Special Operations Medicine* 15(3): 108-113.

Knight, A.C., Holmes, M.E., Chander, H., Kimble, A., and Stewart, J.T. 2016. Assessment of balance among adolescent track and field athletes. *Sports Biomechanics* 15: 169-179.

Knight, E., Stuckey, M.I., and Petrella, R.J. 2014. Validation of the step test and exercise prescription tool for adults. *Canadian Journal of Diabetes* 38: 164-171.

Knight, H., Stetson, B., Krishnasamy, S., and Mokshagundam, S.P. 2015. Diet self-management and readiness to change in underserved adults with type 2 diabetes. *Primary Care Diabetes* 9: 219-215.

Knudson, D. 2001. The validity of recent curl-up tests in young adults. *Journal of Strength and Conditioning Research* 15: 81-85.

Knudson, D., and Johnston, D. 1995. Validity and reliability of a bench trunk-curl test of abdominal endurance. *Journal of Strength and Conditioning Research* 9: 165-169.

Knudson, D.V. 1999. Issues in abdominal fitness: Testing and technique. *Journal of Physical Education, Recreation & Dance* 70(3): 49-55.

Knudson, D.V., Magnusson, P., and McHugh, M. 2000. Current issues in flexibility fitness. *President's Council on Physical Fitness and Sports Research Digest* 3(10): 1-8.

Knuttgen, H.G., and Kraemer, W.J. 1987. Terminology and measurement in exercise performance. *Journal of Applied Sport Science Research* 1: 1-10.

Knutzen, K.M., Brilla, L.R., and Caine, D. 1999. Validity of 1RM prediction equations for older adults. *Journal of Strength and Conditioning Research* 13: 242-246.

Komi, P.V., Viitasalo, J.T., Rauramaa, R., and Vihko, V. 1978. Effect of isometric strength training on mechanical, electrical, and metabolic aspects of muscle function. *European Journal of Applied Physiology* 40: 45-55.

Konrad, A., Stafilidis, S., and Tilp, M. 2017. Effects of acute static, ballistic, and PNF stretching exercise on the muscle and tendon tissue properties. *Scandinavian Journal of Medicine & Science in Sports* 27(10): 1070-1080.

Kosek, D.J., Kim, J.S., Petrella, J.K., Cross, J.M., and Bamman, M.M. 2006. Efficacy of 3 days/wk resistance training on myofiber hypertrophy and myogenic mechanisms in young vs. older adults. *Journal of Applied Physiology* 101: 531-544.

Kostek, M.A., Pescatello, L.S., Seip, R.L., Angelopoulos, T.J., Clarkson, P.M., Gordon, P.M., Moyna, N.M., Visich, P.S., Zoeller, R.F., Thompson, P.D., Hoffman, R.P., and Price, T.B. 2007. Subcutaneous fat alterations resulting from an upper-body resistance training program. *Medicine & Science in Sports & Exercise* 39: 1177-1185.

Kotanidou, E.P., Grammatikopoulou, M.G., Spiliotis, B.E., Kanaka-Gantenbein, C., Tsigga, M., and Galli-Tsinopoulou, A. 2013. Ten-year obesity and overweight prevalence in Greek children: A systematic review and meta-analysis of 2001-2010. *Hormones* 12: 537-549.

Koulmann, N., Jimenez, C., Regal, D., Bolliet, P., Launay, J., Savourey, G., and Melin, B. 2000. Use of bioelectrical impedance analysis to estimate body fluid compartments after acute variations of the body hydration level. *Medicine & Science in Sports & Exercise* 32: 857-864.

Kraemer, W.J. 2003. Strength training basics. *The Physician and Sportsmedicine* 31(8): 39-45.

Kraemer, W.J., and Fleck, S.J. 2007. *Optimizing strength training.* Champaign, IL: Human Kinetics.

Kraemer, W.J., Fleck, S.J., and Evans, W.J. 1996. Strength and power training: Physiological mechanisms of adaptation. In *Exercise and Sport Sciences Reviews,* ed. J.O. Holloszy, 363-397. Baltimore: Williams & Wilkins.

Kraemer, W.J., Gordon, S.J., Fleck, S.J., Marchitelli, L.J., Mello, R., Dziados, J.E., Friedl, K., Harman, E., Maresh, C., and Fry, A.C. 1991. Endogenous anabolic hormonal and growth factor responses to heavy resistance exercise in males and females. *International Journal of Sports Medicine* 12: 228-235.

Kraemer, W.J., Häkkinen, K., Newton, R.U., Nindl, B.C., Volek, J.S., McCormick, M., Gotshalk, L.A., Gordon, S.E., Fleck, S.J., Campbell, W.W., Putukian, M., and Evans, W.J. 1999. Effects of heavy-resistance training on hormonal response patterns in younger vs. older men. *Journal of Applied Physiology* 87: 982-992.

Kraemer, W.J., Hooper, D.R., Szivak, T.K., Kupchak, B.R., Dunn-Lewis, C., Comstock, B.A., Flanagan, S.D., Looney, D.P., Sterczala, A.J., DuPont, W.H., Pryor, J.L., Luk, H.Y., Maladoungdock, J., McDermott, D., Volek, J.S., and Maresh, C.M. 2015. The addition of beta-hydroxy-beta-methylbutyrate and isomaltulose to whey protein improves recovery from highly demanding resistance exercise. *Journal of the American College of Nutrition* 34(2): 91-99.

Kraemer, W.J., Noble, B.J., Clark, M.J., and Culver, B.W. 1987. Physiologic responses to heavy-resistance exercise with very short rest periods. *International Journal of Sports Medicine* 8: 247-252.

Kraemer, W.J., and Ratamess, N.A. 2004. Fundamentals of resistance training: Progression and exercise prescription. *Medicine & Science in Sports & Exercise* 36: 674-688.

Kraemer, W.J., Volek, J.S., Clark, K.L., Gordon, S.E., Puhl, S.M., Koziris, L.P., McBride, J.M., Triplett-McBride, N.T., Putukian, M., Newton, R.U., Häkkinen, K., Bush, J.A., and Sabastianelli, W.J. 1999. Influence of exercise training on physiological and performance changes with weight loss in men. *Medicine & Science in Sports & Exercise* 31: 1320-1329.

Kravitz, L., Heyward, V., Stolarczyk, L., and Wilmerding, V. 1997a. Effects of step training with and without handweights on physiological profiles of women. *Journal of Strength and Conditioning Research* 11: 194-199.

Kravitz, L., and Heyward, V.H. 1995. Flexibility training. *Fitness Management* 11(2): 32-38.

Kravitz, L., Robergs, R., and Heyward, V. 1996. Are all aerobic exercise modes equal? *Idea Today* 14: 51-58.

Kravitz, L., Robergs, R.A., Heyward, V.H., Wagner, D.R., and Powers, K. 1997b. Exercise mode and gender comparisons of energy expenditure at self-selected intensities. *Medicine & Science in Sports & Exercise* 29: 1028-1035.

Kravitz, L., Wax, B., Mayo, J.J., Daniels, R., and Charette, K. 1998. Metabolic response of elliptical exercise training. *Medicine & Science in Sports & Exercise* 30(Suppl.): S169 [abstract].

Kraus, H. 1970. *Clinical treatment of back and neck pain.* New York: McGraw-Hill.

Krause, M.P., Goss, F.L., Robertson, R.J., Kim, K., Elsangedy, H.M., Keinski, K., and da Silva, S.G. 2012. Concurrent validity of an OMNI rating of perceived exertion scale for bench stepping exercise. *Journal of Strength and Conditioning Research* 26: 506-512.

Kreider, R.B., Wilborn, C.D., Taylor, L., Campbell, B., Almada, A.L., Collins, R., Cooke, M., Earnest, C.P., Greenwood, M., Kalman, D.S., Kersick, C.M., Kleiner, S.M., Leutholtz, B., Lopez, H., Lowery, L.M., Mendel, R., Smith, A., Spano, M., Wildman, R., Willoughby, D.S., Ziegenfuss, T.N., and Antonio, J. 2010. ISSN exercise & sport nutrition review: Research & recommendations. *Journal of the International Society of Sports Nutrition* 7: 6-43.

Krieger, J.W. 2010. Single vs. multiple sets of resistance exercise for muscle hypertrophy: A meta-analysis. *Journal of Strength and Conditioning Research* 24: 1150-1159.

Krishnan, S., Tokar, T.N., Boylan, M.M., Griffin, K., McMurry, L., Esperat, C., and Cooper, J.A. 2015. Zumba® dance improves health in overweight/obese or type 2 diabetic women. *American Journal of Health Behavior* 39: 109-120.

Kruger, J., Yore, M.M., and Kohl, H.W. 2007. Leisure-time physical activity patterns by weight control status: 1999-2002 NHANES. *Medicine & Science in Sports & Exercise* 39: 788-795.

Kubo, K., Kaneshisa, H., Takeshita, D., Kawakami, Y., Fukashiro, S., and Fukunaga, T. 2000. In vivo dynamics of human medial gastrocnemius muscle-tendon complex curing stretch-shortening cycle exercise. *Acta Physiologica Scandinavica* 170: 127-135.

Kubo, K., Kawakami, Y., and Fukunaga, T. 1999. Influence of elastic properties of tendon structures on jump performance in humans. *Journal of Applied Physiology* 87: 2090-2096.

Kumar, N., Khunger, M., Gupta, A., and Garg, N. 2015. A content analysis of smartphone-based applications for hypertension management. *Journal of the American Society of Hypertension* 9: 130-136.

Kuramoto, A.K., and Payne, V.G. 1995. Predicting muscular strength in women: A preliminary study. *Research Quarterly for Exercise and Sport* 66: 168-172.

Kurucz, R., Fox, E.L., and Mathews, D.K. 1969. Construction of a submaximal cardiovascular step test. *Research Quarterly* 40: 115-122.

Kushner, R.F. 1992. Bioelectrical impedance analysis: A review of principles and applications. *Journal of the American College of Nutrition* 11: 199-209.

Kushner, R.F., Gudivaka, R., and Schoeller, D.A. 1996. Clinical characteristics influencing bioelectrical impedance analysis measurements. *American Journal of Clinical Nutrition* 64: 423S-427S.

Kushner, R.F., and Schoeller, D.A. 1986. Estimation of total body water in bioelectrical impedance analysis. *American Journal of Clinical Nutrition* 44: 417-424.

Kuukkanen, T., and Malkia, E. 2000. Effects of a three-month therapeutic exercise programme on flexibility in subjects with low back pain. *Physiotherapy Research International* 5: 46-61.

Kwak, D.H., and Ryu, Y.U. 2015. Applying proprioceptive neuromuscular facilitation stretching: Optimal contraction intensity to attain the maximum increase in range of motion in young males. *Journal of Physical Therapy Science* 27: 2129-2032.

Kwon, S., Janz, K.F., Letuchy, E.M., Burns, T.L., and Levy, S.M. 2015. Active lifestyle in childhood and adolescence prevents obesity development in young adulthood: Iowa Bone Development Study. *Obesity (Silver Springs)* 23: 2462-2469.

Kyle, U.G., Genton, L., Karsegard, L., Slosman, D.O., and Pichard, C. 2001. Single prediction equation for bioelectrical impedance analysis in adults aged 20-94 years. *Nutrition* 17: 248-253.

Lacour, J-R., and Bourdin, M. 2015. Factors affecting the energy cost of level running at submaximal speed. *European Journal of Applied Physiology* 115(4): 651-673.

Lake, J.P., and Lauder, M.A. 2012. Kettlebell swing training improves maximal and explosive strength. *Journal of Strength and Conditioning Research* 26: 2228-2233.

Lakhal, K., Ehrmann, S., Martin, M., Faiz, S., Réminiac, F., Cinotti, R., Capdevila, X., Asehnoune, K., Blanloeil, Y., Rozec, B., and Boulain, T. 2015. Blood pressure monitoring during arrhythmia: Agreement between automatic brachial cuff and intra-arterial measurements. *British Journal of Anaesthesia* 115: 540-549.

Lambrick, D., Jakeman, J., Grigg, R., Kaufmann, S., and Faulkner, J. 2017. The efficacy of a discontinuous graded exercise test in measuring peak oxygen update in children aged 8 to 10 years. *Biology of Sport* 34: 57-61.

Landram, M.J., Utter, A.C., Baldari, C., Guidetti, L., McAnulty, S.R., and Collier, S.R. 2016. Differential effects of continuous versus discontinuous aerobic training on blood pressure and hemodynamics. doi:10.1519/JSC.0000000000001661. Accessed July 20, 2017.

Larsen, G.E., George, J.D., Alexander, J.L., Fellingham, G.W., Aldana, S.G., and Parcell, A.C. 2002. Prediction of maximum oxygen consumption from walking, jogging, or running. *Research Quarterly for Exercise and Sport* 73: 66-72.

LaStayo, P., Marcus, R., Dibble, L., Frajacomo, F., and Lindstedt, S. 2014. Eccentric exercise in rehabilitation: Safety, feasibility, and application. *Journal of Applied Physiology* 116: 1426-1434.

Lau, R.W.K., Liao, L-R., Yu, F., Teo, T., Chung, R.C.K., and Pang, M.Y.C. 2011. The effects of whole body vibration therapy on bone mineral density and leg muscle strength in older adults: A systematic review and meta-analysis. *Clinical Rehabilitation* 25: 975-988.

Lauby-Secretan, B., Scoccianti, C., Loomis, D., Grosse, Y., Bianchini, F., and Straif, K. 2016. Body fatness and cancer—Viewpoint of the IARC Working Group. *New England Journal of Medicine* 375(8): 794-798.

Lavie, C.J., McAuley, P.A., Church, T.S., Milani, R.V., and Blair, S.N. 2014. Obesity and cardiovascular diseases: Implications regarding fitness, fatness, and severity in the Obesity Paradox. *Journal of the American College of Cardiology* 63: 1345-1354.

Law, R.Y.W., and Herbert, R.D. 2007. Warm-up reduces delayed-onset muscle soreness but cool-down does not: A randomized controlled trial. *Australian Journal of Physiotherapy* 53: 91-95.

Layne, J.E., and Nelson, M.E. 1999. The effects of progressive resistance training on bone density: A review. *Medicine & Science in Sports & Exercise* 31: 25-30.

Leahy, S., O'Neill, C., Sohun, R., and Jakeman, P. 2012. A comparison of dual energy X-ray absorptiometry and bioelectrical impedance analysis to measure total and segmental body composition in healthy young adults. *European Journal of Applied Physiology* 112: 589-595.

Leal, V.O., Moraes, C., Stockler-Pinto, M.B., Lobo, J.C., Farage, N.E., Velarde, L.G., Fouque, D., and Mafra, D. 2012. Is a body mass index of 23 kg/m^2 a reliable marker of protein-energy wasting in hemodialysis patients? *Nutrition* 28: 973-977.

Leard, J.S., Cirillo, M.A., Katsnelson, E., Kimiatek, D.A., Miller, T.W., Trebincevic, K., and Garbalosa, J.C. 2007. Validity of two alternative systems for measuring vertical jump height. *Journal of Strength and Conditioning Research* 21: 1296-1299.

LeBoeuf, S.F., Aumer, M.E., Kraus, W.E., Johnson, J.L., and Duscha, B. 2014. Earbud-based sensor for the assessment of energy expenditure, HR, and $\dot{V}O_2$max. *Medicine & Science in Sports & Exercise* 46: 1046-1052.

Lee, I-M., Shiroma, E.J., Lobelo, F., Puska, P., Blair, S.N., and Katzmarzyk, P.T. 2012. Impact of physical inactivity on the world's major non-communicable diseases. *Lancet* 380: 219-229. doi:10.1016/S0140-6736(12)61031-9.

Lee, J.A., Williams, S.M., Brown, D.D., and Laurson, K.R. 2015. Concurrent validation of the Actigraph gt3x+, Polar Active accelerometer, Omron HJ-720 and Yamax Digiwalker SW-701 pedometer step counts in lab-based and free-living settings. *Journal of Sports Sciences.* 33: 991-1000.

Lee, M.S., and Ernst, E. 2012. Systematic reviews of t'ai chi: An overview. *British Journal of Sports Medicine* 46: 713-718.

Leger, L.A., Mercier, D., Gadoury, C., and Lambert, J. 1988. The multistage 20-metre shuttle run test for aerobic fitness. *Journal of Sports Sciences* 6: 93-101.

Leighton, J.R. 1955. An instrument and technique for measurement of range of joint motion. *Archives of Physical Medicine and Rehabilitation* 36: 571-578.

Leitzmann, M., Powers, H., Anderson, A.S., Scoccianti, C., Berrino, F., Boutron-Ruault, M-C., Cecchini, M., Espina, C., Key, T.I., Norat, T., Wiseman, M., and Romier, I., 2015. European code against cancer 4th edition: Physical activity and cancer. *Cancer Epidemiology* 39S: S46-S55.

Leonska-Duniec, A., Jastrzebski, Z., Zarebska, A., Maciejewska, A., Ficek, K., and Cieszczyk, P. 2017. Assessing effect of interaction between the FTO A/T polymorphism (rs9939609) and physical activity on obesity-related traits. *Journal of Sport and Health Science.* Advance online publication. doi:10.1016/j.jshs.2016.08.013.

Lesinski, M., Hortobagyi, T., Muehlbauer, T., Gollhofer, A., and Granacher, U. 2015. Dose-response relationships of balance training in healthy young adults: A systematic review and meta-analysis. *Sports Medicine* 45: 557-576.

Lesmes, G.R., Costill, D.L., Coyle, E.F., and Fink, W.J. 1978. Muscle strength and power changes during maximal isokinetic training. *Medicine and Science in Sports* 10: 266-269.

Levine, B., Zuckerman, J., and Cole, C. 1998. Medical complications of exercise. In *ACSM's resource manual for guidelines for exercise testing and prescription*, ed. J.L. Roitman, 488-498. Philadelphia: Lippincott Williams & Wilkins.

Levine, J.A. 2015. Sick of sitting. *Diabetologia* 58: 1751-1758.

Lewis, P.B., Ruby, D., and Bush-Joseph, C.A. 2012. Muscle soreness and delayed-onset muscle soreness. *Clinics in Sports Medicine* 31: 255-262.

Li, S., Zhao, X., Ba, S., He, G., Lam, C.T., Ke, L., Li, N., Yan, L.L., Li, X., and Wu, Y. 2012. Can electronic sphygmomanometers be used for measurement of blood pressure at high altitudes? *Blood Pressure Monitoring* 17: 62-68.

Liang, M.T.C., Su, H., and Lee, N. 2000. Skin temperature and skin blood flow affect bioelectrical impedance study of female fat-free mass. *Medicine & Science in Sports & Exercise* 32: 221-227.

Liang, M.Y., and Norris, S. 1993. Effects of skin blood flow and temperature on bioelectrical impedance after exercise. *Medicine & Science in Sports & Exercise* 25: 1231-1239.

Liebenson, C. 2011. Functional training with the kettlebell. *Journal of Bodywork and Movement Therapies* 15: 542-544.

Lim, S., Kim, J.H., Yoon, J.W., Kang, S.M., Choi, S.H., Park, Y.J., Kim, K.W., Cho, N.H., Shin, H., Park, K.S., and Jang, H.C. 2012. Optimal cut points of waist circumference (WC) and visceral fat area (VFA) predicting for metabolic syndrome (MetS) in elderly population in the Korean Longitudinal Study on Health and Aging (KLoSHA). *Archives of Gerontology and Geriatrics* 54: E29 -E34.

Lin, H-T., Hung, W-C., Hung, J-L., Wu, P.S., Liaw, L-J., and Chang, J-H. 2016. Effects of Pilates on patients with chronic non-specific low back pain: A systematic review. *Journal of Physical Therapy Science* 28: 2961-2969.

Lin, X., Zhang, X., Guo, J., Roberts, C.K., McKenzie, S., Wu, W-C., Liu, S., and Song, Y. 2015. Effects of exercise training on cardiorespiratory fitness and biomarkers of cardiometabolic health: A systematic review and meta-analysis of randomized controlled trials. *Journal of the American Heart Association* 4: e002014. doi:10.1161/JAHA.115.002014.

Litchell, H., and Boberg, J. 1978. The lipoprotein lipase activity of adipose tissue from different sites in obese women and relationship to cell size. *International Journal of Obesity* 2: 47-52.

Liu, S., Brooks, D., Thomas, S., Eysenbach, G., and Nolan, R.P. 2015. Lifesource XL-18 pedometer for measuring steps under controlled and free-living conditions. *Journal of Sports Sciences* 33: 1001-1006.

Liu, H., and Frank, A. 2010. Tai chi as a balance improvement exercise for older adults: A systematic review. *Journal of Geriatric Physical Therapy* 33: 103-109.

Lixandrão, M.E., Damas, F., Chacon-Mikahil, M.P., Cavaglieri, C.R., Ugrinowitsch, C., Bottaro, M., Vechin, F.C., Conceição, M.S., Berton, R., and Libardi, C.A. 2016. Time course of resistance training-induced muscle hypertrophy in the elderly. *Journal of Strength and Conditioning Research* 30(1): 159-163.

Lockner, D., Heyward, V., Baumgartner, R., and Jenkins, K. 2000. Comparison of air-displacement plethysmography, hydrodensitometry, and dual X-ray absorptiometry for assessing body composition of children 10 to 18 years of age. *Annals of the New York Academy of Sciences* 904: 72-78.

Loenneke, J.P., Barnes, J.T., Wagganer, J.D., Wilson, J.M., Lowery, R.P., Green, C.E., and Pujol, T.J. 2014. Validity and reliability of an ultrasound system for estimating adipose tissue. *Clinical Physiology and Functional Imaging* 34: 159-162.

Löffler-Wirth, H., Willscher, E., Ahnert, P., Wirkner, K., Engel, C., Loeffler, M., and Binder, H. 2016. Novel anthropometry based on 3D-bodyscans applied to a large population based cohort. *PLoS One* 11(7): e0159887. doi:10.1371/journal.pone.0159887. Accessed August 5, 2017.

Logghe, I.H.J., Verhagen, A.P., Rademaker, A.C.H.J., Bierma-Zeinstra, S.M.A., van Rossum, E., Faber, M.J., and Koes, B.W. 2010. The effects of tai chi on fall prevention, fear of falling and balance in older people: A meta-analysis. *Preventive Medicine* 51: 222-227.

Lohman, T.G. 1981. Skinfolds and body density and their relation to body fatness: A review. *Human Biology* 53: 181-115.

Lohman, T.G. 1987. *Measuring body fat using skinfolds* [videotape]. Champaign, IL: Human Kinetics.

Lohman, T.G. 1989. Bioelectrical impedance. In *Applying new technology to nutrition: Report of the ninth roundtable on medical issues*, 22-25. Columbus, OH: Ross Laboratories.

Lohman, T.G. 1992. *Advances in body composition assessment. Current issues in exercise science series*. Monograph no. 3. Champaign, IL: Human Kinetics.

Lohman, T.G. 1996. Dual energy X-ray absorptiometry. In *Human body composition*, ed. A.F. Roche, S.B. Heymsfield, and T.G. Lohman, 63-78. Champaign, IL: Human Kinetics.

Lohman, T.G., Boileau, R.A., and Slaughter, M.H. 1984. Body composition in children and youth. In *Advances in pediatric sport sciences*, ed. R.A. Boileau, 29-57. Champaign, IL: Human Kinetics.

Lohman, T.G., Harris, M., Teixeira, P.J., and Weiss, L. 2000. Assessing body composition and changes in body composition: Another look at dual-energy X-ray absorptiometry. *Annals of the New York Academy of Sciences* 904: 45-54.

Lohman, T.G., Pollock, M.L., Slaughter, M.H., Brandon, L.J., and Boileau, R.A. 1984. Methodological factors and the prediction of body fat in female athletes. *Medicine & Science in Sports & Exercise* 16: 92-96.

Lohman, T.G., Roche, A.F., and Martorell, R., eds. 1988. *Anthropometric standardization reference manual*. Champaign, IL: Human Kinetics.

Londeree, B., and Moeschberger, M. 1984. Influence of age and other factors on maximal heart rate. *Journal of Cardiac Rehabilitation* 4: 44-49.

Looker, A.C., Borrud, L.F., Dawson-Hughes, B., and Shepherd, J.A. 2012. Osteoporosis or low bone mass at the femur neck or lumbar spine in older adults: United States, 2005-2008. *NCHS Data Brief. No. 93*. Hyattsville, MD: National Center for Health Statistics. http://inflpro.com/nchs/data/databriefs/db93.pdf. Accessed September 30, 2012.

Loose, B.D., Christiansen, A.M., Smolczyk, J.E., Roberts, K.L., Budziszewska, A., Hollatz, C.G., and Norman, J.F. 2012. Consistency of the counting talk test for exercise prescription. *Journal of Strength and Conditioning Research* 26: 1701-1707.

Loprinzi, P.D. 2015. Dose-response association of moderate-to-vigorous physical activity with cardiovascular biomarkers and all-cause mortality: Considerations by individual sports, exercise and recreational physical activities. *Preventive Medicine* 81: 73-77.

Loprinzi, P.D., Loenneke, J.P., and Blackburn, E.H. 2015. Movement-based behaviors and leukocyte telomere length among U.S. adults. *Medicine & Science in Sports & Exercise* 47: 2347-2352.

Lorant, V., Soto, V.E., Alves, J., Federico, B., Kinnunen, J., Kuipers, M., Moor, I., Perelman, J., Richter, M., Rimpelä, A., Robert, P-O., Roscillo, F., and Kunst, A. 2015. *BMC Research Notes* 8:91. doi:10.1186/s13104-015-1041-z. Accessed April 8, 2016.

Loudon, J.K., Cagle, P.E., Figoni, S.F., Nau, K.L., and Klein, R.M. 1998. A submaximal all-extremity exercise test to predict maximal oxygen consumption. *Medicine & Science in Sports & Exercise* 30: 1299-1303.

Lounana, J., Campion, F., Noakes, T.D., and Medelli, J. 2007. Relationship between %HRmax, %HR reserve, %$\dot{V}O_2$max, and %$\dot{V}O_2$ reserve in elite cyclists. *Medicine & Science in Sports & Exercise* 39: 350-357.

Low, D.C., Walsh, G.S., and Arkesteijn, M. 2017. Effectiveness of exercise interventions to improve postural control in older adults: A systematic review and meta-analysis of centre of pressure measurements. *Sports Medicine* 47: 101-112.

Lowery, R.P., Joy, J.M., Rathmacher, J.A., Baier, S.M., Fuller, J.C. Jr., Shelley, M.C. Jr., Jäger, R., Purpura, M., Wilson, S.M., and Wilson, J.M. 2016. Interaction of beta-hydroxy-beta-methylbutyrate free acid and adenosine triphosphate on muscle mass, strength, and power in resistance trained individuals. *Journal of Strength and Conditioning Research* 30: 1843-1854.

Lowry, D.W., and Tomiyama, A.J. 2015. Air displacement plethysmography versus dual-energy X-ray absorptiometry in underweight, normal-weight, and overweight/obese individuals. *PLoS One* 10(1): e0115086. doi:10.1371/journal.pone.0115086. Accessed August 6, 2017.

Loy, S., Likes, E., Andrews, P., Vincent, W., Holland, G.J., Kawai, H., Cen, S., Swenberger, J., VanLoan, M., Tanaka, K., Heyward, V., Stolarczyk, L., Lohman, T.G., and Going, S.B. 1998. Easy grip on body composition measurements. *ACSM's Health & Fitness Journal* 2(5): 16-19.

Lozano, A., Rosell, J., and Pallas-Areny, R. 1995. Errors in prolonged electrical impedance measurements due to electrode repositioning and postural changes. *Physiological Measurement* 16: 121-130.

Lu, T.W., Chien, H.L., and Chen, H.L. 2007. Joint loading in the lower extremities during elliptical exercise. *Medicine & Science in Sports & Exercise* 39: 1651-1658.

Lu, Y.M., Lin, J.H., Hsiao, S.F., Liu, M.F., Chen, S.M., and Lue, Y.J. 2011. The relative and absolute reliability of leg muscle strength testing by a handheld dynamometer. *Journal of Strength and Conditioning Research* 25: 1065-1071.

Luettengen, M., Foster, C., Doberstein, S., Mikat, R., and Porcari, J. 2012. Zumba®: Is the "fitness-party" a good workout?" *Journal of Sports Science and Medicine* 11: 357-358.

Lukaski, H.C. 1986. Use of the tetrapolar bioelectrical impedance method to assess human body composition. In *Human body composition and fat patterning,* ed. N.G. Norgan, 143-158. Wageningen, Netherlands: Euronut.

Lukaski, H.C., and Bolonchuk, W.W. 1988. Estimation of body fluid volumes using tetrapolar impedance measurements. *Aviation, Space, and Environmental Medicine* 59: 1163-1169.

Lukaski, H.C., Johnson, P.E., Bolonchuk, W.W., and Lykken, G.I. 1985. Assessment of fat-free mass using bioelectric impedance measurements of the human body. *American Journal of Clinical Nutrition* 41: 810-817.

Lundin-Olsson, L., Nyberg, L., and Gustafson, Y. 1997. "Stops walking when talking" as a predictor of falls in elderly people. *Lancet* 349: 617.

Lundqvist, S., Börjesson, M., Larsson, M.E.H., Hagberg, L., and Cider, Å. 2017. Physical activity on prescription (PAP), in patients with metabolic risk factors. A 6-month follow-up study in primary health care. *PLoS One* 12: e0175190. doi:10.1371/journal.pone.0175190.

Lyden, K., Keadle, S.K., Staudenmayer, J., and Freedson, P.S. 2017. The activPAL accurately classifies activity intensity categories in healthy adults. *Medicine & Science in Sports & Exercise* 49: 1022-1028.

Lynch, E., and Barry, S. 2012. The effectiveness of ice water immersion in the treatment of delayed onset muscle soreness in the lower leg. *Physiotherapy Practice and Research* 33: 9-15.

Ma, W-Y., Liu, P-H., Yang, C-Y., Hua, C-H., Shih, S-R., Hsein, Y-C., Hsieh, H-J., Chuang, L-M., Hung, C.S., Lin, J-W., Chiu, F-C., Wei, J-N., Lin, M-S., and Li, H-Y. 2012. *Diabetes Care.* doi:10.2337/dc12-1452.

MacDonald, E.Z., Vehrs, P.R., Fellingham, G.W., Eggett, D., George, J.D., and Hager, R. 2017. Validity and reliability of assessing body composition using a mobile application. *Medicine & Science in Sports & Exercise* [Epub ahead of print]. doi:10.1249/MSS.0000000000001378. Accessed August 13, 2017.

MacDougall, J.D., Sale, D.G., Moroz, J.R., Elder, G.C., Sutton, J.R., and Howalk, H. 1979. Mitochondrial volume density in human skeletal muscle following heavy resistance training. *Medicine and Science in Sports* 11: 164-166.

Macedonio, M.A., and Dunford, M. 2009. *The athlete's guide to making weight.* Champaign, IL: Human Kinetics.

Machado, A., Garcia-Lopez, D., Gonzalez-Gallego, J., and Garatachea, N. 2010. Whole-body vibration training increases muscle strength and mass in older women: A randomized-controlled trial. *Scandinavian Journal of Medicine & Science in Sports* 20: 200-207.

Mackey, A.L., Bojsen-Moller, J., Qvortrup, K., Langberg, H., Suetta, C., Kalliokoski, K.K., Kjaer, M., and Magnusson, S.P. 2008. Evidence of skeletal muscle damage following electrically stimulated isometric muscle contractions in humans. *Journal of Applied Physiology* 105: 1620-1627.

MacRae, I.F., and Wright, V. 1969. Measurement of back movement. *Annals of Rheumatic Diseases* 28: 584-589.

Maddigan, M.E., Peach, A.A., and Behm, D.G. 2012. A comparison of assisted and unassisted proprioceptive neuromuscular facilitation techniques and static stretching. *Journal of Strength and Conditioning Research* 26: 1238-1244.

Maddison, R., Foley, L., Mhurchu, C.N., Jiang, Y., Jull, A., Prapavessis, H., Hohepa, M., and Rodgers, A. 2011. Effects of active video games on body composition: A randomized controlled trial. *American Journal of Clinical Nutrition* 94: 156-163.

Magnan, R.E., Kwan, B.M., Ciccolo, J.T., Gurney, B., Mermier, C.M., and Bryan, A.D. 2013. Aerobic capacity testing with inactive individuals: The role of subjective experience. *Journal of Physical Activity and Health* 10: 271-279.

Magnusdottir, A., Porgilsson, B., and Karlsson, B. 2014. Comparing three devices for jump height measurement in a heterogeneous group of subjects. *Journal of Strength and Conditioning Research* 28: 2837-2844.

Magnusson, S.P. 1998. Passive properties of human skeletal muscle during stretch maneuvers. A review. *Scandinavian Journal of Medicine and Science in Sports* 8(2): 65-77.

Magnusson, S.P., Aagaard, P., Larsson, B., and Kjaer, M. 2000. Passive energy absorption by human muscle-tendon unit is unaffected by increase in intramuscular temperature. *Journal of Applied Physiology* 88: 1215-1220.

Magnusson, S.P., Simonsen, E.B., Aagaard, P., Bueson, J., Johannson, F., and Kjaer, M. 1997. Determinants of musculoskeletal flexibility: Viscoelastic properties, cross-sectional area, EMG and stretch tolerance. *Scandinavian Journal of Medicine and Science in Sports* 7: 195-202.

Magnusson, S.P., Simonsen, E.B., Aagaard, P., Dyhre-Poulsen, P., McHugh, M.P., and Kjaer, M. 1996. Mechanical and physiological responses to stretching with and without pre-isometric contraction in human skeletal muscle. *Archives of Physical Medicine and Rehabilitation* 77: 373-378.

Mahar, M.T., Guerieri, A.M., Hanna, M.S., and Kemble, D. 2011. Estimation of aerobic fitness from 20-M multistage shuttle run test performance. *American Journal of Preventive Medicine* 41: S117-S123.

Mahieu, N.N., McNair, P., DeMuynck, M., Stevens, V., Blanckaert, I., Smits, N., and Witvrouw, E. 2007. Effect of static and ballistic stretching on the muscle-tendon tissue properties. *Medicine & Science in Sports & Exercise* 39: 494-501.

Maksud, M.G., and Coutts, K.D. 1971. Comparison of a continuous and discontinuous graded treadmill test for maximal oxygen uptake. *Medicine and Science in Sports* 3: 63-65.

Malek, M.H., Nalbone, D.P., Berger, D.E., and Coburn, J.W. 2002. Importance of health science education for personal fitness trainers. *Journal of Strength and Conditioning Research* 16: 19-24.

Manini, T.M., and Clark, B.C. 2012. Dynapenia and aging: An update. *Journals of Gerontology, Series A: Biological Sciences and Medical Sciences* 67 A: 28-40.

Mansoubi, M., Pearson, N., Clemes, S.A., Biddle, S.J.H., Bodicoat, D.H., Tolfrey, K., Edwardson, C., and Yates, T. 2015. Energy expenditure during common sitting and standing tasks: Examining the 1.5 MET definition of sedentary behavior. *BMC Public Health* 15: 516. doi:10.1186/s12889-015-1851-x. Accessed July 3, 2017.

Marcus, B.H., Rakowski, W., and Rossi, R.S. 1992. Assessing motivational readiness and decision-making for exercise. *Health Psychology* 11: 257-261.

Markland, D., and Ingledew, L. 1997. The measurement of exercise motives: Factorial validity and invariance across gender of a revised exercise motivation inventory. *British Journal of Health Psychology* 2: 361-376.

Markland, D., and Tobin, V.J. 2004. A modification of the Behavioral Regulation in Exercise Questionnaire to include an assessment of amotivation. *Journal of Sport and Exercise Psychology* 26: 191-196.

Marley, W., and Linnerud, A. 1976. A three-year study of the Åstrand-Ryhming step test. *Research Quarterly* 47: 211-217.

Marocolo, M., Marocolo, I.C., Cunha, F.S.B., Da Mota, G.R., and Maior, A.S. 2016. Influence of percentage of 1RM strength test repetition performance during resistance exercise of upper and lower limbs. *Archivos de Medicina del Deporte* 33: 387-392.

Marsh, C.E. 2012. Evaluation of the American College of Sports Medicine submaximal treadmill running equation for predicting $\dot{V}O_2$max. *Journal of Strength and Conditioning Research* 26: 548-554.

Martin, A.D., Drinkwater, D.T., and Clarys, J.P. 1992. Effects of skin thickness and skinfold compressibility on skinfold thickness measurements. *American Journal of Human Biology* 4: 453-460.

Martin, A.D., Ross, W.D., Drinkwater, D.T., and Clarys, J.P. 1985. Prediction of body fat by skinfold caliper: Assumptions and cadaver evidence. *International Journal of Obesity* 9(Suppl. 1): S31-S39.

Martin, C.A., and McGrath, B.P. 2014. Ambulatory and home blood pressure measurement in the management of hypertension: White-coat hypertension. *Clinical and Experimental Pharmacology and Physiology* 41: 22-29.

Martin, S.B., Jackson, A.W., Morrow, J.R., and Liemohn, W. 1998. The rationale for the sit and reach test revisited. *Measurement in Physical Education and Exercise Science* 2: 85-92.

Martindale, J.L., and Brown, D.F.M. 2017. *A visual guide to ECG interpretation.* 2nd ed. Philadelphia: Wolters Kluwer.

Martuscello, J.M., Nuzzo, J.L., Ashley, C.D., Campbell, B.I., Orriola, J.J., and Mayer, J.M. 2013. Systematic review of core muscle activity during physical fitness exercises. *Journal of Strength and Conditioning Research* 27: 1684-1698.

Marx, J.O., Ratamess, N.A., Nindl, B.C., Gotshalk, L.A., Volek, J.S., Dohi, K., Bush, J.A., Gomez, A.L., Mazzetti, S.A.,

Fleck, S.J., Hakkinen, K., Newton, R.U., and Kraemer, W.J. 2001. Low-volume circuit versus high-volume periodized resistance training in women. *Medicine & Science in Sports & Exercise* 33: 635-643.

Mat, S., Tan, M.P., Kamaruzzaman, S.B., and Ng, C.T. 2015. Physical therapies for improving balance and reducing falls risk in osteoarthritis of the knee: A systematic review. *Age and Ageing* 44: 16-24.

Mauger, A.R., and Sculthorpe, N. 2012. A new $\dot{V}O_2$max protocol allowing self-pacing in maximal incremental exercise. *British Journal of Sports Medicine* 46: 59-63.

Mayer, J. 1968. *Overweight: Causes, costs and control.* Englewood Cliffs, NJ: Prentice Hall.

Mayer, T.G., Tencer, A.F., and Kristoferson, S. 1984. Use of noninvasive technique for quantification of spinal range-of-motion in normal subjects and chronic low back dysfunction patients. *Spine* 9: 588-595.

Mayhew, J.L., Brechue, W.F., Smith, A.E., Kemmler, W., Lauber, D., and Koch, A.J. 2011. Impact of testing strategy on expression of upper-body work capacity and one-repetition maximum prediction after resistance training in college-aged men and women. *Journal of Strength and Conditioning Research* 25: 2796-2807.

Mayhew, J.L., Ball, T.E., Arnold, M.D., and Bowen, J.C. 1992. Relative muscular endurance performance as a predictor of bench press strength in college men and women. *Journal of Applied Sport Science Research* 6: 200-206.

Mayorga-Vega, D., Aguilar-Soto, P., and Viciana, J. 2015. Criterion-related validity of the 20-m shuttle run test for estimating cardiorespiratory fitness: A meta-analysis. *Journal of Sports Science and Medicine* 14: 536-547.

Mayorga-Vega, D., Bocanegra-Parrilla, R., Ornelas, M., and Viciana, J. 2016. Criterion-related validity of the distance and time-based walk/run field tests for estimating cardiorespiratory fitness: A systematic review and meta-analysis. *PLOS One.* doi:10.1371/journal.pone.015167. Accessed June 22, 2016.

Mays, R.J., Boér, N.F., Mealey, L.M., Kim, K.H., and Goss, F.L. 2016. A comparison of practical assessment methods to determine treadmill, cycle and elliptical ergometer $\dot{V}O_2$peak. *Journal of Strength and Conditioning Research* 24: 1325-1331.

Mays, R.J., Goss, F.L., Schafer, M.A., Kim, K.H., Nagle-Stilley, E.F., Robertson, R.J. 2010. Validation of adult OMNI perceived exertion scales for elliptical ergometry. *Perceptual and Motor Skills* 111: 848-862.

Mayson, D.J., Kiely, D.K., LaRose, S.I., and Bean, J.F. 2008. Leg strength or velocity of movement. Which is more influential on the balance of mobility limited elders? *American Journal of Physical Medicine and Rehabilitation* 87: 969-976.

Mazess, R.B., Barden, H.S., and Ohlrich, E.S. 1990. Skeletal and body-composition effects of anorexia nervosa. *American Journal of Clinical Nutrition* 52: 438-441.

McArdle, W.D., Katch, F.I., and Katch, V.L. 1996. *Exercise physiology: Energy, nutrition and human performance,* 4th ed. Baltimore: Williams & Wilkins.

McArdle, W.D., Katch, F.I., and Pechar, G.S. 1973. Comparison of continuous and discontinuous treadmill and bicycle tests for $\dot{V}O_2$max. *Medicine and Science in Sports* 5: 156-160.

McArdle, W.D., Katch, F.I., Pechar, G.S., Jacobson, L., and Ruck, S. 1972. Reliability and interrelationships between maximal oxygen intake, physical working capacity and step-test scores in college women. *Medicine and Science in Sports* 4: 182-186.

McAtee, R.E., and Charland, J. 2014. *Facilitated stretching,* 4th ed. Champaign, IL: Human Kinetics.

McBride, J.M., Nuzzo, J.L., Dayne, A.M., Israetel, M.A., Nieman, D.C., and Triplett, N.T. 2010. Effect of an acute bout of whole body vibration exercise on muscle force output and motor neuron excitability. *Journal of Strength and Conditioning Research* 24: 184-189.

McCarthy, J.P., Agre, J.C., Graf, B.K., Pozniak, M.A., and Vailas, A.C. 1995. Compatibility of adaptive responses with combining strength and endurance training. *Medicine & Science in Sports & Exercise* 27: 429-436.

McConnell, T., and Clark, B. 1987. Prediction of maximal oxygen consumption during handrail-supported treadmill exercise. *Journal of Cardiopulmonary Rehabilitation* 7: 324-331.

McCrory, M.A., Gomez, T.D., Bernauer, E.M., and Mole, P.A. 1995. Evaluation of a new displacement plethysmograph for measuring human body composition. *Medicine & Science in Sports & Exercise* 27: 1686-1691.

McCrory, M.A., Mole, P.A., Gomez, T.D., Dewey, K.G., and Bernauer, E.M. 1998. Body composition by air displacement plethysmography using predicted and measured thoracic gas volumes. *Journal of Applied Physiology* 84: 1475-1479.

McCue, B.F. 1953. Flexibility of college women. *Research Quarterly* 24: 316-324.

McGill, S. 2016. *Low back disorders: Evidence-based prevention and rehabilitation*, 3rd ed. Champaign, IL: Human Kinetics.

McGill, S.M. 2001. Low back stability: From formal description to issues for performance and rehabilitation. *Exercise and Sport Sciences Reviews* 29(1): 26-31.

McGill, S.M., Childs, A., and Liebenson, D.C. 1999. Endurance times for low back stabilization exercises: Clinical targets for testing and training from a normal database. *Archives of Physical Medicine and Rehabilitation* 80: 941-944.

McGill, S.M., and Marshall, L.W. 2012. Kettlebell swing, snatch, and bottoms-up carry: Back and hip muscle activation, motion, and low back loads. *Journal of Strength and Conditioning Research* 26: 16-27.

McGlory, C., Devries, M.C., and Phillips, S.M. 2017. Skeletal muscle and resistance exercise training: The role of protein synthesis in recovery and remodeling. *Journal of Applied Physiology* 122: 541-548.

McGrath, L.J., Hopkins, W.G., and Hinckson, E.A. 2015. Associations of objectively measured built-environment attributes with youth moderate-to-vigorous physical activity: A systematic review and meta-analysis. *Sports Medicine* 45: 841-865.

McHugh, M.P., and Cosgrave, C.H. 2010. To stretch or not to stretch: The role of stretching in injury prevention and performance. *Scandinavian Journal of Medicine and Science in Sports* 20: 169-181.

McHugh, M.P. Kremenic, I.J., Fox, M.B., and Gleim, G.W. 1998. The role of mechanical and neural restraints to joint range of motion during passive stretch. *Medicine & Science in Sports & Exercise* 30: 928-932.

McHugh, M.P., Magnusson, S.P., Gleim, G.W., and Nicholas, J.A. 1992. Viscoelastic stress relaxation in human skeletal muscle. *Medicine & Science in Sports & Exercise* 24: 1375-1382.

McInnis, K., and Balady, G. 1994. Comparison of submaximal exercise responses using the Bruce vs modified Bruce protocols. *Medicine & Science in Sports & Exercise* 26: 103-107.

McKeon, P.O., and Hertel, J. 2008. Systematic review of postural control and lateral ankle instability. Part II: Is balance training clinically effective? *Journal of Athletic Training* 43(3): 305-315.

McMurray, R.G., Butte, N.F., Crouter, S.E., Trost, S.G., Pfeiffer, K.A., Bassett, D.R., Puyay, M.R., Berrigan, D., Watson, K.B., and Fulton, J.E. 2015. Exploring metrics to express energy expenditure of physical activity in youth. *PLoS One*. 10: e0130869. doi:10.1371/journal.pone.0130869. Accessed July 4, 2017.

McRae, G., Payne, A., Zelt, J.G.E., Scribbans, T.D., Jung, M.E., Little, J.P., and Gurd, B.J. 2012. Extremely low volume, whole-body aerobic-resistance training improves aerobic fitness and muscular endurance in females. *Applied Physiology, Nutrition, and Metabolism* 37: 1124-1131.

Mears, J., and Kilpatrick, M. 2008. Motivation for exercise: Applying theory to make a difference in adoption and adherence. *ACSM's Health & Fitness Journal* 12(1): 20-26.

Menant, J.C., Schoene, D., Sarofim, M., and Lord, S.R. 2014. Single and dual task tests of gait speed are equivalent in the prediction of falls in older people: A systematic review and meta-analysis. *Ageing Research Reviews* 16: 83-104.

Mesquita, L.S.A., de Carvalho, F.T., Freire, L.S.A., Neto, O.P., and Zangaro, R.A. 2015. Effects of two exercise protocols on postural balance of elderly women: A randomized controlled trial. *BMC Geriatrics* 15: 61.

Messier, S.P., Royer, T.D., Craven, T.E., O'Toole, M.L., Burns, R., and Ettinger W.H. Jr. 2000. Long-term exercise and its effect on balance in older, osteoarthritic adults: Results from the Fitness, Arthritis, and Seniors Trial (FAST). *Journal of the American Geriatrics Society* 48: 131-138.

Metcalfe, L. 2010. The BEST strength training program for osteoporosis prevention. *ACSM's Certified News* 20(4): 7-8, 11.

Micozzi, M.S., Albanes, D., Jones, Y., and Chumlea, W.C. 1986. Correlations of body mass indices with weight, stature, and body composition in men and women in NHANES I and II. *American Journal of Clinical Nutrition* 44: 725-731.

Midgley, A.W., Bentley, D.J., Luttikholt, H., McNaughton, L.R., and Millet, G.P. 2008. Challenging a dogma of exercise physiology. Does an incremental exercise test for valid $\dot{V}O_2$max determination really need to last between 8 and 12 minutes? *Sports Medicine* 38: 441-447.

Mier, C.M., Alexander, R.P., and Mageean, A.L. 2012. Achievement of $\dot{V}O_2$max criteria during a continuous graded exercise test and a verification stage performed by college-aged athletes. *Journal of Strength and Conditioning Research* 26: 2648-2654.

Mier, C.M., and Feito, Y. 2006. Metabolic cost of stride rate, resistance, and combined use of arms and legs on the elliptical trainer. *Research Quarterly for Exercise and Sport* 77: 507-513.

Mifflin, M.D., St. Jeor, S.T., Hill, L.A., Scott, B.J., Daugherty, S.A., and Koh, Y.O. 1990. A new predictive equation for resting energy expenditure in healthy individuals. *American Journal of Clinical Nutrition* 51: 241-247.

Milani, P., Coccetta, C.A., Rabini, A., Sciarra, T., Massazza, G., and Ferriero, G. 2014. Mobile smartphone applications for body position measurement in rehabilitation: A review of goniometric tools. *PM&R* 6: 1038-1043.

Milanović, Z., Sporiš, G., and Weston, M. 2015. Effectiveness of high-intensity interval training (HIT) and continuous endurance training for $\dot{V}O_2$max improvements: A systematic review and meta-analysis of controlled trials. *Sports Medicine* 45: 1469-1481.

Millard-Stafford, M.L., Collins, M.A., Evans, E.M., Snow, T.K., Cureton, K.J., and Rosskopf, L.B. 2001. Use of air displacement plethysmography for estimating body fat in a four-component model. *Medicine & Science in Sports & Exercise* 33: 1311-1317.

Mills, K.T., Bundy, J.D., Kelly, T.N., Reed, J.E., Kearney, P.M., Reynolds, K., Chen, J., and He, J. 2016. Global disparities on hypertension prevalence and control. *Circulation* 134: 441-450.

Mingji, C., Onakpoya, I.J., Heneghan, C.J., and Ward, A.M. 2016. Assessing agreement of blood pressure-measuring devices in Tibetan areas of China: A systematic review. *Heart Asia* 8: 46-51.

Minkler, S., and Patterson, P. 1994. The validity of the modified sit-and-reach test in college-age students. *Research Quarterly for Exercise and Sport* 65: 189-192.

Miranda, A.B., Simao, F., Rhea, M., Bunker, D., Prestes, J., Leite, R.D., Miranda, H., de Salles, B.F., and Novaes, J. 2011. Effects of linear vs. daily undulating periodized resistance training on maximal and submaximal strength gains. *Journal of Strength and Conditioning Research* 25: 1824-1830.

Mitchell, J.A., Cousminer, D.L., Zemel, B.S., Grant, S.F.A., and Chesi, A. 2016. Genetics of pediatric bone strength. *BoneKEy Reports* 5: article 823. doi:10.1038/bonekey.2016.50. Accessed April 15, 2017.

Mitros, M., Gabriel, K.P., Ainsworth, B., Lee, C.M., Herrmann, S., Campbell, K., and Swan, P. 2011. Comprehensive evaluation of a single-stage submaximal treadmill walking protocol in healthy, middle-aged women. *European Journal of Applied Physiology* 111: 47-56.

Miyachi, M., Yamamoto, K., Ohkawara, K., and Tanaka, S. 2010. METs in adults while playing active video games: A metabolic chamber study. *Medicine & Science in Sports & Exercise* 42: 1149-1153.

Miyazaki, R., Kotani, K., Tszaki, K., Sakane, N., Yonei, Y., and Ishii, K. 2015. Effects of a year-long pedometer-based walking program on cardiovascular disease risk factors in active older people. *Asia-Pacific Journal of Public Health* 27: 155-163.

Mizumura, K., and Taguchi, T. 2016. Delayed onset muscle soreness: Involvement of neurotrophic factors. *Journal of Physiological Sciences* 66: 43-52.

Mizuno, T., and Umemura, Y. 2016. Dynamic stretching does not change the stiffness of the muscle-tendon unit. *International Journal of Sports Medicine* 37: 1044-1050.

Moffatt, R.J., Stamford, B.A., and Neill, R.D. 1977. Placement of tri-weekly training sessions: Importance regarding enhancement of aerobic capacity. *Research Quarterly* 48: 583-591.

Moffroid, M.T., and Whipple, R.H. 1970. Specificity of speed of exercise. *Physical Therapy* 50: 1699-1704.

Moholdt, T., Wisløff, U., Lydersen, S., and Nauman, J. 2014. Current physical activity guidelines for health are insufficient to mitigate long-term weight gain: More data in the fitness versus fatness debate (the HUNT study, Norway). *British Journal of Sports Medicine* 48: 1489-1496.

Mole, P.A., Oscai, L.B., and Holloszy, J.O. 1971. Adaptation of muscle to exercise: Increase in levels of palmityl CoA synthetase, carnitine palmityl-transferase, and palmityl CoA dehydrogenase and the capacity to oxidize fatty acids. *Journal of Clinical Investigation* 50: 2323-2329.

Molnar, D., Jeges, S., Erhardt, E., and Schutz, Y. 1995. Measured and predicted resting metabolic rate in obese and nonobese adolescents. *Journal of Pediatrics* 127: 571-577.

Montalvo, A.M., Shaefer, H., Rodriguez, B., Li, T., Epnere, K., and Myer, G.D. 2017. Retrospective injury epidemiology and risk factors for injury in CrossFit. *Journal of Sports Science and Medicine* 16: 53-59.

Montoye, H.J., and Faulkner, J.A. 1964. Determination of the optimum setting of an adjustable grip dynamometer. *Research Quarterly* 35: 29-36.

Moon, J.R., Stout, J.R., Walter, A.A., Smith, A.E., Stock, M.S., Herda, T.J., Sherk, V.D., Young, K.C., Lockwood, C.M., Kendall, K.L., Fukuda, D.H., Graff, J.L., Cramer, J.T., Beck, T.W., and Esposito, E.N. 2011. Mechanical scale and load cell underwater weighing: A comparison of simultaneous measurements and the reliability of methods. *Journal of Strength and Conditioning Research* 25: 652-661.

Moon, J.R., Tobkin, S.E., Costa, P.B., Smalls, M., Mieding, W.K., O'Kroy, J.A., Zoeller, R.F., and Stout, J.R. 2008. Validity of the Bod Pod for assessing body composition in athletic high school boys. *Journal of Strength and Conditioning Research* 22: 263-268.

Mooney, V., Kron, M., Rummerfield, P., and Holmes, B. 1995. The effect of workplace based strengthening on low back injury rates: A case study in the strip mining industry. *Journal of Occupational Rehabilitation* 5: 157-167.

Moore, D.R., Young, M., and Phillips, S.M. 2012. Similar increases in muscle size and strength in young men after training with maximal shortening or lengthening contractions when matched for total work. *European Journal of Applied Physiology* 112: 1587-1592.

Moore, M.A., and Hutton, R.S. 1980. Electromyographic investigation of muscle stretching techniques. *Medicine & Science in Sports & Exercise* 12: 322-329.

Moore, S.C. 2009. Waist versus weight—which matters more for mortality? *American Journal of Clinical Nutrition* 89: 1003-1004.

Moore, S.C., Lee, I-M., Weiderpass, E., Campbell, P.T., Sampson, J.N., Kitahara, C.M., Keadle, S.K., Arem, J., Berrington de Bonzalez, A., Hartge, P., Adami, H-O, Blair, C.K., Borch, K.B., Boyd, E., Check, D.P., Fournier, A., Freedman, N.D., Gunter, M., Johannson, M., Khaw, K-T., Linet, M.S., Orsini, N., Park, Y., Riboli, E., Robien, K., Schairer, C., Sesso, H., Spriggs, M., Van Dusen, R., Wolk, A., Matthews, C.E., and Patel, A.V. 2016. Association of leisure-time physical activity with risk of 26 types of cancer in 1.44 million adults. *Journal of the American Medical Association: Internal Medicine* 176: 816-825.

Moran, S., Booker, H., Staines, J., and Williams, S. 2017. Rates and risk factors of injury in CrossFit™: A prospective cohort study. *Journal of Sports Medicine and Physical Fitness* 57: 1147-1153.

Morán-Navarro, R., Mora-Rodríguez, R., Rodríguez-Rielves, V., de la Fuente-Pérez, P., and Pallarés, J.G. 2016. Heart rate reserve at ventilator thresholds, maximal lactate steady state and maximal aerobic power in well-trained cyclists: Training application. *European Journal of Human Movement* 36: 150-162.

Morehouse, L.E. 1972. *Laboratory manual for physiology of exercise.* St. Louis: Mosby.

Moritani, T., and deVries, H.A. 1979. Neural factors versus hypertrophy in the time course of muscle strength gain. *American Journal of Physical Medicine* 58: 115-130.

Morrison, S.A., Petri, R.M., Hunter, H.L., Raju, D., and Gower, B. 2016. Comparison of the Lunar Prodigy and iDXA dual-energy X-ray absorptiometers for assessing total and regional body composition. *Journal of Clinical Densitometry: Assessment & Measurement of Musculoskeletal Health* 19: 290-297.

Morrow, J.R., Jackson, A.S., Bradley, P.W., and Hartung, G.H. 1986. Accuracy of measured and predicted residual lung volume on body density measurement. *Medicine & Science in Sport & Exercise* 18: 647-652.

Motalebi, S.A., Iranagh, J.A., Abdollahi, A., and Lim, W.K. 2014. Applying of theory of planned behavior to promote physical activity and exercise behavior among older adults. *Journal of Physical Education and Sport* 14: 562-568.

Muehlbauer, A.B., Roth, T., Mueller, S., and Granacher, U. 2011. Intra and intersession reliability of balance measures during one-leg standing in young adults. *Journal of Strength and Conditioning Research* 25: 2228-2234.

Muir, S.W., Berg, K., Chesworth, B., and Speechley, M. 2008. Use of the Berg Balance Scale for predicting multiple falls in community-dwelling elderly people: A prospective study. *Physical Therapy* 88: 449-459.

Muller, M.J., Bosy-Westphal, A., Klaus, S., Kreymann, G., Luhrmann, P.M., Neuhauser-Berthold, M., Noack, R., Pirke, K.M., Platte, P., Selberg, O., and Steiniger, J. 2004. World Health Organization equations have shortcomings for predicting resting energy expenditure in persons from a modern, affluent population: Generation of a new reference standard from a retrospective analysis of a German database of resting energy expenditure. *American Journal of Clinical Nutrition* 80: 1379-1390.

Müller, W., Lohman, T.G., Stewart, A.D., Maughan, R.J., Meyer, N.L., Sardinha, L.B., Kirihennedige, N., Reguant-Closa, A., Risoul-Salas, V., Sundgot-Borgen, J., Ahammer, H., Anderhuber, F., Fürhapter-Rieger, A., Kainz, P., Matrna, W., Pilsl, U., Pirstinger, W., and Ackland, T.R. 2016. Subcutaneous fat patterning in athletes: Selection of appropriate sites and standardisation of a novel ultrasound measurement technique: Ad hoc working group on body composition, health and performance, under the auspices of the IOC Medical Commission. *British Journal of Sports Medicine* 50(1): 45-54.

Muñoz-Martinez, F.A., Rubio-Arias, J.Á., Ramos-Campo, D.J., and Alcaraz, P.E. 2017. Effectiveness of resistance circuit-based training for maximum oxygen uptake and upper-body one-repetition maximum improvements: A systematic review and meta-analysis. *Sports Medicine* [in press].

Munroe, R.A., and Romance, T.J. 1975. Use of the Leighton flexometer in the development of a short flexibility test battery. *American Corrective Therapy Journal* 29: 22.

Murach, K.A., and Bagley, J.R. 2016. Skeletal muscle hypertrophy with concurrent exercise training: Contrary evidence for an interference effect. *Sports Medicine* 46: 1029-1039.

Murlasits, Z., Kneffel, Z., and Thalib, L. 2017. The physiological effects of concurrent strength and endurance training sequence: A systematic review and meta-analysis. *Journal of Sports Sciences* [in press].

Murphy, E.C.S, Carson, L., Neal, W., Baylis, C., Donley, D., and Yeater, R. 2009. Effects of an exercise intervention using Dance Dance Revolution on endothelial function and other risk factors in overweight children. *International Journal of Pediatric Obesity* 4: 205-214.

Murphy, J.R., Di Santo, M.C., Alkanani, T., and Behm, D.G. 2010. Aerobic activity before and following short-duration static stretching improves range of motion and performance vs. a traditional warm-up. *Applied Physiology, Nutrition, and Metabolism* 35: 679-690.

Muyor, J.M., Vaquero-Cristobal, R., Alacid, F., and Lopez-Minarro, P.A. 2014. Criterion-related validity of sit-and-reach and toe-touch tests as a measure of hamstring extensibility in athletes. *Journal of Strength and Conditioning Research* 28: 546-555.

Myers, J., Forman, D.E., Balady, G.J., Franklin, B.A., Nelson-Worel, J., Martin, B-J. Herbert, W.G., Guazzi, M., and Arena, R. 2014. Supervision of exercise testing by nonphysicians: A scientific statement from the American Heart Association. *Circulation* 130: 1014-1027.

Myers, T.R., Schneider, M.G., Schmale, M.S., and Hazell, T.J. 2015. Whole-body aerobic resistance training circuit improves aerobic fitness and muscle strength in sedentary young females. *Journal of Strength and Conditioning Research* 29: 1592-1600.

Myers, M.G., Valdivieso, M., and Kiss, A. 2009. Use of automated office blood pressure measurement to reduce the white coat response. *Journal of Hypertension* 27: 280-286.

Naclerio, A.B., Rodriguez-Romo, G., Barriopedro-Moro, M.I., Jimenez, A., Alvar, B.A., and Triplett, N.T. 2011. Control of resistance training intensity by the OMNI perceived exertion scale. *Journal of Strength and Conditioning Research* 25: 1879-1888.

Nagle, F.S., Balke, B., and Naughton, J.P. 1965. Gradational step tests for assessing work capacity. *Journal of Applied Physiology* 20: 745-748.

Nakamura, M., Ikezoe, T., Takeno, Y., and Ichihashi, N. 2011. Acute and prolonged effect of static stretching on the passive stiffness of the human gastrocnemius muscle tendon unit in vivo. *Journal of Orthopedic Research* 29: 1759-1763.

Nana, A., Slater, G.J., Hopkins, W.G., and Burke, L.M. 2012. Effects of daily activities on dual-energy X-ray absorptiometry measurements of body composition in active people. *Medicine & Science in Sports & Exercise* 44(1): 180-189.

Nana, A., Slater, G.J., Stewart, A.D., and Burke, L.M. 2015. Methodology review: Using dual-energy X-ray absorptiometry (DXA) for assessment of body composition in athletes and active people. *International Journal of Sport Nutrition and Exercise Metabolism* 25(2): 198-215.

Napolitano, M.A., Lewis, B.A., Whitely, J.A., and Marcus, B.H. 2010. Principles of health behavior change. In *ACSM's resource manual for guidelines for exercise testing and prescription*, 710-723. Philadelphia: Wolters Kluwer/Lippincott Williams & Wilkins.

Nashner, L.M. 1997. In *Handbook of balance function testing*, ed. G.P. Jacobson, C.W. Newman, and J.M. Kartush, 280-307. San Diego: Singular Publishing Group.

National Cholesterol Education Program. 2001. Executive summary of the third report of the National Cholesterol Education Program (NCEP) Expert Panel on detection, evaluation, and treatment of high blood cholesterol in adults (Adult Treatment Panel III). *Journal of the American Medical Association* 285(19): 2486-2497.

National Institutes of Health. 2012. Mad as a hatter campaign for a mercury-free NIH. www.nems.nih.gov/Pages/madhatter.aspx. Accessed October 27, 2012.

National Osteoporosis Foundation. 2004. America's bone health: The state of osteoporosis and low bone mass. www.nof.org/advocacy/prevalence.

National Osteoporosis Foundation. 2017. Bone health basics: Get the facts. www.nof.org/preventing-fractures/general-facts. Accessed April 14, 2017.

National Strength and Conditioning Association. 2017. *Strength training*, 2nd ed. Champaign, IL: Human Kinetics.

National Strength and Conditioning Association. 2016. *Essentials of strength training and conditioning*, 4th ed. Champaign, IL: Human Kinetics.

Naughton, J., Balke, B., and Nagle, F. 1964. Refinement in methods of evaluation and physical conditioning before and after myocardial infarction. *American Journal of Cardiology* 14: 837.

NCD Risk Factor Collaboration. 2017. Worldwide trends in blood pressure from 1975 to 2015: A pooled analysis of 1479 population-based measurement studies with 19.1 million participants. *Lancet* 389: 37-55.

Nelson, A.G., and Kokkonen, J. 2014. *Stretching anatomy, 2nd ed.* Champaign, IL: Human Kinetics.

Nelson, A.G., Kokkonen, J., Arnall, D.A., and Li, L. 2012. Acute stretching increases postural stability in non-balance-trained individuals. *Journal of Strength and Conditioning Research* 26: 3095-3100.

Nelson, M.E., and Folta, S.C. 2009. Further evidence for the benefits of walking. *American Journal of Clinical Nutrition* 89: 15-16.

Nelson, M.E., Rejeski, W.J., Blair, S.N., Duncan, P.W., Judge, J.O., King, A.C., Macera, C.A., and Castaneda-Sceppa, C. 2007. Physical activity and public health in older adults: Recommendations from the American College of Sports Medicine and the American Heart Association. *Medicine & Science in Sports & Exercise* 39(8): 1435-1445.

Neuhauser, H.K., Ellert, U., Thamm, M., and Adler, C. 2015. Calibration of blood pressure data after replacement of the standard mercury sphygmomanometer by an oscillometric device and concurrent change of cuffs. *Blood Pressure Monitoring* 20: 39-42.

Ng, B.K., Hinton, B.J., Fan, B., Kanaya, A.M., and Shepherd, J.A. 2016. Clinical anthropometrics and body composition from 3D whole-body surface scans. *European Journal of Clinical Nutrition* 70: 1265-1270.

Ng, J.K., Kippers, V., Richardson, C.A., and Parnianpour, M. 2001. Range of motion and lordosis of the lumbar spine: Reliability of measurement and normative values. *Spine* 26: 53-60.

Ng, M., Freeman, M.K., Fleming, T.D., Robinson, M., Dwyer-Lindgren, L., Thomson, B., Wollum, A., Sanman, E., Wulf, S., Lopez, A.D., Murray, C.J.L., and Gakidou, E. 2014. Smoking prevalence and cigarette consumption in 187 countries, 1980-2012. *Journal of the American Medical Association* 311: 183-192.

Ng, N. 1995. *Metcalc.* Champaign, IL: Human Kinetics.

NHS Digital. Health survey for England, 2014: Trend tables. http://content.digital.nhs.uk/catalogue/PUB19297. Accessed April 12, 2017.

Ni, M., Mooney, K., Richards, L., Balachandran, A., Sun, M., Harriell, K., Potiaumpai, M., and Signorile, J.F. 2014. Comparative impacts of tai chi, balance training, and a specially-designed yoga program on balance in older fallers. *Archives of Physical Medicine and Rehabilitation* 95(9): 1620-1628.

Nichols, D.L., Sanborn, C.F., and Love, A.M. 2001. Resistance training and bone mineral density in adolescent females. *Journal of Pediatrics* 139: 494-499.

Nichols, J.F., Sherman, C.L., and Abbott, E. 2000. Treading is new and hot: 30 minutes meets the ACSM recommendations for cardiorespiratory fitness and caloric expenditure. *ACSM's Health & Fitness Journal* 4(2): 12-17.

Nick, N., Petramfar, P., Ghodsbin, F., Keshavarzi, S., and Jahanbin, I. 2016. The effect of yoga on balance and fear of falling in older adults. *PM&R* 8: 145-151.

Nicklas, B.J., Wang, X., You, T., Lyles, M.F., Demons, J., Easter, L., Berry, M.J., Lenchik, L., and Carr, J.J. 2009. Effect of exercise intensity on abdominal fat loss during calorie restriction in overweight and obese postmenopausal women: A randomized, controlled trial. *American Journal of Clinical Nutrition* 89: 1043-1052.

Nicklas, J.M., Huskey, K.W., Davis, R.B., and Wee, C.C. 2012. Successful weight loss among obese U.S. adults. *American Journal of Preventive Medicine* 42: 481-485.

Nieman, D.C. 2003. *Exercise testing and prescription: A health related approach.* New York: McGraw-Hill.

Nissen, S.L., and Sharp, R.L. 2003. Effect of dietary supplements on lean mass and gains with resistance training: A meta-analysis. *Journal of Applied Physiology* 94: 651-659.

Noakes, T.D. 2008. How did A V Hill understand the $\dot{V}O_2$max and the "plateau phenomenon"? Still no clarity? *British Journal of Sports Medicine* 42: 574-580.

Noland, M., and Kearney, J.T. 1978. Anthropometric and densitometric responses of women to specific and general exercise. *Research Quarterly* 49: 322-328.

Noreen, E.E., and Lemon, P.W.R. 2006. Reliability of air displacement plethysmography in a large, heterogeneous sample. *Medicine & Science in Sports & Exercise* 38: 1505-1509.

Norkin, C.C., and White, D.J. 1995. *Measurement of joint motion: A guide to goniometry.* Philadelphia: Davis.

Norris, C. 2000. *Back stability.* Champaign, IL: Human Kinetics.

Norris, R.A., Wilder, E., and Norton, J. 2008. The functional reach test in 3- to 5-year-old children without disabilities. *Pediatric Physical Therapy* 20: 47-52.

North American Spine Society. 2009. Exercise for a healthy back. www.spine.org/Pages/ConsumerHealth/Spine-HealthAndWellness/PreventBackPain.

Northey, J.M., Cherbuin, N., Pumpa, K.L., Smee, D.J., and Rattray, B. 2017. Exercise interventions for cognitive function in adults older than 50: A systematic review with meta-analysis. *British Journal of Sports Medicine.* doi:10.1136/bjsports-2016-09658. Accessed April 27, 2017.

Norton, K., Marfell-Jones, M., Whittingham, N., Kerr, D., Carter, L., Saddington, K., and Gore, C. 2000. Anthropometric assessment protocols. In *Physiological tests for elite athletes,* ed. C. Gore, 66-85. Champaign, IL: Human Kinetics.

Nunez, C., Kovera, A., Pietrobelli, A., Heshka, S., Horlick, M., Kehayias, J., Wang, Z., and Heymsfield, S. 1999. Body composition in children and adults by air displacement plethysmography. *European Journal of Clinical Nutrition* 53: 382-387.

Nuri, L., Ghotbi, N., and Faghihzadeh, S. 2013. Acute effects of static stretching, active warm up, or passive warm up on flexibility of the plantar flexors of Iranian professional female taekwondo athletes. *Journal of Musculoskeletal Pain* 21: 263-268.

Nuzzo, J.L., Anning, J.H., and Scharfenberg, J.M. 2011. The reliability of three devices used for measuring vertical jump height. *Journal of Strength and Conditioning Research* 25: 2580-2590.

Nye, N.S., Carnahan, D.H., Jackson, J.D., Covey, C.J., Zarazabal, L.A., Chao, S.Y., Bockhorst, A.D., and Crawford, P.F. 2014. Abdominal circumference is superior to body mass index in estimating musculoskeletal injury risk. *Medicine & Science in Sports & Exercise* 46: 1951-1959.

O'Brien, E., Atkins, N., Stergiou, G., Karpettas, N., Parati, G., Asmar, R., Imai, Y., Want, J., Mengden, T., and Sheenan, A.,

on behalf of the Working Group on Blood Pressure Monitoring of the European Society of Hypertension. 2010. European Society of Hypertension International Protocol revision 2010 for the validation of blood pressure measuring devices in adults. *Blood Pressure Monitoring* 15: 23-38.

O'Brien, R.J., and Drizd, T.A. 1983. Roentgenographic determination of total lung capacity: Normal values from a national population survey. *American Review of Respiratory Diseases* 128: 949-952.

O'Connor, D.M., and Crowe, M.J. 2007. Effects of six weeks of β-hydroxy-β-methylbutyrate (HMB) and HMB/creatine supplementation on strength, power, and anthropometry of highly trained athletes. *Journal of Strength and Conditioning Research* 21: 419-423.

Ogawa, E.F., Leveille, S.G., Write, J.A., Shi, L., Cambi, S.M., and You, T. 2017. Physical activity domains/recommendations and leukocyte telomere length in U.S. adults. *Medicine & Science in Sports & Exercise.* doi:10.1249/MSS.0000000000001253. Accessed March 25, 2017.

Ogden, C.L., Carroll, M.D., Fryar, C.D., and Flegal, K.M. 2015. Prevalence of obesity among adults and youth: United States, 2011-2014. NCHS Data Brief. No. 219. Hyattsville, MD: National Center for Health Statistics.

Ogden, C.L., Carroll, M.D., Kit, B.K., and Flegal, K.M. 2014. Prevalence of childhood and adult obesity in the United States, 2011-2012. *Journal of the American Medical Association* 311: 806-814.

Ogedegbe, G., and Pickering, T. 2010. Principles and techniques of blood pressure measurement. *Cardiology Clinics* 28: 571-586.

Ogedegbe, G., Agyemang, C., and Ravenell, J.E. 2010. Masked hypertension: Evidence of the need to treat. *Current Hypertension Reports* 12: 349-355.

Oh, K.Y., Kim, S.A., Lee, S.Y., and Lee, S.L. 2011. Comparison of manual balance and balance board tests in healthy adults. *Annals of Rehabilitation Medicine* 35: 873-879.

Ohkubo, T., Kikuya, M., Metoki, H., Asayama, K., Obara, T., Hashimoto, J., Totsune, K., Hoshi, H., Satoh, H., and Imai, Y. 2005. Prognosis of "masked" hypertension and "white-coat" hypertension detected by 24-h ambulatory blood pressure monitoring: A 10-year follow-up from the Ohasama study. *Journal of American College of Cardiology* 46: 508-515.

Ohrvall, M., Berglund, L., and Vessby, B. 2000. Sagittal abdominal diameter compared with other anthropometric measurements in relation to cardiovascular risk. *International Journal of Obesity* 24: 497-501.

Oldroyd, B., Treadgold, L., and Hind, K. 2017. Cross calibration of the GE Prodigy and iDXA for the measurement of total and regional body composition in adults. *Journal of Clinical Densitometry: Assessment & Measurement of Musculoskeletal Health* [Epub ahead of print]. doi:10.1016/j.jocd.2017.05.009. Accessed August 6, 2017.

Oliveira, G.B.F., Avezum, A., and Roever, L. 2015. Cardiovascular disease burden: Evolving knowledge of risk factors in myocardial infarction and stroke through population-based research and perspectives in global prevention. *Frontiers in Cardiovascular Medicine* 2: article 32. doi:10.3389/fcvm.2015.00032. Accessed August 14, 2017.

Olmsted, L.C., Carcia, C.R., Hertel, J., and Schultz, S.J. 2002. Efficacy of the star excursion balance tests in detecting reach deficits in subjects with chronic ankle instability. *Journal of Athletic Training* 37: 501-506.

O'Neill, D.C., Cronin, O., O'Neill, S.B., Woods, T., Keohane, D.M., Molloy, M.G., and Falvey, E.C. 2016. Application of a sub-set of skinfold sites for ultrasound measurement of subcutaneous adiposity and percentage body fat estimation in athletes. *International Journal of Sports Medicine* 37: 359-363.

O'Neill, S., and O'Driscoll, L. 2015. Metabolic syndrome: A closer look at the growing epidemic and its associated pathologies. *Obesity Reviews* 16: 1-12.

Opplert, J., Gentry, J.B., and Babault, N. 2016. Do stretch durations affect muscle mechanical and neurophysiological properties? *International Journal of Sports Medicine* 37: 673-679.

Oppliger, R.A., Nielsen, D.H., and Vance, C.G. 1991. Wrestlers' minimal weight: Anthropometry, bioimpedance, and hydrostatic weighing compared. *Medicine & Science in Sports & Exercise* 23: 247-253.

O'Riordan, C.F., Metcalf, B.S., Perkins, J.M., and Wilkin, T.J. 2010. Reliability of energy expenditure prediction equations in the weight management clinic. *Journal of Human Nutrition and Dietetics* 23: 169-175.

Orr, R. 2010. Contribution of muscle weakness to postural instability in the elderly: A systematic review. *European Journal of Physical and Rehabilitation Medicine* 46: 183-220.

Orr, R., de Vos, N.J., Singh, N.A., Ross, D.A., Stavrinos, T.M., and Fiatarone-Singh, M.A. 2006. Power training improves balance in healthy older adults. *Journals of Gerontology, Series A: Biological Sciences and Medical Sciences* 61: 78-85.

Orr, R., Raymond, J., and Singh, M.F. 2008. Efficacy of progressive resistance training on balance performance in older adults. A systematic review of randomized controlled trials. *Sports Medicine* 38: 317-343.

Ortega, F.B., Cadenas-Sánchez, C., Sánchez-Delgado, G., Mora-González, J., Martinez-Téllez, B., Artero, E.G., Castro-Piñero, J., Labayen, I., Chillón, P., Löf, M., and Ruiz, J.R. 2015. Systematic review and proposal of a field-based physical fitness-test battery in preschool children: The PREFIT battery. *Sports Medicine* 45: 533-555.

Ortiz, O., Russell, M., Daley, T.L., Baumgartner, R.N., Waki, M., Lichtman, S., Wang, S., Pierson, R.N., and Heymsfield, S.B. 1992. Differences in skeletal muscle and bone mineral mass between black and white females and their relevance to estimates of body composition. *American Journal of Clinical Nutrition* 55: 8-13.

Osawa, Y., and Oguma, Y. 2013. Effects of vibration on flexibility: A meta-analysis. *Journal of Musculoskeletal Neuronal Interactions* 13: 442-453.

Ostchega, Y., Hughes, J.P., Prineas, R.J., Zhang, G., Nwankwo, T., and Chiappa, M.M. 2014. Mid-arm circumference and recommended blood pressure cuffs for children and adolescents aged between 3 and 19 years: Data from the National Health and Nutrition Examination Survey, 1999-2010. *Blood Pressure Monitoring* 19: 26-31.

Ostchega, Y., Prineas, R.J., Dillon, C., McDowell, M., and Carroll, M. 2004. Estimating equations and tables for adult mid-arm circumference based on measured height and weight: Data from the third National Health and Nutrition Examination Survey (NHANES III) and NHANES 1999-2000. *Blood Pressure Monitoring* 9: 123-131.

Osternig, L.R., Robertson, R.N., Troxel, R.K., and Hansen, P. 1990. Differential responses to proprioceptive neuromuscular facilitation (PNF) stretch techniques. *Medicine & Science in Sports & Exercise* 22: 106-111.

Otto, W.H. III, Coburn, J.W., Brown, L.E., Spiering, B.A. 2012. Effects of weightlifting vs. kettlebell training on vertical jump, strength, and body composition. *Journal of Strength and Conditioning Research* 26: 1199-1202.

Page, P., and Ellenbecker, T. 2011. *Strength band training, 2nd ed.* Champaign, IL: Human Kinetics.

Pajala, S., Era, P., Koskenvuo, M., Kaprio, J., Tormakangas, T., and Rantanen, T. 2008. Force platform balance measures as predictors of indoor and outdoor falls in community-dwelling women 63-76 years. *Journal of Gerontology* 63: 171-178.

Pajunen, P., Heliovaara, M., Rissanen, H., Reunanen, A., Laaksonen, M.A., and Knekt, P. 2013. Sagittal abdominal diameter as a new predictor for incident diabetes. *Diabetes Care* 36(2): 283-288. doi:10.2337/dc11-2451.

Palatini, P., Benetti, E., Fania, C., Malipiero, G., and Saladini, F. 2012. Rectangular cuffs may overestimate blood pressure in individuals with large conical arms. *Journal of Hypertension* 30: 530-536.

Panagiotakos, D.B., Georgousopoulou, E.N., Fitzgerald, A.P., Pitsavos, C., and Stefanadis, C. 2015. Validation of the HellenicSCORE (a calibration of the ESC SCORE Project) regarding 10-year risk of fatal cardiovascular disease in Greece. *Hellenic Journal of Cardiology* 56: 302-308.

Parati, G., and Ochoa, J.E. 2012. Automated-auscultatory (Hybrid) sphygmomanometers for clinic blood pressure measurement: A suitable substitute to mercury sphygmomanometer as reference standard? *Journal of Human Hypertension* 26: 211-213.

Parfitt, G., Evans, H., and Eston, R. 2012. Perceptually regulated training at RPE13 is pleasant and improves physical health. *Medicine & Science in Sports & Exercise* 44: 1613-1618.

Parker, S.B., Hurley, B.F., Hanlon, D.P., and Vaccaro, P. 1989. Failure of target heart rate to accurately monitor intensity during aerobic dance. *Medicine & Science in Sports & Exercise* 21: 230-234.

Parry, I., Carbullido, C., Kawada, J., Baglesy, A., Sen, S., Greenhalgh, D., and Palmieri, T. 2014. Keeping up with video game technology: Objective analysis of Xbox Kinext™ and PlayStation 3 Move™ for use in burn rehabilitation. *Burns* 40: 852-859.

Partridge, S.R., McGeechan, K., Hebden, L., Balestracci, K., Wong, A.T.Y., Denney-Wilson, E., Harris, M.F., Phongsavan, P., Bauman, A., and Allman-Farinelli, M. 2015. Effectiveness of a mHealth lifestyle program with telephone support (TXT2BFIT) to prevent unhealthy weight gain in young adults: Randomized clinical trial. *Journal of Medical Inter-*

net Research 3: e66. doi:10.2196/mhealth.4530. Accessed June 10, 2017.

PAR-Q+ Collaboration. 2017. The new PARQ-X+ and ePARmed-X+: Official website. http://eparmedx.com. Accessed April 19, 2017.

Pata, R.W., Lord, K., and Lamb, J. 2014. The effect of Pilates based exercise on mobility, postural stability, and balance in order to decrease fall risk in older adults. *Journal of Bodywork & Movement Therapies* 18: 361-367.

Pate, R.R., Pratt, M., Blair, S.N., Haskell, W.L., Macera, C.A., Bouchard, C., Buchner, D., Ettinger, W., Heath, G.W., and King, A.C. 1995. Physical activity and public health: A recommendation from the Centers for Disease Control and Prevention and the American College of Sports Medicine. *Journal of the American Medical Association* 273: 402-407.

Patel, R., Sulzberger, L., Li, G., Mair, J., Morley, H., Shing, M.N-W., O'Leary, C., Prakash, A., Robilliard, N., Rutherford, M., Sharpe, C., Shie, C., Sritharan, L., Turnbull, J., Whyte, I. Yu, H., Cleghorn, C., Leung, W., and Wilson, N. 2015. Smartphone apps for weight loss and smoking cessation: Quality ranking of 120 apps [Letter]. 2015. *New Zealand Medical Journal* 128(1421): 73-76.

Patrick, N., Emanski, E., and Knaub, M.A. 2014. Acute and chronic low back pain. *Medical Clinics in North America* 98: 777-789.

Patterson, P., Wiksten, D.L., Ray, L., Flanders, C., and Sanphy, D. 1996. The validity and reliability of the backsaver sit-and-reach test in middle school girls and boys. *Research Quarterly for Exercise and Sport* 67: 448-451.

Pavlou, K.N., Steffee, W.P., Lerman, R.H., and Burrows, B.A. 1985. Effects of dieting and exercise on lean body mass, oxygen uptake, and strength. *Medicine & Science in Sports & Exercise* 17: 466-471.

Payne, N., Gledhill, N., Kazmarzyk, P.T., Jamnik, V., and Keir, P.J. 2000. Canadian musculoskeletal fitness norms. *Canadian Journal of Applied Physiology* 25: 430-442.

Peeters, M.W. 2012. Subject positioning in the BodPod only marginally affects measurement of body volume and estimation of body fat in young adult men. *PLoS One* 7: E32722. doi:10.1371/journal.pone.0032722.

Peeters, M.W., and Claessens, A.L. 2011. Effect of different swim caps on the assessment of body volume and percentage body fat by air displacement plethysmography. *Journal of Sports Sciences* 29: 191-196.

Pekmezi, D., Barbera, B., and Marcus, B.H. 2010. Using the transtheoretical model to promote physical activity. *ACSM's Health & Fitness Journal* 14: 8-13.

Perk, J., DeBacker, G., Gohlke, H., Graham, I., Reiner, Z., Verschuren, W.M.M., Albus, C., Benlian, P., Boysen, G., Cifkova, R., Deaton, C., Ebrahim, S., Fisher, M., Germano, G., Hobbs, R., Hoes, A., Karadeniz, S., Messani, A., Prescott, E., Ryden, L., Scherer, M., Syvänne, M., Scholte, W.J.M., Reimer, O., Vrints, C., Wood, D., Zamorano, J.L., and Zannad, F. 2012. European Guidelines on cardiovascular disease prevention in clinical practice (version 2012). *European Heart Journal* 33: 1635-1701.

Perrier, E.T., Pavol, M.J., and Hoffman, M.A. 2011. The acute effects of a warm-up including static or dynamic stretching on countermovement jump height, reaction time, and flexibility. *Journal of Strength and Conditioning Research* 25: 1925-1931.

Persinger, R., Foster, C., Gibson, M., Fater, D.C.W., and Porcari, J.P. 2004. Consistency of the talk test for exercise prescription. *Medicine & Science in Sports & Exercise* 36: 1632-1636.

Pescatello, L.S., Franklin, B.A., Fagard, R., Farquhar, W.B., Kelley, G.A, and Ray, C.A. 2004. American College of Sports Medicine position stand. Exercise and hypertension. *Medicine & Science in Sports & Exercise* 36: 533-553.

Peters, D., Fox, K., Armstrong, N., Sharpe, P., and Bell, M. 1992. Assessment of children's abdominal fat distribution by magnetic resonance imaging and anthropometry. *International Journal of Obesity* 16(Suppl. 2): S35 [abstract].

Peters, M.J.H., van Nes, S.I., Vanhoutte, E.K., Bakkers, M., van Doorn, P.A., Merkies, I.S.J., and Faber, C.G. 2011. Revised normative values for grip strength with the Jamar dynamometer. *Journal of the Peripheral Nervous System* 16: 47-50.

Peters, S.A.E., Huxley, R.R., and Woodward, M. 2014. Diabetes as risk factor for incident coronary heart disease in women compared with men: A systematic review and meta-analysis of 64 cohorts including 858,507 individuals and 28203 coronary events. *Diabetologia* 57: 1542-1551.

Peterson, M.D. 2010. Resistance exercise for sarcopenic outcomes and muscular fitness in aging adults. *Strength and Conditioning Journal* 32(3): 52-61.

Peterson, M., Chandlee, M., and Abraham, A. 2008. Cost effectiveness analysis of a statewide media campaign to promote adolescent physical activity. *Health Promotion Practice* 9: 126-133.

Peterson, M.D., and Gordon, P.M. 2011. Resistance exercise for the aging adult: Clinical implications and prescription guidelines. *American Journal of Medicine* 124: 194-198.

Peterson, M.D., Rhea, M.R., and Alvar, B.A. 2004. Maximizing strength development in athletes: A meta-analysis to determine the dose-response relationship. *Journal of Strength and Conditioning Research* 18: 377-382.

Peterson, M.D., Rhea, M.R., Sen, A., and Gordon, P.M. 2010. Resistance exercise for muscular strength in older adults: A meta-analysis. *Ageing Research Reviews* 9: 226-237.

Peterson, M.D., Sen, A., and Gordon, P.M. 2011. Influence of resistance exercise on lean body mass in aging adults: A meta-analysis. *Medicine & Science in Sports & Exercise* 43: 249-258.

Petrella, J.K., Kim, J.S., Mayhew, D.L., Cross, J.M., and Bamman, M.M. 2008. Potent myofiber hypertrophy during resistance training in humans is associated with satellite cell-mediated myonuclear addition: A cluster analysis. *Journal of Applied Physiology* 104: 1736-1742.

Petrella, R., Koval, J., Cunningham, D., and Paterson, D. 2001. A self-paced step test to predict aerobic fitness in older adults in the primary care clinic. *Journal of the American Geriatrics Society* 49: 632-638.

Pickering, T.G., Hall, J.E., Appel, L.J., Falkner, B.E., Graves, J., Hill, M.N., Jones, D.W., Kurtz, T., Sheldon, G., and Rocella, E.J. 2005. Recommendations for blood pressure measurement in humans and experimental animals: Part 1: Blood pressure measurement in humans: A statement for professionals from the subcommittee of Professional and Public Education of the American Heart Council on High Blood Pressure Research. *Hypertension* 45(1): 142-161.

Pierce, P., and Herman, S. 2004. Obtaining, maintaining, and advancing your fitness certification. *Journal of Physical Education, Recreation and Dance* 75(7): 50-53.

Pietrobelli, A., Formica, C., Wang, Z., and Heymsfield, S.B. 1996. Dual-energy X-ray absorptiometry body composition model: Review of physical concepts. *American Journal of Physiology* 271: E941-E951.

Pimentel, G.D., Moreto, F., Takahashi, M.M., Portero-Mclellan, K.D., and Burini, R.C. 2011. Sagittal abdominal diameter, but not waist circumference is strongly associated with glycemia, triacylglycerols and HDL-c levels in overweight adults. *Nutricion Hospitalaria* 25: 1125-1129.

Pisani, P., Renna, M.D., Conversano, F., Casciaro, E., Di Paola, M., Quarta, E., Muratore, M., and Casiaro, S. 2016. Major osteoporotic fragility fractures: Risk factor updates and societal impact. *World Journal of Orthopedics* 7: 171-181.

Pi-Sunyer, F.X. 1999. Comorbidities of overweight and obesity: Current evidence and research issues. *Medicine & Science in Sports & Exercise* 31: S602-S608.

Piucco, T., Diefenthaeler, F., Soares, R., Murias, J.M., and Millet, G.Y. 2017. Validation of a maximal incremental skating test performed on a slide board: Comparison with treadmill skating. *International Journal of Sports Physiology and Performance* [Epub ahead of print]. doi:10.1123/ijspp.2016-0613. Accessed July 4, 2017.

Plisky, P.J., Gorman, P.P., Butler, R.J., Kiesel, K.B., Underwood, F.B., and Elkins, B. 2009. The reliability of an instrumented device for measuring components of the star excursion balance test. *North American Journal of Sports Physical Therapy* 4: 92-99.

Plisky, P.J., Rauh, M.J., Kaminski, T.W., and Underwood, F.B. 2006. Star excursion balance test as a predictor of lower extremity injury in high school basketball players. *Journal of Orthopaedic and Sports Physical Therapy* 36: 911-919.

Podsiadlo, D., and Richardson, S. 1991. The timed "up & go": A test of basic functional mobility of frail elderly persons. *Journal of the American Geriatrics Society* 39: 142-148.

Pollock, M.L. 1973. The quantification of endurance training programs. In *Exercise and Sport Sciences Reviews*, ed. J.H. Wilmore, 155-188. New York: Academic Press.

Pollock, M.L., Bohannon, R.L., Cooper, K.H., Ayres, J.J., Ward, A., White, S.R., and Linnerud, A.C. 1976. A comparative analysis of four protocols for maximal treadmill stress testing. *American Heart Journal* 92: 39-46.

Pollock, M.L., Broida, J., and Kendrick, Z. 1972. Validity of the palpation technique of heart rate determination and its estimation of training heart rate. *Research Quarterly* 43: 77-81.

Pollock, M.L., Cureton, T.K., and Greninger, L. 1969. Effects of frequency of training on working capacity, cardiovascular function, and body composition of adult men. *Medicine and Science in Sports* 1: 70-74.

Pollock, M.L., Dimmick, J., Miller, H.S., Kendrick, Z., and Linnerud, A.C. 1975. Effects of mode of training on cardiovascular function and body composition of middle-aged men. *Medicine and Science in Sports* 7: 139-145.

Pollock, M.L., Foster, C., Schmidt, D., Hellman, C., Linnerud, A.C., and Ward, A. 1982. Comparative analysis of physiologic responses to three different maximal graded exercise test protocols in healthy women. *American Heart Journal* 103: 363-373.

Pollock, M.L., Gaesser, G.A., Butcher, J.D., Despres, J.P., Dishman, R.K., Franklin, B.A., and Garber, C.E. 1998. The recommended quantity and quality of exercise for developing and maintaining cardiorespiratory and muscular fitness, and flexibility in healthy adults. *Medicine & Science in Sports & Exercise* 30: 975-991.

Pollock, M.L., Garzarella, L., and Graves, J. 1992. Effects of isolated lumbar extension resistance training on BMD of the elderly. *Medicine & Science in Sports & Exercise* 24: S66 [abstract].

Pollock, M.L., Gettman, L., Milesis, C., Bah, M., Durstine, L., and Johnson, R. 1977. Effects of frequency and duration of training on attrition and incidence of injury. *Medicine and Science in Sports* 9: 31-36.

Pollock, M.L., and Jackson, A.S. 1984. Research progress in validation of clinical methods of assessing body composition. *Medicine & Science in Sports & Exercise* 16: 606-613.

Pollock, M.L., Miller, H.S., Janeway, R., Linnerud, A.C., Robertson, B., and Valentino, R. 1971. Effects of walking on body composition and cardiovascular function of middle-aged men. *Journal of Applied Physiology* 30: 126-130.

Pollock, M.L., Miller, H.S., Linnerud, A.C., and Cooper, K.H. 1975. Frequency of training as a determinant for improvement in cardiovascular function and body composition of middle-aged men. *Archives of Physical Medicine and Rehabilitation* 56: 141-145.

Pollock, M.L., Wilmore, J.H., and Fox, S.M. III. 1978. *Health and fitness through physical activity*. New York: Wiley.

Pondal, M., and del Ser, T. 2008. Normative data and determinants for the timed "up and go" test in a population-based sample of elderly individuals without gait disturbances. *Journal of Geriatric Physical Therapy* 31(2): 57-63.

Poole, D.C., and Jones, A.M. 2017. Measurement of the maximum oxygen uptake $\dot{V}O_2$max: $\dot{V}O_2$peak is no longer acceptable. Journal of Applied Physiology 122: 997-1002.

Pope, R.P., Herbert, R.D., Kirwan, J.D., and Graham, B.J. 2000. A randomized trial of preexercise stretching for prevention of lower-limb injury. *Medicine and Science in Sports and Exercise* 32: 271-277.

Porcari, J., Foster, C., and Schneider, P. 2000. Exercise response to elliptical trainers. *Fitness Management* 16(9): 50-53.

Porszasz, J., Casaburi, R., Somfay, A., Woodhouse, L.J., and Whipp, B.J. 2003. A treadmill ramp protocol using simultaneous changes in speed and grade. *Medicine & Science in Sports & Exercise* 35: 1596-1603.

Porter, G.H. 1988. Case study evaluation for exercise prescription. In *Resource manual for guidelines for exercise testing and prescription*, ed. S.N. Blair, P. Painter, R.R.

Pate, L.K. Smith, and C.B. Taylor, 248-255. Philadelphia: Lea & Febiger.

Porter, M.M. 2006. Power training for older adults. *Applied Physiology, Nutrition and Metabolism* 31: 87-94.

President's Council on Physical Fitness and Sports. 1997. *The presidential physical fitness award program.* Washington, D.C.: Author.

Prevalence of leisure-time physical activity among overweight adults—United States, 1998. 2000. *Morbidity and Mortality Weekly Report* 49(15), April 21.

Price, K., Bird, S.R., Lythgo, N., Raj, I.S., Wong, J.Y.L., and Lynch, C. 2017. Validation of the Fitbit One, Garmin Vivofit and Jawbone UP activity tracker in estimation of energy expenditure during treadmill walking and running. *Journal of Medical Engineering & Technology* 41: 208-215.

Prior, B.M., Cureton, K.J., Modlesky, C.M., Evans, E.M., Sloniger, M.A., Saunders, M., and Lewis, R.D. 1997. In vivo validation of whole body composition estimates from dual-energy X-ray absorptiometry. *Journal of Applied Physiology* 83: 623-630.

Prochaska, J.O., and DiClemente, C.C. 1982. Trans-theoretical therapy: Toward a more integrative model of change. *Psychotherapy: Theory, Research, and Practice* 19: 276-288.

Proske, U., and Morgan, D.L. 2001. Muscle damage from eccentric exercise: Mechanism, mechanical signs, adaptation, and clinical applications. *Journal of Physiology* 537: 333-345.

Province, M.A., Hadley, E.C., Hornbrook, M.C., Lipsitz, L.A., Miller, J.P., Mulrow, C.P., Ory, M.G., Sattin, R.W., Tinetti, M.E., and Wolf, S.L. 1995. The effects of exercise on falls in elderly patients. A preplanned meta-analysis of the FICSIT trials. Frailty and injuries: Cooperative studies of intervention techniques. *Journal of the American Medical Association* 273: 1341-1347.

Psilander, N., Frank, P., Flockhart, M., and Sahlin, K. 2015. Adding strength to endurance training does not enhance aerobic capacity in cyclists. *Scandinavian Journal of Medicine and Science in Sports* 25: e353-e359.

Quatrochi, J.A., Hicks, V.L., Heyward, V.H., Colville, B.C., Cook, K.L., Jenkins, K.A., and Wilson, W. 1992. Relationship of optical density and skinfold measurements: Effects of age and level of body fatness. *Research Quarterly for Exercise and Sport* 63: 402-409.

Quinn, T.J., and Coons, B.A. 2011. Talk test and its relationship with the ventilatory and lactate thresholds. *Journal of Sports Sciences* 29: 1175-1182.

Radaelli, R., Fleck, S.J., Leite, T., Leite, R.D., Pinto, R.S., Fernandes, L., and Simao, R. 2015. Dose-response of 1, 3, and 5 sets of resistance exercise on strength, local muscular endurance, and hypertrophy. *Journal of Strength and Conditioning Research* 29: 1349-1358.

Raffaelli, C., Galvani, C., Lanza, M., and Zamparo, P. 2012. Different methods for monitoring intensity during water-based aerobic exercise. *European Journal of Applied Physiology* 112: 125-134.

Ralston, G.W., Kilgore, L., Wyatt, F.B., and Baker, J.S. 2017. The effect of weekly set volume on strength gain: A meta-analysis. *Sports Medicine* [in press].

Rankinen, T., Rice, T., Teran-Garcia, M., Rao, D.C., and Bouchard, C. 2010. FTO genotype is associated with exercise training-induced changes in body composition. *Obesity* 18: 322-326.

Rapsomaniki, E., Timmis, A., George, J., Pujades-Rodriguez, M., Shah, A.D., Denaxas, S., White, I.R., Caulfield, M.J. Deanfield, J.E., Smeeth, L., Williams, B., Hingorani, A., and Hemingway, H. 2014. Blood pressure and incidence of twelve cardiovascular diseases: Lifetime risks, healthy life-years lost, and age-specific associations in 1.25 million people. *Lancet* 383: 1899-1911.

Ratamess, N.A., Alvar, B.A., Evetoch, T.K., Housh, T.J., Kibler, W.B., Kraemer, W.J., and Triplett, N.T. 2009. ACSM position stand: Progression models in resistance training for healthy adults. *Medicine & Science in Sports & Exercise* 41: 687-708.

Rauch, F., Sievanen, H., Boonen, S., Cardinale, M., Dengens, H., Felsenberg, D., Roth, J., Schoenau, E., Verschueren, S., and Rittweger, J. 2010. Reporting whole-body vibration intervention studies: Recommendations of the International Society of Musculoskeletal and Neuronal Interactions. *Journal of Musculoskeletal and Neuronal Interactions* 10: 193-198.

Raue, U., Trappe, T.A., Estrem, S.T., Qian, H.R., Helvering, L.M., Smith, R.C., and Trappe, S. 2012. Transcriptome signature of resistance training adaptations: Mixed muscle and fiber type specific profiles in young and old adults. *Journal of Applied Physiology* 112: 1625-1636.

Rawson, E.S., and Clarkson, P.M. 2003. Scientifically debatable: Is creatine worth its weight? *Gatorade Sport Science Exchange 91* 16(4): 1-13.

Rebuffe-Scrive, M. 1985. Adipose tissue metabolism and fat distribution. In *Human body composition and fat distribution,* ed. N.G. Norgan, 212-217. Wageningen, Netherlands: Euronut.

Recalde, P.T., Foster, C., Skemp-Arlt, K.M., Fater, D.C.W., Neese, C.A., Dodge, C., and Porcari, J.P. 2002. The talk test as a simple marker of ventilatory threshold. *South African Journal of Sports Medicine* 8: 5-8.

Reed, J.L., and Pipe, A.L. 2014. The talk test: A useful tool for prescribing and monitoring exercise intensity. *Current Opinion in Cardiology* 29: 475-480.

Reed, J.L., and Pipe, A.L. 2016. Practical approaches to prescribing physical activity and monitoring exercise intensity. *Canadian Journal of Cardiology.* 32: 514-522.

Reed-Jones, R.J., Dorgo, S., Hitchings, M.K., and Bader, J.O. 2012. Wii Fit plus balance test scores for the assessment of balance and mobility in older adults. *Gait & Posture* 36: 430-433.

Reese, N.B., and Bandy, W.D. 2003. Use of an inclinometer to measure flexibility of the iliotibial band using the Ober test and the modified Ober test: Differences in magnitude and reliability of measurements. *Journal of Orthopaedic and Sports Physical Therapy* 33: 326-330.

Regnier, S.M., and Sargis, R.M. 2014. Adipocytes under assault: Environmental disruption of adipose physiology. *Biochemica et Biophysica Acta* 1842: 520-533.

Reid, K.F., and Fielding, R.A. 2012. Skeletal muscle power: A critical determinant of physical functioning in older adults. *Exercise and Sport Sciences Reviews* 40: 4-12.

Reiman, M.P., and Manske, R.C. 2009. *Functional testing in human performance.* Champaign, IL: Human Kinetics.

Reiman, M.P., Krier, A.D., Nelson, J.A., Rogers, M.A., Stuke, Z.O., and Smith, B.S. 2010. Reliability of alternative trunk endurance testing procedures using clinician stabilization vs. traditional methods. *Journal of Strength and Conditioning Research* 24: 730-736.

Reinhardt, M., Piaggi, P., DeMers, B., Trinidad, C., and Krakoff, J. 2017. Cross calibration of two dual-energy X-ray densitometers and comparison of visceral adipose tissue measurements by iDXA and MRI. *Obesity* 25: 332-337.

Rhea, M.R., Alvar, B.A., Burkett, L.N., and Ball, S.D. 2003a. A meta-analysis to determine the dose response for strength development. *Medicine & Science in Sports & Exercise* 35: 456-464.

Rhea, M.R., Ball, S.D., Phillips, W.T., and Burkett, L.N. 2002. A comparison of linear and daily undulating periodized programs with equated volume and intensity for strength. *Journal of Strength and Conditioning Research* 16: 250-255.

Rhea, M.R., Phillips, W.T., Burkett, L.N., Stone, W.J., Ball, S.D., Alvar, B.A., and Thomas, A.B. 2003b. A comparison of linear and daily undulating periodized programs with equated volume and intensity for local muscular endurance. *Journal of Strength and Conditioning Research* 17: 82-87.

Ribeiro, A.S., Campos-Filho, M.G.A., Avelar, A., dos Santos, L., Achour Júnior, A., Aguiar, A.F., Fleck, S.J., Serassuelo Júnior, H., and Cyrino, E.S. 2017. Effect of resistance training on flexibility in young adult men and women. *Isokinetics and Exercise Science* 25: 149-155.

Ribeiro, A.S., Schoenfeld, B.J., Fleck, S.J., Pina, F.L.C., Nascimento, M.A., and Cyrino, E.S. 2017. Effects of traditional and pyramidal resistance training systems on muscular strength, muscle mass, and hormonal responses in older women: A randomized crossover trial. *Journal of Strength and Conditioning Research* 31: 1888-1896.

Ribeiro, A.S., Schoenfeld, B.J., Pina, F.L.C., Souza, M.F., Nascimento, M.A., dos Santos, L., Antunes, M., and Cyrino, E.S. 2015. Resistance training in older women: Comparison of single vs. multiple sets on muscle strength and body composition. *Isokinetics and Exercise Science* 23: 53-60.

Ribeiro, A.S., Schoenfeld, B.J., Silva, D.R., Pina, F.L., Guariglia, D.A., Porto, M., Maestá, N., Burini, R.C., and Cyrino, E.S. 2015. Effect of two- versus three-way split resistance training routines on body composition and muscular strength in bodybuilders: A pilot study. *International Journal of Sport Nutrition and Exercise Metabolism* 25(6): 559-565.

Ribeiro, A.S., Schoenfeld, B.J., Souza, M.F., Tomeleri, C.M., Venturini, D., Barbosa, D.S., and Cyrino, E.S. 2016. Traditional and pyramidal resistance training systems improve muscle quality and metabolic biomarkers in older women: A randomized crossover study. *Experimental Gerontology* 79: 8-15.

Richards, J.B., Valdes, A.M., Gardner, J.P., Kato, B.S., Silva, A., Kimura, M., Lu, X., Brown, M.J., Aviv, A., and Spector, T.D. 2008. Homocysteine levels and leukocyte telomere length. *Atherosclerosis* 200: 271-277.

Riddle, D.L., and Stratford, P.W. 1999. Interpreting validity indexes for diagnostic tests: An illustration using the Berg balance test. *Physical Therapy* 79: 939-948.

Ridley, K., Ainsworth, B.E., and Olds, T.S. 2008. Development of a compendium of energy expenditures for youth. *International Journal of Behavioral Nutrition and Physical Activity* 5: 45-52.

Riemann, B.L., Guskiewicz, K.M., and Shields, E.W. 1999. Relationship between clinical and forceplate measures of postural stability. *Journal of Sport Rehabilitation* 8: 71-82.

Rikli, R., Petray, C., and Baumgartner, T. 1992. The reliability of distance run tests for children in grades K-4. *Research Quarterly for Exercise and Sport* 63: 270-276.

Rikli, R.E., and Jones, C.J. 1999. Development and validation of a functional fitness test for community-residing older adults. *Journal of Aging and Physical Activity* 7: 127-159.

Rikli, R.E, and Jones, C.J. 2013. *Senior fitness test manual.* Champaign, IL: Human Kinetics.

Riley, D.A., and Van Dyke, J.M. 2012. The effects of active and passive stretching on muscle length. *Physical Medicine and Rehabilitation Clinics of North America* 23: 51-57.

Ringrose, J., Millay, J., Babwick, S.A., Neil, M., Langkaas, L.A., and Padwal, R. 2015. Effect of overcuffing on the accuracy of oscillometric blood pressure measurements. *Journal of the American Society of Hypertension* 9: 563-568.

Ripka, W.L., Ulbricht, L., Menghin, L., and Gewehr, P.M. 2016. Portable A-mode ultrasound for body composition assessment in adolescents. *Journal of Ultrasound in Medicine* 35: 755-760.

Risérus, U., de Faire, U., Berglund, L., and Hellénius, M-L. 2010. Sagittal abdominal diameter as a screening tool in clinical research: Cutoffs for cardiometabolic risk. *Journal of Obesity* 2010: article 757939. doi:10.1155/2010/757939. Accessed August 14, 2017.

Riva, D., Bianchi, R., Rocca, F., and Mamo, C. 2016. Proprioceptive training and injury prevention in a professional men's basketball team: A six-year prospective study. *Journal of Strength and Conditioning Research* 30: 461-475.

Rixon, K.P., Rehor, P.R., and Bemben, M.G. 2006. Analysis of the assessment of caloric expenditure in four modes of aerobic dance. *Journal of Strength and Conditioning Research* 20: 593-596.

Rizzo, A., Lange, B., Suma, E.A., and Bolas, M. 2011. Virtual reality and interactive digital game technology: New tools to address obesity and diabetes. *Journal of Diabetes Science and Technology* 5: 256-264.

Roberts, H.C., Denison, J.J., Martin, J.J., Patel, H.P., Syddall, H., Cooper, C., and Sayer, A.A. 2011. A review of the measurement of grip strength in clinical and epidemiological studies: Towards a standardized approach. *Age and Ageing* 40: 423-429.

Roberts, J.M., and Wilson, K. 1999. Effect of stretching duration on active and passive range of motion in the lower extremity. *British Journal of Sports Medicine* 33: 259-263.

Robertson, R.J. 2004. *Perceived exertion for practitioners: Rating effort with the OMNI picture system.* Champaign, IL: Human Kinetics.

Robertson, R.J., Goss, F.L., Andreacci, J.L., Dube, J.J., Rutkowski, J.J., Frazee, K.M., Aaron, D.J., Metz, K.F., Kowallis, R.A., and Snee, B.M. 2005. Validation of the children's OMNI-resistance exercise scale of perceived exertion. *Medicine & Science in Sports & Exercise* 37: 819-826.

Robinson, R.H., and Gribble, P.A. 2008. Support for a reduction in the number of trials needed for the star excursion balance test. *Archives of Physical Medicine and Rehabilitation* 89: 364-370.

Roby, R.B. 1962. Effect of exercise on regional subcutaneous fat accumulations. *Research Quarterly* 33: 273-278.

Rochmis, P., and Blackburn, H. 1971. Exercise tests. A survey of procedures, safety and litigation experience in approximately 170,000 tests. *Journal of the American Medical Association* 217: 1061-1066.

Rockport Walking Institute. 1986. *Rockport fitness walking test.* Marlboro, MA: Author.

Rodd, D., Ho, L., and Enzler, D. 1999. Validity of Tanita TBF-515 bioelectrical impedance scale for estimating body fat in young adults. *Medicine & Science in Sports & Exercise* 31(Suppl.): S201 [abstract].

Rodgers, W.M., and Loitz, C.C. 2009. The role of motivation in behavior change: How do we encourage our clients to be active? *ACSM's Health & Fitness Journal* 13(1): 7-12.

Rodriguez, D.A., Brown, A.L., and Troped, P.J. 2005. Portable global positioning units to complement accelerometry-based physical activity monitors. *Medicine & Science in Sports & Exercise* 37(Suppl.): S572-S581.

Rodriguez-Sanchez, N., and Galloway, D.R. 2015. Errors in dual energy X-ray absorptiometry estimation of body composition induced by hypohydration. *International Journal of sport Nutrition and Exercise Metabolism* 25: 60-68.

Roelants, M., Delecluse, C., Goris, M., and Verschueren, S. 2004. Effects of 24 weeks of whole body vibration training on body composition and muscle strength in untrained females. *International Journal of Sports Medicine* 25: 1-5.

Rogan, S., de Bruin, E.D., Radlinger, L., Joehr, C., Wyss, C., Stuck, N.J., Bruelhart, Y., de Bie, R.A., and Hilfiker, R. 2015. Effects of whole-body vibration on proxies of muscle strength in old adults: A systematic review and meta-analysis on the role of physical capacity level. *European Review of Aging and Physical Activity* 12: 12.

Roger, V.L., Go, A.S., Lloyd-Jones, D.M., Benjamin, E.J., Berry, J.D., Borden, W.B., Bravata, D.M., Dai, S., Ford, E.S., Fox, C.S., Fullerton, H.J., Gillespie, C., Jailpern, S.M., Hert, J.A., Howard, V.J., Kissela, B.M., Kittner, S.J., Lackland, D.T., Lichtman, J.H., Lisabeth, L.D., Makue, D.M., Marcus, G.M., Marielli, A., Matchar, D.B., Moy, C.S., Mozaffarian, D., Mussolino, M.E., Nichol, G., Paynter, N.P., Soliman, E.Z., Sorlie, P.D., Sotoodehnia, N.O., Turan, T.N., Virani, S.S., Wong, N.D., Woo, D., and Turner, M.B., on behalf of the American Heart Association Statistics Committee and Stroke Statistics Subcommittee. 2012. Heart disease and stroke statistics—2012 update: A report from the American Heart Association. *Circulation.* doi:10.1161/CIR.0b013e31823ac046.

Rojas, R., Aguilar-Salinas, C.A., Jimenez-Corona, A., Shamah-Levy, T., Rauda, J., Avila-Burgos, L., Villalpando, S., and Ponce, E.L. 2010. Metabolic syndrome in Mexican adults: Results from the National Health and Nutrition Survey 2006. *Salud Publica de Mexico* 52(Suppl. 1): S11-S18.

Rokholm, B., Baker, J.L., and Sorensen, T.I. 2010. The leveling off of the obesity epidemic since the year 1999: A review of evidence and perspectives. *Obesity Reviews* 11: 835-846.

Romo-Perez, V., Schwingel, A., and Chodzko-Zajko, W. 2011. International resistance training recommendations for older adults: Implications for the promotion of healthy aging in Spain. *Journal of Human Sport & Exercise* 6: 639-648.

Ronnestad, B.R., Holden, G., Samnoy, L.E., and Paulsen, G. 2012. Acute effect of whole-body vibration on power, one-repetition maximum, and muscle activation in power lifters. *Journal of Strength and Conditioning Research* 26: 531-539.

Rose, D.J. 2010. *Fall proof: A comprehensive balance and mobility training program, 2nd ed.* Champaign, IL: Human Kinetics.

Rosendale, R.P., and Bartok, C.J. 2012. Air displacement plethysmography for the measurement of body composition in children aged 6-48 months. *Pediatric Research* 71: 299-304.

Ross, J., and Pate, R. 1987. The national children and youth fitness study II: A summary of findings. *Journal of Physical Education, Recreation and Dance* 58: 51-56.

Ross, R., Blair, S.N., Arena, R., Church, T.S., Després, J-P., Franklin, B.A., Haskell, W.L., Kaminsky, L.A., Levine, B.D., Lavie, C.J., Myers, J., Niebauer, J., Sallis, R., Sawada, S.S., Sui, X., and Wisloff, U. 2016. Importance of assessing cardiorespiratory fitness in clinical practice: A case for fitness as a clinical vital sign. *Circulation* 134: e653-e399. doi:10.1161/CIR.0000000000000461. Accessed April 25, 2017.

Ross, R., and Janssen, I. 2001. Physical activity, total and regional obesity: Dose-response considerations. *Medicine & Science in Sports & Exercise* 33(Suppl.): S521-S527.

Ross, W.D., and Marfell-Jones, M.J. 1991. Kinanthropometry. In *Physiological testing of the high-performance athlete,* ed. J.D. MacDougall, H.A. Wenger, and H.J. Green, 75-115, Champaign, IL: Human Kinetics.

Rossi, F.E., Fortaleza, A.C.S., Neves, L.M., Buonani, C., Picolo, M.R., Diniz, T.A. Kalva-Filha, C.A., Papoti, M., Lira, F.S., and Freitas, I.F. Jr. 2016. Combined training (aerobic plus strength) potentiates a reduction in body fat but demonstrates no difference on the lipid profile in postmenopausal women when compared with aerobic training with a similar training load. *Journal of Strength and Conditioning Research* 30: 226-234.

Row, B.S., and Cavanagh, P.R. 2007. Reaching upward is more challenging to dynamic balance than reaching forward. *Clinical Biomechanics* 22: 155-164.

Rowland, M.L. 1990. Self-reported weight and height. *American Journal of Clinical Nutrition* 52: 1125-1133.

Rowlands, A.V., Marginson, V.F., and Lee, J. 2003. Chronic flexibility gains: Effect of isometric contraction duration during proprioceptive neuromuscular facilitation stretching techniques. *Research Quarterly for Exercise and Sport* 74: 47-51.

Roy, J.L.P., Smith, J.F., Bishop, P.A., Hallinan, C., Wang, M., and Hunter, G.R. 2004. Prediction of maximal $\dot{V}O_2$ from a submaximal StairMaster test in young women. *Journal of Strength and Conditioning Research* 18: 92-96.

Roza, A.M., and Shizgal, H.M. 1984. The Harris Benedict equation reevaluated: Resting energy requirements and the body cell mass. *American Journal of Clinical Nutrition* 40: 168-182.

Rubenstein, L.Z., and Josephson, K.R. 2002. The epidemiology of falls and syncope. *Clinics in Geriatric Medicine* 18: 141-158.

Rubini, E.C., Costa, A.L.L., and Gomes, P.S.C. 2007. The effects of stretching on strength performance. *Sports Medicine* 37: 213-224.

Rücker, V., Keil, U., Fitzgerald, A.P., Malzahn, U., Prugger, C., Ertl, G., Heuschmann, P.U., and Neuhauser, H. 2016. Predicting 10-year risk of fatal cardiovascular disease in Germany: An update based on the SCORE-Deutshland risk charts. *PLoS One* 11: e0162188. doi:10.1371/journal.pone.0162188. Accessed April 20, 2017.

Rush, E.C., Plank, L.D., Laulu, M.S., and Robinson, S.M. 1997. Prediction of percentage body fat from anthropometric measurements: Comparison of New Zealand European and Polynesian young women. *American Journal of Clinical Nutrition* 66: 2-7.

Ryan, D., and Heaner, M. 2014. Preface to the full report. *Obesity* 22(Suppl. 2): S1-S3.

Ryan, E.E., Rossi, M.D., and Lopez, R. 2010. The effects of the contract-relax-antagonist-contract form of proprioceptive neuromuscular facilitation stretching on postural stability. *Journal of Strength and Conditioning Research* 24: 1888-1894.

Sahrmann, S. 2002. *Diagnosis and treatment of movement impairment syndromes.* St. Louis: C.V. Mosby.

Saint-Maurice, P.F., Laurson, K.R., Kaj, M., and Csanyi, T. 2015. Establishing normative reference values for standing broad jump among Hungarian youth. *Research Quarterly for Exercise and Sport* 86: S37-S44.

Sale, D. 1988. Neural adaptation to resistance training. *Medicine & Science in Sports & Exercise* 20: S135-S145.

Salem, J.G., Wang, M.Y., and Sigward, S. 2002. Measuring lower extremity strength in older adults: The stability of isokinetic versus 1RM measures. *Journal of Aging and Physical Activity* 10: 489-503.

Sallis, J.F., and Owen, N. 1999. *Physical activity and behavioral medicine.* Thousand Oaks, CA: Sage.

Sallis, J.F., Bull, F., Guthold, R., Heath, G.W., Inoue, S., Kelly, P., Oyeyemi, A.L., Perez, L.G., Richards, J., and Hallal, P.C. 2016. Progress in physical activity over the Olympic quadrennium. *Lancet.* doi:10.1016/S0140-6736(16)30581-5. Accessed March 4, 2017.

Same, R.V., Feldman, D.I., Shah, N., Martin, S.S., Al Rafai, M., Blaha, M.J., Graham, G., and Ahmed, H.M. 2016. Relationship between sedentary behavior and cardiovascular risk. *Current Cardiology Reports* 18. doi:10.1007/s11886-015-0678-5. Accessed March 25, 2017.

Samukawa, M., Hattori, M., Sugama, N., and Takeda, N. 2011. The effects of dynamic stretching on plantar flexor muscle-tendon tissue properties. *Manual Therapy* 16: 618-622.

Sanal, E., Ardic, F., and Kirac, S. 2013. Effects of aerobic or combined aerobic resistance exercise on body composition in overweight and obese adults: Gender differences. A randomized intervention study. *European Journal of Physical and Rehabilitation Medicine* 49: 1-11.

Santos, T.M., Gomes, P.S., Oliveira, B.R.R., Ribeiro, L.G., and Thompson, W.R. 2012. A new strategy for the implementation of an aerobic training session. *Journal of Strength and Conditioning Research* 28: 87-93.

Sanz, C., Gautier, J.F., and Hanaire, H. 2010. Physical exercise for the prevention and treatment of type 2 diabetes. *Diabetes & Metabolism* 36: 346-351.

Saris, W.H.M., Blair, S.N., van Baak, M.A., Eaton, S.B., Davies, P.S.W., Di Pietro, L., Fogelholm, M., Rissanen, A., Schoeller, D., Swinburn, B., Tremblay, A., Westerterp, K.R., and Wyatt, H. 2003. How much physical activity is enough to prevent unhealthy weight gain? Outcome of the IASO 1st Stock Conference and consensus statement. *Obesity Reviews* 4: 101-114.

Sarki, A.M., Nduka, C.U., Stranges, S., Kandala, N-B., and Uthman, O.A. 2015. Prevalence of hypertension in low- and middle-income countries: A meta-analysis. *Medicine* 95: e1959. doi:10.1097/MD.0000000000001959.

Sarzynski, M.A., Schuna, J.M. Jr., Carnethon, M.R., Jacobs, D.R. Jr., Lewis, C.E., Quesenberry, C.P. Jr., Sidney, S., Schreiner, P.J., and Sternfeld, B. 2015. Association of fitness with incident dyslipidemias over 15 years in the Coronary Artery Risk Development in Young Adults study. *American Journal of Preventatitive Medicine* 49: 745-752.

Sasaki, J.E., Hickey, A., Mavilla, M., Tedesco, J., John, D., Keadle, S.K., and Freedson, P.S. 2015. Validation of the Fitbit wireless activity tracker for prediction of energy expenditure. *Journal of Physical Activity and Health* 12: 149-154.

Sattelmair, J., Pertman, J., Ding, E.L., Kohl, H.W. III, Haskell, W., and Lee, I-M. 2011. Dose response between physical activity and risk of coronary heart disease: A meta-analysis. *Circulation* 124: 789-793.

Sawano, M., Kohsaka, S., Okamura, T., Inohara, T., Sugiyama, D., Watanabe, M., Nakamura, Y., Higashiyama, A., Kadota, A., Okud, M., Murakami, Y., Ohkubo, T., Fuhiyoshi, A., Miura, K., Okayama, A., and Ueshima, H., for the National Integrated Project for Prospective Observation of Non-Communicable Disease and its Trends in the Aged (NIPPON DATA 80) research group. 2016. *Atherosclerosis* 252: 116-121.

Saydah, S., Bullard, K.M., Cheng, Y., Ali, M.K., Gregg, E.W., Geiss, L., and Imperatore, G. 2014. Trends in cardiovascular disease risk factors by obesity level in adults in the United States, NHANES 1999-2010. *Obesity* 22: 1888-1895.

Sayers, S.P., Harackiewicz, D.V., Harman, E.A., Frykman, P.N., and Rosenstein, M.T. 1999. Cross-validation of three jump power equations. *Medicine & Science in Sports & Exercise* 31: 572-577.

Schade, M., Hellebrandt, F.A., Waterland, J.C., and Carns, M.L. 1962. Spot reducing in overweight college women: Its influence on fat distribution as determined by photography. *Research Quarterly* 33: 461-471.

Schenk, A.K., Witbrodt, B.C., Hoarty, C.A., Carlson, R.H. Jr., Goulding, E.H., Potter, J.F., and Bonasera, S.J. 2011. Cellular telephones measure activity and lifespace in community-dwelling adults: Proof of principle. *Journal of American Geriatric Society* 59: 345-352.

Scherr, J., Wolfarth, B., Christle, J.W., Pressler, A., Wagenpfeil, S., and Halle, M. 2013. Associations between Borg's rating of perceived exertion and physiological measures of exercise intensity. *European Journal of Applied Physiology* 113: 147-155.

Schleicher, M.M., Wedam, L., and Wu, G. 2012. Review of tai chi as an effective exercise on falls prevention in elderly. *Research in Sports Medicine* 20: 37-58.

Schmidt, C.P., Zwingenberger, S., Walther, A., Reuter, U., Kasten, P., Seifert, J., Gunther, K-P., and Stiehler, M. 2014. Prevalence of low back pain in adolescent athletes: An epidemiological investigation. *International Journal of Sports Medicine* 35(8): 684-689.

Schmidt, P.K., and Carter, J.E.L. 1990. Static and dynamic differences among five types of skinfold calipers. *Human Biology* 62: 369-388.

Schneider, P.J., Jacobs., D.R. Jr., Wong, N.D., and Kiefe, C.I. 2016. Twenty-five year secular trends in lipids and modifiable risk factors in a population-based biracial cohort: The Coronary Artery Risk Development in Young Adults (CARDIA) study, 1985-2011. *Journal of the American Heart Association*. doi:10.1161/JAHA.116.00338. Accessed July 16, 2016.

Schnohr, P., O'Keefe, J.H., Marott, J.L., Lange, P., and Jensen, G.B. 2015. Dose of jogging and long-term mortality: The Copenhagen City Heart Study. *Journal of the American College of Cardiology* 65: 411-419.

Schoenfeld, B.J. 2013. Postexercise hypertrophic adaptations: A reexamination of the hormone hypothesis and its applicability to resistance training program design. *Journal of Strength and Conditioning Research* 27: 1720-1730.

Schoenfeld, B.J., Ogborn, D.I., Vigotsky, A.D., Franchi, M.V., and Krieger, J.W. 2017. Hypertrophic effects of concentric vs. eccentric muscle actions: A systematic review and meta-analysis. *Journal of Strength and Conditioning Research* 31: 2599-2608.

Schot, P.K., Knutzen, K.M., Poole, S.M., and Mrotek, L.A. 2003. Sit-to-stand performance of older adults following strength training. *Research Quarterly for Exercise and Sport* 74: 1-8.

Schrieks, I.C., Barnes, M.J., and Hodges, L.D. 2011. Comparison study of treadmill versus arm ergometry. *Clinical Physiology and Functional Imaging.* 31: 326-331.

Schroeder, M.M., Foster, C., Porcari, J.P., and Mikat, R.P. 2017. Effects of speech passage length on accuracy of predicting metabolic thresholds using the talk test. *Kinesiology* 49: 9-14.

Schutz, Y., and Herren, R. 2000. Assessment of speed of human locomotion using a differential satellite global positioning system. *Medicine & Science in Sports & Exercise* 32: 612-616.

Schwane, J.A., Johnson, S.R., Vandenakker, C.B., and Armstrong, R.B. 1983. Delayed-onset muscular soreness and plasma CPK and LDH activities after downhill running. *Medicine & Science in Sports & Exercise* 15: 51-56.

Scott, S. 2008. *ABLE bodies balance training.* Champaign, IL: Human Kinetics.

Sedentary Behaviour Research Network. 2012. Standardized use of the terms "sedentary" and "sedentary behaviours." *Applied Physiology, Nutrition, and Metabolism* 37: 540-542.

Segal, K.R., Van Loan, M., Fitzgerald, P.I., Hodgdon, J.A., and Van Itallie, T.B. 1988. Lean body mass estimation by bioelectrical impedance analysis: A four-site cross-validation study. *American Journal of Clinical Nutrition* 47: 7-14.

Seidell, J.C., and Halberstadt, J. 2015. The global burden of obesity and the challenges of prevention. *Annals of Nutrition & Metabolism* 66(Suppl. 2): 7-12.

Seip, R., and Weltman, A. 1991. Validity of skinfold and girth based regression equations for the prediction of body composition in obese adults. *American Journal of Human Biology* 3: 91-95.

Sekendiz, B., Altun, O., Korkusuz, F., and Akin, S. 2007. Effects of Pilates exercise on trunk strength, endurance and flexibility in sedentary adult females. *Journal of Bodywork and Movement Therapies* 11: 318-326.

Selassie, M., and Sinha, A.C. 2011. The epidemiology and aetiology of obesity: A global challenge. *Best Practice & Research Clinical Anaesthesiology* 25: 1-9.

Sell, K.E., Verity, T.M., Worrell, T.W., Pease, B.J., and Wigglesworth, J. 1994. Two measurement techniques for assessing subtalar joint position: A reliability study. *Journal of Orthopaedic and Sports Physical Therapy* 19: 162-167.

Sell, K., Lillie, T., and Taylor, J. 2008. Energy expenditure during physically interactive video game playing in male college students with different playing experience. *Journal of American College Health* 56: 505-511.

Sendra-Lillo, J., Sabater-Hernandez, D., Sendra-Ortola, A., and Martinez-Martinez, F. 2011. Comparison of the white-coat effect in community pharmacy versus the physician's office: The Palmera study. *Blood Pressure Monitoring* 16: 62-66.

Seneli, R.M., Ebersole, K.T., O'Connor, K.M., and Snyder, A.C. 2013. Estimated $\dot{V}O_2$max from the Rockport Walk Test on a nonmotorized curved treadmill. *Journal of Strength and Conditioning Research* 27: 3495-3505.

Seynnes, O.R., de Boer, M., and Narici, M.V. 2007. Early skeletal muscle hypertrophy and architectural changes in response to high-intensity resistance training. *Journal of Applied Physiology* 102: 368-373.

Shahbabu, B., Dasgupta, A., Sarkar, K., and Sahoo, S.K. 2016. Which is more accurate in measuring the blood pressure? A digital or an aneroid sphygmomanometer. *Journal of Clinical and Diagnostic Research* 10: LC11-LC14.

Sharkey, B.J., and Gaskill, S.E. 2007. *Fitness and health,* 6th ed. Champaign, IL: Human Kinetics.

Sharman, M.J., Cresswell, A.G., and Riek, S. 2006. Proprioceptive neuromuscular facilitation stretching: Mechanisms and clinical applications. *Sports Medicine* 36: 929-939.

Sharman, J.E., and LaGerche, A. 2015. Exercise blood pressure: Clinical relevance and correct measurement. *Journal of Human Hypertension* 29: 351-358.

Sharman, J.E., La Gerche, A., and Coombes, J.S. 2015. Exercise and cardiovascular risk in patients with hypertension. *American Journal of Hypertension* 28: 147-158.

Shaw, B. 2016. *Beth Shaw's YogaFit,* 3rd ed. Champaign, IL: Human Kinetics.

Shaw, C.E., McCully, K.K., and Posner, J.D. 1995. Injuries during the one repetition maximum assessment in the elderly. *Journal of Cardiopulmonary Rehabilitation* 15: 283-287.

Shaw, K., Gennat, H., O'Rourke, P., and Del Mar, C. 2006. Exercise for overweight or obesity. *Cochrane Database of Systematic Reviews* 4: CD003817. doi:10.1002/14651858. CD003817.pub3.

Shaw, M.P., Robinson, J., and Peart, D.J. 2017. Comparison of a mobile application to estimate percentage body fat to other non-laboratory based measurements. *Biomedical Human Kinetics* 9: 94-98.

Sheard, P.W., and Paine, T.J. 2010. Optimal contraction intensity during proprioceptive neuromuscular facilitation for maximal increase of range of motion. *Journal of Strength and Conditioning Research* 24: 416-421.

Shephard, R.J. 1972. *Alive man: The physiology of physical activity.* Springfield, IL: Charles C Thomas.

Shirato, M., Tsuchiya, Y., Sato, T., Hamano, S., Gushiken, T., Kimura, N., and Ochi, E. 2016. Effects of combined β-hydroxy-β-methylbutyrate (HMB) and whey protein ingestion on symptoms of eccentric exercise-induced muscle damage. *Journal of the International Society of Sports Nutrition* 13: article 7.

Shitara, H., Yamamoto, A., Shimoyama, D., Ichinose, T., Sasaki, T., Hamano, N., Ueno, A., Endo, F., Oshima, A., Sakane, H., Tachibana, M., Tomomatsu, Y., Tajika, T., Kobayashi, T., Osawa, T., Iizuka, H., and Takagishi, K. 2017. Shoulder stretching intervention reduces the incidence of shoulder and elbow injuries in high school baseball players: A time-to-event analysis. *Scientific Reports* 7: 45304.

Shoenhair, C.L., and Wells, C.L. 1995. Women, physical activity, and coronary heart disease: A review. *Medicine, Exercise, Nutrition and Health* 4: 200-206.

Shrier, I., and Gossal, K. 2000. Myths and truths of stretching: Individualized recommendations for healthy muscles. *The Physician and Sportsmedicine* 28: 57-63.

Shubert, T.E. 2011. Evidence-based exercise prescription for balance and falls prevention: A current review of the literature. *Journal of Geriatric Physical Therapy* 34: 100-108.

Shubert, T.E., Schrodt, L.A., Mercer, V.S., Busby-Whitehead, J., and Giuliani, C.A. 2006. Are scores on balance screening tests associated with mobility in older adults? *Journal of Geriatric Physical Therapy* 29(1): 33-39.

Shuger, S.L., Barry, V.W., Sui, X., McClain, A., Hand, G.A., Wilcox, S., Meriwether, R.A., Hardin, J.W., and Blair, S.N. 2011. Electronic feedback in a diet- and physical activity-based lifestyle intervention for weight loss: A randomized controlled trial. *International Journal of Behavioral Nutrition and Physical Activity* 8: 41.

Shumway-Cook, A., Baldwin, M., Polissar, N.L., and Gruber, W. 1997. Predicting the probability for falls in community-dwelling older adults. *Physical Therapy* 77: 812-819.

Shumway-Cook, A., Brauer, S., and Wollacott, M.H. 2000. Predicting the probability of falls in community-dwelling older adults using the timed up and go test. *Physical Therapy* 80: 896-904.

Shumway-Cook, A., and Woollacott, M.H. 1995. *Motor control: Theory and practical applications.* Baltimore: Williams & Wilkins.

Siegel, R.L., Miller, K.D., and Jemal, A. 2016. Cancer statistics, 2016. *CA: Cancer Journal for Clinicians* 66: 7-30.

Simao, R., Spineti, J., Fretas de Salles, B., Matta, T., Ferandes, L., Fleck, S.J., Rhea, M.R., and Strom-Olsen, H.E. 2012. Comparison between nonlinear and linear periodized resistance training: Hypertrophic and strength effects. *Journal of Strength and Conditioning Research* 26: 1389-1395.

Simpson, W.F. 2015. Progress for ACSM Certifications. *ACSM's Health & Fitness Journal* 19(2): 30-31.

Siri, W.E. 1961. Body composition from fluid space and density. In *Techniques for measuring body composition,* ed. J. Brozek and A. Henschel, 223-224. Washington, D.C.: National Academy of Sciences.

Sivén, S.S.E., Niiranen, T.J., Kantola, I.M., and Jula, A.M. 2016. White-coat and masked hypertension as risk factors for progression to sustained hypertension: The Finn-Home study. *Journal of Hypertension* 34: 54-60.

Sjodin, A.M., Forslund, A.H., Westerterp, K.R., Andersson, A.B., Forslund, J.M., and Hambraeus, L.M. 1996. The influence of physical activity on BMR. *Medicine & Science in Sports & Exercise* 28: 85-91.

Sjostrom, M., Lexell, J., Eriksson, A., and Taylor, C.C. 1992. Evidence of fiber hyperplasia in human skeletal muscles from healthy young men? *European Journal of Applied Physiology* 62: 301-304.

Skalski, J., Allison, T.G., and Miller, T.D. 2012. The safety of cardiopulmonary exercise testing in a population with high-risk cardiovascular diseases. *Circulation* 126: 2465-2472.

Skatrud-Mickelson, M., Benson, J., Hannon, J.C., and Askew, W.E. 2011. A comparison of subjective and objective physical exertion. *Journal of Sports Sciences* 29: 1635-1644.

Skinner, J. 1993. *Exercise testing and exercise prescription for special cases.* Philadelphia: Lea & Febiger.

Slaughter, M.H., Lohman, T.G., Boileau, R.A., Horswill, C.A., Stillman, R.J., Van Loan, M.D., and Bemben, D.A. 1988. Skinfold equations for estimation of body fatness in children and youth. *Human Biology* 60: 709-723.

Smith, A.E., Evans, H., Parfitt, G., Eston, R., and Ferrar, K. 2016. Submaximal exercise-based equations to predict maximal oxygen uptake in older adults: A systematic review. *Archives of Physical Medicine and Rehabilitation* 97: 1003-1012.

Smith, L.L. 1991. Acute inflammation: The underlying mechanism in delayed onset muscle soreness? *Medicine & Science in Sports & Exercise* 23: 542-551.

Smith, U., Hammerstein, J., Bjorntorp, P., and Kral, J.G. 1979. Regional differences and effect of weight reduction on human fat cell metabolism. *European Journal of Clinical Investigation* 9: 327-332.

Smith, K.B., and Smith, M.S. 2016. Obesity statistics. *Primary Care: Clinics in Office Practice* 43: 121-135.

Smith-Ryan, A.E., Blue, M.N.M., Trexler, E.T., and Hirsch, K.R. 2016. Utility of ultrasound for body fat assessment: Validity and reliability compared to a multicompartment criterion. *Clinical Physiology and Functional Imaging* [Epub ahead of print]. doi:10.1111/cpf.12402. Accessed August 5, 2017.

Smith-Ryan, A.E., Fultz, S.N., Melvin, M.N., Wingfield, H.L., and Woessner, M.N. 2014. Reproducibility and validity of A-Mode ultrasound for body composition measurement and classification in overweight and obese men and women. *PLoS One* 9(3): e91750. doi:10.1371/journal.pone.0091750. Accessed August 5, 2017.

Smith-Ryan, A.E., Mock, M.G., Ryan, E.D., Gerstner, G.R., Trexler, E.R., and Hirsch, K.R. 2017. Validity and reliability of a 4-compartment body composition model using dual energy X-ray absorptiometry-derived body volume. *Clinical Nutrition* 36: 825-830.

Smutok, M.A., Skrinar, G.S., and Pandolf, K.B. 1980. Exercise intensity: Subjective regulation by perceived exertion. *Archives of Physical Medicine and Rehabilitation* 61: 569-574.

Smye, S.W., Sutcliffe, J., and Pitt, E. 1993. A comparison of four commercial systems used to measure whole-body electrical impedance. *Physiological Measurement* 14: 473-478.

Snarr, R.L., Hallmark, A.V., Nickerson, B.S., and Esco, M.R. 2016. Electromyographical comparison of pike variations performed with and without instability devices. *Journal of Strength and Conditioning Research* 30: 3436-3442.

Snijder, M.B., Kuyf, B.E., and Deurenberg, P. 1999. Effect of body build on the validity of predicted body fat from body mass index and bioelectrical impedance. *Annals of Nutrition and Metabolism* 43: 277-285.

Soileau, L., Bautista, D., Johnson, C., Gao, C., Zhang, K., Li, X., Heymsfield, S.B., Thomas, D., and Zheng, J. 2016. Automated anthropometric phenotyping with novel Kinect-based three-dimensional imaging method: Comparison with a reference laser imaging system. *European Journal of Clinical Nutrition* 70: 475-481.

Spalding, K.L., Arner, E., Westermark, P.O., Bernard, S., Buchholz, B.A., Bergmann, O., Blomqvist, L., Hoffstedt, J., Näslund, E., Britton, T., Concha, H., Hassan, M., Rydén, M., Frisén, J., and Arner, P. 2008. Dynamics of fat cell turnover in humans. *Nature* 453(7196): 783-787.

Spennewyn, K.C. 2008. Strength outcomes in fixed versus free-form resistance equipment. *Journal of Strength and Conditioning Research* 22(1): 75-81.

Sperandei, S., Vieira, M.C., and Reis, A. 2016. Adherence to physical activity in an unsupervised setting: Explanatory variables for high attrition rates among fitness center members. *Journal of Science and Medicine in Sport* 19: 916-920.

Sperlich, P.F., Holmberg, H-C., Reed, J.L., Zinner, C., Mester, J., and Sperlich, B. 2015. Individual versus standardized running protocols in the determination of $\dot{V}O_2$max. *Journal of Sports Science and Medicine* 14: 386-393.

Spierer, D.K., Rosen, Z., Litman, L.L., and Fujii, K. 2015. Validation of photoplethysmography as a method to detect heart rate during rest and exercise. *Journal of Medical Engineering & Technology* 39: 264-271.

Sprey, J.W.C., Ferreira, T., de Lima, M.V., Duarte, A., Jorge, P.B., and Santili, C. 2016. An epidemiological profile of CrossFit Athletes in Brazil. *Orthopaedic Journal of Sports Medicine* 4: 29 August.

Springer, B.A., Marin, R., Cyhan, T., Roberts, H., and Gill, N.W. 2007. Normative values for the unipedal stance test with eyes open and closed. *Journal of Geriatric Physical Therapy* 30: 8-15.

Staiano, A.E., and Flynn, R. 2014. Therapeutic uses of active videogames: A systematic review. *Games for Health Journal* 6: 351-365.

Stark, M., Lukaszuk, J., Prawitz, A., and Salacinski, A. 2012. Protein timing and its effects on muscular hypertrophy and strength in individuals engaged in weight-training. *Journal of the International Society of Sports Nutrition* 9: article 54.

Stark, T., Walker, B., Phillips, J.K., Fejer, R., and Beck, R. 2011. Hand-held dynamometry correlation with the gold standard isokinetic dynamometry: A systematic review. *PM&R: The Journal of Injury, Function, and Rehabilitation* 3: 472-479.

Stathokostas, L., Little, R.M.D., Vandervoort, A.A., and Paterson, D.H. 2012. Flexibility training and functional ability in older adults: A systematic review. *Journal of Aging Research* 2012: article 306818.

Statistics Canada. 2017. Canadian Health Measures Survey: Activity monitor data. http://www.statcan.gc.ca/daily-quotidien/170419/dq170419e-eng.htm. Accessed March 31, 2018.

Steele, J., Fisher, J., Skivington, M., Dunn, C., Arnold, J., Tew, G., Batterham, A.M., Nunan, D., O'Driscoll, J.M., Mann, S., Beedie, C., Jobson, S., Smith, D., Vigotsky, A., Phillips, S., Estabrooks, P., and Winett, R. 2017. A higher effort-based paradigm in physical activity and exercise for public health: Making a case for a greater emphasis on resistance training. *BMC Public Health* 17(1): 300.

Steffens, D., Maher, C.G., Pereira, L.S., Stevens, M.L., Oliveira, V.C., Chapple, M., Teixeira-Salmela, L.F., and Hancock, M.J. 2016. Prevention of low back pain: A systematic review and meta-analysis. *JAMA Internal Medicine* 176(2): 199-208.

Steinberg, S.I., Sammel, M.D., Harrel, B.T., Schembri, A., Policastro, C., Bogner, H.R., Negash, S., and Arnold, S.E. 2015. Exercise, sedentary pastimes, and cognitive performance in healthy older adults. *American Journal of Alzheimer's Disease & Other Dementias* 30: 290-298.

Steinberger, J., Daniels, S.R., Eckel, R.H., Hayman, L., Lustag, R.H., McCrindle, B., and Mietus-Snyder, M. 2009. Progress and challenges in metabolic syndrome in children and adolescents: A scientific statement from the American Heart Association Atherosclerosis, Hypertension and Obesity in the Young Committee of the Council on Cardiovascular Disease in the Young; Council on Cardiovascular Nursing; and Council on Nutrition, Physical Activity, and Metabolism. *Circulation* 119: 628-647.

Stergiou, G.S., Karpettas, N., Atkins, N., and O'Brien, E. 2011. Impact of applying the more stringent validation criteria of the revised European Society of Hypertension International Protocol 2010 on earlier validation studies. *Blood Pressure Monitoring* 16: 67-73.

Stergiou, G.S., Karpettas, N., Kollias, A., Destounis, A., and Tzamouranis, D. 2012a. A perfect replacement for the mercury sphygmomanometer: The case of the hybrid blood pressure monitor. *Journal of Human Hypertension* 26: 220-227.

Stergiou, G.S., Parati, G., Asmar, R., and O'Brien, E. 2012b. Requirements for professional office blood pressure monitors. *Journal of Hypertension* 30: 537-542.

Stiffler, M.R., Bell, D.R., Sanfilippo, J.L., Hetzel, S.J., Pickett, K.A., and Heiderscheit, B.C. 2017. Star excursion balance test anterior asymmetry is associated with injury status in division I collegiate athletes. *Journal of Orthopaedic and Sports Physical Therapy* 47: 339-346.

Stojanovic, M.D., and Ostojic, S.M. 2011. Stretching and injury prevention in football: Current perspectives. *Research in Sports Medicine* 19: 73-91.

Stolarczyk, L.M., Heyward, V.H., Hicks, V.L., and Baumgartner, R.N. 1994. Predictive accuracy of bioelectrical impedance in estimating body composition of Native American women. *American Journal of Clinical Nutrition* 59: 964-970.

Störchle, P., Müller, W., Sengeis, M., Ahammer, H., Fürhapter-Rieger, A., Bachl, N., Lackner, S., Mörkl, S., and Holasek, S. 2017. Standardized ultrasound measurement of subcutaneous fat patterning: High reliability and accuracy in groups ranging from lean to obese. *Ultrasound in Medicine and Biology* 43: 427-438.

Stracciolini, A., Myer, G.D., and Faigenbaum, A.D. 2013. Exercise-deficit disorder in children: Are we ready to make this diagnosis? *The Physician and Sports Medicine* 41. doi:10.3810/psm.2013.02.2003.

Studenski, S., Perera, S., Hile, E., Keller, V., Spadola-Bogard, J., and Garcia, J. 2010. Interactive video dance games for healthy older adults. *Journal of Nutrition, Health, and Aging* 14: 850-852.

Straight, C.R., Lindheimer, J.B., Brady, A.O., Dishman, R.K., and Evans, E.M. 2016. Effects of resistance training on lower-extremity muscle power in middle-aged and older adults: A systematic review and meta-analysis of randomized controlled trials. *Sports Medicine* 46: 353-364.

Strand, S.L., Hjelm, J., Shoepe, T.C., and Fajardo, M.A. 2014. Norms for an isometric muscle endurance test. *Journal of Human Kinetics* 40: 93-1026.

Stuber, K.J., Bruno, P., Sajko, S., and Hayden, J.A. 2014. Core stability exercises for low back pain in athletes: A systematic review of the literature. *Clinical Journal of Sports Medicine* 24: 448-456.

Sturm, R., and Hattori, A. 2012. Morbid obesity rates continue to rise rapidly in the United States. *International Journal of Obesity*. doi:10.1038/ijo.2012.159.

Stutchfield, B.M., and Coleman, S. 2006. The relationships between hamstring flexibility, lumbar flexion, and low back pain in rowers. *European Journal of Sport Science* 6: 255-260.

Sung, R.Y.T., Lau, P., Yu, C.W., Lam, P.K.W., and Nelson, E.A.S. 2001. Measurement of body fat using leg to leg bioimpedance. *Archives of Disease in Childhood* 85: 263-267.

Svendsen, O.L., Hassager, C., Bergmann, I., and Christiansen, C. 1992. Measurement of abdominal and intra-abdominal fat in postmenopausal women by dual energy X-ray absorptiometry and anthropometry: Comparison with computerized tomography. *International Journal of Obesity* 17: 45- 51.

Swain, D.P. 1999. $\dot{V}O_2$ reserve: A new method for exercise prescription. *ACSM's Health & Fitness Journal* 3(5): 10-14.

Swain, D.P., and Leutholtz, B.C. 1997. Heart rate reserve is equivalent to % $\dot{V}O_2$reserve, not to $\dot{V}O_2$max. *Medicine & Science in Sports & Exercise* 29: 410-414.

Swain, D.P., Leutholtz, B.C., King, M.E., Haas, L.A., and Branch, J.D. 1998. Relationship between % heart rate reserve and % $\dot{V}O_2$reserve in treadmill exercise. *Medicine & Science in Sports & Exercise* 30: 318-321.

Swain, D.P., Parrott, J.A., Bennett, A.R., Branch, J.D., and Dowling, E.A. 2004. Validation of a new method for estimating $\dot{V}O_2$max based on $\dot{V}O_2$ reserve. *Medicine & Science in Sports & Exercise* 36: 1421-1426.

Swift, D.L., Johannsen, N.M., Lavie, C.J., Earnest, C.P., and Church, T.S. 2014. The role of exercise and physical activity in weight loss and maintenance. *Progress in Cardiovascular Diseases* 56: 441-447.

Swinburn, B.A., Sacks, G., Hall, K.D., McPherson, L., Finegood, D.T., Moodie, M.L., and Gortmaker, S.L. 2011. The global obesity pandemic: Shaped by global drivers and local environments. *Lancet* 378: 804-814.

Taaffe, D.R., Duret, C., Wheeler, S., and Marcus, R. 1999. Once-weekly resistance exercise improves muscle strength and neuromuscular performance in older adults. *Journal of the American Geriatrics Society* 47: 1208-1214.

Takaishi, T., Ishihara, K., Shima, N., and Hayashi, T. 2014. Health promotion with stair exercise. *Journal of Physical Fitness and Sports Medicine* 3: 173-179.

Takeshima, N., Rogers, M.E., Watanabe, E., Brechue, W.F., Okada, A., Yamada, T., Islam, M.M., and Hayano, J. 2002. Water-based exercise improves health-related aspects of fitness in older women. *Medicine & Science in Sports & Exercise* 34: 544-551.

Talag, T.S. 1973. Residual muscular soreness as influenced by concentric, eccentric, and static contractions. *Research Quarterly* 44: 458-469.

Tanaka, H., Monahan, K.D., and Seals, D.R. 2001. Age-predicted maximal heart rate revisited. *Journal of the American College of Cardiology* 37: 153-156.

Tang, L.H., Zwisler, A-D., Taylor, T.S., Doherty, P., Zangger, G., Berg, S.K., and Langberg, H. 2016. Self-rating level of perceived exertion for guiding exercise intensity during a 12-week cardiac rehabilitation programme and the influence of heart rate reducing medication. *Journal of Science and Medicine in Sport*. 19: 611-615.

Tarleton, H.P., Smith, L.V., Zhang, Z-F., and Kuo, T. 2015. Utility of anthropometric measures in a multiethnic population:

Their association with prevalent diabetes, hypertension and other chronic disease comorbidities. *Journal of Community Health* 39: 471-479.

Taylor, D.C., Dalton, J.D., Seaber, A.V., and Garrett, W.E. 1990. Viscoelastic properties of muscle-tendon units. The biomechanical effects of stretching. *American Journal of Sports Medicine* 18: 300-309.

Taylor, N.A.S., and Wilkinson, J.G. 1986. Exercise-induced skeletal muscle growth: Hypertrophy or hyperplasia? *Sports Medicine* 3: 190-200.

Taylor, W.D., George, J.D., Allsen, P.E., Vehrs, P.R., Hager, R.L., and Roberts, M.P. 2002. Estimation of $\dot{V}O_2max$ from a 1.5-mile endurance test. *Medicine & Science in Sports & Exercise* 35(Suppl.): S257 [abstract].

Tchoukalova, Y.D., Votruba, S.B., Tchkonia, T., Giorgadze, N., Kirkland, J.L., and Jensen, M.D. 2010. Regional differences in cellular mechanisms of adipose tissue gain with overfeeding. *Proceedings of the National Academy of Sciences* 107: 18226-18231.

Tegenkamp, M.H., Clark, R.R., Schoeller, D.A., and Landry, G.L. 2011. Effects of covert subject actions on percent body fat by air-displacement plethysmography. *Journal of Strength and Conditioning Research* 25: 2010-2017.

Teichtahl, A.J., Urquhart, D.M., Wang, Y., Wluka, A.E., O'Sullivan, R., Jones, G., and Cicuttini, F.M. 2015. Physical inactivity is associated with narrower lumbar intervertebral discs, high fat content of paraspinal muscles and low back pain and disability. *Arthritis Research & Therapy* 17: 114-120.

Tesch, P.A. 1988. Skeletal muscle adaptations consequent to long-term heavy resistance exercise. *Medicine & Science in Sports & Exercise* 20: S132-S134.

Tesch, P.A. 1992. Short- and long-term histochemical and biochemical adaptations in muscle. In *Strength and power in sports: The encyclopaedia of sports medicine,* ed. P. Komi, 239-248. Oxford: Blackwell.

Teixeira, P.J., Carraça, E.V., Markland, D., Silva, M.N., and Ryan, R.M. 2012. Exercise, physical activity, and self-determination theory: A systematic review. *Journal of Behavioral Nutrition and Physical Activity* 9: 78. www.ijbnpa.org/content/9/1/78. Accessed June 10, 2017.

Teixeira, P.J., Carraça, E.V., Marques, M.M., Rutter, H., Oppert, J-M., de Bourdeaudhuij, I., Lakerveld, J., and Brug, J. 2015. Successful behavior change in obesity interventions in adults: A systematic review of self-regulation mediators. *BMC Medicine* 13: 84. doi:10.1186/s12916-015-0323-6. Accessed May 3, 2017.

Thacker, S.B., Gilchrist, J., Stroup, D.F., and Kimsey, C.D. 2004. The impact of stretching on sports injury risk: A systematic review of the literature. *Medicine & Science in Sports & Exercise* 36: 371-378.

Thaler, M.S. 2015. *The only EKG book you'll ever need,* 8th ed. Philadelphia: Wolters Kluers.

Tholl, U., Lüders, S., Bramlage, P., Dechend, R., Eckert, S., Mengden, T., Nürnberger, J., Sanner, B., and Anlauf, M. 2016. The German Hypertension League (Deutsche Hochdruck-liga) Quality Seal Protocol for blood pressure-measuring devices: 15-year experience and results from 105 devices for home blood pressure control. *Blood Pressure Monitoring* 21: 197-205.

Thomas, J.F., Larson, K.L., Hollander, D.B., and Kraemer, R.R. 2014. Comparison of two-hand kettlebell exercise and graded treadmill walking: Effectiveness as a stimulus for cardiorespiratory fitness. *Journal of Strength and Conditioning Research* 28: 998-1006.

Thomas, T.R., and Etheridge, G.L. 1980. Hydrostatic weighing at residual volume and functional residual capacity. *Journal of Applied Physiology* 49: 157-159.

Thomas, T.R., Ziogas, G., Smith, T., Zhang, Q., and Londeree, B.R. 1995. Physiological and perceived exertion responses to six modes of submaximal exercise. *Research Quarterly for Exercise and Sport* 66: 239-246.

Thompson, C.J., and Bemben, M.G. 1999. Reliability and comparability of the accelerometer as a measure of muscular power. *Medicine and Science in Sports & Exercise* 31: 897-902.

Thompson, C.J., Cobb, K.M., and Blackwell, J. 2007. Functional training improves club head speed and functional fitness of older golfers. *Journal of Strength and Conditioning Research* 21(1): 131-137.

Thompson, J., Manore, M., and Thomas, J. 1996. Effects of diet and diet-plus-exercise programs on resting metabolic rate: A meta-analysis. *International Journal of Sport Nutrition* 6: 41-61.

Thompson, M., and Medley, A. 2007. Forward and lateral sitting functional reach in younger, middle-aged, and older adults. *Journal of Geriatric Physical Therapy* 30(2): 43-51.

Thompson, P.D. 1993. The safety of exercise testing and participation. In *ACSM's resource manual for guidelines for exercise testing and prescription*, ed. S.N. Blair, P. Painter, R. Pate, L.K. Smith, and C.B. Taylor, 361-370. Philadelphia: Lea & Febiger.

Thompson, W.R. 2017. Worldwide survey of fitness trends for 2018. *ACSM's Health & Fitness Journal* 21(6): 10-19.

Thorstensson, A., Hulten, B., vonDobeln, W., and Karlsson, J. 1976. Effect of strength training on enzyme activities and fibre characteristics in human skeletal muscle. *Acta Physiologica Scandinavica* 96: 392-398.

Thurlow, S., Taylor-Covill, G., Sahota, P., Oldroyd, B., and Hind, K. 2017. Effects of procedure, upright equilibrium time, sex, and BMI on the precision of body fluid measurements using bioelectrical impedance analysis. *European Journal of Clinical Nutrition* [Epub ahead of print]. doi:10.1038/ejcn.2017.110. Accessed August 4, 2017.

Tidstrand, J., and Horneij, E. 2009. Inter-rater reliability of three standardized functional tests in patients with low back pain. *BMC Musculoskeletal Disorders* 10: 58.

Tiedemann, A., Sherrington, C., Close, J.C.T., and Lord, S.R. 2011. Exercise and sports science Australia position statement on exercise and falls prevention in older people. *Journal of Science and Medicine in Sport* 14: 489-495.

Tientcheu, D., Ayers, C., Das, S.R., McGuire, K.K., de Lemos, J.A., Khera, A., Kaplan, N., Victor, R., and Vongpatanasin, W. 2015. Target organ complications and cardiovascular events associated with masked hypertension and white-coat hypertension. *Journal of the American College of Cardiology* 66: 2159-2169.

Timson, B.F., and Coffman, J.L. 1984. Body composition by hydrostatic weighing at total lung capacity and residual volume. *Medicine & Science in Sports & Exercise* 16: 411-414.

Tinetti, M.E. 1986. Performance-oriented assessment of mobility problems in elderly patients. *Journal of the American Geriatric Society* 34: 119-126.

Tinetti, M.E., Speechley, M., and Ginter, S.F. 1988. Risk factors for falls among elderly persons living in the community. *New England Journal of Medicine* 319(26): 1701-1707.

Tinwala, F., Cronin, J., Haemmerle, E., and Ross, A. 2017. Eccentric strength training: A review of the available technology. *Strength and Conditioning Journal* 39: 32-47.

Tipton, C.M., Matthes, R.D., Maynard, J.A., and Carey, R.A. 1975. The influence of physical activity on ligaments and tendons. *Medicine and Science in Sports* 7: 165-175.

Tjønna, A.E., Leinan, I.M., Bartnes, A.T., Jenssen, B., Gibala, M.J., Winett, R.A., and Wisløff. 2013. Low- and high-volume of intensive endurance training significantly improves maximal oxygen update after 10-weeks of training in healthy men. *PLoS One* 8: e65382. doi:10.1371/journal.pone.0065382.g001. Accessed August 2, 2017.

Tognetti, A., Lorussi, F., Carbonaro, N., and de Rossi, D. 2015. Wearable goniometer and accelerometer sensory fusion for knee joint angle measurement in daily life. *Sensors* 15: 28435-28455.

Tognetti, A., Lorussi, F., Dalle Mura, G., Carbonaro, N., Pacelli, M., Paradiso, R., and de Rossi, D. 2014. New generation of wearable goniometers for motion capture systems. *Journal of NeuroEngineering and Rehabilitation* 11: 56.

Tolonen, H., Koponen, P., Naska, A., Männistö, S., Broda, G., Palossari, T., Kuulasmaa, K., and the EHES Pilot Project. 2015. Challenges in standardization of blood pressure measurement at the population level. *BMC Medical Research Methodology* 15: 33. doi:10.1186/s12874-015-0020-3. Accessed April 29, 2017.

Tomiyama, A.J., Hunger, J.M., Nguyen-Cuu, J., and Wells, C. 2016. Misclassification of cardiometabolic health when using body mass index categories in NHANES 2005-2012. *International Journal of Obesity* 40: 883-886.

Toombs, R.J., Ducher, G., Shepherd, J.A., and de Souza, M.J. 2012. The impact of recent technological advancements on the trueness and precision of DXA to assess body composition. *Obesity* 20: 30-39.

Toomey, C.M., McCormack, W.G., and Jakeman, P. 2017. The effect of hydration status on the measurement of lean tissue mass by dual-energy X-ray absorptiometry. *European Journal of Applied Physiology* 117: 567-574.

Toomey, C., McCreesh, K., Leahy, S., and Jakeman, P. 2011. Technical considerations for accurate measurement of subcutaneous adipose tissue thickness using B-mode ultrasound. *Ultrasound* 19: 91-96.

Torbeyns, T., Bailey, S., Bos, I., and Meeusen, R. 2014. Active workstations to fight sedentary behavior. *Sports Medicine* 44: 1261-1273.

Torgan, C.E., and Cousineau, T.M. 2012. Leveraging social media technologies to help clients achieve behavior change goals. *ACSM's Health & Fitness Journal* 16: 18-24.

Torres, R., Ribeiro, F., Duarte, J.A., and Cabri, J.M.H. 2012. Evidence of the physiotherapeutic interventions used currently after exercise-induced muscle damage: Systematic review and meta-analysis. *Physical Therapy in Sport* 13: 101-114.

Torvinen, S., Kannus, P., Sievanen, H., Jarvinen, T.A.H., Pasanen, M., Kontulainen, S., Jarvinen, T.L.N., Jarvinen, M., Oja, P., and Vuori, I. 2002. Effect of four-month vertical whole body vibration on performance and balance. *Medicine & Science in Sports & Exercise* 34: 1523-1528.

Town, G.P., Sol, N., and Sinning, W. 1980. The effect of rope skipping rate on energy expenditure of males and females. *Medicine & Science in Sports & Exercise* 12: 295-298.

Townsend, N., Rutter, H., and Foster, C. 2012. Evaluating the evidence that the prevalence of childhood obesity is plateauing. *Pediatric Obesity* 7: 343-346.

Townsend, N., Wildon, L., Bhatnagar, P., Wickramasinghe, K., Rayner, M., and Nichols, M. 2016. Cardiovascular disease in Europe: Epidemiological update 2016. *European Heart Journal* 37: 3232-3245.

Tran, Z.V., and Weltman, A. 1988. Predicting body composition of men from girth measurements. *Human Biology* 60: 167-175.

Tran, Z.V., and Weltman, A. 1989. Generalized equation for predicting body density of women from girth measurements. *Medicine & Science in Sports & Exercise* 21: 101-104.

Trapp, E.G., Chisholm, D.J., Freund, J., and Boutcher, S.H. 2008. The effects of high-intensity intermittent exercise training on fat loss and fasting insulin levels of young women. *International Journal of Obesity* 32: 684-691.

Tremblay, M.S., Warburton, D.E.R., Janssen, I., Paterson, D.H., Latimer, A.E., Rhodes, R.E., Kho, M.E., Hicks, A., LeBlanc, A.G., Zehr, L., Murumets, K., and Duggan, M. 2011. New Canadian physical activity guidelines. *Applied Physiology, Nutrition, and Metabolism* 36: 36-46.

Troped, P.J., Oliveira, M.S., Matthews, C.E., Cromley, E.K., Melly, S.J., and Craig, B.A. 2008. Prediction of activity mode with global positioning system and accelerometer data. *Medicine & Science in Sports & Exercise* 10: 972-978.

Trost, S.G., Owen, N., Bauman, A.E., Sallis, J.F., and Brown, W. 2002. Correlates of adults' participation in physical activity: Review and update. *Medicine & Science in Sports & Exercise* 34: 1996-2001.

Tseng, K., Tseng, W., Lin, M., Chen, H., Nosaka, K., and Chen, T.C. 2016. Protective effect by maximal isometric contractions against maximal eccentric exercise-induced muscle damage of the knee extensors. *Research in Sports Medicine* 24: 243-256.

Tsukamoto, H., Takenaka, S., Suga, T., Tanaka, D., Takeuchi, T., Hamaoka, T., Isaka, T., and Hashimoto, T. 2017. Effect of exercise intensity and duration on postexercise executive function. *Medicine & Science in Sports & Exercise* 49: 774-784.

Tucker, L.A., Lechiminant, J.D., and Bailey, B.W. 2014. Test re-test reliability of the BodPod: The effect of multiple assessments. *Perceptual and Motor Skills: Physical Development and Movement* 118: 563-570.

Tudor-Locke, C., Bassett, D.R., Shipe, M.F., and McClain, J.J. 2011. Pedometry methods for assessing free-living adults. *Journal of Physical Activity and Health* 8: 445-453.

Tudor-Locke, C., Pangrazi, R.P., Corbin, C.B., Rutherford, W.J., Vincent, S.D., Raustorp, A., Tomson, L.M., and Cuddihy, T.F. 2004. BMI-referenced standards for recommended pedometer-determined steps/day in children. *Preventive Medicine* 38: 857-864.

Turcato, E., Bosello, O., Francesco, V.D., Harris, T.B., Zoico, E., Bissoli, L., Fracassi, E., and Zamboni, M. 2000. Waist circumference and abdominal sagittal diameter as surrogates of body fat distribution in the elderly: Their relation with cardiovascular risk factors. *International Journal of Obesity* 24: 1005-1010.

Tyrrell, V.J., Richards, G., Hofman, P., Gillies, G.F., Robinson, E., and Cutfield, W.S. 2001. Foot-to-foot bioelectrical impedance analysis: A valuable tool for the measurement of body composition in children. *International Journal of Obesity* 25: 273-278.

Urwin, S.G., Kader, D.F., Caplan, N., St. Clair Gibson, A., and Stewart, S. 2013. Validation of an electrogoniometry system as a measure of knee kinematics during activities of daily living. *Journal of Musculoskeletal Research* 16: article 1350005.

U.S. Department of Health and Human Services. 1996. *Physical activity and health: A report of the Surgeon General—At a glance*. Atlanta: U.S. Department of Health and Human Services, Centers for Disease Control and Prevention, National Center for Chronic Disease Prevention and Health Promotion.

U.S. Department of Health and Human Services. 2007. *The Surgeon General's call to action to prevent overweight and obesity in children and adolescents*. Washington, DC: Author. www.surgeongeneral.gov/topics/obesity/calltoaction/fact_adolescents.html.

U.S. Department of Health and Human Services. 2008. Physical activity guidelines for Americans. At-a-glance: A fact sheet for professionals. www.health.gov/paguidelines/factsheet-prof.aspx.

U.S. Department of Health and Human Services, Centers for Disease Control and Prevention. 2015. How much physical activity do adults need? www.cdc.gov/physicalactivity/basics/adults/index.htm. Accessed June 27, 2017.

U.S. Department of Health and Human Services. 2010. *Dietary guidelines for Americans 2010*. Washington, D.C.: Author.

U.S. Department of Health and Human Services. 2012. *Healthy People 2020*. www.healthypeople.gov/2020. Accessed June 15, 2012.

U.S. Environmental Protection Agency. 2017. Minata Convention on Mercury. www.epa.gov/international-cooperation/minamata-convention-mercury. Accessed April 30, 2017.

Utter, A.C., Nieman, D.C., Ward, A.N., and Butterworth, D.E. 1999. Use of the leg-to-leg bioelectrical impedance method in assessing body-composition change in obese women. *American Journal of Clinical Nutrition* 69: 603-607.

Vaisman, N., Corey, M., Rossi, M.F., Goldberg, E., and Pencharz, P. 1988. Changes in body composition during refeeding of patients with anorexia nervosa. *Journal of Pediatrics* 113: 925-929.

Vaisman, N., Rossi, M.F., Goldberg, E., Dibden, L.J., Wykes, L.J., and Pencharz, P.B. 1988. Energy expenditures and body composition in patients with anorexia nervosa. *Journal of Pediatrics* 113: 919-924.

Van Adrichem, J.A.M., and van der Korst, J.K. 1973. Assessment of flexibility of the lumbar spine: A pilot study in children and adolescents. *Scandinavian Journal of Rheumatology* 2: 87-91.

van den Beld, W.A., van der Sanden, G.A.C., Sengers, R.C.A., Verbeek, A.L.M., and Gabreels, F.J.M. 2006. Validity and reproducibility of hand-held dynamometry in children aged 4-11 years. *Journal of Rehabilitation Medicine* 38: 57-64.

van der Kooy, K., Leenen, R., Seidell, J.C., Deurenberg, P., Droop, A., and Bakker, C.J.G. 1993. Waist-hip ratio is a poor predictor of changes in visceral fat. *American Journal of Clinical Nutrition* 57: 327-333.

van Genugten, L., Dusseldorp, E., Webb, T.L., and van Empelan, P. 2016. Which combinations of techniques and modes of delivery in Internet-based interventions effectively change health behavior? A meta-analysis. *Journal of Medical Internet Research*. 18: e155. doi:10.2196/jmir.4218. Accessed June 11, 2017.

Vanhelder, W.P., Radomski, M.W., and Goode, R.C. 1984. Growth hormone responses during intermittent weight lifting exercise in men. *European Journal of Applied Physiology* 53: 31-34.

Van Loan, M.D., and Mayclin, P.L. 1987. Bioelectrical impedance analysis: Is it a reliable estimator of lean body mass and total body water? *Human Biology* 59: 299-309.

Van Mechelen, W., Holbil, H., and Kemper, H.C. 1986. Validation of two running tests as estimates of maximal aerobic power in children. *European Journal of Applied Physiology and Occupational Physiology* 55: 503-506.

Van Remoortel, H., Giavedoni, S., Raste, Y., Burtin, C., Louvaris, Z., Gimeno-Santos, E., Langer, D., Glendenning, A., Hopkinson, N.S., Vogiatzis, I., Peterson, B.T., Wilson, F., Mann, B., Rabinovich, R., Puhan, M.A., and Troosters, T. 2012. Validity of activity monitors in health and chronic disease: A systematic review. *International Journal of Behavioral Nutrition and Physical Activity* 9: 84.

VanWormer, J.J., Martinez, A.M., Martinson, B.C., Crain, A.L., Benson, G.A., Cosentino, D.L., and Pronk, N.P. 2009. Self-weighing promotes weight loss for obese adults. *American Journal of Preventive Medicine* 36: 70-73.

Vehrs, P.R., Drummond, M., Fellingham, D.K., and Brigham, G.W. 2002. Accuracy of five heart rate monitors during exercise. *Medicine & Science in Sports & Exercise* 34(Suppl.): S272 [abstract].

Velthuis, M.J., Schuit, A.J., Peeters, P.H.M., and Monninkhof, E.M. 2009. Exercise program affects body composition but not weight in postmenopausal women. *Menopause: The Journal of the North American Menopause Society* 16: 777-784.

Vera-Garcia, F.J., Grenier, S.G., and McGill, S.M. 2000. Abdominal muscle responses during curl-ups on both stable and labile surfaces. *Physical Therapy* 80: 564-569.

Vescovi, J.D., Zimmerman, S.L., Miller, W.C., Hildebrandt, L., Hammer, R.L., and Fernhall, B. 2001. Evaluation of the Bod Pod for estimating percentage body fat in a heterogeneous group of adult humans. *European Journal of Applied Physiology* 85: 326-332.

Větrovska, R., Vilikus, Z., Klaschka, J., Stránská, Z., Svačina, Š., Svobodova, Š., and Matoulek, M. 2014. Does impedance measure a functional state of body fat? *Physiological Research* 63(Suppl. 2): S309-S320.

Vikmoen, O., Ronnestad, B.R., Ellefsen, S., and Raastad, T. 2017. Heavy strength training improves running and cycling performance following prolonged submaximal work in well-trained female athletes. *Physiological Reports* 5: article e13149.

Vincent, K.R., Braith, R.W., Feldman, R.A., Magyari, P.M., Cutler, R.B., Persin, S.A., Lennon, S.L., Gabr, A.H., and Lowenthal, D.T. 2002. Resistance exercise and physical performance in adults aged 60 to 83. *Journal of the American Geriatrics Society* 50: 1100-1107.

Vohralik, S.L., Bowen, A.R., Burns, J., Hiller, C.E., and Nightingale, E.J. 2015. Reliability and validity of a smartphone app to measure joint range. *American Journal of Physical Medicine and Rehabilitation* 94: 325-330.

von Stengel, S., Kemmler, W., Bebenek, M., Engelke, K., and Kalender, W.A. 2011. Effects of whole-body vibration training on different devices on bone mineral density. *Medicine & Science in Sports & Exercise* 43: 1071-1079.

von Stengel, S., Kemmler, W., Engelke, K., and Kalender, W.A. 2011. Effects of whole body vibration on bone mineral density and falls: Results of the randomized controlled ELVIS study with postmenopausal women. *Osteoporosis International* 22: 317-325.

von Stengel, S., Kemmler, W., Engelke, K., and Kalender, W.A. 2012. Effect of whole-body vibration on neuromuscular performance and body composition for females 65 years and older: A randomized-controlled trial. *Scandinavian Journal of Medicine & Science in Sports* 22: 119-127.

Wagner, D.R., 2013. Ultrasound as a tool to assess body fat. *Journal of Obesity* 2013: article 280713. doi:10.1155/2013/280713. Accessed August 1, 2014.

Wagner, D.R. 2014. Exercise physiologists in the United States: A 2012 national survey. *Journal of Exercise Physiology* [online]. www.asep.org/asep/asep/JEPonlineOCTOBER2014_Wagner.pdf.

Wagner, D.R. 2015. Predicted versus measured thoracic gas volumes of collegiate athletes made by Bod Pod air displacement plethysmography system. *Applied Physiology, Nutrition, and Metabolism* 10: 1075-1077.

Wagner, D.R., Cain, D.L., and Clark, N.W. 2016. Validity and reliability of A-mode ultrasound for body composition assessment of NCAA Division I athletes. *PLoS One* 11(4): e0153146. doi:10.1371/journal.pone.0153146.

Wagner, D.R., and Heyward, V.H. 2001. Validity of two-component models of estimating body fat of Black men. *Journal of Applied Physiology* 90: 649-656.

Wagner, D., Heyward, V., and Gibson, A. 2000. Validation of air displacement plethysmography for assessing body composition. *Medicine & Science in Sports & Exercise* 32: 1339-1344.

Wagner, K.H., and Brath, H. 2012. A global view on the development on non communicable diseases. *Preventive Medicine* 54: s38-s41.

Wallick, M.E., Porcari, J.P., Wallick, S.B., Berg, K.M., Brice, G.A., and Arimond, G.R. 1995. Physiological responses to in-line skating compared to treadmill running. *Medicine & Science in Sports & Exercise* 27: 242-248.

Wallman, H.W. 2001. Comparison of elderly nonfallers and fallers on performance measures of functional reach, sensory organization, and limits of stability. *Journal of Gerontology* 56: M589-M583.

Wallman, K., Plant, L.A., Rakimov, B., and Maiorana, A.J. 2009. The effects of two modes of exercise on aerobic fitness and fat mass in an overweight population. *Research in Sports Medicine* 17: 156-170.

Walts, C.T., Hanson, E.D., Delmonico, M.J., Yao, L., Wang, M.W., and Hurley, B.F. 2008. Do sex or race differences influence strength training effects on muscle or fat? *Medicine & Science in Sports & Exercise* 40: 669-676.

Wan, Y., Henegghan, C., Stevens, R., McManus, R.J., Ward, A., Perera, R., Thompson, M., Tarassenko, L., and Mant, D. 2010. Determining which automatic digital blood pressure device performs adequately: A systematic review. *Journal of Human Hypertension* 24: 431-438.

Wang, J., Thornton, J.C., Russell, M., Burastero, S., Heymsfield, S., and Pierson, R.N. 1994. Asians have lower body mass index (BMI) but higher percent body fat than do whites: Comparison of anthropometric measurements. *American Journal of Clinical Nutrition* 60: 23-28.

Wang, J-G., Zhang, Y., Chen, H-E., Li, Y., Cheng, X-G., Xu, L., Guo, Z., Zhao, X-S., Sato, T., Cao, Q-Y., Chen, K-M., and Li, B. 2013. Comparison of two bioelectrical impedance analysis devices with dual energy X-ray absorptiometry and magnetic resonance imaging in the estimation of body composition. *Journal of Strength and Conditioning Research* 27: 236-243.

Wang, R., Wu, M.J., Ma, X.Q., Zhao, Y.F., Yan, X.Y., Gao, Q.B., and He, J. 2012. Body mass index and health-related quality of life in adults: A population based study in five cities of China. *European Journal of Public Health* 22(4): 497-502.

Wang, X.Q., Zheng, J.J., Yu, Z.W., Bi, X., Lou, S.J., Liu, J., Cai, B., Hua, Y.H., Wu, M., Wei, M.L., Shen, H.M., Chen, Y., Pan, Y.J., Xu, G.H., and Chen, P.J. 2012. A meta-analysis of core stability exercise versus general exercise for chronic low back pain. *PLoS One* 7(1): e52082.

Warburton, D.E.R., and Breden, S.S.D. 2016. Reflections on physical activity and health: What should we recommend? *Canadian Journal of Cardiology* 32: 495-504.

Warburton, D.E.R., Sarkany, D., Johnson, M., Rhodes, R.E., Whitford, W., Esch, B.T.A., Scott, J.M., Wong, S.C., and Bredin, S.S.D. 2009. Metabolic requirements of interactive video game cycling. *Medicine & Science in Sports & Exercise* 41: 920-926.

Ward, R., and Anderson, G.S. 1998. Resilience of anthropometric data assembly strategies to imposed error. *Journal of Sports Sciences* 16: 755-759.

Ward, R., Rempel, R., and Anderson, G.S. 1999. Modeling dynamic skinfold compression. *American Journal of Human Biology* 11: 521-537.

Wathen, D. 1994. Load assignment. In *Essentials of strength testing*, ed. T.R. Baechle, 435-446. Champaign, IL: Human Kinetics.

Watson, L.P.E., Venables, M.C., and Murgatroyd, P.R. 2017. An investigation into the differences in bone density and body composition measurements between 2 GE Lunar densitometers and their comparison to a 4-component model. *Journal of Clinical Densitometry: Assessment & Management of Musculoskeletal Health* [Epub ahead of print]. doi:10.1016/j.jocd.2017.06.029. Accessed August 6, 2017.

Watson, S.L., Weeks, B.K., Weis, L.J., Horan, S.A., and Beck, B.R. 2015. Heavy resistance training is safe and improves bone, function, and stature in postmenopausal women with low to very low bone mass: Novel early findings from the LIFTMOR trial. *Osteoporosis International* 26: 2889-2894.

Weakley, J.J.S., Till, K., Read, D.B., Roe, G.A.B., Darrall-Jones, J., Phibbs, P.J., and Jones, B. 2017. The effects of traditional, superset, and tri-set resistance training structures on perceived intensity and physiological responses. *European Journal of Applied Physiology* 117: 1877-1889.

Weaver, T.B., Ma, C., and Laing, A.C. 2017. Use of the Nintendo Wii balance board for studying standing static balance control: Technical considerations, force-plate congruency, and the effect of battery life. *Journal of Applied Biomechanics* 33: 48-55.

Webb, C., Vehrs, P.R., George, J.D., and Hager, R. 2014. Estimating $\dot{V}O_2$max using a personalized step test. *Measurement in Physical Education and Exercise Science* 18: 184-197.

Webb, T.L., Joseph, J., Yardley, L., and Michie, S. 2010. Using the Internet to promote health behavior change: A systematic review and meta-analysis of the impact of theoretical basis, use of behavior change techniques, and mode of delivery on efficacy. *Journal of Medicine and Internet Research* 12:e4. doi:10.2196/jmir.1376. Accessed November 4, 2012.

Wei, N., Pang, M.Y.C., Ng, S.S.M., and Ng, G.Y.F. 2016. Optimal frequency/time combination of whole-body vibration training for improving muscle size and strength of people with age-related muscle loss (sarcopenia): A randomized controlled trial. *Geriatrics and Gerontology International* [in press].

Weier, A.T., and Kidgell, D.J. 2012. Strength training with superimposed whole body vibration does not preferentially modulate cortical plasticity. *Scientific World Journal* 2012: 876328.

Weiglein, L., Herrick, J., Kirk, S., and Kirk, E.P. 2011. The 1-mile walk test is a valid predictor of $\dot{V}O_2$max and is a reliable alternative fitness test to the 1.5-mile run in U.S. Air Force males. *Military Medicine* 176: 669-673.

Weijs, P.J.M. 2008. Validity of predictive equations for resting energy expenditure in U.S. and Dutch overweight and obese class I and II adults aged 18-65 y. *American Journal of Clinical Nutrition* 88: 959-970.

Weinheimer, E.M., Sands, L.P., and Campbellnure, W.W. 2010. A systematic review of the separate and combined effects of energy restriction and exercise on fat-free mass in middle-aged and older adults: Implications for sarcopenic obesity. *Nutrition Reviews* 68: 375-388.

Weisenthal, B.M., Beck, C.A., Maloney, M.D., DeHaven, K.E., and Giordano, B.D. 2014. Injury rate and patterns among CrossFit athletes. *Orthopaedic Journal of Sports Medicine* 2: article 2325967114531177.

Weiss, E.C., Galuska, D.A., Khan, L.K., and Serdula, M.K. 2006. Weight-control practices among U.S. adults, 2001-2002. *American Journal of Preventive Medicine* 31: 18-24.

Weiss, L.W., Cureton, K.J., and Thompson, F.N. 1983. Comparison of serum testosterone and androstenedione responses to weight lifting in men and women. *European Journal of Applied Physiology* 50: 413-419.

Weits, T., Van der Beek, E.J., Wedel, M., and Ter Haar Romeny, B.M. 1988. Computed tomography measurement of abdominal fat deposition in relation to anthropometry. *International Journal of Obesity* 12: 217-225.

Wellmon, R.H., Gulick, D.T., Paterson, M.L., and Gulick, C.N. 2016. Validity and reliability of 2 goniometric mobile apps: Device, application, and examiner factors. *Journal of Sport Rehabilitation* 25: 371-379.

Weltman, A., Levine, S., Seip, R.L., and Tran, Z.V. 1988. Accurate assessment of body composition in obese females. *American Journal of Clinical Nutrition* 48: 1179-1183.

Weltman, A., Seip, R.L., and Tran, Z.V. 1987. Practical assessment of body composition in adult obese males. *Human Biology* 59: 523-535.

Wen, C.P., Wai, J.P., Tsai, M.K., Yang, Y.C., Cheng, T.Y., Lee, M.C., Chan, H.T., Tsao, C.K., Tsai, S.P., and Wu, X. 2011. Minimum amount of physical activity for reduced mortality and extended life expectancy: A prospective cohort study. *Lancet* 378: 1244-1253.

Wessel, H.U., Strasburger, J.F., and Mitchell, B.M. 2001. New standards for Bruce treadmill protocol in children and adolescents. *Pediatric Exercise Science* 13: 392-401.

Wewege, M., van den Berg, R., Ward, R.E., and Keech, A. 2017. The effects of high-intensity interval training vs. moderate-intensity continuous training on body composition in overweight and obese adults: A systematic review and meta-analysis. *Obesity Reviews* 18: 635-646.

Whaley, M., Kaminsky, L., Dwyer, G., Getchell, L., and Norton, J. 1992. Predictors of over- and underachievement of age-predicted maximal heart rate. *Medicine & Science in Sports & Exercise* 24: 1173-1179.

Whelton, P.K., Carey, R.M., Aronow, W.S., Casey, D.E. Jr., Collins, K.J., Himmelfarb, C.D., DePalma, S.M., Gidding, S., Jamerson, K.A., MacLaughlin, E.J., Muntner, P., Ovbiagele,

B., Smith, S.C. Jr., Stafford, R.S., Taler, S.J., Thomas, R.J., Williams Sr., K.A., Williamson, J.D., and Wright, J.T. Jr. 2017. 2017 ACC/AHA/AAPA/ABC/ACPM/AGS/APhA/ ASH/ASPC/NMA/PCNA guideline for the prevention, detection, evaluation, and management of high blood pressure in adults. *Journal of the American College of Cardiology* [e-pub ahead of print]. doi:10.1016/j.jacc.2017.11.006. Accessed November 14, 2017.

Whitmer, T.D., Fry, A.C., Forsythe, C.M., Andre, M.J., Lane, M.T., Hudy, A., and Honnold, D.E. 2015. Accuracy of a vertical jump contact mat for determining jump height and flight time. *Journal of Strength and Conditioning Research* 29: 877-881.

Whitney, S.L., Poole, J.L., and Cass, S.P. 1998. A review of balance instruments for older adults. *American Journal of Occupational Therapy* 52: 666-671.

Wibner, T., Doering, K., Kropf-Sanshen, C., Rüdger, S., Blanta, I., Stoiber, K.M., Rottbauer, W., and Schumann, C. 2014. Pulse transit time and blood pressure during cardiopulmonary exercise tests. *Physiological Research* 63: 287-296.

Wild, D., Nayak, U.S.L., and Isaacs, B. 1981. Prognosis of falls in old people at home. *Journal of Epidemiology and Community Health* 35: 200-204.

Wild, S., Hanley, J., Lewis, S., McKnight, J., McCloughan, L., Padfield, P., Paterson, M., Pinnock, H., and McKinstry, B. 2013. The impact of supported telemetric monitoring in people with type 2 diabetes: Study protocol for a randomised controlled trial. *Trials* 14: 198.

Wilkin, L.D., Cheryl, A., and Haddock, B.L. 2012. Energy expenditure comparison between walking and running in average fitness individuals. *Journal of Strength and Conditioning Research* 26: 1039-1044.

Willardson, J.M. 2008. A periodized approach for core training. *ACSM's Health & Fitness Journal* 12(1): 7-13.

Willey, J.Z., Gardener, H., Caunca, M.R., Moon, Y.P., Dong, C., Cheung, Y.K., Sacco, R.L., Elkind, M.S.V., and Wright, C.B. 2016. Leisure-time physical activity associates with cognitive decline: The Northern Manhattan Study. *Neurology.* 86: 1897-1903.

Williams, D.P., Going, S.B., Massett, M.P., Lohman, T.G., Bare, L.A., and Hewitt, M.J. 1993. Aqueous and mineral fractions of the fat-free body and their relation to body fat estimates in men and women aged 49-82 years. In *Human body composition: In vivo methods, models and assessment,* ed. K.J. Ellis and J.D. Eastman, 109-113. New York: Plenum Press.

Williams, M.A. 2001. Exercise testing in cardiac rehabilitation: Exercise prescription and beyond. *Cardiology Clinics* 19: 415-431.

Williams, P.T. 2001. Physical fitness and activity as separate heart disease risk factors: A meta-analysis. *Medicine & Science in Sports & Exercise* 33: 754-761.

Williams, R., Binkley, J., Bloch, R., Goldsmith, C.H., and Minuk, T. 1993. Reliability of the modified-modified Schober and double inclinometer methods for measuring lumbar flexion and extension. *Physical Therapy* 73: 26-37.

Williams, T.D., Tolusso, D.V., Fedewa, M.V., and Esco, M.R. 2017. Comparison of periodized and non-periodized resistance training on maximal strength: A meta-analysis. *Sports Medicine* 47: 2083-2100.

Willson, J.D., Dougherty, C.P., Ireland, M.L., and Davis, I.M. 2005. Core stability and its relationship to lower extremity function and injury. *Journal of the American Academy of Orthopaedic Surgery* 13: 316-325.

Willson, T., Nelson, S.D., Newbold, J., Nelson, R.E., and LaFleur, J. 2015. The clinical epidemiology of male osteoporosis: A review of the recent literature. *Clinical Epidemiology* 7: 65-75.

Wilmore, J.H. 1974. Alterations in strength, body composition, and anthropometric measurements consequent to a 10-week weight training program. *Medicine and Science in Sports* 6: 133-138.

Wilmore, J.H., and Behnke, A.R. 1969. An anthropometric estimation of body density and lean body weight in young men. *Journal of Applied Physiology* 27: 25-31.

Wilmore, J.H., and Behnke, A.R. 1970. An anthropometric estimation of body density and lean body weight in young women. *American Journal of Clinical Nutrition* 23: 267-274.

Wilmore, J.H., Davis, J.A., O'Brien, R.S., Vodak, P.A., Walder, G.R., and Amsterdam, E.A. 1980. Physiological alterations consequent to 20-week conditioning programs of bicycling, tennis and jogging. *Medicine & Science in Sports & Exercise* 12: 1-9.

Wilmore, J.H., Frisancho, R.A., Gordon, C.C., Himes, J.H., Martin, A.D., Martorell, R., and Seefeldt, R.D. 1988. Body breadth equipment and measurement techniques. In *Anthropometric standardization reference manual,* ed. T.G. Lohman, A.F. Roche, and R. Martorell, 27-38. Champaign, IL: Human Kinetics.

Wilmore, J.H., Parr, R.B., Girandola, R.N., Ward, P., Vodak, P.A., Barstow, T.J., Pipes, T.V., Romero, G.T., and Leslie, P. 1978. Physiological alterations consequent to circuit weight training. *Medicine and Science in Sports* 10: 79-84.

Wilmore, J.H., Royce, J., Girandola, R.N., Katch, F.I., and Katch, V.L. 1970. Body composition changes with a 10-week program of jogging. *Medicine and Science in Sports* 2: 113-119.

Wilms, B., Schmid, S.M., Ernst, B., Thurnheer, M., Mueller, M.J., and Schultes, B. 2010. Poor prediction of resting energy expenditure in obese women by established equations. *Metabolism Clinical and Experimental* 59: 1181-1189.

Wilson, J.M., Lowery, R.P., Joy, J.M., Andersen, J.C., Wilson, S.M., Stout, J.R., Duncan, N., Fuller, J.C., Baier, S.M., Naimo, M.A., and Rathmacher, J. 2014. The effects of 12 weeks of beta-hydroxy-beta-methylbutyrate free acid supplementation on muscle mass, strength, and power in resistance-trained individuals: A randomized, double-blind, placebo-controlled study. *European Journal of Applied Physiology* 114(6): 1217-1227.

Wilson, J.M., Marin, P.J., Rhea, M.R., Wilson, S.M.C., Loenneke, J.P., and Anderson, J.C. 2012. Concurrent training: A meta-analysis examining interference of aerobic and resistance exercises. *Journal of Strength and Conditioning Research* 26: 2293-2307.

Wilson, P.K., Winga, E.R., Edgett, J.W., and Gushiken, T.J. 1978. *Policies and procedures of a cardiac rehabilitation program—immediate to long term care.* Philadelphia: Lea & Febiger.

Withers, R.T., LaForgia, J., Pillans, R.K., Shipp, N.J., Chatterton, B.E., Schultz, C.G., and Leaney, F. 1998. Comparisons of two-, three-, and four-compartment models of body composition analysis in men and women. *Journal of Applied Physiology* 85: 238-245.

Witten, C. 1973. Construction of a submaximal cardiovascular step test for college females. *Research Quarterly* 44: 46-50.

Woei-Ni Hwang, P., and Braun, K.L. 2015. The effectiveness of dance interventions to improve older adults' health: A systematic literature review. *Alternative Therapies in Health and Medicine* 21: 64-70.

Women's Exercise Research Center. 1998. Based on figures published by Brown, D.A., and Miller, W.C. 1998. Normative data for strength and flexibility of women throughout life. *European Journal of Applied Physiology* 78: 77-82.

Wolpern, A.E., Burgos, D.J., Janot, J.M., and Dalleck, L.C. 2015. Is a threshold-based model a superior method to the relative percent concept for establishing individual exercise intensity? A randomized controlled trial. *BMC Sports Science, Medicine and Rehabilitation* 7: 16. doi:10.1186/s13102-015-0011-z. Accessed July 3, 2017.

World Health Organization. 1998. Obesity: Preventing and managing a global epidemic. *Report of a WHO Consultation on Obesity.* Geneva: Author.

World Health Organization. 2002a. Reducing risks, promoting healthy life. *World Health Report 2002.* www.who.int/whr/2002/chapter4/en/index4.html.

World Health Organization. 2002b. Smoking statistics. www.wpro.who.int/public/press_release/press_view.asp?id=219.

World Health Organization. 2010. Global recommendations on physical activity for health. http://whqlibdoc.who.int/publications/2010/9789241599979_eng.pdf. Accessed July 5, 2012.

World Health Organization. 2011. Global atlas on cardiovascular disease prevention and control. http://whqlibdoc.who.int/publications/2011/9789241564373_eng.pdf. Accessed September 9, 2012.

World Health Organization. 2012a. Childhood obesity. www.who.int/dietphysicalactivity/childhood/Childhood_obesity_Tool.pdf. Accessed October 5, 2012.

World Health Organization. 2012b. Global database on body mass index. http://apps.who.int/bmi/index.jsp. Accessed on September 8, 2012.

World Health Organization. 2013. Global action plan for the prevention and control of noncommunicable diseases 2013-2020. http://apps.who.int/iris/bitstream/10665/94384/1/9789241506236_eng.pdf?ua=1. Accessed March 19, 2017.

World Health Organization. 2014. Global status report on NCDs 2014. http://apps.who.int/iris/bitstream/10665/148114/1/9789241564854_eng.pdf. Accessed March 24, 2017.

World Health Organization. 2016a. Cardiovascular diseases. www.who.int.libproxy.unm.edu/mediacentre/factsheets/fs317/en. Accessed April 2, 2017.

World Health Organization. 2016b. Global report on diabetes. http://apps.who.int/iris/bitstream/10665/204871/1/9789241565257_eng.pdf. Accessed April 9, 2017.

World Health Organization. 2016c. Obesity and overweight fact sheet. www.who.int/mediacentre/factsheets/fs311/en. Accessed June 25, 2017.

World Health Organization. 2016d. *World health statistics 2016: Monitoring health for the SDGs.* Geneva, Switzerland: WHO Press.

World Health Organization. 2018a. Cancer Fact Sheet. http://www.who.int/mediacentre/factsheets/fs297/en/. Accessed March 31, 2018.

World Health Organization. 2018b. Obesity and Overweight Fact Sheet. http://www.who.int/mediacentre/factsheets/fs311/en/ Accessed March 31, 2018.

World Health Organization. 2018c. Physical Activity Fact Sheet. http://www.who.int/mediacentre/factsheets/fs385/en/ Accessed March 31, 2018.

World Medical Association. 2017. Non-communicable diseases. www.wma.net/en/20activities/30publichealth/10noncommunicablediseases. Accessed March 16, 2017.

Wright, N.C., Sang, K.G., Dawson-Hughes, B., Khosla, S., and Siris, E.S. 2017. The impact of the new National Bone Health Alliance (NBHA) diagnostic criteria on the prevalence of osteoporosis in the USA. *Osteoporosis International* 28: 1225-1232.

Wysocki, A., Butler, M., Shamilyan, T., and Kane, R.L. 2011. Whole-body vibration therapy for osteoporosis: State of the Science. *Annals of Internal Medicine* 155: 680-686.

Xian, H., Vasilopoulos, T., Liu, W., Hanger, R.L. Jacobson, K.C., Lyons, M.J., Panizzon, M., Reynolds, C.A., Vuoksimua, E., Kremen, W.S., and Franz, C.E. 2017. Steeper change in body mass across four decades predicts poorer cardiometabolic outcomes at midlife. *Obesity* 25: 773-780.

Xu, J., Lombardi, G., Jiao, W., and Banfi, G. 2016. Effects of exercise on bone status in female subjects, from young girls to postmenopausal women: An overview of systematic reviews and meta-analyses. *Sports Medicine* 46: 1165-1182.

Xu, W., Chafi, H., Guo, B., Heymsfield, S.B., Murray, K.B., Zheng, J., and Jie, G. 2016. Quantitative comparison of 2 dual-energy X-ray absorptiometry systems in assessing body composition and bone mineral measurements. *Journal of Clinical Densitometry* 19: 298-304.

Yamanoto, K. 2002. Omron Institute of Life Science [personal communication].

Yamato, T.P., Maher, C.G., Saragiotto, B.T., Hancock, M.J., Ostelo, R.W., Cabral, C.M., Costa, L.C., and Costa, L.O. 2016. Pilates for low back pain: Complete republication of a Cochrane review. *Spine* 41(12): 1013-1021.

Yang, Q., Cogswell, M.E., Flanders, W.D., Hong, Y., Zhang, Z., Loustalot, F., Gillespie, C., Merritt, R., and Hu, F.B. 2012. Trends in cardiovascular health metrics and associations with all-cause and CVD mortality among U.S. adults. *Journal of the American Medical Association* 307: 1273-1283.

Yee, A.J., Fuerst, T., Salamone, L., Visser, M., Dockrell, M., Van Loan, M., and Kern, M. 2001. Calibration and validation of an air-displacement plethysmography method for estimating percentage body fat in an elderly population: A comparison among compartmental models. *American Journal of Clinical Nutrition* 74: 637-642.

Yee, S.Y., and Gallagher, D. 2008. Assessment methods in human body composition. *Current Opinion in Clinical Nutrition and Metabolic Care* 11: 566-572.

Yessis, M. 2003. Using free weights for stability training. *Fitness Management* 19(11): 26-28.

Yim-Chiplis, P.K., and Talbot, L.A. 2000. Defining and measuring balance in adults. *Biological Research for Nursing* 1(4): 321-331.

YMCA of the USA. 2000. *YMCA fitness testing and assessment manual*, 4th ed. Champaign, IL: Human Kinetics.

Yoke, M., and Kennedy, C. 2004. *Functional exercise progressions*. Monterey, CA: Healthy Learning.

Yoon, B.K., Kravitz, L., and Robergs, R. 2007. $\dot{V}O_2$max, protocol duration, and the $\dot{V}O_2$ plateau. *Medicine & Science in Sports & Exercise* 39: 1186-1192.

Yoon, Y.S., and Oh, S.W. 2014. Optimal waist circumference cutoff values for the diagnosis of abdominal obesity in Korean adults. *Endocrinology and Metabolism* 29: 418-426.

Youkhana, S., Dean, C.M., Wolff, M., Sherrington, C., and Tiedemann, A. 2016. Yoga-based exercise improves balance and mobility in people aged 60 and over: A systematic review and meta-analysis. *Age and Ageing* 45: 21-29.

Yu, J-H., and Lee, G-C. 2012. Effect of core stability training using Pilates on lower extremity muscle strength and postural stability in healthy subjects. *Isokinetics and Exercise Science* 20: 141-146.

Zakas, A., Balaska, P., Grammatikopoulou, M.G., Zakas, N., and Vergou, A. 2005. Acute effects of stretching duration on the range of motion of elderly women. *Journal of Bodywork and Movement Therapies* 9: 270-276.

Zamboni, M., Turcato, E., Armellini, F., Kahn, H.S., Zivelonghi, A., Santana, H., Bergamo-Andreis, I.A., and Bosello, O. 1998. Sagittal abdominal diameter as a practical predictor of visceral fat. *International Journal of Obesity and Related Metabolic Disorders* 22: 655-660.

Zampieri, S., Pietrangelo, L., Loefler, S., Fruhmann, H., Vogelauer, M., Burggraf, S., Pond, A., Grim-Stieger, M., Cvecka, J., Sedliak, M., Tirpáková, V., Mayr, W., Sarabon, N., Rossini, K., Barberi, L., DeRossi, M., Romanello, V., Boncompagni, S., Musarò, A., Sandri, M., and Protasi, F. 2015. Lifelong physical exercise delays age-associated skeletal muscle decline. *Journals of Gerontology: Biological Sciences and Medical Sciences* 70: 163-173.

Zancanaro, C., Milanese, C., Lovato, C., Sandri, M., and Giachetti, A. 2015. Reliability of three-dimensional photonic scanner anthropometry performed by skilled and naïve operators. *International Journal of Ergonomics* 5: 1-11.

Zanchi, N.E., Gerlinger-Romero, F., Guimaraes-Ferreira, L., de Siqueira Filho, M., Felitti, V., Lira, F.S., Seelaender, M., and Lancha, A.H. Jr. 2011. HMB supplementation: Clinical and athletic performance-related effects and mechanisms of action. *Amino Acids* 40: 1015-1025.

Zanetti, J.R., Gonçalves da Cruz, L., Lourenço, C.L.M., Ribeiro, G.C., Ferreira de Jusus Leite, M.A., Neves, F.F., Sivla-Vergara, M.L., and Mendes, E.L. 2016. Nonlinear resistance training enhances the lipid profile and reduces inflammation marker in people living with HIV: A randomized clinical trial. *Journal of Physical Activity and Health* 12: 765-770. Zeni, A.I., Hoffman, M.D., and Clifford, P.S. 1996. Energy expenditure with indoor exercise machines. *Journal of the American Medical Association* 275: 1424-1427.

Zhu, S., Heshka, S., Wang, Z., Shen, W., Allison, D.B., Ross, R., and Heymsfield, S.B. 2004. Combination of BMI and waist circumference for identifying cardiovascular risk factors in whites. *Obesity Research* 12: 633-645.

Zhu, S., Heymsfield, S.B., Toyoshima, H., Wang, Z., Petrobelli, A., and Heshka, S. 2005. Race-ethnicity-specific waist circumference cutoffs for identifying cardiovascular disease risk factors. *American Journal of Clinical Nutrition* 81: 409-415.

Zhu, W. 2008. Promoting physical activity using technology. *President's Council on Physical Fitness and Sports Research Digest* 9(3): 1-8.

Zhuang, J., Huang, L., Wu, Y., and Zhang, Y. 2014. The effectiveness of a combined exercise intervention on physical fitness factors related to falls in community-dwelling older adults. *Clinical Interventions in Aging* 9: 131-140.

Zwald, M.L, Akinbami, L.J., Fakhouri, T.H.I., and Fryar, C.D. 2017. Prevalence of low high-density lipoprotein cholesterol among adults, by physical activity: United States, 2011-2014. NCHS Data Brief. No. 276. www-cdc-gov.libproxy.unm.edu/nchs/data/databriefs/db276.pdf. Accessed April 3, 2017.

Index

Note: Page numbers followed by italic *f* and *t* refer to figures and tables, respectively.

graded 81-82, 84, 86
recumbent stepper 111
rowing ergometer 111, 112*f*
stair climbing 110-111
treadmill 101-103
super circuit resistance training 145
supersetting 195
SuperTracker (U.S. Department of Agriculture) 295
supplements 217
suspension training 212
Swain cycle ergometer submaximal test 106-107, 107*f*, 394
swimming tests 115
Swinburn, B.A. 287, 288
switch mats 174
systolic blood pressure (SBP) 11, 12, 37, 45-48

T

tachycardia 49
Tae Bo 142
tai chi 56, 130, 364, 365, 366*t*, 367-368
talk tests 135-136
Tanita analyzers 261-266, 262*f*
tare weight 234*f*, 235
TBW. *See* total body water (TBW)
TC. *See* total cholesterol (TC)
TE (total error) 59*t*, 61, 61*f*
technician skill 177-178, 250-252, 258, 268, 277
technology. *See also* dynamometers
accelerometers 73, 74, 167, 176, 286, 301
active video games 74-75
activity trackers 286, 301
blood pressure smartphone apps 39
calipers 253-254, 253-254*f*, 255*t*
electrocardiogram 50-52, 51-52*f*
goniometers 312-318, 313-314*f*, 315-316*t*, 318*f*
GPS 74, 116
heart rate monitors 50, 73-74, 115
pedometers 72-73, 72*t*, 137
persuasive 75-76
social networking 76
telemonitoring scales 288
ultrasound 256-257*f*, 256-260
virtual reality 75, 365-366
wearable 72-74, 72*t*, 301, 317
for workplace physical activity 2
TEE. *See* total energy expenditure (TEE)
Tegenkamp, M.H. 242
telemonitoring scales 288
telomeres 24-25
Tendo Weightlifting Analyzer System 167
terminal digit bias 44
test anxiety 57
testosterone 222, 300, 306
TGV (thoracic gas volume) 239, 241, 242
theory of planned behavior 70
theory of reasoned action 69-70
thigh extensions 412
30 sec chair stand test 183-185, 184*f*, 184*t*
Thompson, M. 359
thoracic gas volume (TGV) 239, 241, 242
three-dimensional (3D) body surface scanners 246
thyroxine 286
timed one-leg stance test 354-355, 354*t*
timed up and go tests 359-360*t*, 359-361, 361*f*

TLC (total lung capacity) 236, 237
TMS (transcranial magnetic stimulation) 223
tobacco use 16
tonic vibration reflex 213-214
Toomey, C. 258-259
total body water (TBW) 231, 237, 260-261, 267, 268
total cholesterol (TC) 14, 15, 34*t*, 36, 36*t*. *See also* cholesterol
total energy expenditure (TEE) 87-88, 96, 285, 285*t*, 291, 294-295
total error (TE) 59*t*, 61, 61*f*
total lung capacity (TLC) 236, 237
training volume 64, 190, 193, 196, 203
transcranial magnetic stimulation (TMS) 223
transcriptome signature of resistance exercise 220-221
transtheoretical model 69
treading workouts 144-145
treadmill desks 2
treadmills 87*f*
treadmill tests
Balke protocol for 91-92*t*, 91*f*, 92, 93*f*, 103, 394
Bruce protocol for 90*f*, 91-92*t*, 92-93, 93*f*, 94*t*, 102, 394
for children and adolescents 115-116, 117*t*
duration of 85
maximal 87-95
metabolic equations for 87-89, 88*t*, 92, 92*t*, 93, 102
modified Balke protocol for 116, 117*t*, 119, 394
modified Bruce protocol for 91*f*, 91*t*, 93, 116, 394
multistage model 102
Naughton protocol for 90*f*, 91-92*t*, 394
for older adults 119
oxygen uptake in 87-89, 88*t*, 92*t*, 93*f*
ramp protocols for 94-95, 94*t*
running/jogging 88, 88*t*, 89, 103
self-paced protocols for 93-94
single-stage model 103
submaximal 101-103
unit conversions in 89
walking 88-89, 88*t*, 103
triaxial joints 310, 310*t*
triceps extension 171*t*, 411
triglycerides
classification of 34*t*
guidelines on 36*t*, 37
physical activity and 7, 7*f*
tri-sets 195, 206-208
trunk curl tests 173
trunk endurance tests 165-166
trunk extensor flexibility exercises 448-449
trunk flex exercise 343, 456
trunk flexor flexibility exercises 446, 449-450
T wave 50
12 min cycling test 115
12 min run test 109*t*, 113, 395
12 min swimming test 115
twelve-lead electrocardiogram 50-52, 51-52*f*
20 m shuttle run test 114, 117, 395
two-component model of body composition 231, 232*t*
2 min step test 121-122, 121*t*

type A, B, C, and D aerobic activities 127-128, 132, 139, 142-143, 150
type 1 diabetes 17
type 2 diabetes 3, 6, 7, 13*t*, 17-18, 21

U

ultrasound 256-257*f*, 256-260
undercuffing 47
underwater weight (UWW) 233-236, 234*f*
underweight. *See also* weight management
BMI classification of 270-271, 272*t*
defined 282
health risks related to 281, 282
undulating periodization (UP) 196, 206-208, 211
uniaxial joints 310, 310*t*
unipedal stance test 354-355, 354*t*
unit conversions 89
United States
cancer in 21
cardiovascular disease in 10, 11
diabetes mellitus in 17
dietitian and nutritionist regulation in 297, 298*t*
falls and fall risk in 349
hypertension in 12
kettlebell training in 215
metabolic syndrome in 20-21
obesity in 18, 19, 282-283, 287
osteoporosis in 22
physical activity trends in 1, 4, 67
preferred test modalities in 87
tobacco use in 16
universal goniometers 312-314, 313*f*, 315-316*t*, 318
UP (undulating periodization) 196, 206-208, 211
upper body analyzers 263-265
upper body obesity 284
USDHHS (U.S. Department of Health and Human Services) 4-6, 5*t*, 126, 299*t*
UWW (underwater weight) 233-236, 234*f*

V

validity
of arm curl test 182
of balance assessments 354, 355, 357, 363
of cardiorespiratory fitness tests 103, 105, 107, 113-116
of countermovement jump 176
of flexibility assessments 314, 318
of Myotest accelerometer 167
of OMNI RPE scales 83
of physical fitness tests 57-58, 58*f*
of prediction equations 61-62, 61*f*
of sit-and-reach tests 58, 59, 319-320, 322-324, 327
of 6 min walking test 120
of step tests 119, 121-122
of Tendo system 167
of 30 sec chair stand test 183, 185
validity coefficient 57-58, 61, 62
variable-resistance exercise 166-171, 168-171*t*
variable-resistance muscle action 160-161, 160*f*
VAT. *See* visceral adipose tissue (VAT)
ventilatory threshold (VT) 135
Vera-Garcia, F.J. 213
verification bout 80, 82
Vertec device 174, 176

About the Authors

Ann L. Gibson, PhD, FACSM, is an associate professor and researcher in exercise science at the University of New Mexico, with research interests in body composition and physiological responses to exercise. She developed the ancillary materials for the sixth edition of *Advanced Fitness Assessment and Exercise Prescription* in addition to coauthoring the seventh edition.

Gibson has presented internationally in the area of obesity research and has published original research in journals such as *Medicine & Science in Sports & Exercise, American Journal of Clinical Nutrition, International Journal of Sport Nutrition & Exercise Metabolism, Research Quarterly for Exercise and Sport,* and *Journal of Bone and Joint Surgery.* She is a member of the American College of Sports Medicine, National Strength and Conditioning Association, and the Clinical Exercise Physiology Association.

Gibson resides in New Mexico, where she enjoys spending time outdoors hiking, biking, snowshoeing, cross-country skiing, and gardening.

Dale R. Wagner, PhD, EPC, ACSM-CEP, CSCS, is a professor of exercise physiology at Utah State University (USU). His research interests include body composition assessment and exercise physiology at high altitude. He has been an active researcher for 20 years and has authored over 60 peer-reviewed research publications. He is a coauthor of *Applied Body Composition Assessment* (Human Kinetics, 2004) with Vivian Heyward.

Wagner is a past president of the Southwest Chapter of the American College of Sports Medicine (SWACSM) and of the American Society of Exercise Physiologists. He is a research council member of the Wilderness Medical Society and a member of the National Strength and Conditioning Association, the International Society for Mountain Medicine, and the International Society for Body Composition Research.

In his spare time, Wagner enjoys mountaineering, cycling (both road and mountain), and international travel.

Vivian H. Heyward, PhD, is a regents' professor emerita at the University of New Mexico, where she taught physical fitness assessment and exercise prescription courses for 26 years. In addition to the previous editions of this book, she has authored two editions of *Applied Body Composition Assessment* (Human Kinetics, 1996, 2004) as well as numerous articles in research and professional journals dealing with various aspects of physical fitness assessment and exercise prescription. Heyward has received many professional awards, including the SWACSM Recognition Award for distinguished professional achievement and the Distinguished Alumni Award from the University of Illinois and the State University of New York at Cortland.

In her free time, she enjoys hiking, nature photography, golfing, and snowshoeing. Heyward resides in Albuquerque, New Mexico.

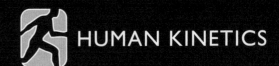